Immunotherapy in Transplantation

Immunotherapy in Transplantation

Principles and Practice

EDITED BY

Bruce Kaplan MD

Kathy and Harry Jentsch Professor of Medicine
Professor of Surgery and Pharmacology
Chief, Division of Nephrology
Medical Director of Abdominal Transplant
University of Arizona Medical Center
Tucson, AZ, USA;
Adjunct Professor of Medicine, Applied Genomics Center
University of Alberta
Edmonton, AB, Canada

Gilbert J. Burckart PharmD

Associate Director, Office of Clinical Pharmacology
Center for Drug Evaluation and Research
US Food and Drug Administration
Silver Spring, MD, USA

Fadi G. Lakkis MD

Professor of Surgery, Immunology and Medicine
Frank & Athena Sarris Chair in Transplantation Biology
Scientific Director, Thomas E. Starzl Transplantation Institute
University of Pittsburgh
Pittsburgh, PA, USA

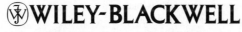

WILEY-BLACKWELL

A John Wiley & Sons, Ltd., Publication

Library of Congress Cataloging-in-Publication Data

Immunotherapy in transplantation : principles and practice / edited by Bruce Kaplan, Gilbert J. Burckart, Fadi G. Lakkis.
       p. ; cm.
   Includes bibliographical references and index.
   ISBN 978-1-4051-8271-3 (hard cover : alk. paper)
I. Kaplan, Bruce, 1958–   II. Burckart, Gilbert J.   III. Lakkis, Fadi G.
[DNLM: 1. Transplantation Immunology–drug effects.   2. Transplantation Immunology–physiology.
3. Immunosuppressive Agents–pharmacology.   4. Immunotherapy–methods.   5. Pharmacology, Clinical–methods.
6. Transplantation–physiology. WO 680]
   615.3'7–dc23

                                  2011035464

A catalogue record for this book is available from the British Library.

Wiley also publishes its books in a variety of electronic formats. Some content that appears in print may not be available in electronic books.

Set in 9/12pt Meridien by SPi Publisher Services, Pondicherry, India
Printed and bound in Singapore by Markono Print Media Pte Ltd

1   2012

Contents

List of Contributors

Avinash Agarwal MD
Department of Surgery and the Emory Transplant Center
Emory University
Atlanta, GA, USA

Muna Alnimri MD
Instructor in Medicine
University of California
San Francisco Transplant Service
San Francisco, CA, USA

Christian Bloy PhD
Senior Director R&D
Genzyme Corporation
Lyon, France

Olivia R. Blume PA-C
Abdominal Transplant Service
University of Arizona Medical Center
Tucson, AZ, USA

Lyndsey J. Bowman PharmD
Clinical Pharmacist, Abdominal Transplant
Barnes-Jewish Hospital
St. Louis, MO, USA

Daniel C. Brennan MD, FACP
Professor of Medicine
Washington University in St. Louis;
Director, Transplant Nephrology
St. Louis, MO, USA

Barry J. Browne MD, MS, FACS
Director, Abdominal Transplantation
Balboa Institute of Transplantation
San Diego, CA, USA

David Bruno MD
Department of Surgery and the Emory Transplant Center
Emory University
Atlanta, GA, USA

Gilbert J. Burckart PharmD
Associate Director, Office of Clinical Pharmacology
Center for Drug Evaluation and Research
US Food and Drug Administration
Silver Spring, MD, USA

Bryna Burrell PhD
Postdoctoral Fellow
Mount Sinai School of Medicine
New York, NY, USA

Gary Chan PharmD, MS
Senior Director
Clinical Development
Specialty Care Business Unit
Pfizer
Groton, CT, USA

Paul S. Changelian PhD
Vice President, Biology
Lycera Corporation
Plymouth, MI, USA

Anita S. Chong PhD
Professor of Surgery
Department of Surgery / Section of Transplantation
University of Chicago
Chicago, IL, USA

Robert B. Colvin MD
Professor of Pathology
Massachusetts General Hospital;
Professor of Pathology
Harvard Medical School
Boston, MA, USA

John J. Curtis MD
Professor of Medicine and Surgery
Endowed Professor of Transplant Nephrology
Division of Nephrology
University of Alabama at Birmingham
Birmingham, AL, USA

Arjang Djamali MD, MS, FASN
Associate Professor of Medicine-Surgery
Chief, Nephrology Division
University of Wisconsin-Madison
Madison, WI, USA

John L. Dzuris PhD
Assistant Director
Transplant and Immunology Research
Genzyme Corporation
Framingham, MA, USA

William E. Fitzsimmons PharmD, MS
Senior Vice President
Astellas Pharma Global Development, Inc.
Deerfield, IL, USA

Jogarao V.S. Gobburu PhD
Professor
University of Maryland School of Pharmacy
Baltimore, MD, USA

Daniel R. Goldstein PhD
Associate Professor of Internal Medicine and Immunobiology
Yale University School of Medicine
New Haven, CT, USA

David Hager PharmD, CNSC
Clinical Pharmacist in Transplantation
University of Wisconsin Hospital and Clinics
Madison, WI, USA

Peter S. Heeger MD
Professor of Medicine
Division of Nephrology
Recanati/Miller Transplantation Institute
Mount Sinai School of Medicine
New York, NY, USA

Stanley C. Jordan MD
Professor of Pediatrics & Medicine
David Geffen School of Medicine at UCLA;
Medical Director, Renal Transplant Program
Director, Nephrology and Transplant Immunology
Cedars-Sinai Medical Center
Los Angeles, CA, USA

Barry D. Kahan PhD, MD
Emeritus Professor
Division of Immunology and Organ Transplantation
The University of Texas Medical School at Houston
Houston, TX, USA

Joseph Kahwaji MD
Kidney and Transplant Program
Cedars-Sinai Medical Center;
Assistant Clincial Professor
David Geffen School of Medicine at UCLA
Los Angeles, CA, USA

Bruce Kaplan MD, PhD
Kathy and Harry Jentsch Professor of Medicine
Professor of Surgery and Pharmacology
Chief, Division of Nephrology
Medical Director of Abdominal Transplant
University of Arizona Medical Center
Tucson, AZ, USA;
Adjunct Professor of Medicine, Applied Genomics Center
University of Alberta
Edmonton, AB, Canada

Paul A. Keown MD, DSc, MBA, FACP, FASN, FRCP, FRCPC, FRCPath, FRSC, FIBiol
Professor of Medicine and Director of Immunology
Departments of Medicine and Pathology and Laboratory Medicine
University of British Columbia
Vancouver, BC, Canada

Allan D. Kirk MD, PhD, FACS
Professor of Surgery and Pediatrics
Scientific Director, Emory Transplant Center
Emory University School of Medicine
Atlanta, GA, USA

Stuart J. Knechtle MD, PhD
Professor of Surgery and Pediatrics
Chief, Division of Transplantation
Emory University School of Medicine
Atlanta, GA, USA

Fadi G. Lakkis MD
Professor of Surgery and Immunology
Scientific Director, Thomas E. Starzl Transplantation Institute
University of Pittsburgh
Pittsburgh, PA, USA

Mallika Lala PhD
Division of Pharmacometrics
Office of Clinical Pharmacology
Center for Drug Evaluation and Research
US Food and Drug Administration
Silver Spring, MD, USA

Richard D. Mamelok MD
Mamelok Consulting
Palo Alto, CA, USA

Didier A. Mandelbrot, MD
Medical Director, BIDMC Living Kidney Donor Program
Director of Clinical Trials, The Transplant Institute, BIDMC
Associate Professor of Medicine, Harvard Medical School
Boston, MA, USA

Beata Mierzejewska MD
Senior Research Scholar
University of Toledo College of Medicine
Toledo, OH, USA

Michael C. Milone MD, PhD
Assistant Professor of Pathology and Laboratory Medicine
Associate Director, Toxicology and Therapeutic Drug
Monitoring Laboratory
Hospital of the University of Pennsylvania
Philadelphia, PA, USA

Martin H. Oberbarnscheidt MD, PhD
Research Assistant Professor
Thomas E. Starzl Transplantation Institute
University of Pittsburgh
Pittsburgh, PA, USA

Edward C. Parkin BS
Doctoral Student, Physciological Sciences
Research Specialist
Center for Cellular Research
Department of Surgery
University of Arizona
Tucson, AZ, USA

Alice Peng MD
Medical Director, Kidney/Pancreas Transplant Program
Program Director, Nephrology Fellowship Program
Cedars-Sinai Medical Center;
Assistant Professor of Medicine
David Geffen School of Medicine at UCLA
Los Angeles, CA, USA

Mark D. Pescovitz MD *(deceased)*
Professor of Surgery and Microbiology/Immunology
Indiana University Medical Center
Indianapolis, IN, USA

Venkateswaran C. Pillai PhD
Research Associate
Clinical Pharmacokinetics Laboratory
Department of Pharmaceutical Sciences
School of Pharmacy
University of Pittsburgh
Pittsburgh, PA, USA

Horacio L. Rodriguez Rilo MD
Professor of Surgery
Director, Center for Cellular Transplantation
Associate Director
Arizona Diabetes Center
Tucson, AZ, USA

Melanie Ruzek PhD
Principal Scientist
Genzyme Corporation
Framingham, MA, USA

Mohamed H. Sayegh MD
Director, Schuster Family Transplantation Research Center
Brigham and Women's Hospital & Children's Hospital Boston
Visiting Professor of Medicine and Pediatrics
Harvard Medical School
Boston, MA, USA;
Raja N. Khuri Dean, Faculty of Medicine
Vice President of Medical Affairs
American University of Beirut
Beirut, Lebanon

Roger Sciammas PhD
Research Associate/Assistant Professor
Department of Surgery/Section of Transplantation
University of Chicago
Chicago, IL, USA

Leslie M.J. Shaw PhD, DABCC
Professor of Pathology and Laboratory Medicine
Director, Toxicology and Therapeutic Drug Monitoring
Laboratory
Hospital of the University of Pennsylvania
Philadelphia, PA, USA

Swetha K. Srinivasan MD
Research Fellow
Department of Surgery
Emory Transplantation Center
Emory University
Atlanta, GA, USA

Stanislaw M. Stepkowski DVM, PhD, DSc
Professor, Departments of Medical Microbiology & Immunology
and Surgery
University of Toledo College of Medicine
Toledo, OH, USA

Bradford Strijack MD
Renal Transplant Fellow
Division of Nephrology, Department of Medicine
University of British Columbia
Vancouver, BC, Canada

Terry B. Strom MD
Professor of Medicine, Harvard Medical School
Co-director, Transplant Institute at Beth Israel Deaconess
Medical Center
Boston, MA, USA

Mieko Toyoda PhD
Director, Transplant Immunology Laboratory
Cedars-Sinai Medical Center;
Professor
David Geffen School of Medicine at UCLA
Los Angeles, CA, USA

Helen L. Triemer PharmD
Transplant Center Pharmacist
Emory Transplantation Center
Emory University
Atlanta, GA, USA

Laurence A. Turka MD
Professor of Medicine
Co-Director, Harvard Institute
of Translational Immunology
Harvard Medical School
Co-Research Director, The Transplant Institute
Co-Chief, Division of Transplantation Immunology
Beth Israel Deaconess Medical Center
Boston, MA, USA

Marina Vardanyan MD, PhD
Research Associate
Center for Cellular Transplantation
Department of Surgery
University of Arizona
Tucson, AZ, USA

Raman Venkataramanan PhD
Professor of Pharmaceutical Sciences
School of Pharmacy
Professor of Pathology, School of Medicine
Associate Director TDM and Toxicology
Director of Clinical Pharmacokinetics Laboratory
Thomas Starzl Transplantation Institute
Magee Womens Research Institute
McGowan Institute for Regenerative Medicine
Pittsburgh, PA, USA

Flavio Vincenti MD
Professor of Clinical Medicine
University of California
Transplant Service
San Francisco, CA, USA

Ashley A. Vo PharmD
Administrative Director
Transplant Immunotherapy Program
Cedars-Sinai Medical Center;
Assistant Clinical Professor
David Geffen School of Medicine at UCLA
Los Angeles, CA, USA

Richard M. Watanabe PhD
Associate Professor
Division of Biostatistics
Preventive Medicine and Physiology & Biophysics
Keck School of Medicine
University of Southern California
Los Angeles, CA, USA

John M. Williams PhD
Vice President
Transplant and Immunology Research
Genzyme Corporation
Framingham, MA, USA

Kathryn J. Wood DPhil, FMedSci
Professor of Immunology
Transplantation Research Immunology Group
Nuffield Department of Surgical Sciences
University of Oxford
John Radcliffe Hospital
Oxford, UK

Sarah E. Yost PharmD
Clinical Pharmacist in Abdominal Transplantation
University of Arizona Medical Center
Tucson, AZ, USA

Preface

The discipline of transplantation has always been inextricably linked to our ability to pharmacologically modulate and suppress the immune system, while at the same time avoiding infections, malignancy, and other side effects. By virtue of this, transplant physicians must excel not only as diagnosticians and surgeons, but also as pharmacologists. Perhaps in no other field of medicine is there such a close association between the basic field of pharmacology and clinical practice.

This textbook is not intended as an all-inclusive treatise on clinical pharmacology and immunology, nor on all the agents utilized to modulate the immune system. Rather, it is our hope that this textbook will serve as an introductory text to better understand the general principles of pharmacologic interventions of the immune system.

The book is divided into three parts. Part 1 is an overview of transplantation immunology. Particular attention is paid to the mechanisms by which pharmacologic agents may exert their effect. Part 2 is an overview of pharmacologic principles and drug development. Part 3 concentrates on individual agents, with an emphasis on how Parts 1 and 2 intersect to produce their clinical effects. It should be noted that this part does not include all agents utilized, but rather highlights certain agents to serve as examples of the principles we hope to cover.

A tremendous amount of work went into this text and we thank the authors for their selfless contributions.

Bruce Kaplan MD, PhD
Tucson, AZ, USA

Gilbert J. Burckart PharmD
Silver Spring, MD, USA

Fadi G. Lakkis MD
Pittsburgh, PA, USA

March 2012

PART 1
Transplantation Immunobiology

CHAPTER 1

The Immune Response to a Transplanted Organ: An Overview

Fadi G. Lakkis

Thomas E. Starzl Transplantation Institute, Departments of Surgery, Immunology, and Medicine, University of Pittsburgh, Pittsburgh, PA, USA

Basic definitions

Organs transplanted between two members of the same species are rejected unless the donor and recipient are genetically indistinguishable (identical twins in the case of humans). Rejection is caused by the recipient's immune response to foreign elements present on the transplanted organ. These elements are usually proteins that differ between the donor and recipient and are called "alloantigens." The transplanted organ itself is referred to as the "allograft" and the immune response mounted against it as the "alloimmune response" or "alloimmunity." The prefix "xeno," on the other hand, is used to denote the transplantation of organs between members of different species, as in the terms xeno-antigens, xenografts, and xenotransplantation.

The principal players

The T lymphocyte is the principal mediator of the alloimmune response [1, 2]. Experimental animals devoid of T cells do not reject tissue or organ allografts [3, 4]. Similarly, T cell depletion in humans prevents rejection effectively until T cells return to the circulation [5]. T cells cause direct injury to the allograft through a variety of cytotoxic molecules or cause damage indirectly by activating macrophages and other inflammatory cells (Chapter 3). T cells also provide help to B lymphocytes to produce a host of antibodies that recognize alloantigens ("alloantibodies"). Alloantibodies inflict injury on the transplanted organ by activating the complement cascade or by activating macrophages and natural killer cells (Chapter 4). An exception to the T cell requirement for allograft rejection is the rapid rejection of organs transplanted between ABO blood-group-incompatible individuals. In this case, allograft destruction is mediated by preformed anti-ABO antibodies that are produced by B-1 lymphocytes, a subset of B cells that are activated independent of help from T cells. Another potential mechanism of T-cell-independent rejection is graft dysfunction mediated by monocytes. This has been observed in renal transplant recipients after profound T cell depletion [5], but it is unlikely that monocytes lead to full-blown rejection in the absence of T cells or preformed antibodies.

The principal alloantigens recognized by T cells, B cells, and antibodies are the human leukocyte antigens (HLAs). These are cell-surface proteins that are highly variable (polymorphic) between unrelated individuals. Two main classes of HLA proteins have been identified. Class I molecules (HLA-A, -B, and -C) are expressed on all nucleated cells, whereas class II molecules (HLA-DP, -DQ, and -DR) are present on cells of the immune system that process and present foreign proteins to T cells;

Immunotherapy in Transplantation: Principles and Practice, First Edition. Edited by Bruce Kaplan, Gilbert J. Burckart and Fadi G. Lakkis.
© 2012 Blackwell Publishing Ltd. Published 2012 by Blackwell Publishing Ltd.

these are referred to as antigen-presenting cells (APCs) and include B cells, dendritic cells, macrophages, and other phagocytic cells (Chapter 2). In humans, activated T cells and inflamed endothelial cells also express class II molecules. Since HLA inheritance is codominant, any given individual shares one haplotype (one set of alleles) with either biological parent and has a 25 % chance of being HLA-identical (sharing both haplotypes) with a sibling. The chance that two unrelated individuals are HLA-identical is less than 5 %, because of the highly polymorphic nature of the HLA. Although HLA matching between donor and recipient confers long-term survival advantage on grafts [6], it does not in any way obviate the need for immunosuppression. The immune system is, in fact, capable of recognizing any non-HLA protein that differs between the donor and recipient as foreign and of mounting an alloimmune response to it that is sufficient to cause rejection. Non-HLA proteins that trigger an alloimmune response and are targeted during allograft rejection are referred to as "minor histocompatibility antigens" (Chapter 2). It is likely that a large number of minor antigens exist, making it very difficult to match for them.

Types of rejection

Pathologists have traditionally divided allograft rejection into three groups based on the tempo of allograft injury: hyperacute, acute, and chronic. Hyperacute rejection is a very rapid form of rejection that occurs within minutes to hours after transplantation and destroys the allograft in an equally short period of time. It is triggered by preformed anti-ABO or anti-HLA antibodies present in the recipient [7, 8]. Blood typing and clinical cross-matching, whereby preformed anti-HLA antibodies are screened for by mixing recipient serum with donor cells, or more commonly nowadays by sensitive flow-cytometric methods, has virtually eliminated hyperacute rejection. Acute rejection, in contrast, leads to allograft failure over a period of several days rather than minutes or hours. It usually occurs within a few days or weeks after transplantation, but it could happen at much later time points if the immune system is "awakened" by infection or by significant reduction in immunosuppression. Chronic rejection is a slow form of rejection that primarily affects the graft vasculature (or the bronchioles and bile ducts in the case of lung and liver transplants respectively) and causes graft fibrosis. Chronic rejection may become manifest during the first year after transplantation, but more often progresses gradually over several years, eventually leading to the demise of the majority of transplanted organs, with the exception perhaps of liver allografts. Since acute and chronic rejections are caused by T cells, antibodies, or both, it is increasingly common to label rejection by its predominant immunological mechanism, cellular or antibody mediated, in addition to its temporal classification (Chapters 3 and 4). Rejection is also graded according to agreed-upon criteria known collectively as the Banff classification [9]. These are important advances in transplantation pathology, as they often guide the choice of anti-rejection treatment and are used as prognosticators of long-term allograft outcome.

Distinguishing features of the alloimmune response

Although alloimmune responses resemble antimicrobial immune responses in many ways, they are distinguishable by several salient features. These features are highlighted here, as they have direct implications for the development of anti-rejection therapies.

Alloimmune responses are vigorous responses that involve a relatively large proportion of the T cell repertoire

Humans carry a large repertoire of T lymphocytes that recognize and react to virtually any foreign protein with a high degree of specificity. The diversity of T cell reactivity is attributed to the random rearrangement during T cell ontogeny of genes that code for components of the T cell receptor (TCR) for antigen (Chapter 3). The same applies to B cells, leading to an immense variety of antibodies that detect almost any conceivable foreign antigen (Chapter 4). The high specificity of T cells is explained by the fact that TCRs do not recognize whole antigens; instead, they recognize small peptides derived from foreign proteins and presented in the context of HLA molecules on antigen-presenting or infected cells (Chapter 2). This leads to fine molecular specificity in which only a very small proportion of T cells react to a non-self peptide. It is estimated that only 1 in 10 000 or less of all T cells in a human being recognize peptides derived from any given microbe. The small proportion (or precursor frequency) of microbe-specific T cells is nevertheless sufficient to eliminate the infection because of the ability of T lymphocytes to proliferate exponentially (a phenomenon referred to as clonal expansion) before differentiating into effector cells. In sharp contrast, the immune response to an allograft involves anywhere between 1 and 10 % of the T cell repertoire [10, 11] – essentially 10–100 times more than an antimicrobial response. The large-scale participation of T cells in the alloimmune response can be readily demonstrated in the mixed lymphocyte reaction (MLR), a laboratory test in which coculturing recipient peripheral blood mononuclear cells (PBMCs) with donor PBMCs results in conspicuous proliferation of recipient T lymphocytes. Detecting T cell proliferation against microbial antigens, on the other hand, is a much more difficult feat because of the low precursor frequency of microbe-specific lymphocytes. Alloimmune responses, therefore, are especially vigorous responses because of the participation of a significant proportion of T cells with a wide range of specificities. The reasons for this phenomenon, perhaps the dominant obstacle to improving allograft survival without unduly compromising the recipient's immune system, are explained next.

T cell alloreactivity is cross-reactivity

The immune system has evolved to protect animals against infection. It is not surprising, therefore, that humans and most other vertebrate species are armed with T cells that recognize microbial antigens. Why is it, then, that we also carry a disproportionately large proportion of T cells that react to alloantigens? Based on cellular and molecular studies in humans and experimental animals, it has become evident that TCRs specific for a microbial peptide (presented in the context of self-HLA) are also capable of recognizing allogeneic, non-self HLA [11]. This phenomenon is known as cross-reactivity or heterologous immunity and has been best demonstrated for T cells specific to Epstein–Barr virus (EBV) antigens [12]. The same is likely to be true of T cells specific to other viruses. The inherent ability of developing T cells to bind to HLA molecules also contributes to the high precursor frequency of alloreactive T cells in the mature T cell repertoire [13]. The inherent bias to generate TCRs that "see" HLA is attributed to the fact that T cell education in the thymus and the ultimate development of a mature cellular immune system are dependent on recognition of peptides bound to HLA (Chapter 3). Therefore, alloreactivity is an unintended side effect of an immune system that has evolved to effectively fend off foreign, generally microbial, antigens.

T cell alloreactivity is in large part a memory response, even in naive individuals not previously exposed to alloantigens

The primary immune response to a foreign antigen not previously encountered by the host is mediated by naive T lymphocytes (Chapter 3). Naive T cells specific to the foreign antigen are present at a low precursor frequency, have a relatively high stimulation threshold (e.g., stringent dependence on costimulatory molecules), can only be activated within secondary lymphoid tissues (e.g., the spleen and lymph nodes) [14], and are, therefore, slow to respond. In contrast, the secondary immune response to an antigen previously encountered by an individual (e.g., after vaccination or infection) is mediated by memory T cells and is significantly stronger and faster than a primary response. Antigen-specific memory T cells are long-lived lymphocytes that exist at a greater precursor frequency than their naive counterparts, have a low stimulation threshold and high proliferative capacity, and can be activated within secondary lymphoid tissues or at non-lymphoid sites – for example, the site of infection or in the allograft itself [15]. Memory B cells and plasma cells share some of the properties of memory T cells thus, endowing vaccinated individuals with the ability to rapidly produce high titers of antigen-specific antibodies upon reinfection (Chapter 4). Immunological memory, therefore, provides humans with optimal protection against microbes.

Humans for the most part are not exposed to alloantigens, with the exception of mothers who may have been sensitized to paternal antigens during pregnancy or individuals who had prior transfusions or organ transplants. Yet all humans, including those presumably never exposed to allogeneic cells or tissues, harbor alloreactive memory T cells. Accurate quantitation of alloreactive T cells has demonstrated that approximately 50 % of the alloreactive T cell repertoire in humans is made up of memory T lymphocytes [11, 16, 17]. This finding can again be explained by the phenomenon of cross-reactivity, whereby memory T cells specific to microbial antigens also recognize alloantigens and contribute to the high precursor frequency of alloreactive T cells. Therefore, the extent of one's alloreactivity is intimately shaped by one's immunological memory to foreign antigens not necessarily related to the graft.

The distinguishing features of alloimmunity summarized above have important implications for both the immunological monitoring of transplant recipients and the development of anti-rejection therapies. It is becoming increasingly clear that measuring anti-donor memory T cells or donor-specific antibodies either before or after transplantation could predict rejection incidence and graft outcomes [18]. Moreover, T-lymphocyte-depleting agents used to prevent rejection invariably skew T cells that repopulate the host towards memory [19, 20]. These memory T cells arise from antigen-independent, homeostatic proliferation of undepleted naive or memory T cells – a phenomenon known as lymphopenia-induced proliferation [21]. Lymphopenia-induced T cell proliferation is responsible for early and late acute rejection episodes in lymphocyte-depleted transplant recipients and creates an obstacle to minimizing immunosuppression [22]. Another clinical implication of alloreactive

memory T cells is that anti-rejection agents that inhibit naive lymphocyte activation or migration are not expected to be as effective as those that suppress both naive and memory lymphocytes. Targeting memory T or B cells, therefore, is desirable but leads to the important conundrum of how to inhibit alloreactivity without compromising beneficial antimicrobial memory. Overcoming this challenge could pave the path towards developing the next generation of immunotherapeutic agents in transplantation.

Immune regulation

The alloimmune response is subject to regulatory mechanisms common to all immune responses. Four principal regulatory mechanisms have been described: activation-induced cell death (AICD), regulation by specialized lymphocyte subsets known as T_{REG} and B_{REG}, anergy, and exhaustion. These mechanisms ensure that "collateral damage" to the host is kept to a minimum during or after a productive immune response.

Primary and secondary T cell responses are characterized by exponential proliferation of antigen-specific T cells followed by a "crash" phase in which the majority of activated or effector T cells die by apoptosis (Plate 1.1). This process prevents unnecessary immunopathology while allowing T cells that escape apoptosis to become memory lymphocytes. The same is true for B cells, where the process of expansion followed by death allows for the selection of B lymphocytes with the highest affinity to their target antigens (affinity maturation) (Chapter 4). Most immunusuppressive drugs available for clinical use target lymphocyte proliferation and in some cases (e.g., calcineurin inhibitors) prevent AICD [23], leaving the possibility of developing agents that selectively enhance the apoptosis of activated T cells open. Such a strategy would be more specific than pan-T-cell depletion, as only T cells that have been activated by alloantigens are killed.

The isolation of T and B cell subpopulations that downregulate immune responses in vitro and in vivo has led to a resurgence of studies on regulatory lymphocytes (Chapter 6). T_{REG} and B_{REG} populations have been identified in rodents and, in the case of the former, in humans as well. Regulatory lymphocytes suppress mixed lymphocyte reactions in vitro and prolong allograft survival in rodent transplantation models. The mechanisms by which T_{REG} suppress immune responses are varied. They include cytokines (e.g., IL-10 and TGFβ), inhibitory membrane molecules (e.g., CTLA-4), and possibly direct cytotoxicity to naive or effector lymphocytes. In addition to interest in isolating and expanding T_{REG} for adoptive cell therapy in transplant recipients, there has been an important focus on developing or exploiting existing immunosuppressive drugs that spare or enhance regulatory lymphocytes. One example is the mTOR inhibitor rapamycin, which in mice generates a favorable T_{REG} to effector T cell ratio that may contribute to long-term allograft survival. It is not certain, however, whether the salutary effects of rapamycin on T_{REG} in rodents will translate to longer allograft survival in humans because of the pleiotropic functions of mTOR signaling in different cells of the immune system.

Anergy and exhaustion refer to the state in which T cells or B cells become unresponsive to restimulation with antigen. Anergy occurs when naive lymphocytes encounter antigen in the absence of critical costimulatory signals necessary for their full activation. A prime example of costimulation is the B7–CD28 pathway (Chapter 3). B7 molecules expressed on antigen-presenting cells engage CD28 on T cells concurrent with T cell stimulation through the TCR. Blocking B7-CD28 interaction renders T cells anergic and/or induces their apoptosis [24, 25]. CTLA4-Ig, a fusion protein that binds B7 molecules and prevents them from engaging CD28, is currently approved for use in renal transplant recipients. Published data suggest that CTLA4-Ig may be an effective substitute for calcineurin inhibitors. Finally, exhaustion occurs when effector or memory T cells repeatedly encounter a persistent antigen, as would occur during chronic viral infection or in the case of an allograft. Repeated antigenic stimulation induces the expression of inhibitory molecules that keep T cells hypo- or un-responsive. One example of such inhibitory molecules is PD-1, shown in rodents to suppress alloreactive effector T cells [26]. These regulatory pathways provide interesting opportunities for developing novel strategies to inhibit T cells that have been activated by alloantigens. By targeting activated but not naive T cells, these strategies may prove more selective than currently available immunosuppressive therapies.

The innate immune system in transplantation

The mammalian immune system consists of two integrated arms: the innate and adaptive.

The adaptive immune system (the subject of discussion of this chapter so far) consists of T and B lymphocytes which express diverse and highly specific antigen receptors brought about by gene rearrangement, expand clonally, and generate immunological memory. Unlike the adaptive system, the innate immune system is made up of inflammatory cells (dendritic cells, monocytes, macrophages, neutrophils, eosinophils, basophils, and other cells) that do not express rearranging receptors, have limited proliferative capacity, and, for the most part, do not generate memory. Cells of the innate immune system instead express nonrearranging, germ-line-encoded receptors that detect conserved molecular patterns present in microbes but not shared by mammalian cells [27]. A representative example of innate receptors is toll-like receptor (TLR)-4, which recognizes lipopolysaccharide on Gram-negative bacteria (Chapter 5). It should be noted that the innate immune system also encompasses noncellular mediators capable of microbial recognition – for example, complement proteins. Activation of the innate immune system by microbial ligands causes inflammation, the first line of defense against infection, but more importantly induces the maturation and migration of antigen-presenting cells to secondary lymphoid tissues where they trigger primary T cell and B cell responses. The latter function of the innate immune system is critical for initiating adaptive immunity to infection and vaccines in the naive host. The innate immune system, therefore, is responsible for the first self–non-self recognition event that ultimately leads to productive T and B cell immunity.

Although the innate recognition pathways required for establishing antimicrobial immunity have been uncovered for many infectious diseases, how the innate immune system triggers the adaptive alloimmune response is not as straightforward. Several endogenous ligands released by dying cells in the graft participate in ischemia–reperfusion injury (Chapter 6), but it is not clear whether any single ligand has a dominant role or whether any are critical for triggering either naive or memory T cell activation. These uncertainties could be due to the release of myriads of redundant activators of the innate immune system by the graft at the time of transplantation or due to the possibility that memory T cell activation, an important component of the alloimmune response, could occur independent of innate immune activation. Nevertheless, it is generally accepted that inflammation influences the migration of effector and memory T cells to the transplanted organ and increases the intensity of rejection [28]. Prolonged cold or warm ischemia not only predisposes allografts to delayed function after transplantation, but also to increased risk of acute and chronic rejection [29]. Recent studies have suggested that the innate immune system may be capable of distinguishing between self and allogeneic non-self [30, 31], akin to its role in detecting microbial non-self. This intriguing possibility could imply that an innate allorecognition system that precedes allorecognition of HLA by the adaptive immune system maintains immunity against allografts long after the early inflammatory phase has subsided. The nature of such innate allorecognition and whether it contributes to either acute or chronic rejection remains to be determined.

Concluding remarks

The immune system is composed of rich layers of cellular and humoral mediators that work in concert to protect humans against potentially fatal infections. One price that humans pay for this highly developed defense system is the rejection of life-saving organ transplants. Better understanding of the regulatory mechanisms embedded in the immune system and of the subtle distinctions between antimicrobial and alloimmunity should pave the path towards selective immunotherapies that prevent rejection but preserve beneficial immunity against infection. Studying the immune system is like peeling an onion: beneath each layer we find another; "chopping the onion will bring tears … only during peeling does it speak the truth" [32].

References

1 Hall BM, Dorsch S, Roser B. The cellular basis of allograft rejection in vivo. II. The nature of memory cells mediating second set heart graft rejection. *J Exp Med* 1978;148:890–902.

2 Hall BM, Dorsch S, Roser B. The cellular basis of allograft rejection in vivo. I. The cellular requirements for first-set rejection of heart grafts. *J Exp Med* 1978;148:878–889.

3 Miller JFAP. Effect of neonatal thymectomy on the immunological responsiveness of the mouse. *Proc R Soc Lond B* 1962;156:415–428.

4 Bingaman AW, Ha J, Waitze S-Y *et al*. Vigorous allograft rejection in the absence of danger. *J Immunol* 2000;164:3065–3071.

5 Kirk AD, Hale DA, Mannon RB *et al*. Results from a human renal allograft tolerance trial evaluating the humanized CD52-specific monoclonal antibody alemtuzumab (CAMPATH-1H). *Transplantation* 2003;76: 120–129.

6 Takemoto S, Terasaki PI, Cecka JM *et al*. Survival of nationally shared, HLA-matched kidney transplants from cadaveric donors. The UNOS Scientific Renal Transplant Registry. *N Engl J Med* 1992;327:834–839.

7 Starzl TE, Lerner RA, Dixon FJ *et al*. Shwartzman reaction after human renal homotransplantation. *N Engl J Med* 1968;278:642–648.

8 Patel R, Terasaki PI. Significance of the positive crossmatch test in kidney transplantation. *N Engl J Med* 1969;280:735–739.

9 Solez K, Colvin RB, Racusen LC *et al*. Banff 07 classification of renal allograft pathology: updates and future directions. *Am J Transplant* 2008;8:753–760.

10 Suchin EJ, Langmuir PB, Palmer E *et al*. Quantifying the frequency of alloreactive T cells in vivo: new answers to an old question. *J Immunol* 2001;166:973–981.

11 Macedo C, Orkis EA, Popescu I *et al*. Contribution of naïve and memory T-cell populations to the human alloimmune response. *Am J Transplant* 2009;9: 2057–2066.

12 Burrows S, Khanna R, Burrows J, Moss D. An alloresponse iln humans is dominated by cytotoxic T lymphocytes (CTL) cross-reactive with a single Epstein–Barr virus CTL epitope: implications for graft-versus-host disease. *J Exp Med* 1994;179:1155–1161.

13 Zerrahn J, Held W, Raulet DH. The MHC reactivity of the T cell repertoire prior to positive and negative selection. *Cell* 1997;88:627–636.

14 Lakkis FG, Arakelov A, Konieczny BT, Inoue Y. Immunologic "ignorance" of vascularized organ transplants in the absence of secondary lymphoid tissue. *Nature Med.* 2000;6:686–688.

15 Chalasani G, Dai Z, Konieczny BT *et al.* Recall and propagation of allospecific memory T cells independent of secondary lymphoid organs. *Proc Natl Acad Sci U S A* 2002;99:6175–6180.

16 Merkenschlager M, Terry L, Edwards R, Beverley PC. Limiting dilution analysis of proliferative responses in human lymphocyte populations defined by the monoclonal antibody UCHL1: implications for differential CD45 expression in T cell memory formation. *Eur J Immunol* 1988;18:1653–1661.

17 Lombardi G, Sidhu S, Daly M *et al.* Are primary alloresponses truly primary? *Int Immunol* 1990;2:9–13.

18 Dinavahi R, Heeger PS. T-cell immune monitoring in organ transplantation. *Curr Opin Organ Transplant* 2008;13:419–424.

19 Pearl J, Parris J, Hale D *et al.* Immunocompetent T-cells with a memory-like phenotype are the dominant cell type following antibody-mediated T-cell depletion. *Am J Transplant* 2005;5:465–474.

20 Toso C, Edgar R, Pawlick R *et al.* Effect of different induction strategies on effector, regulatory and memory lymphocyte sub-populations in clinical islet transplantation. *Transpl Int* 2009;22:182–191.

21 Surh CD, Sprent J. Homeostasis of naive and memory T cells. *Immunity* 2008;29:848–862.

22 Wu Z, Bensinger SJ, Zhang J *et al.* Homeostatic proliferation is a barrier to transplantation tolerance. *Nat Med* 2004;10:87–92.

23 Li Y, Li XC, Zheng XX *et al.* Blocking both signal 1 and signal 2 of T-cell activation prevents apoptosis of alloreactive T cells and induction of peripheral allograft tolerance. *Nat Med* 1999;5:1298–1302.

24 Dai Z, Konieczny BT, Baddoura FK, Lakkis FG. Impaired alloantigen-mediated T cell apoptosis and failure to induce long-term allograft survival in IL-2-deficient mice. *J Immunol* 1998;161:1659–1663.

25 Wells AD, Li XC, Li Y *et al.* Requirement for T-cell apoptosis in the induction of peripheral transplantation tolerance. *Nat Med* 1999;5:1303–1307.

26 Habicht A, Kewalaramani R, Vu MD *et al.* Striking dichotomy of PD-L1 and PD-L2 pathways in regulating alloreactive CD4$^+$ and CD8$^+$ T cells in vivo. *Am J Transplant* 2007;7:2683–2692.

27 Palm NW, Medzhitov R. Pattern recognition receptors and control of adaptive immunity. *Immunol Rev* 2009;227:221–233.

28 Chalasani G, Li Q, Konieczny BT *et al.* The allograft defines the type of rejection (acute versus chronic) in the face of an established effector immune response. *J Immunol* 2004;172:7813–7820.

29 Murphy SP, Porrett PM, Turka LA. Innate immunity in transplant tolerance and rejection. *Immunol Rev* 2011;241:39–48.

30 Fox A, Mountford J, Braakhuis A, Harrison LC. Innate and adaptive immune responses to nonvascular xenografts: evidence that macrophages are direct effectors of xenograft rejection. *J Immunol* 2001;166:2133–2140.

31 Zecher D, van Rooijen N, Rothstein D *et al.* An innate response to allogeneic nonself mediated by monocytes. *J Immunol* 2009;183:7810–7816.

32 Grass G. *Peeling the Onion.* New York: Harcourt; 2007.

CHAPTER 2
Antigen Presentation in Transplantation

Martin H. Oberbarnscheidt and Fadi G. Lakkis

Thomas E. Starzl Transplantation Institute, Departments of Surgery, Immunology, and Medicine, University of Pittsburgh, Pittsburgh, PA, USA

Transplantation antigens

Transplantation of organs between genetically disparate individuals of the same species (allogeneic individuals) leads to recognition and rejection of the allogeneic tissue by the recipient's immune system. The immune process of discriminating between self- and non-self-tissues is called allorecognition. The principal transplantation antigens, or alloantigens, recognized during this process are genetically encoded polymorphic proteins that are expressed on tissues of individuals. These polymorphic determinants are the major histocompatibility complex (MHC) antigens (in humans known as human leukocyte antigens or HLAs) and the minor histocompatibility antigens (mHAgs). MHC antigens are glycoproteins expressed by polymorphic multigene clusters located on chromosome 17 in mice and chromosome 6 in humans (Figure 2.1), whereas mHAgs can be any other polymorphic protein that is encoded virtually anywhere in the genome.

MHC molecules

The MHC is polygenic, polymorphic and codominantly expressed. All of these features contribute to the large inter-individual variability – at least 300 HLA alleles have been identified in the human population. There are two classes of MHC molecules, class I and II, that differ in their structure, function, and tissue distribution. MHC class I proteins are expressed on all nucleated cells, whereas MHC class II expression is restricted to antigen-presenting cells (APCs), activated T cells, and endothelial cells. APCs include B cells, dendritic cells (DCs), macrophages, and other phagocytic cells described in more detail later in this chapter. An individual can express at least three different MHC class I (HLA-A, -B and -C) and class II (HLA-DR, -DP and -DQ) proteins (Figure 2.1). Typically, most individuals will be heterozygous at the MHC locus, and the MHC class II HLA-DR cluster will contain an additional β chain (HLA-DRB), resulting in the expression of six different MHC class I and eight different MHC class II molecules on cells.

The primary function of MHC molecules is to bind short peptides that are derived from proteins processed by the cell. The cellular and biochemical mechanisms of antigen processing are reviewed elsewhere [1]. Briefly, exogenous antigens are processed into small peptides in endosomes and lysosomes, whereas endogenous (cytosolic) antigens are processed by proteosomes. Peptide loading onto MHC molecules occurs in the Golgi apparatus

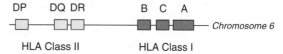

Figure 2.1 *HLAs*. Organization of the genes coding for the HLA on human chromosome 6.

Immunotherapy in Transplantation: Principles and Practice, First Edition. Edited by Bruce Kaplan, Gilbert J. Burckart and Fadi G. Lakkis.
© 2012 Blackwell Publishing Ltd. Published 2012 by Blackwell Publishing Ltd.

with the help of specialized transporter proteins. Peptide:MHC complexes then translocate to the cell membrane where they can be surveyed by the immune system. Non-self-peptide:MHC complexes expressed by APCs trigger T cell activation by binding the T cell receptor (TCR) for antigen (Chapter 3). In the case of non-APCs, non-self-peptide:MHC complexes serve as a target for T cells specific for the presented antigenic peptide. The MHC, therefore, ensures that foreign antigens, especially those derived from infecting organisms, are detected and eliminated by the immune system with great specificity. The high degree of polymorphism (diversity) of the MHC guarantees that virtually any microbial-derived peptide can be presented to the immune system.

Peptides presented by MHC class I molecules are usually derived from endogenous, cytosolic proteins (either self or foreign), although exogenous antigens may also be presented. The presentation of exogenous proteins in the context of MHC class I is referred to as cross-presentation or cross-priming [2, 3]. MHC class I complexes interact with the TCR on CD8 T cells. They are comprised of a heavier glycosylated α chain and a lighter β2-microglobulin chain. The α chain contains a transmembrane domain and three extracellular domains: α-1, α-2, and α-3. The variable α-1 and α-2 helices form a groove, which is closed at the ends, that serves as the binding site for processed peptides. The specificity of the peptide-binding groove is determined by the different alleles encoding the α-1 and α-2 helices. The peptide and surrounding amino acids of the α-1 and α-2 helices are recognized by the TCR. α-3 is not variable and interacts with CD8 to increase the binding of the MHC:peptide complex to the TCR. β2-Microglobulin is also not variable and is encoded on a different chromosome (chromosome 15) than the α chain.

MHC class II molecules generally present peptides derived from exogenous proteins, which are taken up by APCs and processed in the vesicular compartment (endosomes and lysomes), but MHC class II molecules can also present endogenous, cytosolic peptides [4–6]. MHC class II complexes interact with the TCR on CD4 T cells. They are heterodimers composed of an α and a β chain – both of which are polymorphic. The variable α-1 and β-1 domains of each of these chains form the peptide-binding pocket, which is open so that longer peptides can be presented than those of MHC class I. The bound peptide in conjunction with surrounding amino acids is then recognized by the TCR. CD4 interacts with the nonvariable α-2 domain of MHC class II molecules to strengthen the binding of the MHC:peptide complex to the TCR.

Although the principal function of MHC molecules is to present microbial peptides to T cells, they are also the most prominent transplantation antigens. Non-self-MHC is recognized by 1–10 % of the T cells of an individual (Chapter 1). Since T cells are selected to recognize foreign peptides in the context of self-MHC, it is thought that cross-reactivity of TCRs allows allorecognition by T cells. Allorecognition by T cells, therefore, includes the recognition of self-peptide:non-self-MHC, non-self-peptide:self-MHC or non-self-peptide:non-self-MHC complexes. The different models proposed to explain TCR cross-reactivity are reviewed by Yin & Mariuzza [7].

mHAgs

The mHAgs play an important role in allorecognition and account for the rejection of HLA-matched organs and graft versus host disease (GvHD) after hematopoietic stem cell (bone marrow) transplantation. An example of a clinically relevant mHAg is the H-Y antigen present in male mice and humans. In mice, transplantation of skin from a male to an otherwise syngeneic female recipient will result in rejection of the graft in most strains [8]. Recent reports reviewed the role of H-Y and other mHAgs in solid organ transplantation [9, 10]. In humans, Gratwohl *et al.* [9] showed in a retrospective multivariate analysis that female recipients of male kidney transplants have a higher risk of graft failure, suggesting an immunological effect of H-Y in kidney transplantation. The effect of sex-mismatched hematopoietic stem cell transplantation (female donor to male recipient) leading to GvHD has been well described [11, 12]. Antigen-specific T cells and antibodies against H-Y-encoded gene products could be detected in these recipients [13–15]. So far, more than 50 mHAgs in mice and humans have been described, with differences between donor and recipient ranging from single amino acid residues to extensive variation, but it is estimated that there may be hundreds more. mHAgs are presented in the context of recipient MHC class I and II. How subtle differences in mHAgs influence their presentation by MHC molecules and lead to TCR recognition is an area of active investigation.

Other transplantation antigens

No discussion of transplantation antigen is complete without underscoring the fact that the first alloantigens to be discovered were those that define blood groups in humans, the ABO system being the most prominent. ABO antigens are carbohydrate determinants expressed on red blood cells, as well as in other cells and tissues. Since they do not evoke T cell responses, they are not classified as mHAgs. Matching for ABO blood types made both blood transfusion and organ transplantation possible – as transplantation across ABO-incompatibility without prior desensitization led to the hyperacute rejection of organ allografts. Hyperacute rejection is caused by preformed IgM antibodies produced during infancy by B-1 lymphocytes, so-called innate B cells, independent of T cell help (Chapter 4).

APCs

An important link between the innate and adaptive immune system are professional APCs. APCs take up, process, and present antigens in the context of MHC molecules and, in addition, possess the necessary molecules to activate or inhibit the adaptive immune system through a variety of cell-surface proteins; these include adhesion molecules (e.g., integrins) and costimulatory molecules (e.g., B7 family members CD80 and CD86) (Chapter 3). DCs, macrophages, and B cells are the main populations of professional APCs. Other APCs include subtypes of phagocytic cells, such as Kupfer and stellate cells in the liver.

DCs

DCs were first described morphologically by Steinman and colleagues and were found to be potent stimulators of the mixed leukocyte reaction (MLR) [16, 17], an in vitro test that measures T cell alloreactivity. All DCs originate from myeloid precursors in the bone marrow and are distributed throughout most tissues of the body. DCs are specialized in antigen uptake through a variety of different mechanisms, which include phagocytosis, macropinocytosis, and receptor-mediated endocytosis (e.g., via Fc, C-type lectin, scavenger, and complement receptors). They also process antigens into small peptides that are presented in the context of MHC molecules. DCs are highly migratory. Activated DCs that have taken up antigen and have received innate activation signals (e.g., from microbes) mature and migrate to secondary lymphoid tissue where they present antigen to T cells.

DCs are often divided into lymphoid tissue DCs (CD8$^+$ and CD8$^-$ DC) and non-lymphoid tissue DCs (tissue-specific subsets, like Langerhans cells in the skin or intestinal CD103$^+$ and CD103$^-$ DC) [18, 19]. Non-lymphoid tissue DC subsets differ in their migratory properties, although in general they migrate to secondary lymphoid tissue after antigen uptake and innate activation. While most DCs originate from pre-DCs in the bone marrow (these DCs are increasingly referred to as conventional DCs or cDCs), there is increasing evidence that monocytes are the precursors of certain non-lymphoid tissue DC subsets under steady-state conditions and, more importantly, upon inflammation. DCs play a twofold role in transplantation: donor DCs that accompany the allograft can be directly recognized by the recipient's T cells (direct allorecognition), whereas recipient's DCs take up donor alloantigen, process it, and present it to recipient T cells (indirect allorecognition) (see next section).

DCs also include a distinct but small subset known as plasmacytoid DCs (pDCs) because of their plasma cell-like morphology [20]. Despite their name, pDCs derive from a myeloid precursor in the bone marrow; but unlike other DCs, they express CD4 and produce large amounts of type I interferons in response to viral infection. They are capable of presenting alloantigen to T cells, but recent evidence suggests that pDCs may play a role in tolerance induction in transplantation [21].

Macrophages and monocytes

Macrophages are phagocytic cells that engulf pathogens and clear dying cells. They are equipped with a variety of receptors, such as mannose, scavenger, and complement receptors. Macrophages, like DCs, process antigen and present it in the context of MHC molecules, but they are not as potent activators of the MLR as DCs. Because macrophages scavenge dead cells, expression of costimulatory molecules is tightly regulated and thought to be only upregulated in the context of non-self recognition. Monocytes are rapidly recruited to sites of inflammation and are thus also a prominent cell type in allograft rejection. Although their main role has been seen as pro-inflammatory effector cells that differentiate into macrophages and contribute to graft destruction, there is increasing evidence that they differentiate into either DCs or immunregulatory cells sometimes referred to as myeloid-derived suppressor cells [22]. The role of host monocyte-derived DCs in transplantation is currently under investigation.

B lymphocytes

B cells can bind specific soluble antigens through their cell surface immunoglobulin, internalize them, and present peptides in the context of MHC class II. B cells constitutively express high levels of MHC class II, but require induction of costimulatory molecules for efficient T cell priming upon activation. Antigen presentation by B cells has been shown to be relevant in autoimmunity [23–25] and microbial immunity [26], as well as in transplantation [27, 28]. In the latter case, antigen presentation by B cells has been shown to potentiate the alloimmune response, leading to increased generation of memory T cells.

Antigen presentation pathways

Three pathways of antigen presentation have been described in the context of transplantation: direct, indirect, and semi-direct (Figure 2.2). In direct presentation, recipient T cells recognize self- or non-self-peptides presented in the context of allogeneic, donor MHC molecules expressed on donor APCs [29, 30]. In indirect presentation, alloantigens are taken up and processed by recipient APCs and presented in the context of recipient MHC molecules to recipient T cells. Semi-direct presentation refers to the acquisition of intact donor MHC:peptide complexes by recipient APCs and their presentation to recipient T cells.

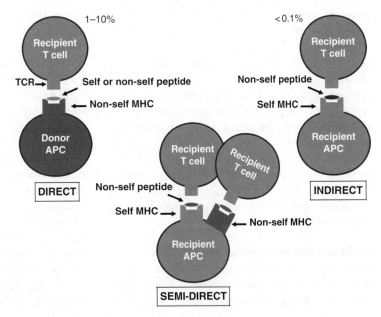

Figure 2.2 *Pathways of alloantigen presentation.* The three pathways of alloantigen presentation (direct, indirect, and semi-direct) are shown. The frequency (%) of T cells that react to a specific pathway is indicated where known. APC: antigen-presenting cell; MHC: major histocompatibility complex molecule; TCR: T cell receptor for antigen.

Direct alloantigen presentation

Direct presentation has historically been viewed as the major pathway involved in acute allograft rejection. This view is supported by the strong T cell proliferation observed in the MLR, as well as by the original studies of Lafferty and coworkers showing that depletion of APCs (so-called passenger leukocytes) from thyroid allografts by culturing prior to transplantation results in prolonged graft survival in the absence of immunosuppression [31, 32]. Another early study by Lechler *et al.* showed that retransplantation of renal allografts "parked" in an intermediate, immunosuppressed host (causing depletion of donor APCs) leads to graft acceptance in rats [33]. Pietra *et al.* showed that CD4 T cells adoptively transferred to severe combined immunodeficiency (SCID) or recombination-activating-gene-deficient (Rag$^{-/-}$) mice were not able to reject MHC class II deficient cardiac allografts [34]. Conversely, Rag$^{-/-}$ MHC class II$^{-/-}$ recipients were able to reject the cardiac allografts after the adoptive transfer of CD4 T cells, indicating that CD4 T cells with direct allorecognition are sufficient to mediate allograft rejection. The high precursor frequency of "directly" alloreactive T cells is most likely due to cross-reactivity [35]. Supportive of this hypothesis are the findings that in humans a large number of alloreactive T cells have a memory phenotype [36, 37]. Human memory T cell populations contributing to the alloresponse contain virus-specific T cells (e.g., reactivity against EBV) that cross-react with specific alloantigens (e.g., HLA-B44) [38]. Since direct recognition is dependent on the presence of donor APCs in the allograft, it is thought to dominate T cell priming in the immediate post-transplantation period. After donor APC frequency declines by means of apoptosis and rejection by the recipient's immune response, the number of direct recognition recipient T cells also declines. Therefore, it is presumed that direct antigen presentation is particularly relevant to acute rejection.

Indirect alloantigen presentation

Indirect antigen presentation is in fact the default pathway of T cell priming outside of transplantation, as T cells are selected to recognize antigens in the context of self-MHC. In transplantation, it was suggested as a pathway of allograft rejection after the observation that donor-leukocyte-depleted renal allografts in rats were still rejected, although much more slowly than nondepleted allografts [39]. Accelerated allograft rejection was demonstrated by Fabre and coworkers by immunizing recipients with peptides of allogeneic donor MHC antigens [40]. More evidence came from experiments using skin grafts from MHC class II$^{-/-}$ mice, which fail to initiate direct recognition by CD4 T cells and were still rejected in a CD4 T-cell-dependent manner by MHC class I$^{-/-}$ recipients (these recipients lack CD8 T cells) [41]. Indirect allorecognition, therefore, is largely host CD4 T cell dependent and MHC class II dependent. This could be further demonstrated in murine cardiac allograft experiments using combinations of MHC class I, class II, and double knock-out mice as donors or recipients [42]. Here, MHC class II deficiency of the cardiac allograft was necessary to obtain indefinite graft survival, and a corresponding experiment resulted in prolonged graft survival only if the recipient lacked CD4 T cells (MHC class II$^{-/-}$ recipient). Because donor-derived APCs (passenger leukocytes) are eliminated within a short period after transplantation, it is thought that indirect allorecognition is the principal alloantigen presentation pathway that leads to chronic rejection. There is ample evidence to support this in mice and humans, but it is also increasingly recognized that indirect allorecognition is sufficient and perhaps critical for acute rejection.

Like CD4 T cells, CD8 T cells are also capable of indirect recognition, a phenomenon known as cross-priming. Cross-priming refers to the process of presenting peptides derived from exogenous donor alloantigens in the context of recipient MHC class I molecules on recipient APCs. One study provided evidence that recipient endothelium can indirectly cross-present donor skin graft antigens in the context of MHC class I to TCR-transgenic CD8 T cells, which resulted in skin graft rejection [43]. However, the same group showed that, in a cardiac allograft model, indirectly primed CD8 T cells are nonpathogenic bystanders [44]. The significance of the indirect CD8 T cell pathway (cross-priming) in organ transplantation is, therefore, not completely understood.

Semi-direct alloantigen presentation

Semi-direct presentation has been described as a novel pathway of alloantigen presentation by APCs [45]. Herrera *et al.* reported that mouse DCs acquire allogeneic MHC:peptide complexes after in vitro incubation with allogeneic DCs but also in vivo upon migration of donor APCs to regional lymph nodes. The semi-direct antigen presentation model proposed would link T cells with direct and indirect allospecificity. The traditional model of CD4 T cell help for generating cytotoxic CD8 T cells requires priming by the same APCs. In transplantation, this could unlink the direct from the indirect presentation pathway. The semi-direct presentation model allows a recipient APC to present processed allopeptide:self-MHC complexes as well as acquired allopeptide:donor MHC complexes, linking both the direct and indirect presentation pathway (Figure 2.2). This model also helps explain the finding that embryonic thymic epithelium, which lacks APCs, is rejected in the absence of indirect allorecognition [46] and that costimulation-deficient cardiac allografts (CD80$^{-/-}$CD86$^{-/-}$ donors) are acutely rejected by MHC class II$^{-/-}$ recipients lacking the indirect pathway [47]. The significance of the semi-direct pathway in vivo has not yet been fully determined.

Migration of APCs and sites of interaction with T cells

APC trafficking in organ transplantation encompasses the migration of donor DCs from the graft to the secondary lymphoid tissues (e.g., spleen and lymph nodes) where they interact with host naive and memory T cells, and the migration of host monocytes and other DC precursors to the graft. The latter migration pattern leads to repopulation of the graft with host-derived DCs, which interact with effector and memory T cells in the graft or migrate back to the secondary lymphoid tissues after picking up donor alloantigens. It is important to note that naive T cell activation by APCs occurs within the organized structures of secondary lymphoid tissues, whereas memory T cells can be activated in lymphoid and non-lymphoid tissues (e.g., within the graft itself) [48–50]. One exception to this rule is the activation of naive T cells within the graft if ectopic lymphoid tissues, also known as tertiary lymphoid tissues, are present, as is the case in organs undergoing chronic inflammation/rejection [51–54]. Naive T cell activation by resident APCs also occurs in lung allografts, which contain broncho-alveolar lymphoid tissues (BALT), and in small-bowel allografts, which contain Peyer's patches [55, 56]. Since naive and memory T cells are both involved in initiating and propagating the alloimmune response in humans (Chapter 1), all three sites of T cell activation (the graft, secondary lymphoid tissues, and tertiary lymphoid tissues) are important in the rejection process.

DC migration from sites of inflammation to secondary lymphoid tissues occurs via the blood or afferent lymphatic channels [57]. The principal mechanism responsible for DC migration to lymph nodes is the chemokine receptor CCR7. CCR7 is a G protein-coupled receptor that binds CCL19 and CCL21, chemokines present in high concentration on high endothelial venules in lymph nodes. The adhesion molecules involved in adhesion and transendothelial migration of DCs into lymph nodes are L-selectin and possibly other molecules, such as the C-type lectin receptor DC-SIGN (CD209). Monocyte migration from the bone marrow, spleen, and blood into sites of inflammation, such as the graft, is dependent on the chemokine receptors CCR2 and/or CX3CR1 (fractalkine receptor) [58].

Relevance to immunotherapy

Although immunosuppressive agents currently in clinical use for solid organ transplantation are not viewed as immunotherapies that target antigen presentation, some do influence APC function. Prime examples are corticosteroids and the mammalian target of rapamycin (mTOR) inhibitor, rapamycin. There is evidence that corticosteroids suppress the maturation of and MHC class II and inflammatory cytokine expression by monocytes, macrophages, and DCs, making them less effective at presenting antigen and activating T cells. Rapamycin, on the other hand, has contrasting effects on APCs [59]. It inhibits the maturation of in-vitro-generated DCs but surprisingly also increases antigen presentation by enhancing autophagy in monocytes, macrophages, and DCs. The complex effects of rapamycin on the immune system could explain its pleiotropic effects in humans and may underlie its less than predictable effects on long-term allograft survival.

Further elucidation of the types of APC and antigen-presentation pathways involved in allograft rejection promises to yield novel immunotherapies in transplantation. Potential strategies include (a) specific targeting of APC subsets by monoclonal antibodies or pharmacological agents, (b) inhibition of APC migration from or to the graft, and (c) manipulating DCs in vitro to render them "tolerogenic." "Tolerogenic" DCs can then be administered to humans at the time of transplantation to downmodulate the alloimmune response by a process known as "negative vaccination" [60]. APCs, therefore, provide an attractive target for immunotherapy in transplantation.

References

1 Cresswell P. Antigen processing and presentation. *Immunol Rev* 2005;207:5–7.

2 Bevan MJ. Cross-priming for a secondary cytotoxic response to minor H antigens with H-2 congenic cells which do not cross-react in the cytotoxic assay. *J Exp Med* 1976;143(5):1283–1288.

3 Bevan MJ. Cross-priming. *Nat Immunol* 2006;7(4): 363–365.

4 Dissanayake SK, Tuera N, Ostrand-Rosenberg S. Presentation of endogenously synthesized MHC class II-restricted epitopes by MHC class II cancer vaccines is independent of transporter associated with Ag processing and the proteasome. *J Immunol* 2005;174(4):1811–1819.

5 Nimmerjahn F, Milosevic S, Behrends U *et al.* Major histocompatibility complex class II-restricted presentation of a cytosolic antigen by autophagy. *Eur J Immunol* 2003; 33(5):1250–1259.

6 Paludan C, Schmid D, Landthaler M *et al.* Endogenous MHC class II processing of a viral nuclear antigen after autophagy. *Science* 2005;307(5709):593–596.

7 Yin Y, Mariuzza RA. The multiple mechanisms of T cell receptor cross-reactivity. *Immunity* 2009;31(6):849–851.

8 Eichwald EJ, Silmser CR. Skin. *Transplant Bull* 1955;2:148–149.

9 Gratwohl A, Dohler B, Stern M, Opelz G. H-Y as a minor histocompatibility antigen in kidney transplantation: a retrospective cohort study. *Lancet* 2008;372(9632): 49–53.

10 Dierselhuis M, Goulmy E. The relevance of minor histocompatibility antigens in solid organ transplantation. *Curr Opin Organ Transplant* 2009;14(4):419–425.

11 Miklos DB, Kim HT, Miller KH *et al.* Antibody responses to H-Y minor histocompatibility antigens correlate with chronic graft-versus-host disease and disease remission. *Blood* 2005;105(7):2973–2978.

12 Stern M, Passweg JR, Locasciulli A *et al.* Influence of donor/recipient sex matching on outcome of allogeneic hematopoietic stem cell transplantation for aplastic anemia. *Transplantation* 2006;82(2):218–226.

13 Goulmy E, van Leeuwen A, Blokland E *et al.* Major histocompatibility complex-restricted H-Y-specific antibodies and cytotoxic T lymphocytes may recognize different self determinants. *J Exp Med* 1982; 155(5):1567–1572.

14 Voogt PJ, Fibbe WE, Marijt WA *et al.* Rejection of bone-marrow graft by recipient-derived cytotoxic T lymphocytes against minor histocompatibility antigens. *Lancet* 1990;335(8682):131–134.

15 Spierings E, Vermeulen CJ, Vogt MH *et al.* Identification of HLA class II-restricted H-Y-specific T-helper epitope evoking CD4+ T-helper cells in H-Y-mismatched transplantation. *Lancet* 2003;362(9384):610–615.

16 Steinman RM, Witmer MD. Lymphoid dendritic cells are potent stimulators of the primary mixed leukocyte reaction in mice. *Proc Natl Acad Sci U S A* 1978; 75(10):5132–5136.

17 Steinman RM, Cohn ZA. Identification of a novel cell type in peripheral lymphoid organs of mice. I. Morphology, quantitation, tissue distribution. *J Exp Med* 1973;137(5):1142–1162.

18 Liu K, Nussenzweig MC. Origin and development of dendritic cells. *Immunol Rev* 2010;234(1):45–54.

19 Helft J, Ginhoux F, Bogunovic M, Merad M. Origin and functional heterogeneity of non-lymphoid tissue dendritic cells in mice. *Immunol Rev* 2010;234(1):55–75.

20 Swiecki M, Colonna M. Unraveling the functions of plasmacytoid dendritic cells during viral infections, autoimmunity, and tolerance. *Immunol Rev* 2010; 234(1):142–162.

21 Ochando JC, Homma C, Yang Y *et al.* Alloantigen-presenting plasmacytoid dendritic cells mediate

tolerance to vascularized grafts. *Nat Immunol* 2006; 7(6):652–662.

22 Geissmann F, Manz MG, Jung S *et al.* Development of monocytes, macrophages, and dendritic cells. *Science* 2010;327(5966):656–661.

23 O'Neill SK, Shlomchik MJ, Glant TT *et al.* Antigen-specific B cells are required as APCs and autoantibody-producing cells for induction of severe autoimmune arthritis. *J Immunol* 2005;174(6):3781–3788.

24 Chan OT, Hannum LG, Haberman AM *et al.* A novel mouse with B cells but lacking serum antibody reveals an antibody-independent role for B cells in murine lupus. *J Exp Med* 1999;189(10):1639–1648.

25 Noorchashm H, Lieu YK, Noorchashm N *et al.* I-Ag7-mediated antigen presentation by B lymphocytes is critical in overcoming a checkpoint in T cell tolerance to islet beta cells of nonobese diabetic mice. *J Immunol* 1999;163(2):743–750.

26 Lund FE, Hollifield M, Schuer K *et al.* B cells are required for generation of protective effector and memory CD4 cells in response to Pneumocystis lung infection. *J Immunol* 2006;176(10):6147–6154.

27 Noorchashm H, Reed AJ, Rostami SY *et al.* B cell-mediated antigen presentation is required for the pathogenesis of acute cardiac allograft rejection. *J Immunol* 2006;177(11):7715–7722.

28 Ng YH, Oberbarnscheidt MH, Chandramoorthy HC *et al.* B cells help alloreactive T cells differentiate into memory T cells. *Am J Transplant* 2010;10(9):1970–1980.

29 Warrens AN, Lombardi G, Lechler RI. Presentation and recognition of major and minor histocompatibility antigens. *Transpl Immunol* 1994;2(2):103–107.

30 Whitelegg A, Barber LD. The structural basis of T-cell allorecognition. *Tissue Antigens* 2004;63(2):101–108.

31 Talmage DW, Dart G, Radovich J, Lafferty KJ. Activation of transplant immunity: effect of donor leukocytes on thyroid allograft rejection. *Science* 1976; 191(4225):385–388.

32 Lafferty KJ, Cooley MA, Woolnough J, Walker KZ. Thyroid allograft immunogenicity is reduced after a period in organ culture. *Science* 1975;188(4185):259–261.

33 Batchelor JR, Welsh KI, Maynard A, Burgos H. Failure of long surviving, passively enhanced kidney allografts to provoke T-dependent alloimmunity. I. Retransplantation of (AS X AUG)F1 kidneys into secondary AS recipients. *J Exp Med* 1979;150(3):455–464.

34 Pietra BA, Wiseman A, Bolwerk A *et al.* CD4 T cell-mediated cardiac allograft rejection requires donor but not host MHC class II. *J Clin Invest* 2000;106(8):1003–1010.

35 Gras S, Kjer-Nielsen L, Chen Z *et al.* The structural bases of direct T-cell allorecognition: implications for T-cell-mediated transplant rejection. *Immunol Cell Biol* 2011;89(3):388–395.

36 Merkenschlager M, Ikeda H, Wilkinson D *et al.* Allorecognition of HLA-DR and-DQ transfectants by human CD45RA and CD45R0 CD4 T cells: repertoire analysis and activation requirements. *Eur J Immunol* 1991;21(1):79–88.

37 Lombardi G, Sidhu S, Daly M *et al.* Are primary alloresponses truly primary? *Int Immunol* 1990;2(1):9–13.

38 Macedo C, Orkis EA, Popescu I *et al.* Contribution of naive and memory T-cell populations to the human alloimmune response. *Am J Transplant* 2009;9(9): 2057–2066.

39 Lechler RI, Batchelor JR. Immunogenicity of retransplanted rat kidney allografts. Effect of inducing chimerism in the first recipient and quantitative studies on immunosuppression of the second recipient. *J Exp Med* 1982;156(6):1835–1841.

40 Benham AM, Sawyer GJ, Fabre JW. Indirect T cell allorecognition of donor antigens contributes to the rejection of vascularized kidney allografts. *Transplantation* 1995;59(7):1028–1032.

41 Auchincloss H, Jr, Lee R, Shea S *et al.* The role of "indirect" recognition in initiating rejection of skin grafts from major histocompatibility complex class II-deficient mice. *Proc Natl Acad Sci U S A* 1993;90(8):3373–3377.

42 Campos L, Naji A, Deli BC *et al.* Survival of MHC-deficient mouse heterotopic cardiac allografts. *Transplantation* 1995;59(2):187–191.

43 Valujskikh A, Lantz O, Celli S *et al.* Cross-primed CD8⁺ T cells mediate graft rejection via a distinct effector pathway. *Nat Immunol* 2002;3(9):844–851.

44 Valujskikh A, Zhang Q, Heeger PS. CD8 T cells specific for a donor-derived, self-restricted transplant antigen are nonpathogenic bystanders after vascularized heart transplantation in mice. *J Immunol* 2006;176(4): 2190–2196.

45 Herrera OB, Golshayan D, Tibbott R *et al.* A novel pathway of alloantigen presentation by dendritic cells. *J Immunol* 2004;173(8):4828–4837.

46 Pimenta-Araujo R, Mascarell L, Huesca M *et al.* Embryonic thymic epithelium naturally devoid of APCs is acutely rejected in the absence of indirect recognition. *J Immunol* 2001;167(9):5034–5041.

47 Mandelbrot DA, Kishimoto K, Auchincloss H, Jr *et al.* Rejection of mouse cardiac allografts by costimulation in trans. *J Immunol* 2001;167(3):1174–1178.

48 Lakkis FG, Arakelov A, Konieczny BT, Inoue Y. Immunologic 'ignorance' of vascularized organ transplants in the absence of secondary lymphoid tissue. *Nat Med* 2000;6:686–688.

49 Chalasani G, Dai Z, Konieczny BT *et al.* Recall and propagation of allospecific memory T cells independent of secondary lymphoid organs. *Proc Natl Acad Sci U S A* 2002;99:6175–61780.

50 Lakkis F. Where is the alloimmune response initiated? *Am J Transplant* 2003;3:241–242.

51 Baddoura FK, Nasr IW, Wrobel B *et al.* Lymphoid neogenesis in murine cardiac allografts undergoing chronic rejection. *Am J Transplant* 2005;5(3):510–516.

52 Nasr IW, Reel M, Oberbarnscheidt MH *et al.* Tertiary lymphoid tissues generate effector and memory T cells that lead to allograft rejection. *Am J Transplant* 2007;7(5):1071–1079.

53 Kerjaschki D, Regele HM, Moosberger I *et al.* Lymphatic neoangiogenesis in human kidney transplants is associated with immunologically active lymphocytic infiltrates. *J Am Soc Nephrol* 2004;15(3):603–612.

54 Thaunat O, Field A-C, Dai J *et al.* Lymphoid neogenesis in chronic rejection: evidence for a local humoral alloimmune response. *Proc Natl Acad Sci U S A* 2005; 102:14723–14728.

55 Gelman AE, Li W, Richardson SB *et al.* Cutting edge: acute lung allograft rejection is independent of secondary lymphoid organs. *J Immunol* 2009;182(7): 3969–3973.

56 Wang J, Dong Y, Sun JZ *et al.* Donor lymphoid organs are a major site of alloreactive T-cell priming following intestinal transplantation. *Am J Transplant* 2006;6(11): 2563–2571.

57 Randolph GJ, Ochando J, Partida-Sanchez S. Migration of dendritic cell subsets and their precursors. *Annu Rev Immunol* 2008;26:293–316.

58 Gelman AE, Okazaki M, Sugimoto S *et al.* CCR2 regulates monocyte recruitment as well as CD4 T1 allorecognition after lung transplantation. *Am J Transplant* 2010;10(5):1189–1199.

59 Thomson AW, Turnquist HR, Raimondi G. Immunoregulatory functions of mTOR inhibition. *Nat Rev Immunol* 2009;9(5):324–337.

60 Thomson AW. Tolerogenic dendritic cells: all present and correct? *Am J Transplant* 2010;10(2):214–219.

CHAPTER 3

The T Cell Response to Transplantation Antigens

Didier A. Mandelbrot[1], Bryna Burrell[2], Mohamed H. Sayegh[3], and Peter S. Heeger[4]

[1]The Transplant Institute and Harvard Medical School, Boston, MA, USA
[2]Mount Sinai School of Medicine, Recanati/Miller Transplantation Institute, New York, NY, USA
[3]Brigham and Women's Hospital, Boston, MA, USA
[4]Mount Sinai School of Medicine, Recanati/Miller Transplantation Institute, New York, NY, USA

Basic T cell lexicon

T lymphocytes are a critical component of immune responses. Using their T cell receptors (TCRs), they recognize specific peptide antigens presented in the context of major histocompatibility (MHC) molecules expressed on antigen-presenting cells (APCs). The two main types of mature T cells are CD4-expressing T helper (Th) lymphocytes, which recognize peptides expressed on class II MHC, and the CD8-expressing cytolytic T lymphocytes (CTLs), which recognize peptides expressed on class I MHC. CD4 T cells regulate immune responses both by directly engaging signaling receptors on APCs and by secreting cytokines, which act locally to regulate additional T cells, B cells and other leukocytes. CD4 T cells are important in both stimulating and downregulating various specific immune responses. CD8 T lymphocytes can kill cells expressing foreign antigens, such as cells infected with microbes or transplanted cells that express alloantigens, but also produce cytokines. While circulating T cells express either CD4 or CD8, during thymic development T cell precursors can express one, neither (double negative, DN), or both (double positive, DP) of these molecules.

T cell activation requires two signals. The first signal is provided by cognate interactions between the Ag/MHC complex on APCs and the TCRs on T cells. The second, or costimulatory, signal is provided by ligands on APCs such as B7-1 and B7-2 to receptors on T cells, such as CD28. Further activation signals are provided by cytokines such as IL-2 and by numerous intracellular signaling pathways. For example, the calcineurin and target of rapamycin (TOR) pathways transmit and integrate signals from cell-surface receptors, resulting in T cell proliferation and differentiation. Activation of naive T cells, which occurs predominantly in secondary lymphoid organs (LN and spleen), induces proliferation, differentiation, and an ability to migrate to peripheral organs where, upon re-encounter of their specific antigen, they mediate effector functions. Thus, CD4 T cells serve to regulate both the afferent and efferent limbs of the immune response: they both recognize the transplanted graft antigens and mediate the effector mechanisms that reject grafts. CD4 cells can differentiate into Th1, Th2, and Th17 cells, which have distinct phenotypes and functions in immune responses. CD4 cells can also differentiate into regulatory T cells (Tregs), which are important for downregulating immune responses, and into memory cells. In the effector phase of the alloresponse, helper CD4 cells provide direct cellular signals as well as cytokine signals to other

Immunotherapy in Transplantation: Principles and Practice, First Edition. Edited by Bruce Kaplan, Gilbert J. Burckart and Fadi G. Lakkis.
© 2012 Blackwell Publishing Ltd. Published 2012 by Blackwell Publishing Ltd.

CD4 cells, CD8 cells, B cells, and macrophages. Interactions between APCs and T cells, as well as leukocyte trafficking in general, are regulated by a number of adhesion molecules, such as leukocyte factor antigen (LFA)-1 and intercellular adhesion molecule (ICAM)-1.

Anti-rejection therapies in clinical use target both cell-surface molecules, such as CD3 and CD25, and intracellular signaling pathways. Therapies that are likely to be used in the future target B7, CD28, CD40, and other costimulatory molecules, as well as adhesion molecules [1].

T cell development and maintenance

Origins of T cell precursors

T cells originate in the fetal liver prenatally and in the bone marrow as hematopietic stem cells (HSCs) postnatally [2]. HSC lymphoid progenitors were initially described as Thy-1.1^{lo}, Lineage (Lin)$^-$ and stem cell antigen-1 (Sca-1)$^+$ [3]. Although only 0.02–0.06 % of mouse bone marrow cells fit this phenotype, reconstitution by as few as 30 of these cells results in the rescue and viability of half of syngeneic irradiated mice [3]. Further characterization shows these cells to fall into one of three groups: long-term HSCs possessing unlimited self-renewal capacity, short-term HSCs with some degree of self-renewal capacity, and multipotent progenitors that cannot self-renew [4]. These groups can be further differentiated based on low versus negative expression of Mac-1 and CD4. In irradiated recipients, HSCs negative for these markers provide long-term reconstitution, whereas low expression of these markers on HSCs correlates with transient reconstitution [5]. Additionally, HSCs are delineated by CD34 expression in humans [6] and are CD117 (c-kit)$^+$ and CD34$^{lo/-}$ in mice [7]. Lymphoid progenitors are thought to be Lin$^-$c-kit^{lo}IL-7Rα^+ [4].

T cell maturation

T cells mature in the thymus, and at least six T cell populations are exported from the thymus: γ/δ T cells, naive CD4$^+$ and CD8$^+$ α/β T cells, NKT cells, regulatory T cells, and intraepithelial lymphocytes [2]. Thymocyte precursors have only a limited self-

renewal capacity [2], and primitive lymphoid cells are continually imported into the thymic medullary cortex [8] from the circulation to varying degrees throughout life [9]. As these cells progressively develop through stages of maturation, their progeny lose their differentiation potential. Once in the thymus, this CD4 and CD8 negative (DN) precursor population migrates through the thymus and progresses through the DN stages [8], DN2 (CD25$^+$CD44$^+$), DN3 (CD25$^+$CD44$^-$), and DN4 (CD25$^-$CD44$^-$), as cells migrate across the cortex to the subcapsular zone (SCZ) [8] (Figure 3.1). Rearrangement of the TCR β-chain locus occurs during the DN2 to DN3 progression. DN3 T cells are highly proliferative, but as they lose CD25 their

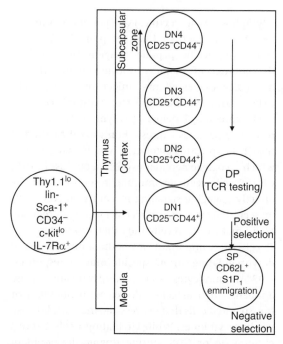

Figure 3.1 T cell maturation. Lymphocyte precursors enter the thymus via the cortex. Double negative (CD4$^-$CD8$^-$, DN) cells progress through the cortex as they mature until they reach the subcapsular zone. Double positive (CD4$^+$CD8$^+$, DP) cells migrate back into the cortex towards the medulla while undergoing TCR testing. Single positive (CD4$^+$CD8$^-$ or CD4$^-$CD8$^+$, SP) cells complete their maturation in the medulla before export to the periphery. Cell-surface markers are notated for each developmental step. Arrows denote direction of cell migration.

division rate slows and they become DN4 T cells. DN4 T cells eventually stop dividing and transform to DP thymocytes that express both CD4 and CD8.

DP thymocytes begin rearranging the TCR α-chain locus, migrate from the SCZ to the thymic cortex [2] and undergo rounds of positive selection, where randomly generated α/β TCRs are tested for their ability to interact with self-MHC [10]. This test of MHC reactivity may not exclude reactivity with foreign MHC and would allow self-derived T cells to react with donor-derived APCs. If T cells cannot engage self-MHC then they undergo programmed cell death, or "death by neglect," allowing only T cells with potentially MHC-reactive TCRs to survive. These DP cells can engage both class II and class I MHC molecules, since both CD4 and CD8 are expressed. By binding to class II or I MHC, extracellular CD4 [11] or CD8 cells [12] bring the protein tyrosine kinase LCK associated with their intracellular domains in proximity to the TCRs, allowing for TCR signaling [10, 13].

DP cells that are positively selected continue to mature into single-positive (SP) cells and are guided to the medulla by CCR7 [14]. Historically, various models have been used to describe the maturation of DP precursors to SP cells with matching coreceptor and TCR-MHC specificity. The stochastic model suggests that complementary coreceptor and TCR-MHC specificity is a random event, whereby the coreceptors are expressed randomly and are rescued by a later TCR signal [10]. In the strength-of-signal model, the strength of the TCR interaction with class I or II MHC determines if cells become either CD8+ or CD4+ SP respectively [15]. More recently, the kinetic model suggests that the length of TCR engagement and presence of the cytokine IL-7 determines of coreceptor specificity [10, 16].

After coreceptor commitment, these SP cells are maintained in the medulla for several (four to five) days before emigrating from the thymus [17]. Here, potentially self-reactive cells are deleted in a process known as negative selection, the main component of central tolerance [18, 19]. This process is dependent upon the presentation of tissue-specific antigens (TSAs) by medullary thymic epithelial cells (mTECs) and/or dendritic cells (DCs) [20]. Under the direction of the autoimmune regulator protein (AIRE), these cells present antigens located throughout the body to ensure tolerance to a wide range of self-antigens [18]. Before leaving the thymus as naive T cells through the medulla or corticomedullary junction [21], these SP cells gain homing markers such as CD62L (required for migration into lymph nodes) and upregulate the sphingosine-1 phosphate receptor (S1P$_1$) [17]. Inhibitors of S1P receptor function, such as FTY720, sequester T cells in the lymph nodes and thymus by blocking egress [21, 22].

T cell maintenance

Once in the periphery, T cells require various signals to remain viable and in circulation. For both CD4+ and CD8+ T cells, basal or tonic TCR engagement by self-MHC is required for homeostasis [23]. Indeed, precursor populations decay in the absence of TCR signaling [24] or in the presence of high precursor frequency [25]. In both mice [26] and humans [27], IL-7 serves to maintain naive T cells and increase the number of naive T cells in the circulation in lymphopenic conditions. Tan *et al.* [28] proposed that basal levels of IL-7 and TCR signaling maintain T cell numbers. However, less IL-7 is consumed in lymphopenic environments. The elevated basal level of IL-7 augments TCR signaling and expands the pool of naive T cells. Additionally, high levels of both the cytokines IL-2 [29] and IL-15 [30] in lymphopenic animals drive the expansion of naive T cells (IL-15 drives CD8+ T cells), favoring the generation of effector and memory T cells respectively [23].

T cell recognition of alloantigen

T cells are central mediators of allograft rejection [31]. Lymphocytes and monocytes were first described as entering inflamed skin grafts through graft vessels shortly following transplantation in a highly graft-specific fashion by Medawar in 1944 [32]. Later, adoptive immunity to grafts was described by transferring cells from the regional lymph nodes of recipients rejecting grafts to a naive recipient; these secondary recipients went on to reject grafts at an accelerated rate [33]. It was concluded that the transferred cells themselves, not transferred donor antigen or donor-reactive antibodies, were responsible for this accelerated response [33]. Conversely, mice lacking T cells (either due to neonatal thymectomy or genetic mutation) fail to reject grafts unless reconstituted with T cells [34].

Alloreactive T cells

Alloreactivity is defined as "the response of T cells to MHC molecules not encountered during thymic development" [35]. Indeed, research regarding causative mechanisms of skin or tumor transplant rejection resulted in the discovery of MHC molecules [36]. Encoded by the MHC (HLA in humans, H2 in mice [37]), alloantigens are present on virtually all nucleated cells. Class I MHC is present on all nucleated cells, whereas class II expression is restricted to professional APCs: B cells, DCs, and macrophages – but is induced on endothelial cells during inflammation [37]. After microbial infection, CD8+ and/or CD4+ T cells recognize foreign antigens that are presented by class I MHC and class II MHC respectively [37, 38]. Following transplantation, however, the foreign MHC itself and antigen shed by the graft are recognized by recipient T cells. As expected, matching donor and recipient MHC results in decreased alloreactivity and prolonged graft survival [39].

High frequencies of recipient T cells, estimated to be 1–10 % of T cells [36], react to allogeneic MHC

[40]. In contrast, the typical frequency of T cells reactive to microbial antigens that have not been previously encountered is 1 in 10^6 [41]. The relatively large proportion of alloreactive T cells is attributed to cross-reactivity (T cells specific to microbial peptides presented by self-MHC cross-react with non-self-MHC) and due to the ability of alloreactive TCRs to respond in a highly specific fashion to multiple ligands, leading to "polyspecificity" of alloreactive T cells [35].

Allorecognition

T cells can recognize alloantigen either directly or indirectly (Figure 3.2). Direct recognition of the graft occurs when recipient T cells are cross-reactive with donor allogeneic MHC [42]. Following transplantation, donor-derived DCs migrate out of the graft and into the spleen where they can directly prime recipient T cells [43]. A potent T cell response is generated when either donor or recipient peptide is presented in the context of allogeneic MHC [36]. Indirect recognition occurs when recipient T cells recognize donor antigen that has been processed by recipient APCs and presented upon recipient MHC [42, 44]. This antigen can either be shed by the graft itself or result from the relatively short-lived donor DCs being phagocytosed following

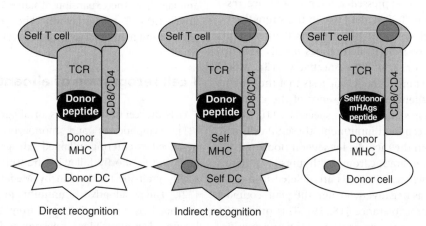

Figure 3.2 Recognition of alloantigen. Direct recognition of alloantigen occurs when the self-T cells cross-react with the MHC molecule of the donor DC. Indirect recognition occurs when self-T cells recognize donor peptide that has been processed and presented by recipient DCs. An alloantigen response is also generated when self-T cells recognize self-peptide presented by donor-cell MHC or minor histocompatibility antigens (mHAgs).

their migration to the spleen [44]. Semidirect recognition occurs when donor-derived MHC is acquired, possibly through membrane transfer, by recipient DCs [45]. These "cross-dressed" APCs can now directly activate recipient T cells and induce graft pathology.

Both direct and indirect alloantigen recognition account for graft pathology. Direct recognition has been implicated in acute graft rejection [42], defined as grafts rejected days or weeks after transplantation. Indirect recognition can also lead to acute rejection, but may be more important for chronic rejection – the rejection of grafts months or years after transplantation [42]. While donor APCs present antigen in the spleen and activate T cells, cells of the graft expressing MHC can serve as direct targets for T-cell-mediated rejection [46].

In addition to the recognition of allogeneic MHC complexes, recognition of mHAgs can induce anti-donor T cell responses. These mHAgs are peptides derived from polymorphic proteins presented by MHC molecules [47]. While better described in priming graft versus host responses following stem cell transplantation [48] and host versus tumor responses [49], mHAgs can trigger T-cell-mediated rejection, an issue particularly relevant to recipients of HLA-matched solid organ transplants [47].

T cell activation, proliferation, and differentiation

T cell activation: two-signal model
Signal 1: TCR engagement
Naive T cells express CD62L and CCR7, which allows them to traffic to the T cell areas of secondary lymphoid tissues [50]. In the periphery, immature DCs acquire antigen and receive "danger signals," such as those transmitted via toll-like receptor ligation under inflammatory or necrotic conditions. The DCs then mature and carry their antigen to secondary lymphoid tissues [51]. In the T cell areas of draining lymph nodes or other secondary lymphoid tissues [51], T cell activation begins with the engagement of the TCR/CD3 complex with the

MHC:peptide complex present on the DCs [52]. Classically, class I MHC molecules present peptides derived from cytosolic intracellular sources to CD8 T cells, whereas class II MHC molecules present antigens derived from endolysosomal compartments (generally exogenous) to CD4 T cells [53]. TCR interactions with MHC:peptide complexes are stabilized by coreceptors present on the T cell surface; CD4 binding to class II MHC and CD8 binding to class I MHC dictate the types of antigen to which CD4$^+$ and CD8$^+$ T cells respond [37, 53]. "Helper" CD4$^+$ T cells aid in the activation of CD8$^+$ T cells by producing IL-2 and providing CD40 signals to the DCs, which in turn facilitates CD8$^+$ T cell activation [54].

Naive T cells require approximately 20 h of DC stimulation to begin proliferation [55], whereas effector T cells require approximately 30 min of TCR engagement to proliferate as their TCR signaling machinery has been fully coupled [51]. T cells continue to divide roughly every 10 h following activation [51].

Signal 2: costimulation
Originally, one signal transmitted via an antigen receptor was hypothesized to be sufficient for T cell activation. In 1969, Lafferty and Jones postulated that the "stimulator" cell provided strong proliferative stimulus [56], later termed "allogeneic stimulus" in the setting of transplantation antigens [57]. The observations that the APCs need to be viable [58] and provide additional "costimulatory" signals in response to "danger" signals indicating damage of host cells [59] resulted in current dogma: multiple signals are needed to activate T cells. Indeed, signal 1 in the absence of signal 2 leads to T cell anergy (inability to respond) [60] or death [61].

Two well-characterized costimulatory interactions in transplantation are the CD40/CD154 and the B7/CD28 pathways. CD40 is a transmembrane protein belonging to the TNFR superfamily [62] expressed by APCs and endothelial cells [63]. CD154 (CD40L, gp39) is expressed on activated CD4$^+$ T cells, CD8$^+$ T cells, NK cells, and eosinophils [63]. Engagement of CD154 enhances T cell production of IL-10 [64], IFNγ [64], and IL-4 [65], and engagement of CD40 results in IL-12 secretion [66] and increased

	Costimulatory molecule	Cognate T cell receptor	Stimulatory (+) or inhibitory (–) of T cells
B7/CD28 family	B7-1/B7-2	CD28	+
	B7-1/B7-2	CTLA-4	–
	ICOSL	ICOS	+
	PDL-1/2	PD-1	–
TNF/TNF-R family	CD40	CD154	+
	4-1BBL	4-1BB	+
	OX40L	OX40	+

Table 3.1 Major costimulatory molecules.

B7-1/B7-2 (CD80/CD86) expression [67] by the APCs, both of which provide activation signals for T cells. Indeed, the CD40–CD154 interaction has been termed the "master switch" for costimulation, as ligation induces the upregulation of other costimulatory molecules [68]. In addition, CD40 ligation on B cells is required for immunoglobulin isotype switching from IgM to IgG. Of relevance to transplantation, blocking CD154 in mice serves to significantly prolong cardiac allograft survival and inhibit APC B7-1/B7-2 expression [69].

CD28 is constitutively expressed by resting human and murine T cells and belongs to the Ig superfamily [70]. Ligation of CD28 by B7-1/B7-2 on the APC surface results in T cell production of IL-2, IFNγ, GM-CSF, TNFα, IL-1, IL-3, and IL-4 [71]. Similar to CD40 ligation, the cytokines IFNγ and IL-4 upregulate B7-1/B7-2 expression [52]. Signaling through CD28 promotes T cell activation by decreasing the number of TCR engagements necessary for T cell activation [72] and activating transcription factors such as NFkB, NFAT, and AP-1 [73]. Additionally, CD28 costimulation serves to inhibit T cell apoptosis by upregulating bcl-x$_L$, offering protection from cell death mediated by Fas [74]. Naive T cells activated through TCR and CD28 engagement differentiate into effector T cells, which lose their CCR7 expression and upregulate receptors needed to enter areas of inflammation [51].

Following activation, T cells upregulate cytotoxic T-lymphocyte-associated antigen 4 (CTLA-4), which engages B7-1/B7-2 molecules with a greater affinity than CD28 [75]. Signaling through CTLA-4 induces T cell death by blocking progression through the cell cycle [75] and serves as a brake to the T cell response.

Other costimulatory molecules belonging to both the Ig and TNF/TNFR families have also been described and deliver both positive and negative signals to activated T cells (Table 3.1 [76]). In the Ig superfamily, the ICOS/ICOSL pathway has been described as augmenting the Th2 pathway, and blocking this interaction results in prolonged graft survival in mice [77]. Interactions between OX40 and OX40L, additional members of the TNF/TNFR superfamily, result in prolonged activated T cell survival and memory generation. Importantly, OX40 stimulation of regulatory T cells inhibits their suppressive function. Also members of the TNF/TNFR superfamily, 4-1BB/4-1BBL interact and augment both cytotoxic T lymphocyte responses and CD4$^+$ T cell responses. Blocking this pathway promotes graft survival in mice [76]. In contrast, one set of Ig superfamily members, the PD-1/PDL-1/2 pathway, inhibits activation of antigen-specific T cells [78]. By activating PD-1 on T cells, graft rejection is inhibited in mice when administered with additional immunosuppressive agents [76].

Recent work indicates that the complement cascade, traditionally considered a component of innate immunity, participates in T cell costimulation. Several reports [79–83] showed that during cognate T cell–APC interactions both cell types produce alternative pathway complement components (C3, factor B, factor D) following CD40/CD154 and CD28/B7 costimulation. The resultant cleavage products, C3a and C5a, bind to their respective receptors on T cells, C3aR and C5aR, and act as essential downstream mediators of costimulatory interactions required for T cell activation. The transmitted C5aR and C3aR (G-protein-coupled receptors) signals activate phosphoinositide 3-kinase gamma (PI3Kγ), leading to phosphorylation of the central intracellular signaling molecule AKT. Activated AKT upregulates the anti-apoptotic gene Bcl2 and downregulates the pro-apoptotic molecule Fas, resulting in an augmented effector T effector response. The locally produced C3a and C5a also affect C3aR/C5aR-expressing APCs, inducing cytokine production (e.g. IL-12, IL-23) and costimulatory molecule upregulation (e.g. B7), amplifying and inducing differentiation of effector T cell responses [79–83]. Studies performed using bone marrow chimeric animals revealed that these effects on T cell immunity are entirely mediated by immune cell-derived complement and are independent of serum complement [80–82].

Intracellular signaling in T cells

Complex machinery transduces surface molecular events to the T cell nucleus, modifying the expression of genes regulating cell function. Engagement of the TCR induces phosphorylation of TCR-associated proteins such as the ζ (zeta) chain, as well as a variety of adapter proteins. These phosphorylation events lead to the activation of several biochemical pathways, including the calcineurin pathway, the protein kinase C pathway, and the Ras– and Rac–mitogen-activated protein (MAP) kinase pathways. Within minutes of TCR engagement, phosphorylation of ZAP-70 (ζ-associated protein of 70 kDa) leads to the phosphorylation of PLCγ1 (phospholipase C γ1), which hydrolyzes a membrane phospholipid phosphatidylinositol 4,5-bisphosphate (PIP_2) into inositol 1,4,5-trisphosphate (IP_3) and diacylglycerol (DAG). IP_3 leads to an increase in cytosolic calcium, which binds calmodulin, forming a complex that activates several enzymes, including the phosphatase calcineurin [84]. Calcineurin dephosphorylates NFAT (nuclear factor of activated T cells), allowing NFAT to translocate from the cytoplasm to the nucleus. Once in the nucleus, NFAT binds to regulatory sequences and increases the transcription of genes for several cytokines, including the T-cell growth factor IL-2 [85].

Binding of IL-2 to the IL-2 receptor further activates T cells through a number of pathways, including the TOR pathway. Activation of TOR leads to increased synthesis of proteins important for cell growth and proliferation, including IL-2. TOR also induces G1 to S phase progression through the cell cycle.

Generation of T cell effector and memory responses

After receiving activation signals, naive CD4+ and CD8+ T cells become effector and memory cells. CD4+ T cells can mature into one of multiple lineages, including T helper 17 (Th17), Th1, or Th2 cells that employ distinct patterns of cytokines to destroy pathogens, or regulatory T cells, which limit or prevent effector T cell responses. CD8+ T cells can also mature into Tc17, Tc1, Tc2, cytotoxic or regulatory T cells. Signals from the microenvironment, the type of APC, concentration of antigen, and costimulatory pathways involved all dictate to which lineage these cells commit [86]. Most effector T cells undergo apoptosis after the immune response reaches its peak, but some primed T cells survive as long-lived memory cells which can be quickly reactivated upon re-exposure to antigen [87, 88].

Th1

Th1 T cells are characterized by the production of IFNγ, as well as IL-2, TNFα, and lymphotoxin. CD8α+ DCs and macrophages produce IL-12 in response to T-cell-produced early T lymphocyte activation-1 (Eta-1, osteopontin) [89] or following the recognition of foreign ligands [90]. IL-12 then synergizes with macrophage-derived IL-18, resulting in IFNγ production by several cell types, including T cells [91]. IFNγ binds to IFNγ receptors on the T cell surface, resulting in STAT-1 translocation to the nucleus [92] and T-bet transcription [93] (Figure 3.3).

T-bet (T-box expressed in T cells) induces and supports IFNγ production [94] by remodeling the IFNγ gene [95] and inducing T cell IL-12Rβ2 expression. CD4+ T cells are completely dependent upon T-bet for Th1 commitment, whereas CD8+ T

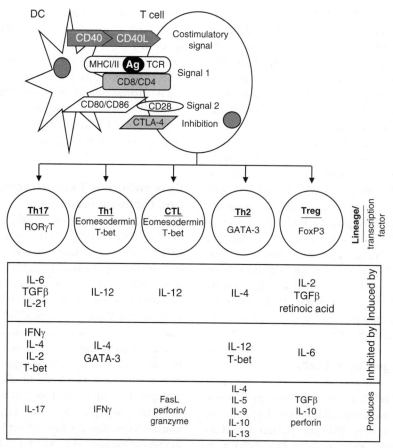

Figure 3.3 T cell activation and differentiation. In the T cell zone of the secondary lymphoid tissues, mature DCs present antigen to T cells. Following costimulation and the second activation signal, T cells can proliferate and differentiate into a variety of lineages. Cytokines/molecules that both induce and inhibit the lineage commitments, the transcription factors required, and the cytokines/molecules produced by the lineages are depicted.

cells can utilize eomesodermin, a T-bet homologue and alternative Th1 transcription factor [96]. T-bet also negatively regulates Th17 cells [90]. Th1 commitment is inhibited by GATA-3, the Th2 transcription factor [97]. In addition to stimulating Th1 responses, IL-12 inhibits Th2 responses by repressing the expression of GATA-3 [90].

Of relevance to transplantation, Th1 responses correlate with episodes of acute graft rejection [98]. Further, MHC upregulation is induced by IFNγ, increasing the number of potential targets for the TCR/CD3 complex to bind [99]. IFNγ also induces complement-fixing IgG2a production by B cells [86, 100] and helps prime cytotoxic lymphocyte responses [101].

Th2

Following TCR engagement with CD8α-DC MHC class II, T cells produce IL-4, the signature cytokine of Th2 cells [102]. IL-4 engages the T cell IL-4 receptor and induces STAT-6 translocation to the nucleus [103], resulting in expression of the IL-4 receptor and the Th2 transcription factor GATA-3 [97, 104]. Similar to the inhibition of Th1 differentiation by Th2 cells, Th2 differentiation is negatively regulated by IL-12 [97] and the Th1 transcription factor T-bet [105]. The Th2 response (and the associated cytokines IL-4, IL-5, IL-9, IL-10, and IL-13) results in B cell production of IgG1 and IgE [106] and is critical in the response to extracellular pathogens and allergens [105]. Th2 responses are relevant to transplantation, as they can induce an alternative form of graft rejection characterized by granulocytic recruitment and vascular involvement [107, 108]. Further, by inducing antibody production, Th2 responses can result in graft pathology. Donor-reactive antibody can result in hyperacute rejection occurring minutes after transplant and both early and chronic graft loss, depending on when the antibody is formed [109].

Th17

The Th17 lineage is named for production of its signature cytokine, IL-17. The six members of the IL-17 family (IL-17A–F) are produced by CD4$^+$ T cells, CD8$^+$ T cells, eosinophils, neutrophils, and monocytes [110]. The five known receptors (IL-17R, IL-17RB-RE) are expressed in a wide variety of tissues [110]. STAT-3 [111], the transcription factor RORγT, and the cytokines TGF-β (transforming growth factor-β), IL-6, and IL-21 induce IL-17 secretion, whereas IL-23 is necessary for its continued production [112, 113]. Negative regulators of Th17 include IFNγ [114], IL-4 [114], IL-2 [115], and the Th1 transcription factor T-beta [116].

IL-17 stimulates production of the chemokines IL-8, MCP-1, and Gro-α, resulting in chemotaxis of monocytes and neutrophils to sites of inflammation [117]. This influx provides immediate protection at sites of acute infection, giving the adaptive immune response the necessary time to generate a more tailored response while minimizing host tissue damage [118]. IL-17 is detrimental to graft survival as it primes DCs to present donor antigens to T cells [119] and upregulates CD40 expression [120]. Clinically, Th17 responses have been correlated with lung graft rejection in humans [121].

Cytotoxic T lymphocytes

Once exposed to antigen, CD8$^+$ CTLs rapidly proliferate [122] and memory CTLs are programmed [123]. To induce this rapid (1–2 days post-exposure) response, both CD4$^+$ T cells [122] and antigen presentation by DCs [124] are integral. CD4$^+$ T cell "licensing" [122] and TLR agonists [125] induce DCs to produce IL-12 and prime CTLs. Subsequent TCR engagement of the primed CTLs results in release of perforin/granzyme and/or upregulation of Fas Ligand (FasL) on the CTL surface, which induces apoptosis of the target cell [126].

Regulatory T cells

Regulatory T cells (Tregs) are generated in both the thymus and in the periphery and serve to limit immune responses and prevent autoimmunity [127]. In the thymus, regulatory cells (or tTregs) are thought to evolve before the CD4$^+$ CD8$^+$ step of cell selection [128]. While the exact mechanism of Treg commitment remains to be elucidated, high-affinity TCRs, IL-2, and CD28 signaling may play an important role [127]. Tregs generated in the peripheral lymphoid tissues (also called induced, or iTreg [127]) may arise in response to the amount of antigen [129], method of antigen presentation [129], and presence of TGFβ [130] and retinoic acid [127]. Regardless of point of origin, Tregs are reported to express the coreceptors CD4 or CD8, the activation marker/IL-2 receptor α-chain CD25, and the costimulatory molecules GITR, OX40, and/or CLTA-4 on their cell surface [131]. However, this heterogeneous population has a common link, in that all Tregs rely on the transcription factor FoxP3 [132]. In the absence of FoxP3, both mice [132] and humans [133] develop autoimmune disorders.

Tregs mediate a number of functions that serve to limit effector cell damage to healthy tissue and cells, including prevention of transplant rejection [134]. Treg-derived TGFβ, IL-10, perforin, and FasL may suppress effector T cell function [135–137]. Much of the exact mechanism by which Tregs down-modulate immune responses remains undefined. Instances of Tregs suppressing effector cells via modulation of cytokine production, costimulatory molecule expression, inhibition of proliferation, conversion to a regulatory phenotype, and induction of anergy have all been described [138] (see Chapter 6).

Memory

Development of memory cells is dependent upon dose and duration of antigenic stimulation [139]. Memory cells are segregated based on homing receptors expressed and function. Central memory T cells express CD62L and/or CCR7, which directs them towards lymph nodes. They proliferate rapidly and produce IL-2 upon restimulation [140]. Effector memory T cells express CCR5 and CCR6 that draw these cells to peripheral tissues [141].

These cells proliferate poorly but are immediately cytolytic following antigen re-exposure [141]. Memory cells derived from Th1 and Th2 responses maintain their Th phenotype upon restimulation [141] and provide a quick defense upon antigen re-exposure [51]. CD4+ T cells [142] and the transcription factors T-bet and eomesodermin are thought to be necessary for memory CTL generation [143], while IL-7 and IL-15 are necessary in maintaining memory CTLs [122].

Memory cells provide a major barrier to transplant tolerance. They are refractive to costimulatory blockade, cell depletion, and regulatory-cell-mediated suppression [139]. These memory cells may be generated in response to previous transplantation, blood transfusion, pregnancy, or lymphopenia [139]. Further, memory cells generated in response to infection may be alloreactive, a phenomenon termed heterologous immunity [144].

How T cells reject an organ

Acute and chronic rejection

Graft rejection is traditionally classified by the timing of the rejection event with respect to the transplantation procedure. Hyperacute rejection occurs within minutes or hours of transplantation and is mediated by preformed antibodies. These antibodies are directed against ABO blood group antigens or MHC molecules. Hyperacute rejection is rare in current clinical practice because of careful pre-transplant blood typing and in vitro screening for donor-specific antibodies. T cells do not play a significant role in hyperacute rejection, which is characterized by complement activation and intravascular thrombosis.

Acute cellular rejection usually develops a week or more after transplantation, with CD4 T cells playing a critical role in the regulation of various effector mechanisms that destroy a graft [107]. The initial inflammatory response to transplantation-associated injury is antigen independent and mediated by innate immunity (Chapter 5). It contributes to T cell activation and the recruitment of T cells to the graft. The antigen-specific activation of CD4 T cells leads to expression of cell-surface molecules and production of cytokines, which

further stimulate monocytes. This cooperation between CD4 T cells and monocytes, or DTH response, plays an important role in graft destruction [145]. Additionally, CD4 T cells can directly reject grafts [146].

The activation of CD4 T cells also stimulates the activation and proliferation of cytolytic CD8 T cells. Upon recognition of class I MHC molecules on graft cells, CD8 T cells cause cell death by two main mechanisms. CD8 T cells can release soluble cytotoxic factors such as granzymes and perforin, which are potential markers for the noninvasive diagnosis of rejection [147]. CD8 T cells also upregulate Fas ligand that binds Fas (CD95) on target cells [148]. When Fas is engaged on cells of a graft, these cells undergo apoptosis, or programmed cell death. While these cytolytic pathways all contribute to graft damage, none of them is necessary for rejection [149]. There is also evidence that allografts can directly stimulate CD8 cells to destroy allografts [150], and that acute rejection by CD8 cells can occur in the absence of CD4 cells [151].

Cytokines produced by CD4 T cells also stimulate B cells. Upon binding of specific antigen by the B cell receptor, or cell surface immunoglobulin, B cells proliferate and differentiate into plasma cells. Plasma cells release soluble immunoglobulins, or antibodies, which can bind allogeneic cells. Antibodies can cause cell damage by fixing complement or by mediating antibody-dependent cellular cytotoxicity (ADCC). This humoral response contributes to graft damage in acute rejection and is described in detail in Chapter 4.

Chronic rejection usually refers to processes that occur more than a year after transplantation. While the indirect pathway appears to be less important than the direct pathway in acute rejection, indirect antigen presentation becomes particularly important in chronic rejection [152]. In general, mechanisms that are important in acute rejection are also important in chronic rejection. These mechanisms include both humoral and cellular responses, including DTH reactions by CD4 T cells. Cytokines such as IFNγ and TNF stimulate both the endothelial and smooth muscle cells of the graft as well as macrophages. Additionally, factors such as FGF (fibroblast growth factor) and TGF-β have been implicated in graft fibrosis [153]. Most grafts eventually develop a chronic vasculopathy characterized by the proliferation of intimal smooth muscle cells, leading to narrowed arteries, ischemia, and scarring. The importance of IFNγ in this process is highlighted by studies demonstrating that IFNγ leads to vasculopathy even in the absence of leukocytes [154]. In addition, residual scarring from episodes of acute rejection contributes to chronic graft failure. Not surprisingly, episodes of acute rejection are associated with worse long-term graft outcome [155].

While allospecific T cells contribute to chronic rejection, antibody does as well. This is supported by the finding that patients who develop donor-specific antibodies after transplantation are at higher risk of chronic rejection than those who do not (please see Chapter 4). Also, numerous antigen-independent factors contribute to chronic vasculopathy and graft failure [156]. For example, in kidney transplantation the nephrotoxicity of calcineurin inhibitors, hypertension, diabetes, and recurrence of primary renal disease can all contribute to chronic graft failure.

Leukocyte recruitment

For leukocytes to exit a blood vessel and enter a site of tissue injury, such as an allograft, a complex series of interactions between adhesion molecules must take place [157]. Leukocyte homing can be divided into three steps. In the first, endothelial cells are activated, leading to the expression of selectins. The binding of selectins to their ligands on leukocytes slows their travel through the blood vessel and the leukocytes start rolling along the endothelium, allowing circulating cells to sample various environments. The second step involves the secretion of chemokines (chemotactic cytokines), which attract more leukocytes to the site of inflammation and lead to the firm attachment of leukocytes to the endothelium. This firm adhesion is mediated by integrins on leukocytes binding to their ligands, either on the endothelial cell surface or in the extracellular matrix. The third step is the extravasation (transendothelial migration) of leukocytes into surrounding tissue. One of the most extensively

studied adhesive interactions occurs between the integrin LFA-1 (CD11a/CD18) and ICAM-1 (CD54). In addition to their role in leukocyte extravasation, LFA-1 and ICAM-1 are also important in antigen-specific immune responses as they mediate firm adhesion between T cells and APCs [158].

Many of the steps involved in leukocyte recruitment have been studied specifically in the context of transplantation. Ischemic injury causes increased production of several cytokines, including interleukin (IL)-1, which upregulates expression of selectins. Cytokines produced following the surgical trauma of transplantation also induce expression of several other adhesion molecules, including E-selectin, ICAM-1, and vascular cell adhesion molecule (VCAM)-1 [159]. Chemokines are also upregulated in the context of graft ischemia–reperfusion injury and infiltration with leukocytes [160].

Relevance to therapy

Relevance to mechanisms of action of current agents

One of the most specific markers of T cells is the cell-surface marker CD3, which is associated with the TCR. Monoclonal antibodies to CD3 are potent immunosuppressants. By binding to CD3, these antibodies induce T cell apoptosis. All subtypes of T cells are affected, including naive and memory CD4 and CD8 cells [161]. To more specifically target activated T cells, monoclonal antibodies to the IL-2 receptor were developed. Resting T cells express the β and γ subunits of the IL-2 receptor, and activated T cells additionally express the α subunit (CD25). Antibodies to the IL-2 receptor bind the α subunit, and work by blocking the binding of IL-2, not by causing cell death [162]. Anti-thymocyte globulin is a polyclonal rabbit antiserum which includes specificities to numerous T cell markers such as CD3, CD4 and CD8, costimulatory molecules such as CD28, B7-1 and B7-2 and adhesion molecules such as LFA-1, ICAM-1 [163]. ATG works both by antibody mediated cell lysis and by inducing programmed cell death of T cells.

Several times in the history of transplant immunology the empiric discovery of immunosuppressive agents pre-dated knowledge about their mechanisms of action. Subsequently, these immunosuppressive agents were used as important tools to understand basic mechanisms of T cell activation. For example, the discovery of cyclosporine eventually led to a detailed understanding of the calcineurin pathway. Cyclosporine exerts its immunosuppressant effect by binding to an intracellular protein, cyclophilin (CYP), and the cyclosporine–cyclophilin complex inhibits the activity of calcineurin (Figure 3.4). Tacrolimus (originally known as FK506) binds to FK-binding protein (FKBP) and the tacrolimus–FKBP complex similarly inhibits the activity of calcineurin. Tacrolimus does not bind to cyclophilin, but the FKBP also binds to sirolimus (formerly known as rapamycin), which has a similar molecular structure to tacrolimus. However, the sirolimus–FKBP complex does not interact at all with calcineurin. Rather, it binds and inhibits the TOR, resulting in decreased transcription of cytokine genes and decreased cell cycling and growth [164]. The anti-metabolites azathioprine

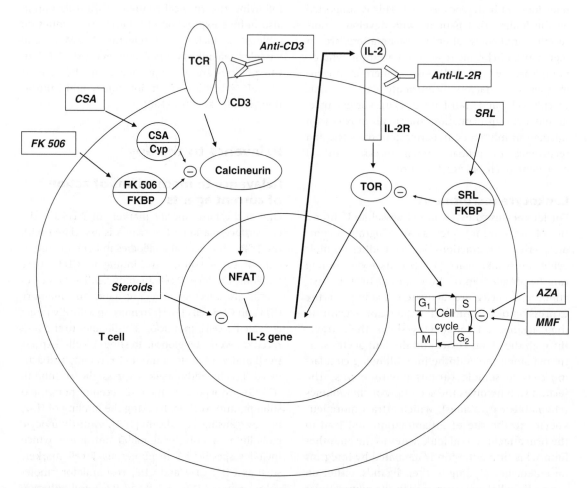

Figure 3.4 Mechanisms of action of current immunosuppressive agents (shown in boxed italics). Abbreviations: CSA (cyclosporine), FK506 (tacrolimus), Cyp (cyclophilin), FKBP (FK binding protein), TCR (T cell receptor), NFAT (nuclear factor of activation of T cells), SRL (sirolimus), AZA (azathioprine), MMF (mycophenolate mofetil), TOR (target of rapamycin).

(AZA) and mycophenolate mofetil (MMF) work by inhibiting the nucleotide synthesis that is required for DNA replication and cell division [165]. Steroids, the first drugs used clinically to prevent transplant rejection, work by a number of mechanisms, including the inhibition of cytokine gene transcription and the inhibition of cell adhesion.

Relevance to future therapies

The immunosuppressive drugs in current use are extremely potent in blocking transplant rejection. However, as none of these drugs is antigen specific they also suppress immune responses to infections and tumors. Targeting costimulatory molecules as an approach to anti-rejection therapy has generated great interest. Timing costimulatory blockade to occur at the time of transplantation, thus allowing engagement of signal 1 but not signal 2, holds the promise of specifically blocking responses to transplantation antigens without producing global immunosuppression. This approach has proven successful in animal models and is currently in phase III trials in humans. For example, using CTLA-4-Ig to block the interaction between CD28 and B7-1/B7-2 and using anti-CD154 to block CD40/CD154 interactions are effective in preventing rejection in primates [166]. In combination they are particularly potent [166]. A CTLA-4-Ig preparation, abatacept (Orencia), has been approved to treat rheumatoid arthritis [167]. A modified version of CTLA-4-Ig with increased avidity for B7-1 and B7-2 [168], LEA29Y (belatacept), shows promise in human trials of renal transplantation [169].

Early clinical trials of the anti-CD154 antibody hu5c8 showed promise in preventing rejection but were rapidly terminated due to thromboembolic complications due to the expression of CD154 on platelets. Typically, CD154 plays an important role in stabilizing arterial thrombi [170]. In an attempt to avoid the thromboembolic complications from hu5c8, new anti-CD154 antibodies in development target different epitopes of CD154 [171]. Other antibodies in development target the CD40 molecule itself [172]. In addition to the classical costimulatory pathways involving CD28/B7 and CD40/CD154, numerous additional costimulatory pathways have been described as critical for T cell responses and

potential targets for anti-rejection therapy [76]. Additionally, adhesion molecules serve as potential therapeutic targets. For example, the anti-LFA-1 (CD11) monoclonal antibody efalizumab (Raptiva) is FDA approved for the treatment of psoriasis and is under investigation for renal transplantation [173]. Recent nonhuman primate studies suggest that the anti-CD2 antibody (alefacept) could further prolong allograft survival in combination with belatacept by targeting effector memory T cells [174].

References

1 Halloran PF. Immunosuppressive drugs for kidney transplantation. *N Engl J Med* 2004;351(26):2715–29.
2 Petrie HT. Cell migration and the control of post-natal T-cell lymphopoiesis in the thymus. *Nat Rev* 2003;3(11): 859–866.
3 Spangrude GJ, Heimfeld S, Weissman IL. Purification and characterization of mouse hematopoietic stem cells. *Science (New York, NY)* 1988;241(4861):58–62.
4 Kondo M, Weissman IL, Akashi K. Identification of clonogenic common lymphoid progenitors in mouse bone marrow. *Cell* 1997;91(5):661–672.
5 Morrison SJ, Weissman IL. The long-term repopulating subset of hematopoietic stem cells is deterministic and isolatable by phenotype. *Immunity* 1994;1(8):661–673.
6 Baum CM, Weissman IL, Tsukamoto AS *et al*. Isolation of a candidate human hematopoietic stem-cell population. *Proc Natl Acad Sci U S A* 1992;89(7):2804–2808.
7 Osawa M, Hanada K, Hamada H, Nakauchi H. Long-term lymphohematopoietic reconstitution by a single CD34-low/negative hematopoietic stem cell. *Science* 1996;273(5272):242–245.
8 Lind EF, Prockop SE, Porritt HE, Petrie HT. Mapping precursor movement through the postnatal thymus reveals specific microenvironments supporting defined stages of early lymphoid development. *J Exp Med* 2001;194(2):127–134.
9 Scollay R, Smith J, Stauffer V. Dynamics of early T cells: prothymocyte migration and proliferation in the adult mouse thymus. *Immunol Rev* 1986;91:129–157.
10 Singer A, Adoro S, Park JH. Lineage fate and intense debate: myths, models and mechanisms of CD4- versus CD8-lineage choice. *Nat Rev Immunol* 2008;8(10): 788–801.
11 Doyle C, Strominger JL. Interaction between CD4 and class II MHC molecules mediates cell adhesion. *Nature* 1987;330(6145):256–259.

12 Norment AM, Salter RD, Parham P *et al.* Cell-cell adhesion mediated by CD8 and MHC class I molecules. *Nature* 1988;336(6194):79–81.

13 Turner JM, Brodsky MH, Irving BA *et al.* Interaction of the unique N-terminal region of tyrosine kinase p56lck with cytoplasmic domains of CD4 and CD8 is mediated by cysteine motifs. *Cell* 1990;60(5):755–65.

14 Ueno T, Saito F, Gray DH *et al.* CCR7 signals are essential for cortex–medulla migration of developing thymocytes. *J Exp Med* 2004;200(4):493–505.

15 Teh HS, Kisielow P, Scott B *et al.* Thymic major histocompatibility complex antigens and the alpha beta T-cell receptor determine the CD4/CD8 phenotype of T cells. *Nature* 1988;335(6187):229–233.

16 Brugnera E, Bhandoola A, Cibotti R *et al.* Coreceptor reversal in the thymus: signaled CD4+8+ thymocytes initially terminate CD8 transcription even when differentiating into CD8+ T cells. *Immunity* 2000;13(1):59–71.

17 McCaughtry TM, Wilken MS, Hogquist KA. Thymic emigration revisited. *J Exp Med* 2007;204(11):2513–2520.

18 Peterson P, Org T, Rebane A. Transcriptional regulation by AIRE: molecular mechanisms of central tolerance. *Nat Rev* 2008;8(12):948–957.

19 Anderson G, Lane PJ, Jenkinson EJ. Generating intrathymic microenvironments to establish T-cell tolerance. *Nat Rev* 2007;7(12):954–963.

20 Palmer E. Negative selection – clearing out the bad apples from the T-cell repertoire. *Nat Rev* 2003; 3(5):383–391.

21 Weinreich MA, Hogquist KA. Thymic emigration: when and how T cells leave home. *J Immunol* 2008;181(4):2265–2270.

22 Rosen H, Alfonso C, Surh CD, McHeyzer-Williams MG. Rapid induction of medullary thymocyte phenotypic maturation and egress inhibition by nanomolar sphingosine 1-phosphate receptor agonist. *Proc Natl Acad Sci U S A* 2003;100(19):10907–10912.

23 Surh CD, Sprent J. Homeostasis of naive and memory T cells. *Immunity* 2008;29(6):848–862.

24 Seddon B, Zamoyska R. TCR signals mediated by Src family kinases are essential for the survival of naive T cells. *J Immunol* 2002;169(6):2997–3005.

25 Hataye J, Moon JJ, Khoruts A *et al.* Naive and memory CD4+ T cell survival controlled by clonal abundance. *Science (New York, NY)* 2006;312(5770):114–116.

26 Broers AE, Posthumus-van Sluijs SJ, Spits H *et al.* Interleukin-7 improves T-cell recovery after experimental T-cell-depleted bone marrow transplantation in T-cell-deficient mice by strong expansion of recent thymic emigrants.;102(4):1534–1540.

27 Sportes C, Hakim FT, Memon SA *et al.* Administration of rhIL-7 in humans increases in vivo TCR repertoire diversity by preferential expansion of naive T cell subsets. *J Exp Med* 2008;205(7):1701–1714.

28 Tan JT, Dudl E, LeRoy E *et al.* IL-7 is critical for homeostatic proliferation and survival of naive T cells. *Proc Natl Acad Sci U S A* 2001;98(15):8732–8737.

29 Cho JH, Boyman O, Kim HO *et al.* An intense form of homeostatic proliferation of naive CD8+ cells driven by IL-2. *J Exp Med* 2007;204(8):1787–1801.

30 Ramsey C, Rubinstein MP, Kim DM *et al.* The lymphopenic environment of CD132 (common gamma-chain)-deficient hosts elicits rapid homeostatic proliferation of naive T cells via IL-15. *J Immunol* 2008;180(8):5320–5326.

31 Rocha PN, Plumb TJ, Crowley SD, Coffman TM. Effector mechanisms in transplant rejection. *Immunol Rev* 2003;196:51–64.

32 Medawar PB. The behaviour and fate of skin autografts and skin homografts in rabbits: a report to the War Wounds Committee of the Medical Research Council. *J Anat* 1944;78(Pt 5):176–199.

33 Billingham RE, Brent L, Medawar PB. Quantitative studies on tissue transplantation immunity. II. The origin, strength and duration of actively and adoptively acquired immunity. *Proc R Soc Lond B Biol Sci* 1954; 143(910):58–80.

34 Hall BM. Cells mediating allograft rejection. *Transplantation* 1991;51(6):1141–1151.

35 Felix NJ, Donermeyer DL, Horvath S *et al.* Alloreactive T cells respond specifically to multiple distinct peptide–MHC complexes. *Nat Immunol* 2007;8(4):388–397.

36 Sherman LA, Chattopadhyay S. The molecular basis of allorecognition. *Annu Rev Immunol* 1993;11:385–402.

37 Trivedi HL. Immunobiology of rejection and adaptation. *Transpl Proc* 2007;39(3):647–652.

38 Barrett AJ, Rezvani K, Solomon S *et al.* New developments in allotransplant immunology. *Hematol Am Soc Hematol Educ Program* 2003:350–371.

39 Gould DS, Auchincloss H, Jr. Direct and indirect recognition: the role of MHC antigens in graft rejection. *Immunol Today* 1999;20(2):77–82.

40 Merkenschlager M, Ikeda H, Wilkinson D *et al.* Allorecognition of HLA-DR and -DQ transfectants by human CD45RA and CD45R0 CD4 T cells: repertoire analysis and activation requirements. *Eur J Immunol* 1991;21(1):79–88.

41 Suchin EJ, Langmuir PB, Palmer E *et al.* Quantifying the frequency of alloreactive T cells in vivo: new answers to an old question. *J Immunol* 2001;166(2):973–981.

42 Game DS, Lechler RI. Pathways of allorecognition: implications for transplantation tolerance. *Transpl Immunol* 2002;10(2–3):101–108.

43 Larsen CP, Morris PJ, Austyn JM. Migration of dendritic leukocytes from cardiac allografts into host spleens. A novel pathway for initiation of rejection. *J Exp Med* 1990;171(1):307–314.

44 Inaba K, Turley S, Yamaide F *et al*. Efficient presentation of phagocytosed cellular fragments on the major histocompatibility complex class II products of dendritic cells. *J Exp Med* 1998;188(11):2163–2173.

45 Herrera OB, Golshayan D, Tibbott R *et al*. A novel pathway of alloantigen presentation by dendritic cells. *J Immunol* 2004;173(8):4828–4837.

46 Grazia TJ, Pietra BA, Johnson ZA *et al*. A two-step model of acute CD4 T-cell mediated cardiac allograft rejection. *J Immunol* 2004;172(12):7451–7458.

47 Dierselhuis M, Goulmy E. The relevance of minor histocompatibility antigens in solid organ transplantation. *Curr Opin Organ Transpl* 2009;14(4):419–425.

48 Mattsson J. Recent progress in allogeneic stem cell transplantation. *Curr Opin Mol Ther* 2008;10(4):343–349.

49 Goulmy E. Minor histocompatibility antigens: allo target molecules for tumor-specific immunotherapy. *Cancer J* 2004;10(1):1–7.

50 Cyster JG. Chemokines and cell migration in secondary lymphoid organs. *Science* 1999;286(5447):2098–2102.

51 Lanzavecchia A, Sallusto F. Dynamics of T lymphocyte responses: intermediates, effectors, and memory cells. *Science* 2000;290(5489):92–97.

52 Rothstein DM, Sayegh MH. T-cell costimulatory pathways in allograft rejection and tolerance. *Immunol Rev* 2003;196:85–108.

53 Janeway CA, Jr. The T cell receptor as a multicomponent signalling machine: CD4/CD8 coreceptors and CD45 in T cell activation. *Annu Rev Immunol* 1992;10:645–674.

54 Csencsits KL, Bishop DK. Contrasting alloreactive CD4+ and CD8+ T cells: there's more to it than MHC restriction. *Am J Transpl* 2003;3(2):107–115.

55 Iezzi G, Karjalainen K, Lanzavecchia A. The duration of antigenic stimulation determines the fate of naive and effector T cells. *Immunity* 1998;8(1):89–95.

56 Lafferty KJ, Jones MA. Reactions of the graft versus host (GVH) type. *Aust J Exp Biol Med Sci* 1969;47(1):17–54.

57 Lafferty KJ, Misko IS, Cooley MA. Allogeneic stimulation modulates the in vitro response of T cells to transplantation antigen. *Nature* 1974;249(454):275–276.

58 Jenkins MK, Schwartz RH. Antigen presentation by chemically modified splenocytes induces antigen-specific T cell unresponsiveness in vitro and in vivo. *J Exp Med* 1987;165(2):302–319.

59 Matzinger P. Tolerance, danger, and the extended family. *Annu Rev Immunol* 1994;12:991–1045.

60 Schwartz RH. A cell culture model for T lymphocyte clonal anergy. *Science* 1990;248(4961):1349–1356.

61 Ferguson TA, Green DR. T cells are just dying to accept grafts. *Nat Med* 1999;5(11):1231–1232.

62 Xu Y, Song G. The role of CD40–CD154 interaction in cell immunoregulation. *J Biomed Sci* 2004;11(4):426–438.

63 Clarkson MR, Sayegh MH. T-cell costimulatory pathways in allograft rejection and tolerance. *Transplantation* 2005;80(5):555–563.

64 Blair PJ, Riley JL, Harlan DM *et al*. CD40 ligand (CD154) triggers a short-term CD4+ T cell activation response that results in secretion of immunomodulatory cytokines and apoptosis. *J Exp Med* 2000;191(4):651–660.

65 Blotta MH, Marshall JD, DeKruyff RH, Umetsu DT. Cross-linking of the CD40 ligand on human CD4+ T lymphocytes generates a costimulatory signal that up-regulates IL-4 synthesis. *J Immunol* 1996;156(9):3133–3140.

66 Cella M, Scheidegger D, Palmer-Lehmann K *et al*. Ligation of CD40 on dendritic cells triggers production of high levels of interleukin-12 and enhances T cell stimulatory capacity: T–T help via APC activation. *J Exp Med* 1996;184(2):747–752.

67 Ranheim EA, Kipps TJ. Activated T cells induce expression of B7/BB1 on normal or leukemic B cells through a CD40-dependent signal. *J Exp Med* 1993;177(4):925–935.

68 Watts TH. TNF/TNFR family members in costimulation of T cell responses. *Annu Rev Immunol* 2005;23:23–68.

69 Hancock WW, Sayegh MH, Zheng XG *et al*. Costimulatory function and expression of CD40 ligand, CD80, and CD86 in vascularized murine cardiac allograft rejection. *Proc Natl Acad Sci U S A* 1996;93(24):13967–13972.

70 Lenschow DJ, Walunas TL, Bluestone JA. CD28/B7 system of T cell costimulation. *Annu Rev Immunol* 1996;14:233–258.

71 Linsley PS, Ledbetter JA. The role of the CD28 receptor during T cell responses to antigen. *Annu Rev Immunol* 1993;11:191–212.

72 Sharpe AH, Freeman GJ. The B7-CD28 superfamily. *Nat Rev* 2002;2(2):116–126.

73 Acuto O, Michel F. CD28-mediated co-stimulation: a quantitative support for TCR signalling. *Nat Rev Immunol* 2003;3(12):939–951.

74 Boise LH, Minn AJ, Noel PJ *et al.* CD28 costimulation can promote T cell survival by enhancing the expression of Bcl-XL. *Immunity* 1995;3(1):87–98.

75 Greenwald RJ, Latchman YE, Sharpe AH. Negative co-receptors on lymphocytes. *Curr Opin Immunol* 2002;14(3):391–396.

76 Li XC, Rothstein DM, Sayegh MH. Costimulatory pathways in transplantation: challenges and new developments. *Immunol Rev* 2009;229(1):271–293.

77 Ozkaynak E, Gao W, Shemmeri N *et al.* Importance of ICOS-B7RP-1 costimulation in acute and chronic allograft rejection. *Nat Immunol* 2001;2(7):591–596.

78 Brown JA, Dorfman DM, Ma FR *et al.* Blockade of programmed death-1 ligands on dendritic cells enhances T cell activation and cytokine production. *J Immunol* 2003;170(3):1257–1266.

79 Heeger PS, Lalli PN, Lin F *et al.* Decay-accelerating factor modulates induction of T cell immunity. *J Exp Med* 2005;201(10):1523–1530.

80 Lalli PN, Strainic MG, Lin F *et al.* Decay accelerating factor can control T cell differentiation into IFN-gamma-producing effector cells via regulating local C5a-induced IL-12 production. *J Immunol* 2007; 179(9):5793–5802.

81 Lalli PN, Strainic MG, Yang M *et al.* Locally produced C5a binds to T cell-expressed C5aR to enhance effector T-cell expansion by limiting antigen-induced apoptosis. *Blood* 2008;112(5):1759–1766.

82 Pavlov V, Raedler H, Yuan S *et al.* Donor deficiency of decay-accelerating factor accelerates murine T cell-mediated cardiac allograft rejection. *J Immunol* 2008; 181(7):4580–4589.

83 Strainic MG, Liu J, Huang D *et al.* Locally produced complement fragments C5a and C3a provide both costimulatory and survival signals to naive CD4⁺ T cells. *Immunity* 2008;28(3):425–435.

84 Clipstone NA, Crabtree GR. Identification of calcineurin as a key signalling enzyme in T-lymphocyte activation. *Nature* 1992;357(6380):695–697.

85 Rao A, Luo C, Hogan PG. Transcription factors of the NFAT family: regulation and function. *Annu Rev Immunol* 1997;15:707–747.

86 Szabo SJ, Sullivan BM, Peng SL, Glimcher LH. Molecular mechanisms regulating Th1 immune responses. *Annu Rev Immunol* 2003;21:713–758.

87 MacLeod MK, Clambey ET, Kappler JW, Marrack P. CD4 memory T cells: what are they and what can they do? *Semin Immunol* 2009;21(2):53–61.

88 D'Cruz LM, Rubinstein MP, Goldrath AW. Surviving the crash: transitioning from effector to memory CD8⁺ T cell. *Semin Immunol* 2009;21(2):92–98.

89 Ashkar S, Weber GF, Panoutsakopoulou V *et al.* Eta-1 (osteopontin): an early component of type-1 (cell-mediated) immunity. *Science (New York, NY)* 2000; 287(5454):860–864.

90 Reiner SL. Development in motion: helper T cells at work. *Cell* 2007;129(1):33–36.

91 Yoshimoto T, Takeda K, Tanaka T *et al.* IL-12 up-regulates IL-18 receptor expression on T cells, Th1 cells, and B cells: synergism with IL-18 for IFN-gamma production. *J Immunol* 1998;161(7):3400–3407.

92 Leonard WJ, O'shea JJ. Jaks and STATs: biological implications. *Annu Rev Immunol* 1998;16:293–322.

93 Lighvani AA, Frucht DM, Jankovic D *et al.* T-bet is rapidly induced by interferon-gamma in lymphoid and myeloid cells. *Proc Natl Acad Sci U S A* 2001; 98(26):15137–15142.

94 Peng SL. The T-box transcription factor T-bet in immunity and autoimmunity. *Cell Mol Immunol* 2006;3(2):87–95.

95 Grogan JL, Mohrs M, Harmon B *et al.* Early transcription and silencing of cytokine genes underlie polarization of T helper cell subsets. *Immunity* 2001; 14(3):205–215.

96 Pearce EL, Mullen AC, Martins GA *et al.* Control of effector CD8⁺ T cell function by the transcription factor eomesodermin. *Science* 2003;302(5647):1041–1043.

97 Ouyang W, Ranganath SH, Weindel K *et al.* Inhibition of Th1 development mediated by GATA-3 through an IL-4-independent mechanism. *Immunity* 1998;9(5): 745–755.

98 Atalar K, Afzali B, Lord G, Lombardi G. Relative roles of Th1 and Th17 effector cells in allograft rejection. *Curr Opin Organ Transplant* 2009;14(1):23–29.

99 Boehm U, Klamp T, Groot M, Howard JC. Cellular responses to interferon-gamma. *Annu Rev Immunol* 1997;15:749–795.

100 Hussain R, Dawood G, Abrar N *et al.* Selective increases in antibody isotypes and immunoglobulin G subclass responses to secreted antigens in tuberculosis patients and healthy household contacts of the patients. *Clin Diagn Lab Immunol* 1995;2(6):726–732.

101 Mackey MF, Barth RJ, Jr, Noelle RJ. The role of CD40/CD154 interactions in the priming, differentiation, and effector function of helper and cytotoxic T cells. *J Leukoc Biol* 1998;63(4):418–428.

102 Glimcher LH, Murphy KM. Lineage commitment in the immune system: the T helper lymphocyte grows up. *Genes Dev* 2000;14(14):1693–1711.

103 Lederer JA, Perez VL, DesRoches L *et al.* Cytokine transcriptional events during helper T cell subset differentiation. *J Exp Med* 1996;184(2):397–406.

104 Kaplan MH, Schindler U, Smiley ST, Grusby MJ. Stat6 is required for mediating responses to IL-4 and for development of Th2 cells. *Immunity* 1996;4(3): 313–319.

105 Abbas AK, Murphy KM, Sher A. Functional diversity of helper T lymphocytes. *Nature* 1996;383(6603): 787–793.

106 Kuhn R, Rajewsky K, Muller W. Generation and analysis of interleukin-4 deficient mice. *Science (New York, NY)* 1991;254(5032):707–710.

107 Le Moine A, Flamand V, Demoor FX *et al*. Critical roles for IL-4, IL-5, and eosinophils in chronic skin allograft rejection. *J Clin Invest* 1999;103(12): 1659–1667.

108 Piccotti JR, Chan SY, Goodman RE *et al*. IL-12 antagonism induces T helper 2 responses, yet exacerbates cardiac allograft rejection. Evidence against a dominant protective role for T helper 2 cytokines in alloimmunity. *J Immunol* 1996;157(5):1951–1957.

109 Pescovitz MD. B cells: a rational target in alloantibody-mediated solid organ transplantation rejection. *Clin Transplant* 2006;20(1):48–54.

110 Dong C. Regulation and pro-inflammatory function of interleukin-17 family cytokines. *Immunol Rev* 2008;226:80–86.

111 Nishihara M, Ogura H, Ueda N *et al*. IL-6-gp130-STAT3 in T cells directs the development of IL-17+ Th with a minimum effect on that of Treg in the steady state. *Int Immunol* 2007;19(6):695–702.

112 Miossec P, Korn T, Kuchroo VK. Interleukin-17 and type 17 helper T cells. *N Engl J Med* 2009;361(9):888–898.

113 Aggarwal S, Ghilardi N, Xie MH *et al*. Interleukin-23 promotes a distinct CD4 T cell activation state characterized by the production of interleukin-17. *J Biol Chem* 2003;278(3):1910–1914.

114 Harrington LE, Hatton RD, Mangan PR *et al*. Interleukin 17-producing CD4+ effector T cells develop via a lineage distinct from the T helper type 1 and 2 lineages. *Nat Immunol* 2005;6(11):1123–1132.

115 Lohr J, Knoechel B, Wang JJ *et al*. Role of IL-17 and regulatory T lymphocytes in a systemic autoimmune disease. *J Exp Med* 2006;203(13):2785–2791.

116 Mathur AN, Chang HC, Zisoulis DG *et al*. T-bet is a critical determinant in the instability of the IL-17-secreting T-helper phenotype. *Blood* 2006;108(5): 1595–1601.

117 Miyamoto M, Prause O, Sjostrand M *et al*. Endogenous IL-17 as a mediator of neutrophil recruitment caused by endotoxin exposure in mouse airways. *J Immunol* 2003;170(9):4665–4672.

118 McKenzie BS, Kastelein RA, Cua DJ. Understanding the IL-23–IL-17 immune pathway. *Trends Immunol* 2006;27(1):17–23.

119 Antonysamy MA, Fanslow WC, Fu F *et al*. Evidence for a role of IL-17 in organ allograft rejection: IL-17 promotes the functional differentiation of dendritic cell progenitors. *J Immunol* 1999;162(1):577–584.

120 Woltman AM, de Haij S, Boonstra JG *et al*. Interleukin-17 and CD40-ligand synergistically enhance cytokine and chemokine production by renal epithelial cells. *J Am Soc Nephrol* 2000;11(11): 2044–2055.

121 Vanaudenaerde BM, Dupont LJ, Wuyts WA *et al*. The role of interleukin-17 during acute rejection after lung transplantation. *Eur Respir J* 2006;27(4): 779–787.

122 Williams MA, Bevan MJ. Effector and memory CTL differentiation. *Annu Rev Immunol* 2007;25:171–192.

123 Kaech SM, Ahmed R. Memory CD8+ T cell differentiation: initial antigen encounter triggers a developmental program in naive cells. *Nat Immunol* 2001;2(5): 415–422.

124 Zammit DJ, Cauley LS, Pham QM, Lefrancois L. Dendritic cells maximize the memory CD8 T cell response to infection. *Immunity* 2005;22(5):561–570.

125 Iwasaki A, Medzhitov R. Toll-like receptor control of the adaptive immune responses. *Nat Immunol* 2004; 5(10):987–995.

126 Russell JH, Ley TJ. Lymphocyte-mediated cytotoxicity. *Annu Rev Immunol* 2002;20:323–370.

127 Josefowicz SZ, Rudensky A. Control of regulatory T cell lineage commitment and maintenance. *Immunity* 2009;30(5):616–625.

128 Pennington DJ, Silva-Santos B, Silberzahn T *et al*. Early events in the thymus affect the balance of effector and regulatory T cells. *Nature* 2006;444(7122): 1073–1077.

129 Apostolou I, von Boehmer H. In vivo instruction of suppressor commitment in naive T cells. *J Exp Med* 2004;199(10):1401–1408.

130 Huber S, Schramm C, Lehr HA *et al*. Cutting edge: TGF-beta signaling is required for the in vivo expansion and immunosuppressive capacity of regulatory CD4+CD25+ T cells. *J Immunol* 2004;173(11): 6526–6531.

131 Yi H, Zhen Y, Jiang L *et al*. The phenotypic characterization of naturally occurring regulatory CD4+CD25+ T cells. *Cell Mol Immunol* 2006;3(3):189–195.

132 Hori S, Nomura T, Sakaguchi S. Control of regulatory T cell development by the transcription factor Foxp3. *Science (New York, NY)* 2003;299(5609):1057–1061.

133 Chatila TA, Blaeser F, Ho N *et al*. JM2, encoding a fork head-related protein, is mutated in X-linked autoimmunity-allergic disregulation syndrome. *J Clin Invest* 2000;106(12):R75–R81.

134 Afzali B, Lombardi G, Lechler RI, Lord GM. The role of T helper 17 (Th17) and regulatory T cells (Treg) in human organ transplantation and autoimmune disease. *Clin Exp Immunol* 2007;148(1):32–46.

135 Marks L, Levy RB. The cytotoxic potential of regulatory T cells: what has been learned from gene knockout model systems? *Transplantation* 2004;77(1 Suppl):S19–S22.

136 Schramm C, Huber S, Protschka M *et al*. TGFβ regulates the CD4+CD25+ T-cell pool and the expression of Foxp3 in vivo. *Int Immunol* 2004;16(9):1241–1249.

137 Shevach EM. Mechanisms of foxp3+ T regulatory cell-mediated suppression. *Immunity* 2009;30(5):636–645.

138 Wood KJ, Ushigome H, Karim M *et al*. Regulatory cells in transplantation. *Novartis Found Symp* 2003;252:177–188; discussion 88–93, 203–210.

139 Ford ML, Kirk AD, Larsen CP. Donor-reactive T-cell stimulation history and precursor frequency: barriers to tolerance induction. *Transplantation* 2009;87(9 Suppl):S69–S74.

140 Sallusto F, Geginat J, Lanzavecchia A. Central memory and effector memory T cell subsets: function, generation, and maintenance. *Annu Rev Immunol* 2004;22:745–763.

141 Bouneaud C, Garcia Z, Kourilsky P, Pannetier C. Lineage relationships, homeostasis, and recall capacities of central- and effector-memory CD8 T cells in vivo. *J Exp Med* 2005;201(4):579–590.

142 Sun JC, Bevan MJ. Defective CD8 T cell memory following acute infection without CD4 T cell help. *Science* 2003;300(5617):339–342.

143 Intlekofer AM, Takemoto N, Wherry EJ *et al*. Effector and memory CD8+ T cell fate coupled by T-bet and eomesodermin. *Nat Immunol* 2005;6(12):1236–1244.

144 Adams AB, Williams MA, Jones TR *et al*. Heterologous immunity provides a potent barrier to transplantation tolerance. *J Clin Invest* 2003;111(12):1887–1895.

145 Bogman MJ, Dooper IM, van de Winkel JG *et al*. Diagnosis of renal allograft rejection by macrophage immunostaining with a CD14 monoclonal antibody, WT14. *Lancet* 1989;2(8657):235–238.

146 Bishop DK, Chan S, Li W *et al*. CD4-positive helper T lymphocytes mediate mouse cardiac allograft rejection independent of donor alloantigen specific cytotoxic T lymphocytes. *Transplantation* 1993;56(4):892–897.

147 Li B, Hartono C, Ding R *et al*. Noninvasive diagnosis of renal-allograft rejection by measurement of messenger RNA for perforin and granzyme B in urine. *N Engl J Med* 2001;344(13):947–954.

148 Hahn S, Gehri R, Erb P. Mechanism and biological significance of CD4-mediated cytotoxicity. *Immunol Rev* 1995;146:57–79.

149 Selvaggi G, Ricordi C, Podack ER, Inverardi L. The role of the perforin and Fas pathways of cytotoxicity in skin graft rejection. *Transplantation* 1996;62(12):1912–1915.

150 Kreisel D, Krupnick AS, Gelman AE *et al*. Non-hematopoietic allograft cells directly activate CD8+ T cells and trigger acute rejection: an alternative mechanism of allorecognition. *Nat Med* 2002;8(3):233–239.

151 Rosenberg AS, Singer A. Cellular basis of skin allograft rejection: an in vivo model of immune-mediated tissue destruction. *Annu Rev Immunol* 1992;10:333–358.

152 Gokmen MR, Lombardi G, Lechler RI. The importance of the indirect pathway of allorecognition in clinical transplantation. *Curr Opin Immunol* 2008;20(5):568–574.

153 Spriewald BM, Ensminger SM, Billing JS *et al*. Increased expression of transforming growth factor-beta and eosinophil infiltration is associated with the development of transplant arteriosclerosis in long-term surviving cardiac allografts. *Transplantation* 2003;76(7):1105–1111.

154 Tellides G, Tereb DA, Kirkiles-Smith NC *et al*. Interferon-gamma elicits arteriosclerosis in the absence of leukocytes. *Nature* 2000;403(6766):207–211.

155 Cosio FG, Pelletier RP, Falkenhain ME *et al*. Impact of acute rejection and early allograft function on renal allograft survival. *Transplantation* 1997;63(11):1611–1615.

156 Tullius SG, Tilney NL. Both alloantigen-dependent and -independent factors influence chronic allograft rejection. *Transplantation* 1995;59(3):313–318.

157 Springer TA. Traffic signals for lymphocyte recirculation and leukocyte emigration: the multistep paradigm. *Cell* 1994;76(2):301–314.

158 Sims TN, Dustin ML. The immunological synapse: integrins take the stage. *Immunol Rev* 2002;186:100–117.

159 Dedrick RL, Bodary S, Garovoy MR. Adhesion molecules as therapeutic targets for autoimmune diseases and transplant rejection. *Expert Opin Biol Ther* 2003;3(1):85–95.

160 Hancock WW. Chemokine receptor-dependent alloresponses. *Immunol Rev* 2003;196:37–50.

161 Norman DJ, Kahana L, Stuart FP, Jr *et al.* A randomized clinical trial of induction therapy with OKT3 in kidney transplantation. *Transplantation* 1993;55(1):44–50.

162 Vincenti F, Kirkman R, Light S *et al.* Interleukin-2-receptor blockade with daclizumab to prevent acute rejection in renal transplantation. Daclizumab Triple Therapy Study Group. *N Engl J Med* 1998;338(3): 161–165.

163 Ballen K. New trends in transplantation: the use of thymoglobulin. *Expert Opin Drug Metab Toxicol* 2009;5(3):351–355.

164 Huang S, Bjornsti MA, Houghton PJ. Rapamycins: mechanism of action and cellular resistance. *Cancer Biol Ther* 2003;2(3):222–232.

165 Elion GB. The George Hitchings and Gertrude Elion Lecture. The pharmacology of azathioprine. *Ann N Y Acad Sci* 1993;685:400–407.

166 Kirk AD, Harlan DM, Armstrong NN *et al.* CTLA4-Ig and anti-CD40 ligand prevent renal allograft rejection in primates. *Proc Natl Acad Sci U S A* 1997;94(16):8789–8794.

167 Kremer JM, Westhovens R, Leon M *et al.* Treatment of rheumatoid arthritis by selective inhibition of T-cell activation with fusion protein CTLA4Ig. *N Engl J Med* 2003;349(20):1907–1915.

168 Larsen CP, Pearson TC, Adams AB *et al.* Rational development of LEA29Y (belatacept), a high-affinity variant of CTLA4-Ig with potent immunosuppressive properties. *Am J Transpl* 2005;5(3):443–453.

169 Vincenti F, Larsen C, Durrbach A *et al.* Costimulation blockade with belatacept in renal transplantation. *N Engl J Med* 2005;353(8):770–781.

170 Inwald DP, McDowall A, Peters MJ *et al.* CD40 is constitutively expressed on platelets and provides a novel mechanism for platelet activation. *Circ Res* 2003;92(9):1041–1048.

171 Kanmaz T, Fechner JJ, Jr, Torrealba J *et al.* Monotherapy with the novel human anti-CD154 monoclonal antibody ABI793 in rhesus monkey renal transplantation model. *Transplantation* 2004; 77(6):914–920.

172 Adams AB, Shirasugi N, Jones TR *et al.* Development of a chimeric anti-CD40 monoclonal antibody that synergizes with LEA29Y to prolong islet allograft survival. *J Immunol* 2005;174(1):542–550.

173 Vincenti F, Mendez R, Pescovitz M *et al.* A phase I/II randomized open-label multicenter trial of efalizumab, a humanized anti-CD11a, anti-LFA-1 in renal transplantation. *Am J Transpl* 2007;7(7): 1770–1777.

174 Weaver TA, Charafeddine AH, Agarwal A *et al.* Alefacpt promotes co-stimulation blockade based allograft survival in non-human prmates. *Nat Med* 2009;15(7):746–749.

CHAPTER 4

The B Cell Response to Transplantation Antigens

Roger Sciammas[1], Anita S. Chong[1], and Robert B. Colvin[2]

[1]Department of Surgery/Section of Transplantation, University of Chicago, Chicago, IL, USA
[2]Massachusetts General Hospital, Boston, MA, USA

Basic B cell biology, lexicon, and definitions

The production of B cells capable of humoral immunity involves a developmental progression marked by quality control checkpoints. B cells arise from the fetal liver or the adult bone marrow from a hematopoietic stem cell and, once committed to a B cell fate, assemble a B cell receptor (BCR) via the process of V–D–J recombination such that each B cell expresses a unique receptor, consistent with the one-cell/one-receptor/one-antigen specificity paradigm. Quality control mechanisms ensure that the receptor is properly expressed and that it is harmless to the organism or "self," thus preventing autoreactivity. B cells that pass this checkpoint are considered immature and are allowed to exit the fetal liver or bone marrow to seed the secondary lymphoid organs, where they develop into mature B cells. At this stage, B cells wait for their chance to respond to their cognate antigens. If their receptor recognizes a "non-self" antigen, it will undergo a process of cellular activation that leads to proliferation (clonal expansion) and the acquisition of effector functions that form the basis of humoral immunity. Antibody production, secretion of immunoregulatory cytokines, and cellular communication with T or dendritic cells constitute protective effector functions. Several principles guide the developmental progression of B cells, including the integrity of BCR expression, the ability to properly integrate survival cues, and the ability to undergo clonal expansion. All of these features are critical for humoral protection against pathogenic infections, but pose a barrier to successful transplantation. In this chapter we will describe how B cells are produced and how they participate in the immune response with a particular emphasis on how these features impact organ rejection.

How B cells see alloantigen: formation and use of the BCR

Unique to B cells is their ability to form an antibody molecule, also known as the BCR or immunoglobulin (Ig). The receptor is a protein heterodimer formed by two pairs of one heavy chain and one light chain. The structure comprises a characteristic α-helical and β-barrel fold that constitutes the founding member of the Ig superfamily. The amino-terminus encodes the antigen recognition module, whereas the carboxy-terminus comprises the "constant" domain, also known as the Fc. Everything about the biology of B cells is ruled by the formation, expression, and use of its BCR, and this section will highlight its many facets.

Immunotherapy in Transplantation: Principles and Practice, First Edition. Edited by Bruce Kaplan, Gilbert J. Burckart and Fadi G. Lakkis.

Rearrangement and diversity

BCRs are capable of recognizing a universe of antigens. This is due to a library of gene segments encoded in mammalian genomes that are randomly recombined to create unique receptors [1]. Three segments of the heavy-chain gene, termed variable (VH), diversity (DH), and joining (JH) and two segments of the light-chain gene (VL and JL) are spliced together. The heavy-chain locus is on the order of one megabase of DNA and encodes a large repertoire of VH genes, DH genes, and JH genes. There are two light-chain loci, κ and λ, which also encode a large repertoire of VL and JL genes. Table 4.1 compares the features encoded by the mouse and human Ig locus. Thus, this library of segments in the pair of the heavy- and light-chain segments can theoretically produce $\geq 10^{11}$ different combinations – which correspond to different antigen specificities. Furthermore, rearrangement of the VH–DH–JH or VL–JL junction is imprecise owing to random nucleotide excision and addition, resulting in further diversification of the repertoire of BCRs, specifically within the interface that experiences the greatest antigen contact – the active site.

Antigen recognition

Each VH and VL segment is unique and encodes two regions of high variability, termed complementarity determining regions (CDRs) 1 and 2. CDR 3 corresponds to the junction of the VH–DH–JH or VL–JL segments, and is also highly variable [7]. In the tertiary structure, the CDRs from the heavy and light chain come together and form the active site surface that is used to recognize antigen.

Somatic hypermutation

After the BCR has been formed and during the immune response, B cell clones with an initial affinity for antigen have the potential to improve their affinity by the process of somatic hypermutation [8]. This is a highly controlled, antigen-driven, process that predominantly occurs in specialized lymphoid structures known as germinal centers. Single residues in the V genes are randomly mutated and can confer increased affinity to the BCR. The highest concentration of mutations occurs in the CDR 1, 2, and 3 regions and is associated with sequence motifs, termed hotspots. Once mutated, the new BCRs are tested: if the affinity is abolished (most often), the cell dies; if the affinity is increased, the cell re-enters the immune response with a competitive advantage.

Class switch recombination

Antibodies can be subdivided into several subclasses distinguished by the structure of the constant domain. While, all BCRs start off with the μ and δ constant domains, they can be exchanged for alternate constant regions during the immune response, through a process termed class switch recombination [9]. The Ig locus encodes at least six constant domains (see Table 4.1). Each of these constant domains imparts different immune functionalities. For instance, the μ domains are able

Table 4.1 Differences in B cell biology between mice and humans.

Property	Mouse	Human	Ref.
Well-defined marginal zone in spleen with metallophilic and sialoadhesin + macrophages and a marginal sinus	Yes	No, only mantle zone	[2]
CD27 expression as a marker for memory B cells	No	Yes	[3]
Circulating memory B cells	5 %	40 %	[4, 5]
Constant region genes	8 (μ, δ, γ3, γ1, γ2b, γ2a, ε, α)	9 (μ, δ, γ3, γ1, α1, γ2, γ4, ε, α2)	
Germline heavy-chain variable gene repertoire	~130	~50	[6]

to pentamerize and thus increase the avidity of the antibody–antigen interaction. The γ domains have varied functions that enable different inflammatory reactions, such as the fixation of complement and interactions with inflammatory cells bearing Fcγ receptors. The α domain can interact with inflammatory cells that express the Fcε receptor, which plays a role in allergic reactions. Lastly, the α domains can dimerize and interact with the polymeric Igα receptor and cross into luminal spaces. The recombination event occurs during the immune response and links different immune functionalities to the same antigen recognition module. Importantly, the recombination event is deletional, preventing a recombined receptor reverting to its original constant domain.

Antibody secretion

B cells have the capability to differentiate into plasma cells and secrete their antibodies into the blood and lymph. This process is highly controlled and occurs only during an immune response [10]. Each of the constant domain genes encode two terminal 3′ exons that are differentially utilized. The downstream exon encodes the transmembrane and cytoplasmic tail segment important for anchoring to the membrane, whereas the upstream exon lacks these regions and the corresponding protein product is destined to be secreted. The decision to make a membrane or secretory receptor is executed at the post-transcriptional level and is the result of both alternative splicing and poly-adenylation. This is in contrast to the aforementioned uses of the antibody genes which all occur at the level of DNA.

It is clear that the BCR genes are highly evolved and have incorporated multiple facets for their use. The identity of each B cell is determined by its BCR specificity and, correspondingly, the immune system checks each B cell by insuring that its BCR is functional.

B cell development and maintenance

The function of B cells is ruled by the formation, expression, and antigen recognition by its BCR. The pre-antigen phase of development insures that the

BCR has been properly assembled and is not detrimental to the host (autoreactive). Antigen recognition marks the transition to the post-antigen phase of B cell development when cellular activation leads to the elaboration of germinal center and antibody-secreting plasma cells. The intermediates of the pre- and post-antigen phases are highlighted in Plate 4.1. Maturation through each of these intermediate stages requires integration of external cues from cellular interactions or soluble cytokines (IL-4, IL-6, IL-21) with programmed gene expression mediated by transcription factors (Ebf, Pax5, Bach2, Bcl6, Irf4, Blimp-1, Xbp1, Obf).

Pre-antigen phase of development

B cells get their name from the bursa of Fabricius, the site of B cell development in birds. Once B cell identity is committed from the hematopoietic stem cell [11], B cells turn on the expression of the recombination activating genes (RAG 1 and 2). This enables each B cell, at the pro-B cell stage, to undergo go VH–DH–JH recombination of the heavy-chain gene. The product of this reaction is the pre-BCR, a rearranged heavy-chain gene complexed with surrogate light-chain proteins λ5 and VpreB. Unsuccessful pre-BCR formation results in further attempts at rearrangement or cell death. In contrast, successful pre-BCR formation signals the extinction of RAG gene expression and progression to pre-B cells [12], whereupon the RAG genes are re-expressed and VL–JL rearrangement of the light chain occurs. Again, the BCR is checked against improper formation by confirming that the light chain has rearranged in-frame. In addition, an immunological checkpoint is encountered that checks against self-reactivity. Depending on the intensity of self-reactivity, the cells are signaled to die or to reinitiate light-chain recombination in order to assemble a new receptor that is less self-reactive – a process referred to as "editing" [13]. It has been estimated that, in the mouse, 10–20 million B cells are produced in the bone marrow daily but that only 10 % reach the periphery – the bottleneck being censoring of autoreactive cells. Passage through this checkpoint is followed by migration from the bone marrow into the blood and eventually the secondary lymphoid organs, where they will comprise the naive B cell repertoire.

The majority (85%) of naive B cells reside in B cell follicles, whereas the remainder reside in the marginal zone in the mouse [14]. Numerous differences exist between the follicular and marginal-zone B cells, including anatomical location, propensity for activation, phenotype, and repertoire; however, their capacity for differentiating into antibody-secreting plasma cells or for class switch recombination and/or affinity maturation is conserved. This indicates that the "core" effector functions are shared by each subset, but that modulation of the "core" effector functions can be adjusted by details intrinsic to each subset. Importantly, access to these regions is controlled by a competition mechanism for BCRs that are not self-reactive. Part of this mechanism includes crosstalk with Baff/BLys that functions as an important survival signal [15]. Indeed, excess Baff/BLys signaling predisposes to autoimmune conditions, while the absence of Baff/BLys signals leads to a paucity of mature B cells.

The marginal zone, which is rich in metallophilic macrophages in the mouse, is positioned to filter the incoming blood in the spleen and is thus poised to react with blood-borne pathogens [16]. Hence, the marginal-zone B cells express a skewed repertoire reactive to carbohydrate antigens expressed by many bacteria. In contrast, follicular B cells access antigens via sub-capsular regions where antigen from the afferent lymph has been captured. Immune complexes are also displayed by follicular dendritic cells, which play a major role in activating B cells and for selecting high-affinity B cells. The ability of an antigen to promote a secondary response is highly dependent on the ability of the initial antibody to fix complement in the complex and the binding of this complex via C3b/C3d receptors on dendritic cells [17]. With regard to transplantation, intact major histocompatibility complex (MHC) antigens would most likely be recognized directly on the transplant or on migrating donor cells that reach the secondary lymphoid organs. In the former case, ischemia-dependent inflammation would lead to chemokine cues that recruit antigen-presenting cells (APCs), including B cells, while in the latter case the most likely migrating population would be donor dendritic cells resident in the transplanted tissue. Alternatively, cell constituents shed from the graft can reach the lymph node via draining lymphatics or blood.

In the human a well-defined marginal zone, with metallophilic and sialoadhesin-positive macrophages separated by a marginal sinus from the B and T cell areas, does not exist (see Ref. [2] and Table 4.1). Rather, the human has a perifollicular mantle zone with a mixture of B cells, including a subset that express markers similar to mouse marginal-zone B cells (IgM^{hi}, IgD^{lo}, $CD21^+$, $CD23^-$, $CD1^+$).

Post-antigen phase of development

Naive B cells that are stimulated by incoming antigen become activated and exit from the G0 phase of the cell cycle, which is a non-dividing and metabolically minimally consumptive state [18]. Entry into G1 integrates multiple signaling pathways that emanate from the BCR, CD19 coreceptor, CD22, and other receptors which then initiate post-translational signals that stabilize the D-type cyclins, modulate the cyclin-dependent kinases, and phosphorylate the retinoblastoma protein. These pathways lead to the control cell of survival, increased translational output, and increased metabolic fitness and are regulated by mammalian target of rapamycin (mTOR), PI3K, and LXR. Cumulatively, these events serve to prepare the cells for a proliferative burst that is the basis of clonal expansion. The immunosuppressive drug rapamycin used in transplantation operates by blocking the activity of mTOR and subsequent B cell clonal expansion.

B cells migrate to different areas of the secondary lymphoid structures to communicate with other cell types [19]. First, by upregulating the CCR7 gene, B cells move to the T–B border and initiate cognate interactions with antigen-specific T cells. During this interaction, B cells present processed antigen on MHC class II molecules and activate peptide/MHC-specific T cells. Both B and T cells profit from this interaction: B cells present antigen and costimulate T cells via CD28–B7 interactions; in turn, T cell help is provided to the B cells via signals through CD40.

Plasma cells

Coupled with clonal expansion, B cells face a major developmental branch point and decide between differentiating either into plasma cells or into germinal center B cells [20]. Separation of these two functional states is necessary for maintaining self-tolerance by preventing cells from simultaneously secreting and mutating the BCR. This branchpoint is influenced by a number of mechanisms, including affinity for antigen, the degree of T cell help, the cytokine milieu, as well as innate signals [21]. Overall, it is thought that higher affinity clones preferentially differentiate into IgM-secreting plasmablasts, while lower affinity clones seed the germinal center to undergo somatic hypermutation that can lead to enhanced affinity. Lastly, this branchpoint results in differential migration and seeding of plasma cells in the extrafollicular regions and germinal center B cells in the follicle.

Differentiation into plasma cells has long been known to be highly regulated, since the cell expands its cytoplasmic volume manifold, coincident with an enlargement of the endoplasmic reticulum [22]. The genetic program that controls plasma cell differentiation requires the sequential action of the Irf4, Blimp-1, and Xbp1 transcription factors. While Irf4 upregulates Blimp-1 expression, it is the activity of Blimp-1 that commits B cells to the plasma cell fate [23]. Lastly, Xbp1 activity facilitates antibody secretion by controlling the expression of many ER resident gene products [24]. Interestingly, the plasma cell gene program results in the suppression of many B-cell-specific genes that modulate BCR signaling and B cell function. In this regard, phenotypic characterization of plasma cells does not include the use of many B cell markers but, rather, depends on the upregulation of Syndecan-1 extracellular matrix protein, CD138 [25]. The majority of plasma cells early in the response are plasmablasts, in that they are short-lived, cycling, and antibody secreting [26]. Plasmablasts are also dependent on Baff/BLys signals presented by extrafollicular dendritic cells, and it is thought that the magnitude of the initial plasmablast response is regulated by the availability of Baff/BLys. Plasma cell differentiation and survival are also controlled by IL-21 produced by T-follicular helper cells [27]. The plasmablast response contracts at the termination of the immune response, but it is thought that a few cells are selected to become long lived.

Long-lived plasma cells reside in the sinusoids of the secondary lymphoid organs or in the bone marrow. In these niches, they are highly dependent on interactions with stromal cells that provide adhesive and survival signals through BCMA and the IL-6 cytokine that maintain up to life-long antibody secretion [28]. Long-lived plasma cell production results in persistent high titers of antigen-specific antibodies that are crucial for protection against secondary infections. Importantly, these high titers can also be a barrier to transplantation if a transplant recipient has already been exposed to an alloantigen due to previous transplants, blood transfusions, or in mothers that have been sensitized to the father's allo-antigens.

Germinal center

Differentiation into germinal center B cells is highly regulated owing to the activity of the mutating enzyme activation-induced cytidine deaminase (AID) [29]. This enzyme is induced specifically within germinal center B cells, where its activity is responsible for affinity maturation. Since both point mutations and double-strand breaks of genomic DNA have to occur for somatic hypermutation and class switch recombination respectively, B cells at this stage also express a battery of genes associated with the DNA-damage response. The BCR that is altered by somatic hypermutation in germinal center B cells undergoes two selection mechanisms [30]. First, the cells are censored against gaining reactivity to "self" antigen, which is controlled by Fas–FasLigand (FasL) interactions. Second, the cells are selected for high-affinity BCRs via a two-step process. In the first step, mutated clones compete for antigen that is trapped on follicular dendritic cells. Then, BCR-internalized antigen is presented to T-follicular helper cells. Productive interactions with T cells results in the cessation of affinity maturation and exit from the germinal center.

Exit from the germinal center represents a second critical branchpoint in B cell development.

High-affinity B cells that successfully become high-affinity plasmablast cells migrate to the extrafollicular region or they become memory B cells [31]. The regulation of this decision is poorly understood, but is thought to be dependent on both antigen affinity and T cell interactions. Furthermore, since differentiation into plasmablast cells is irreversible, an area of active research investigates how the system is able to preserve B cells with the same specificity in two functionally dissimilar cellular pools – plasma and memory.

Memory B cells

Memory B cells are long-lived B cells that have been selected from the primary response to antigen [32]. These cells are nondividing and quiescent – similar to naive B cells. In a secondary response, memory B cells respond to cognate antigen and participate in the same developmental decisions as a naive B cell. However, in contrast to naive B cells, they respond much more efficiently on a per cell basis. It is not known if this augmented activation is fundamentally quantitative (greater expression of the pre-existing set of signaling molecules), qualitative (exclusive expression of a highly efficacious signaling molecule(s)), or both. To date, no unique markers have enabled a comprehensive analysis of memory B cells in mice, and the identification of memory B cells has been defined by markers associated with the progression through an immune response, such as having mutated variable genes or switched constant regions. However, this approach is limited, as it is appreciated that not all memory B cells are products of the germinal center. In humans, expression of CD27, a member of the TNF family of receptors that includes CD40 and Baff/BLys, is expressed on a subset of memory but not naive B cells [33]. Although this has been an important marker, it has also been problematic because CD27 expression does not capture all memory cells and because nonmemory B cells, such as those in the mantle zone, can express CD27.

Memory B cells can be a barrier in transplantation as recipients that have been exposed to alloantigens due to previous transplants, blood transfusions, or pregnancies often generate accelerated alloreactive B cell responses [34]. The ability to control memory B cell reactivation would address an important barrier to the successful transplantation of pre-sensitized patients.

Reciprocal regulation by T and B cells

Although there is a rich literature implicating T-regulatory cell (Treg)-mediated suppression of T cell responses, it is also clear that Tregs can suppress antibody production [35]. Reciprocal regulation of T cells by B cells is gaining increased attention [36,37]. In this context, the mechanism of counter-repression appears to be through the secretion of the IL-10 cytokine, which exhibits negative effects on T cell activation. A novel population of CD5 and CD1d double-positive B cells that are poised to produce IL-10 during immune responses has been identified as the major regulatory B cell subset in mice. The human counterpart of this population remains to be identified. Thus, in thinking of immunosuppressive therapy, as with T cells, the optimal drugs to control allograft rejection will control effector B cells but preserve these regulatory B cell subsets.

Preclinical studies on B cells and antibodies in transplantation rejection

B cells and antibodies can induce transplantation rejection by at least three distinct mechanisms: (1) direct effects of antibody on graft parenchymal cells (especially endothelial cells, so-called humoral rejection), (2) promotion of a T cell response by B cell presentation of antigen or (3) stimulation of an alloimmune response by the generation of immune complexes that bind to Fc receptor-expressing antigen presenting cells (Plate 4.2). We will consider first the role of antibodies in mediating direct graft injury, through fixation of complement, Fc receptors on NK or macrophages or possibly by the cross-linking of cell surface molecules [38]. The major target of these effects is considered to be the endothelial cell, although other graft cells may also serve as targets (vascular smooth muscle cells, epithelial cells, cardiac myocytes).

Hyperacute rejection

When sufficient levels of antibodies reactive to the graft endothelium are present before a vascularized organ is transplanted, hyperacute rejection ensues. The classical features are rapid loss of graft function within minutes to hours of transplantation and characteristic changes in the microvasculature, including neutrophil accumulation, complement (C4d) deposition, hemorrhage, platelet thrombi, and necrosis of the endothelium. An association between preoperative cytotoxic antibody titers in the recipient serum and hyperacute rejection of canine heart and kidney allografts was initially described by Kuwahara et al. [39]. It was difficult to demonstrate any effect of antibody on murine skin grafts (in contrast to lymphoid cells), in part because of the relative cytotoxic weakness of the mouse complement system and also because of the transient expression of donor antigens on the endothelium of the skin. However, Gerlag et al. [40] reported that immediate rejection of skin allografts in mouse could be precipitated by the transfer of alloantibody and rabbit complement, and that the presence of a functioning vascular network was a prerequisite for the occurrence of hyperacute rejection. Further studies indicated that the graft vascular bed is sensitive only during a window in which the skin vessels have restored circulation, but then becomes progressively more resistant due to replacement of the endothelium by recipient cells after 14 days [41, 42]. In contrast, primarily vascularized organ grafts, such as the heart, remain sensitive to antibody indefinitely [43].

The role for recipient complement in hyperacute rejection was initially demonstrated by studies with cobra venom factor, which depleted hemolytic C3 activity [44]. Subsequently, the contribution of terminal complement components to hyperacute rejection was confirmed using reagents that block C5 or by using C6-deficient recipients [45]. In the case of xenografts, absence of the complement regulatory protein decay-accelerating factor (DAF) in the donor heart increases the susceptibility considerably to hyperacute or acute antibody-mediated rejection [46].

Recent studies by Yin et al. [47] suggest the existence of a second type of hyperacute rejection that is dependent on complement activation as well as FcγR-mediated interactions. This type of hyperacute rejection is induced with antibodies that are poorly complement-fixing but are able to bind to FcγRs. Using a panel of anti-Gal monoclonal antibodies of different IgG subclass, Ding et al. [48] demonstrated that hyperacute rejection can be variably dependent on both FcγRI and FcγRIII: mouse IgG1 being most dependent and IgG2a and IgG3 least dependent on FcγRIII; and IgG1, IgG2a, and IgG2b, but not IgG3, being dependent on FcγRI. Those studies illustrated an unappreciated but critical role for FcγRs, in addition to the well-established role for complement, in antibody-mediated hyperacute rejection.

Based on these observations, antibodies and complement fixation are necessary and sufficient to mediate hyperacute rejection and that, in some circumstances, cells with Fc receptors can have additive effects.

Acute antibody-mediated rejection

The ability of alloantibodies to elicit acute humoral or antibody-mediated rejection in the mouse is best illustrated using models of allograft transplantation into CCR5$^{-/-}$ recipients [49–51]. CCR5$^{-/-}$ recipients have enhanced alloantibody responses and acutely rejected MHC-mismatched allografts have low T cell infiltration but intense deposition of C3d in the large vessels and capillaries of the graft, characteristics of antibody-mediated rejection. Furthermore, the transfer of serum from CCR5$^{-/-}$ recipients into RAG1$^{-/-}$ recipients resulted in the acute vascular rejection of allografts that was characterized by C3d deposition and intense neutrophil and macrophage infiltration. These observations confirm that alloantibodies can mediate T-independent antibody-mediated acute rejection.

Acute rejection can be facilitated by alloantibodies binding to graft endothelium and synergizing with alloreactive T cells to induce acute allograft rejection. This notion that complement activation can contribute to the acute rejection of MHC-incompatible cardiac allografts was initially demonstrated by Qian *et al.* [52]. The importance of antibodies, upstream of complement activation, to acute rejection was reported by Wasawska *et al.* [53], whereby the delayed rejection of allogeneic hearts in B-cell-deficient mice was restored to normal kinetics by the administration of alloantibodies. Passive transfer of complement-activating IgG2b alloantibodies, but not non-complement-activating IgG1 alloantibodies, to B cell-deficient recipients reconstituted acute rejection of cardiac allografts, while the combination of both complement-fixing and nonfixing alloantibodies cooperated to induce acute graft rejection [54, 55]. Collectively, these experiments confirmed the contribution of antibodies and complement to acute allograft rejection and led to the mechanistic delineation of antibodies binding to vascular endothelium, stimulating the production chemokines, monocyte chemotactic protein 1 (MCP-1) and neutrophil chemoattractant growth-related oncogene alpha (KC), which then attract macrophages, monocytes, basophils, neutrophils and T cells into the graft.

Interactions with T cells

In addition to the effects directly arising from antibodies binding to the allografts, B cells and antibody may affect the priming of alloreactive T cells. Engagement of the BCR with antigen results in B cell activation and the shuttling of the BCR–Ag complex to the endosomal and lysosomal compartments where MHC class II processing and presentation occur. Thus, in contrast to passive antigen uptake via macropinocytosis that occurs in dendritic cells, BCR-mediated internalization of antigen facilitates antigen-specific presentation, perhaps most efficiently under low antigen concentrations, when B cells can effectively acquire high amounts of the antigen and present specific peptide–MHC complexes at high density. Coupled with the ability of B cells to present a high density of specific peptide–MHC complexes is the ability of B cells to undergo clonal expansion thereby increasing the frequency of cells presenting alloantigen. Antigen-specific B cells can expand their numbers and outnumber other types of

antigen-presenting cells such as dendritic cells, later in the adaptive immune response. Thus, T–B cell interactions may be an important event that maximizes the T cell response and/or drives late rejection of transplants.

B cells can express high levels of the B7-family of costimulatory ligands necessary for efficient T cell activation and can be an important source of many cytokines, such as interferon-γ, TGFβ, and interleukins 2, 4, 6, and 10 that T cells and other immune cells utilize. In fact, during T–B interactions, focused secretion of cytokines produced by B cells into the immunological synapse has been shown to be effective for T cell activation. These feature of B cells suggest their ability to facilitate many aspects of immunological "cross-talk" critical for coordinating the allospecific immune response.

Initial observations suggesting a role for B cells and/or alloantibodies in acute allograft rejection come from studies using B-cell-deficient mice that show delayed acute allograft rejection [53, 56]. However, interpretations from the use of B-cell-deficient mice are constrained by a number of caveats because B-cell-deficient mice exhibit secondary immunological consequences arising from the role of B cells in patterning proper cellular architecture via lymphotoxin signaling during lymph node organogenesis [57–59]. Recent observations of the ability of the B-cell-depleting antibody Rituximab® in conjunction with rapamycin to significantly outperform conventional T-cell-directed therapy in a nonhuman primate model of islet transplantation have lent credence to the hypothesis that B cells can play a critical role in allograft rejection [60]. While mechanistic studies on the role of B cells could not be easily performed in those nonhuman primate studies, they underscored the contribution of B cells, and possibly alloantibodies, to the induction of T-dependent allograft rejection.

The ability of alloreactive B cells to produce antibodies of the IgG isotype is dependent on cognate interactions with CD4+ T cells. The importance of this T–B interaction was elegantly illustrated by studies that used recipients which harbored B cells lacking the expression of MHC class II, and thus cognate B cell–CD4⁺ T cell interactions were prevented [61]. These mice had significantly reduced allo-IgG production and delayed rejection kinetics with cardiac allografts, but were able to reject skin allografts with normal kinetics. These observations suggest that the rejection of heart allografts is more dependent on the presence of alloantibodies, compared with skin allografts. An alternative interpretation is that skin grafts are able to stimulate sufficient alloreactive T cells to induce skin graft rejection independently of T–B interactions and/or alloantibodies.

Opsonization of antigen

Antibodies may facilitate the development of acute T-cell-mediated rejection by binding to graft cells or shed alloantigens to generate opsonins or multivalent antibody–antigen complexes. The binding of antibody to graft-derived cells or antigens enhances their internalization by macrophage and dendritic cells expressing Fc receptors, and ultimately their presentation of alloantigen to alloreactive T cells [62]. Also, immune complex activation of Fc receptors on APCs may lead to their maturation and acquisition of costimulatory molecules that allow for more effective alloantigen presentation to T cells. The ability of alloantibodies to generate immune complexes and opsonins in the context of transplantation was recently suggested by Burns et al. [63], in which alloantibodies and memory allospecific B cells, but not naive or nonspecific memory B cells, facilitated the rejection of cardiac allografts in recipients treated with anti-CD154.

Collectively, experimental data support a role for B cells and alloantibodies in mediating acute humoral rejection, synergizing with alloreactive T cells to mediate mixed humoral and cellular rejection, or generating opsonins to elicit cellular rejection. However, the relative contributions of B cells, serving as APCs versus alloantibody-producing cells, to the process of acute allograft rejection remains to be evaluated.

Chronic antibody-mediated rejection

Early studies by Russell et al. [64] indicated that the arteriopathic lesions that occurred in heart transplants were more severe in the mouse strain combinations known to produce detectable humoral antibodies to donor antigens than in the strain combinations that did not produce antibodies. Infusion of class I MHC donor-specific antiserum significantly increased coronary lesions in a dose-dependent fashion, confirming that alloantibodies can instigate vascular changes that occur in transplanted hearts. Subsequent studies using B-cell-deficient recipients demonstrating that fully developed, fibrous, chronic allograft vasculopathy was observed only in the presence of alloantibodies [65] further confirmed a contribution of alloantibodies in chronic allograft rejection. Uehara et al. [66] went on to demonstrate that even transient alloantibody and C4d deposition can be sufficient to trigger the inexorable decline of the allograft to chronic allograft vasculopathy. Those studies emphasized the importance of serial monitoring to determine the full extent of the role of alloantibodies in chronic allograft rejection. Endothelial response to anti-MHC antibody can be identified in vivo in the graft by detection of phosphorylation of signaling proteins, such as AKT and mTOR, by immunohistochemistry [67]. The activation of these pro-survival signaling pathways may contribute to the development of chronic antibody-mediated rejection.

More recent studies have focused on whether complement fixation is required for antibody-mediated chronic rejection, analogous to its necessity in acute and hyperacute rejection. In a study of rat heart allografts, Qian et al. [68] showed that the severity and onset of graft arteriosclerosis was reduced in cyclosporine-treated recipients deficient in C6 (affecting the terminal components of complement, C5b–C9). Because these recipients had an intact T cell function, it was difficult to determine the site of action of the C6 (whether related to T cell immunity, macrophage function or complement fixation in the graft endothelium). Studies by Hirohashi et al. [69], in the mouse, showed that passive transfer of class I MHC donor reactive antibodies into RAG1 KO recipients of heart allografts leads to the induction of chronic allograft arteriopathy, irrespective of whether the alloantibodies fix complement or not (IgG2a versus IgG1) and whether the recipient is deficient in C3 (C3 and RAG1 double KO) or not. Further experiments revealed that antibody-mediated chronic arteriopathy required NK cells, as judged by the ability of NK depletion (anti-NK1.1) to block chronic arteriopathy caused by passive transfer of alloantibody [70]. These observations where antibody-mediated chronic rejection can occur in the absence of C4d deposition may have relevance to C4d negative, donor alloantibody positive, chronically rejected grafts in humans.

Accommodation

The ability of grafts to function in the presence of graft-specific antibodies and complement is referred to as "graft accommodation." Graft accommodation has been demonstrated in the presence of antibodies that recognize carbohydrate residues on the graft, including anti-ABO as well as anti-Gal antibodies [71, 72] in the context of xenotransplantation [73]. While anti-MHC antibodies may also elicit at least temporary accommodation [74], clinical data suggest that this state of accommodation may be less stable and results ultimately in late graft deterioration.

The mechanism of accommodation is not resolved but appears to involve the expression of "protective" genes by endothelial cells. In accommodated xenografts, expression of A20 and bcl-2, as well as hemeoxygenase (HO-1), are upregulated and demonstrated to be important to the development and maintenance of the accommodated state [73, 75]. In other models of xenograft accommodation, the upregulated expression of complement regulatory proteins has been implicated in the accommodated state [71].

Studies in humans

Alloantibodies are widely appreciated as an important mediator of acute and chronic rejection in humans [76]. Four forms of antibody-mediated graft injury have been defined, corresponding to those described above in the mouse: namely hyperacute rejection, acute humoral rejection, chronic humoral rejection and accommodation. These categories are well documented in kidney allografts, and are being increasingly recognized in heart, pancreas, lung, and liver allografts. Appreciation of the clinical relevance of alloantibodies has rested on a new diagnostic technique (C4d) that permits a definitive diagnosis of antibody-mediated rejection and the wide application of solid-phase assays for donor reactive HLA antibodies.

Complement (C4d) is widely and characteristically deposited in the capillary endothelium in acute antibody-mediated rejection, arguing that complement fixation is important in the pathogenesis [76]. Supportive evidence comes from the demonstration that alloantibodies that fix complement (C4d or C1q on luminex beads) are associated with a worse outcome than alloantibodies that do not fix complement [77, 78]. Furthermore, preliminary studies suggest that acute humoral rejection is completely inhibited by anti-C5 [79].

While the primary targets of antibody-mediated rejection are the conventional HLA class I and II antigens, other MHC-related alloantigens (MICA) [80] and even autoantigens, such as the angiotensin type II receptor [81] and parenchymal cell antigens [82], are considered potentially relevant. Since IgG subclasses differ in their ability to fix complement there has been some interest in whether the distribution of subclasses of donor reactive alloantibodies has an effect on outcome. Indeed, patients who had donor reactive complement fixing IgG1 were more likely to lose their renal allograft [83]. Anti-donor antibodies of the strongest complement fixing subclass, IgG3, were present in patients with acute rejection, but not in stable patients, whereas the latter had an increase in the noncomplement fixing, IgG4 subclass [84]. Noncomplement fixing anti-donor antibodies of the IgG2 and IgG4 subclasses can be eluted from a minority of rejected renal allografts; whether they have a protective or injurious role is unclear [85].

B cells are not commonly abundant in acute rejection, but in the chronic setting they become quite apparent, often concentrated in nodular aggregates. Early studies by Sarwal et al. suggested that renal allografts with dysfunction had a worse prognosis if B cells were prominent in the infiltrate [86]. However, subsequent studies have not found a consistent correlation [87–92]. It is notable that B cells in nodules express AID [93], suggesting that they are undergoing hypermutation and selection within the graft itself. Indeed, there is evidence that lymphoid neogenesis occurs in some grafts late after transplant [94] and the possibility is raised that a self-sustaining, entirely local immune reaction can promote long-term graft injury. In the heart, nodules of B cells are commonly found under the endocardium, known as the Quilty lesion [95]. This is generally regarded as not pathologic (i.e., not rejection); however, its significance is still unclear.

Plasma cells have long been noted in renal allografts and sometimes been associated with a more adverse outcome. Careful studies by Meehan *et al.* showed that plasma-cell-rich acute rejection in the first year had a worse prognosis than acute rejection without prominent plasma cells [96]. However, late acute rejection had a poor prognosis whether or not plasma cells were abundant. Others have shown an association of plasma cells with C4d deposition and donor-specific antibody [87, 97]. Gene expression studies by Einecke *et al.* [98] showed that B cell and plasma cell (Ig) transcripts increase with time after transplant in biopsies taken for graft dysfunction. One could argue that this means that they are incidental and passive, or that the later the graft dysfunction, the more likely it is to be due to B cells or plasma cells. Studies by Thaunat *et al.* in two patients have shown that the plasma cells in rejecting renal allografts secrete donor-specific alloantibody [93]. This fits with the notion that a local immune response can be generated, possibly without detectable circulating antibodies. The allograft thereby can become a niche for plasma cells, as has been described in other sites of chronic inflammation [99].

In chronic rejection the evidence is not so clear that complement fixation is necessary. First, the C4d pattern may be focal and not widespread in the capillaries [100]. Second, a substantial number of cases studied by Sis *et al.* [101] showed that evidence of endothelial injury and reaction could be detected by gene expression analysis (microarray) in patients with donor reactive HLA antibodies, even if C4d was not detectable in the graft. Capillaritis can also be a manifestation of early chronic antibody mediated rejection, even without detectable C4d deposition [102]. These authors concluded that C4d was not sufficiently sensitive to detect chronic antibody-mediated injury. Alternatively, some of these lesions may be related to noncomplement fixing antibodies. It is known that chronic vascular rejection in the mouse is complement independent, and it is possible that this also applies to humans. Further studies will be needed to test this hypothesis.

Therapies directed at B cells and antibodies to prevent transplantation rejection

Accumulating evidence supports a predominantly pathogenic role for B cells and alloantibodies in allograft transplantation. The reduction of circulating alloantibodies is currently achieved through the use of plasmapheresis or intravenous immunoglobulin (IVIG). However, effectiveness is limited by transient and variable efficacy, prompting the notion that targeting the cellular source of antibody may be a more effective strategy for controlling B cells and antibody-mediated allograft rejection (summarized in Table 4.2). To this end, an

Table 4.2 B cell, plasma cell and antibody-directed immunosuppressive strategies.

Drug	Species	Efficacy
Plasmapheresis	Humans	Immediate, but temporary benefit
IVIG	Humans	Beneficial, potential longer term effects
Rituximab (anti-CD20)	Humans	Variable, uncontrolled trials
Bortezomib	Humans	Early noncontrolled studies suggest benefit
Anti-BAFF, TACI-Ig	Nonhuman primates	In development
Anti-C5	Humans	In development

important strategy aimed at depleting B cells via the use of rituximab (Rituxan®), a B-cell-depleting antibody that targets the B lineage marker CD20, is currently under investigation to control antibody-mediated rejection. This treatment was initially used for non-Hodgkin's lymphoma with great success, and was shown to have surprising efficacy in type 1 diabetes and multiple sclerosis, auto-immune diseases that have traditionally been considered T cell driven [103, 104]. Likewise, rituximab, in conjunction with rapamycin, significantly outperformed conventional T-cell-directed therapy in a nonhuman primate model of islet transplantation [60]. These reports, along with the clinical success of rituximab to treat acute humoral or steroid- and antilymphocyte-resistant humoral rejection [105, 106], reinforce the centrality of B cells in immune responses and generate excitement for the use of rituximab in inhibiting transplant rejection – a reaction that is generally considered to be T cell driven.

The major limitation with the use of rituximab is that it fails at targeting plasma cells due to their low-level CD20 expression, and suggests that this therapy could be markedly improved with a drug or reagent that can target plasma cells. Two recent studies describing the treatment of humoral rejection have used the proteosome inhibitor borte-zomib, a drug approved for the effective treatment of multiple myeloma, a plasma cell malignancy [107]. Bortezomib was shown to successfully deplete plasma cells and depress alloantibody titers in vitro and in a limited number of patients under-going humoral rejection, raising the possibility that it may be an effective new agent for the removal of alloantibodies [108].

Another novel strategy that is currently in preclinical and clinical development that is generating excitement is the targeting of the BAFF receptor system (BAFF/BLYS and APRIL interacting with the common ligands, BCMA, TACI, or BAFF-R). Targeting of this system should preferentially limit mature B cell, short-lived plasma cells and long-lived plasma cell survival [109]. Four different BAFF antagonists are being developed for clinical use. Anti-Baff/BLys (belimumab) is a recombinant IgG1λ monoclonal

antibody derived from a human phage display library that targets only soluble human BAFF protein, BR3-Fc is a fully human fusion protein of the extracellular domain of human BAFF-R with the Fc of human IgG, and anti-BAFF-R is a monoclonal antibody to BAFF-R. These agents caused reductions in naive and activated CD69[+] B cells and circulating plasmablasts, while anti-BAFF-R additionally depleted B cells expressing the BAFF-R. None of these agents affected plasma cell numbers. TACI-Ig (atacicept), the fourth antagonist in development for clinical use, is a fully human fusion protein of the extracellular domain of human TACI with the Fc of human IgG1 [105]. It also depleted B cells, but it induced a more profound depletion of circulating Igs than the agonists targeting the Baff/BLys pathways. The impact of these agents in the context of transplantation has yet to be defined.

Conclusion

The ability of the B cell system to produce alloantibody is dependent on "help" cues from T cells and survival cues from T and dendritic cells. The resulting alloantibody drives the ongoing alloresponse by (i) cytotoxicity mediated by ADCC and/or complement; (ii) regulatory effects mediated by antigen opsonization and Fc receptor signaling and/or subsequent antigen presentation. Attempts to control B cells and antibody-mediated effects of graft rejection have focused on the control of B cells and alloantibodies in patients with B-cell-depleting reagents, IVIG, and plasmapheresis. There are limitations to these therapies, and second-generation strategies focused on controlling effector and memory B cells, as well as plasma cells, are warranted. An optimal therapy, of course, would be one that targets pathogenic B cells and plasma cells while sparing regulatory B cells. The elucidation of basic mechanisms that promote B cell activation and survival are heralding a new set of biologicals that have the potential for improved control of alloantibody production and antibody-mediated injury during transplantation.

References

1 Hunkapiller T, Goverman J, Koop BF, Hood L. Implications of the diversity of the immunoglobulin gene superfamily. *Cold Spring Harb Symp Quant Biol* 1989;54(Pt 1):15–29.

2 Steiniger B, Timphus EM, Jacob R, Barth PJ. CD27+ B cells in human lymphatic organs: re-evaluating the splenic marginal zone. *Immunology* 2005;116:429–442.

3 Xiao Y, Hendriks J, Langerak P *et al*. CD27 is acquired by primed B cells at the centroblast stage and promotes germinal center formation. *J Immunol* 2004;172: 7432–7441.

4 Schittek B, Rajewsky K. Natural occurrence and origin of somatically mutated memory B cells in mice. *J Exp Med* 1992;176:427–438.

5 Klein U, Rajewsky K, Kuppers R. Human immunoglobulin (Ig)M+IgD+ peripheral blood B cells expressing the CD27 cell surface antigen carry somatically mutated variable region genes: CD27 as a general marker for somatically mutated (memory) B cells. *J Exp Med* 1998;188:1679–1689.

6 De Bono B, Madera M, Chothia C. VH gene segments in the mouse and human genomes. *J Mol Biol* 2004;342:131–143.

7 Padlan EA. Anatomy of the antibody molecule. *Mol Immunol* 1994;31:169–217.

8 Teng G, Papavasiliou FN. Immunoglobulin somatic hypermutation. *Annu Rev Genet* 2007;41:107–120.

9 Chaudhuri J, Alt FW. Class-switch recombination: interplay of transcription, DNA deamination and DNA repair. *Nat Rev Immunol* 2004;4:541–552.

10 Sciammas R, Davis MM. Blimp-1; immunoglobulin secretion and the switch to plasma cells. *Curr Top Microbiol Immunol* 2005;290:201–224.

11 Medina KL, Singh H. Gene regulatory networks orchestrating B cell fate specification, commitment, and differentiation. *Curr Top Microbiol Immunol* 2005;290:1–14.

12 Melchers F, Rolink A, Grawunder U *et al*. Positive and negative selection events during B lymphopoiesis. *Curr Opin Immunol* 1995;7:214–227.

13 Nemazee D, Weigert M. Revising B cell receptors. *J Exp Med* 2000;191:1813–1817.

14 Allman D, Pillai S. Peripheral B cell subsets. *Curr Opin Immunol* 2008;20:149–157.

15 Stadanlick JE, Cancro MP. BAFF and the plasticity of peripheral B cell tolerance. *Curr Opin Immunol* 2008;20:158–161.

16 Batista FD, Harwood NE. The who, how and where of antigen presentation to B cells. *Nat Rev Immunol* 2009;9:15–27.

17 Carroll MC. The role of complement and complement receptors in induction and regulation of immunity. *Annu Rev Immunol* 1998;16:545–568.

18 Richards S, Watanabe C, Santos L *et al*. Regulation of B-cell entry into the cell cycle. *Immunol Rev* 2008; 224:183–200.

19 Okada T, Cyster JG. B cell migration and interactions in the early phase of antibody responses. *Curr Opin Immunol* 2006;18:278–285.

20 McHeyzer-Williams MG. B cells as effectors. *Curr Opin Immunol* 2003;15:354–361.

21 Brink R, Phan TG, Paus D, Chan TD. Visualizing the effects of antigen affinity on T-dependent B-cell differentiation. *Immunol Cell Biol* 2008;86:31–39.

22 Ma Y, Hendershot LM. The stressful road to antibody secretion. *Nat Immunol* 2003;4:310–311.

23 Sciammas R, Shaffer AL, Schatz JH *et al*. Graded expression of interferon regulatory factor-4 coordinates isotype switching with plasma cell differentiation. *Immunity* 2006;25:225–236.

24 Shaffer AL, Shapiro-Shelef M, Iwakoshi NN *et al*. XBP1, downstream of Blimp-1, expands the secretory apparatus and other organelles, and increases protein synthesis in plasma cell differentiation. *Immunity* 2004;21:81–93.

25 Sanderson RD, Lalor P, Bernfield M. B lymphocytes express and lose syndecan at specific stages of differentiation. *Cell Regul* 1989;1:27–35.

26 MacLennan IC, Toellner KM, Cunningham AF *et al*. Extrafollicular antibody responses. *Immunol Rev* 2003;194:8–18.

27 Konforte D, Simard N, Paige CJ. IL-21: an executor of B cell fate. *J Immunol* 2009;182:1781–1787.

28 McHeyzer-Williams MG, Ahmed R. B cell memory and the long-lived plasma cell. *Curr Opin Immunol* 1999;11:172–179.

29 Honjo T, Muramatsu M, Fagarasan S. AID: how does it aid antibody diversity? *Immunity* 2004;20:659–668.

30 Allen CD, Okada T, Cyster JG. Germinal-center organization and cellular dynamics. *Immunity* 2007; 27:190–202.

31 Benson MJ, Erickson LD, Gleeson MW, Noelle RJ. Affinity of antigen encounter and other early B-cell signals determine B-cell fate. *Curr Opin Immunol* 2007;19:275–280.

32 Tarlinton D. B-cell memory: are subsets necessary? *Nat Rev Immunol* 2006;6:785–790.

33 Klein U, Goossens T, Fischer M *et al.* Somatic hypermutation in normal and transformed human B cells. *Immunol Rev* 1998;162:261–280.

34 Zarkhin V, Li L, Sarwal M. "To B or not to B?" B-cells and graft rejection. *Transplantation* 2008;85: 1705–1714.

35 Zheng Y, Chaudhry A, Kas A *et al.* Regulatory T-cell suppressor program co-opts transcription factor IRF4 to control T$_H$2 responses. *Nature* 2009;458: 351–356.

36 Bouaziz JD, Yanaba K, Tedder TF. Regulatory B cells as inhibitors of immune responses and inflammation. *Immunol Rev* 2008;224:201–214.

37 Mizoguchi A, Bhan AK. A case for regulatory B cells. *J Immunol* 2006;176:705–710.

38 Colvin RB, Smith RN. Antibody-mediated organ-allograft rejection. *Nat Rev Immunol* 2005;5:807–817.

39 Kuwahara O, Kondo Y, Kuramochi T *et al.* Organ specificity in hyperacute rejection of canine heart and kidney allografts. *Ann Surg* 1974;180:72–79.

40 Gerlag PG, Koene RA, Hagemann JF, Wijdeveld PG. Hyperacute rejection of skin allografts in the mouse. Sensitivity of ingrowing skin grafts to the action of alloantibody and rabbit complement. *Transplantation* 1975;20:308–313.

41 Jooste SV, Colvin RB, Soper WD, Winn HJ. The vascular bed as the primary target in the destruction of skin grafts by antiserum. I. Resistance of freshly placed xenografts of skin to antiserum. *J Exp Med* 1981; 154:1319–1331.

42 Jooste SV, Colvin RB, Winn HJ. The vascular bed as the primary target in the destruction of skin grafts by antiserum. II. Loss of sensitivity to antiserum in long-term xenografts of skin. *J Exp Med* 1981;154: 1332–1341.

43 Burdick JF, Russell PS, Winn HJ. Sensitivity of long standing xenografts of rat hearts to humoral antibodies. *J Immunol* 1979;123:1732–1735.

44 Forbes RD, Pinto-Blonde M, Guttmann RD. The effect of anticomplementary cobra venom factor on hyperacute rat cardiac allograft rejection. *Lab Invest* 1978;39: 463–470.

45 Brauer RB, Lam TT, Wang D *et al.* Extrahepatic synthesis of C6 in the rat is sufficient for complement-mediated hyperacute rejection of a guinea pig cardiac xenograft. *Transplantation* 1995;59:1073–1076.

46 Shimizu I, Smith NR, Zhao G *et al.* Decay-accelerating factor prevents acute humoral rejection induced by low levels of anti-alphaGal natural antibodies. *Transplantation* 2006;81:95–100.

47 Yin D, Zeng H, Ma L *et al.* Cutting Edge: NK cells mediate IgG1-dependent hyperacute rejection of xenografts. *J Immunol* 2004;172:7235–7238.

48 Ding JW, Zhou T, Seng H, *et al.* Hyperacute rejection by anti-Gal IgG1, IgG2a and IgG2b is dependent on complement and Fc-gamma receptors. *J Immunol* 2008; 180:261–268.

49 Amano H, Bickerstaff A, Orosz CG *et al.* Absence of recipient CCR5 promotes early and increased allospecific antibody responses to cardiac allografts. *J Immunol* 2005;174:6499–6508.

50 Bickerstaff A, Nozaki T, Wang JJ *et al.* Acute humoral rejection of renal allografts in CCR5$^{-/-}$ recipients. *Am J Transplant* 2008;8:557–566.

51 Nozaki T, Amano H, Bickerstaff A *et al.* Antibody-mediated rejection of cardiac allografts in CCR5-deficient recipients. *J Immunol* 2007;179:5238–5245.

52 Qian Z, Jakobs FM, Pfaff-Amesse T *et al.* Complement contributes to the rejection of complete and class I major histocompatibility complex-incompatible cardiac allografts. *J Heart Lung Transplant* 1998;17:470–478.

53 Wasowska BA, Qian Z, Cangello DL *et al.* Passive transfer of alloantibodies restores acute cardiac rejection in IgKO mice. *Transplantation* 2001;71:727–736.

54 Murata K, Fox-Talbot K, Qian Z *et al.* Synergistic deposition of C4d by complement-activating and non-activating antibodies in cardiac transplants. *Am J Transplant* 2007;7:2605–2614.

55 Rahimi S, Qian Z, Layton J *et al.* Non-complement- and complement-activating antibodies synergize to cause rejection of cardiac allografts. *Am J Transplant* 2004;4:326–334.

56 Brandle D, Joergensen J, Zenke G *et al.* Contribution of donor-specific antibodies to acute allograft rejection: evidence from B cell-deficient mice. *Transplantation* 1998;65:1489–1493.

57 Endres R, Alimzhanov MB, Plitz T *et al.* Mature follicular dendritic cell networks depend on expression of lymphotoxin beta receptor by radioresistant stromal cells and of lymphotoxin beta and tumor necrosis factor by B cells. *J Exp Med* 1999;189:159–168.

58 Fu YX, Huang G, Wang Y, Chaplin DD. B lymphocytes induce the formation of follicular dendritic cell clusters in a lymphotoxin alpha-dependent fashion. *J Exp Med* 1998;187:1009–1018.

59 Gonzalez M, Mackay F, Browning JL *et al.* The sequential role of lymphotoxin and B cells in the development of splenic follicles. *J Exp Med* 1998;187:997–1007.

60 Liu C, Noorchashm H, Sutter JA *et al.* B lymphocyte-directed immunotherapy promotes long-term islet

allograft survival in nonhuman primates. *Nat Med* 2007;13:1295–1298.

61 Noorchashm H, Reed AJ, Rostami SY *et al*. B cell-mediated antigen presentation is required for the pathogenesis of acute cardiac allograft rejection. *J Immunol* 2006;177:7715–7722.

62 Nimmerjahn F, Ravetch JV. Fcgamma receptors as regulators of immune responses. *Nat Rev Immunol* 2008;8:34–47.

63 Burns AM, Ma L, Li Y *et al*. Memory alloreactive B cells and alloantibodies prevent anti-CD154-mediated allograft acceptance. *J Immunol* 2009;182:1314–1324.

64 Russell PS, Chase CM, Winn HJ, Colvin RB. Coronary atherosclerosis in transplanted mouse hearts. II. Importance of humoral immunity. *J Immunol* 1994; 152:5135–5141.

65 Russell PS, Chase CM, Colvin RB. Alloantibody- and T cell-mediated immunity in the pathogenesis of transplant arteriosclerosis: lack of progression to sclerotic lesions in B cell-deficient mice. *Transplantation* 1997;64:1531–1536.

66 Uehara S, Chase CM, Cornell LD *et al*. Chronic cardiac transplant arteriopathy in mice: relationship of alloantibody, C4d deposition and neointimal fibrosis. *Am J Transplant* 2007;7:57–65.

67 Jindra PT, Hsueh A, Hong L *et al*. Anti-MHC class I antibody activation of proliferation and survival signaling in murine cardiac allografts. *J Immunol* 2008;180:2214–2224.

68 Qian Z, Hu W, Liu J *et al*. Accelerated graft arteriosclerosis in cardiac transplants: complement activation promotes progression of lesions from medium to large arteries. *Transplantation* 2001;72:900–906.

69 Hirohashi T, Uehara S, Chase CM *et al*. Complement independent antibody-mediated endarteritis and transplant arteriopathy in mice. *Am J Transplant* 2010;10:510–517.

70 Hirohashi T, Chase CM, Alessandrini A *et al*. A novel pathway of chronic allograft rejection mediated by NK cells and alloantibody. *Am J Transplant* 2011; in press.

71 Ding JW, Zhou T, Ma L *et al*. Expression of complement regulatory proteins in accommodated xenografts induced by anti-alpha-Gal IgG1 in a rat-to-mouse model. *Am J Transplant* 2008;8:32–40.

72 Fan X, Ang A, Pollock-Barziv SM *et al*. Donor-specific B-cell tolerance after ABO-incompatible infant heart transplantation. *Nat Med* 2004;10:1227–1233.

73 Bach FH, Ferran C, Candinas D *et al*. Accommodation of xenografts: expression of "protective genes" in endothelial and smooth muscle cells. *Transplant Proc* 1997;29:56–58.

74 Wang H, Arp J, Liu W *et al*. Inhibition of terminal complement components in presensitized transplant recipients prevents antibody-mediated rejection leading to long-term graft survival and accommodation. *J Immunol* 2007;179:4451–4463.

75 Rother RP, Arp J, Jiang J *et al*. C5 blockade with conventional immunosuppression induces long-term graft survival in presensitized recipients. *Am J Transplant* 2008;8:1129–1142.

76 Colvin RB. Antibody-mediated renal allograft rejection: diagnosis and pathogenesis. *J Am Soc Nephrol* 2007;18:1046–1056.

77 Smith JD, Hamour IM, Banner NR, Rose ML. C4d fixing, luminex binding antibodies – a new tool for prediction of graft failure after heart transplantation. *Am J Transplant* 2007;7:2809–2815.

78 Wahrmann M, Exner M, Schillinger M *et al*. Pivotal role of complement-fixing HLA alloantibodies in presensitized kidney allograft recipients. *Am J Transplant* 2006;6:1033–1041.

79 Stegall MD, Diwan T, Raghavaiah S *et al*. Terminal complement inhibition decreases antibody-mediated rejection in sensitized renal transplant recipients. *Am J Transplant* 2011;11: 2405–2413.

80 Zou Y, Stastny P, Susal C *et al*. Antibodies against MICA antigens and kidney-transplant rejection. *N Engl J Med* 2007;357:1293–1300.

81 Dragun D, Muller DN, Brasen JH *et al*. Angiotensin II type 1-receptor activating antibodies in renal-allograft rejection. *N Engl J Med* 2005;352:558–569.

82 Li L, Wadia P, Chen R *et al*. Identifying compartment-specific non-HLA targets after renal transplantation by integrating transcriptome and "antibodyome" measures. *Proc Natl Acad Sci U S A* 2009;106:4148–4153.

83 Griffiths EJ, Nelson RE, Dupont PJ, Warrens AN. Skewing of pretransplant anti-HLA class I antibodies of immunoglobulin G isotype solely toward immunoglobulin G1 subclass is associated with poorer renal allograft survival. *Transplantation* 2004;77:1771–1773.

84 Gao ZH, McAlister VC, Wright JR, Jr, *et al*. Immunoglobulin-G subclass antidonor reactivity in transplant recipients. *Liver Transpl* 2004;10:1055–1059.

85 Heinemann FM, Roth I, Rebmann V *et al*. Immunoglobulin isotype-specific characterization of anti-human leukocyte antigen antibodies eluted from explanted renal allografts. *Hum Immunol* 2007;68: 500–506.

86 Sarwal M, Chua MS, Kambham N *et al*. Molecular heterogeneity in acute renal allograft rejection identified by DNA microarray profiling. *N Engl J Med* 2003;349:125–138.

87 Zarkhin V, Kambham N, Li L *et al.* Characterization of intra-graft B cells during renal allograft rejection. *Kidney Int* 2008;74:664–673.

88 Scheepstra C, Bemelman FJ, van der Loos C *et al.* B cells in cluster or in a scattered pattern do not correlate with clinical outcome of renal allograft rejection. *Transplantation* 2008;86:772–778.

89 Segerer S, Schlondorff D. B cells and tertiary lymphoid organs in renal inflammation. *Kidney Int* 2008;73:533–537.

90 Heller F, Lindenmeyer MT, Cohen CD *et al.* The contribution of B cells to renal interstitial inflammation. *Am J Pathol* 2007;170:457–468.

91 Stuht S, Gwinner W, Franz I *et al.* Lymphatic neoangiogenesis in human renal allografts: results from sequential protocol biopsies. *Am J Transplant* 2007;7:377–384.

92 Muorah MR, Brogan PA, Sebire NJ *et al.* Dense B cell infiltrates in paediatric renal transplant biopsies are predictive of allograft loss. *Pediatr Transplant* 2009;13:217–222.

93 Thaunat O, Patey N, Gautreau C *et al.* B cell survival in intragraft tertiary lymphoid organs after rituximab therapy. *Transplantation* 2008;85:1648–1653.

94 Kerjaschki D, Regele HM, Moosberger I *et al.* Lymphatic neoangiogenesis in human kidney transplants is associated with immunologically active lymphocytic infiltrates. *J Am Soc Nephrol* 2004;15:603–612.

95 Smith RN, Chang Y, Houser S *et al.* Higher frequency of high-grade rejections in cardiac allograft patients after Quilty B lesions or grade 2/4 rejections. *Transplantation* 2002;73:1928–1932.

96 Meehan SM, Domer P, Josephson M *et al.* The clinical and pathologic implications of plasmacytic infiltrates in percutaneous renal allograft biopsies. *Hum Pathol* 2001;32:205–215.

97 Poduval RD, Kadambi PV, Josephson MA, Cohn RA, Harland RC, Javaid B *et al.* Implications of immunohistochemical detection of C4d along peritubular capillaries in late acute renal allograft rejection. *Transplantation* 2005;79:228–235.

98 Einecke G, Reeve J, Mengel M *et al.* Expression of B cell and immunoglobulin transcripts is a feature of inflammation in late allografts. *Am J Transplant* 2008;8:1434–1443.

99 Huard B, McKee T, Bosshard C *et al.* APRIL secreted by neutrophils binds to heparan sulfate proteoglycans to create plasma cell niches in human mucosa. *J Clin Invest* 2008;118:2887–2895.

100 Colvin RB. Pathology of chronic humoral rejection. *Contrib Nephrol* 2009;162:75–86.

101 Sis B, Jhangri GS, Bunnag S *et al.* Endothelial gene expression in kidney transplants with alloantibody indicates antibody-mediated damage despite lack of C4d staining. *Am J Transplant* 2009;9:2312–2323.

102 Loupy A, Hill GS, Suberbielle C *et al.* Significance of C4d Banff scores in early protocol biopsies of kidney transplant recipients with preformed donor-specific antibodies (DSA). *Am J Transplant* 2011; 11:56–65.

103 Cree B. Emerging monoclonal antibody therapies for multiple sclerosis. *Neurologist* 2006;12:171–178.

104 Hu CY, Rodriguez-Pinto D, Du W *et al.* Treatment with CD20-specific antibody prevents and reverses autoimmune diabetes in mice. *J Clin Invest* 2007; 117:3857–3867.

105 Pena-Rossi C, Nasonov E, Stanislav M *et al.* An exploratory dose-escalating study investigating the safety, tolerability, pharmacokinetics and pharmacodynamics of intravenous atacicept in patients with systemic lupus erythematosus. *Lupus* 2009;18:547–555.

106 Venetz JP, Pascual M. New treatments for acute humoral rejection of kidney allografts. *Expert Opin Investig Drugs* 2007;16:625–633.

107 Obeng EA, Carlson LM, Gutman DM *et al.* Proteasome inhibitors induce a terminal unfolded protein response in multiple myeloma cells. *Blood* 2006;107:4907–4916.

108 Perry DK, Burns JM, Pollinger HS *et al.* Proteasome inhibition causes apoptosis of normal human plasma cells preventing alloantibody production. *Am J Transplant* 2009;9:201–209.

109 Ramanujam M, Davidson A. BAFF blockade for systemic lupus erythematosus: will the promise be fulfilled? *Immunol Rev* 2008;223:156–174.

CHAPTER 5

The Innate Response to a Transplanted Organ

Daniel R. Goldstein[1] and Laurence A. Turka[2]
[1]Yale University School of Medicine, New Haven, CT, USA
[2]Beth Israel Deaconess Medical Center, Harvard Medical School, Boston, MA, USA

Overview of the innate immune system

Discovery of the innate immune system

Over the last decade there has been a growing appreciation of the importance of the innate immune system in different clinical scenarios. The innate immune system is typically activated by pathogens, although stimulation by noninfectious substances occurs. The innate system, as opposed to the adaptive one, is considered more ancient in its origins and is found in organisms which do not possess adaptive immunity, for example the sea urchin [1]. Classically, the innate system is activated in an antigen-independent fashion without evidence of immune memory. This is in contrast to adaptive immunity, which is characterized by the response of clonally selected lymphocytes that respond to molecular details of antigenic structure with high specificity, leading to robust immunological memory. The Russian scientist Elie Metchnikoff was one of the first to discover the innate immune system by examining the importance of phagocytic cells of invertebrate organisms in "digesting" invading microbes. This work led to the Nobel Prize in 1908 [2]. Since this discovery, the phagocytic macrophage has been noted to be one of the most important cellular components of the innate system, rapidly producing a variety of inflammatory mediators in response to injury [3]. Other cellular components of the innate system include dendritic cells (DCs), which are also mediators of inflammation but possess key antigen-presentation functions [4]. Neutrophils also rapidly respond to injury and secrete host defense molecules in order to eradicate the invading pathogen and contain the infection [5]. However, the innate immune system is not confined to hematopoietic or myeloid cells: epithelial cells carry out important host defense functions, by producing antimicrobial peptides, for example defensins [6]. Clearly, the innate system evolved as a first line of defense against invading pathogens.

Identification of pathogen recognition receptors on innate immune cells

Janeway was the first to propose a conceptual link between the innate and the adaptive immune systems, when he advocated that conserved components of pathogens possess adjuvant properties, suggesting that the innate system could activate the adaptive one [7]. Evidence supporting this concept was subsequently provided by the discovery of the Toll receptors several years later. The first discovery of these receptors was reported in *Drosophila*. Originally known as a gene that controlled dorsoventral orientation, it was subsequently determined that the Toll receptor was vital for antifungal host

Immunotherapy in Transplantation: Principles and Practice, First Edition. Edited by Bruce Kaplan, Gilbert J. Burckart and Fadi G. Lakkis.
© 2012 Blackwell Publishing Ltd. Published 2012 by Blackwell Publishing Ltd.

Table 5.1 Toll-like receptors and a representative list of known exogenous and endogenous TLR agonists [12]. With permission from the American Society of Nephrology, from *J Am Soc Nephrol* 2008;19:1444–1450.

Toll-like receptor	Ligand	
	Exogenous	Endogenous
TLR1+TLR2	Triacyl lipopeptides, Lipoarabinomannan	
TLR2	Peptidoglycan, Zymosan	HSP 70, HMGB1, Hyaluronic Acid
TLR2+TLR6	Diacyl lipopeptides, Lipoteichoic acid	
TLR3	dsRNA, siRNA	mRNA
TLR4	LPS, peptidoglycan, taxol	Tamm–Horsfall glycoprotein
		Hyaluronic acid
		HMGB1
		Heparan sulfate
		Fibronectin domain A
		Surfactant protein A
		Modified LDL
TLR5	Flagellin	
TLR7	ssRNA, imiquimod	RNA
TLR8	ssRNA	
TLR9	CpG DNA (dsDNA)	Chromatin complex
TLR10	Unknown	
TLR11	Profilin-like molecule	

defense, by activating a kinase-mediated protease cascade, leading to the production of the antifungal peptide drosomycin [8]. However, *Drosophila* that were deficient for the Toll receptor exhibited intact host defense to Gram-negative bacteria [8]. At the time, the first mammalian Toll-like receptor (TLR) was discovered but its immune functions were not appreciated [9]. This was subsequently realized by the discovery that overexpression of this receptor (TLR4) in mammalian cells activated NFκB, a signaling pathway that is critical for many inflammatory immune responses [9, 10]. TLR4 was subsequently found by positional cloning to be responsible for the lipopolysaccharide (LPS or endotoxin) hyporesponsive phenotype of the C3H/HEJ mouse, clearly establishing the role of TLRs in immune responses and inflammation [11].

Thirteen TLRs have been discovered in mice and humans so far (see Plate 5.1 and Table 5.1). Mice lack TLR10 but express all others, whereas humans do not express TLRs 11, 12, and 13. TLRs are members of a larger group of innate immune receptors, termed pattern recognition receptors (PRRs), which are classically activated by conserved motifs on invading pathogens [13, 14]. TLRs are type 1 integral glycoprotein transmembrane receptors which contain leucine-rich repeats in their extracellular domains. The cytoplasmic domains of TLRs are homologous to the IL-1 receptor, as both groups of receptors contain a Toll/IL-1R (TIR) domain. TLRs are either expressed on the cell surface (e.g., TLRs 2, 4, and 5) or within endosomes (e.g., TLRs 3, 7, 8, and 9). Cell-surface receptors typically respond to bacterial products, such as TLR4, which is activated by LPS in a complex with CD14 and MD2 [13, 15]. In contrast, endosomal TLRs are activated by viral products, such as single-stranded RNA or unmethylated CpG sequences [16]. However, there is firm evidence that TLRs are also activated by endogenous products released during sterile inflammation, for example fragmented hyaluronan (HA), a component of the extracellular matrix, which activates TLRs 2 and 4 [17, 18]. Other putative ligands include heparan sulfate, high-mobility group box-1 protein (HGMB-1), heat shock proteins, mammalian chromatin, uric acid, fibrinogen, and surfactant [12].

Other PRRs include the NOD-like receptors (NLRs) that lead to the activation of the inflammasome and production of IL-1 beta in several inflammatory disorders, including familial Mediterranean fever [19]. Furthermore, uric acid, which is the mediator that induces gouty inflammation, activates this innate pathway. Emerging evidence indicates that viral infection can also stimulate this pathway. RNA viruses, for example influenza, are sensed by cytosolic receptors, the RNA helicase pathway that transduces signals via adaptors retinoic acid-inducible gene (RIG)-1 and MDA [14]. Furthermore, recent evidence indicates a cytosolic viral DNA sensing pathway, which signals via IRF-3 [20, 21]. In sum, the complexity of the innate immune system is only just emerging and it is evident that there are many complementary signaling pathways that sense the presence of infections or sterile inflammation.

TLR signaling pathways

Five signal adaptor proteins that transduce TLR signals have been identified. These are myeloid differentiation factor 88 (MyD88), MyD88 adaptor-like MAL (also known as TIRAP), TIR-domain containing adaptor protein inducing IFNβ, TRIF (also known as TICAM-1) and TRIF-related adaptor molecule (TRAM, also known as TICAM-2), and sterile α- and armadillo-motif-containing protein [13, 22]. With the exception of TLR3, which signals exclusively via TRIF, all TLRs signal via MyD88. TLR4 is a unique receptor as it signals via two independent pathways: TRIF dependent and MyD88 dependent. Initially, it was found that TRIF-dependent signaling was critical for the upregulation of costimulatory molecules (e.g., CD40 and CD86), which are important for antigen presentation on DCs, whereas MyD88 was critical for the production of certain inflammatory cytokines after TLR4 activation (e.g., IL-6 and TNF-α) [23]. Furthermore, type I IFN production was found to be completely TRIF dependent but independent of MyD88. However, a later study determined that these responses are cell specific: in macrophages the upregulation of costimulatory molecules are TRIF

dependent, whereas this was not the case in DCs [24]. Differential sensitivity of these cells to type I interferons explained these differences between the cell types [24]. Generally, TLR signal transduction leads to switching inflammatory responses on, which occur via several transcription factors including the NF-κB, mitogen-activated protein kinase and the IFN regulatory factor pathway. Additionally, negative regulatory pathways are present, which act in a negative feedback loop to dampen the inflammatory process once they are initiated. IRAK-M, SOCS1, and MyD88 short are a few examples of TLR signal adaptors with inhibitory properties [25].

The innate immune response in transplantation

There are a number of ways by which the innate immune system can be activated during transplantation. Broadly, these fall into two categories: the result of ischemia reperfusion injury (IRI) itself and the response to the engrafted organ.

PRRs and IRI

IRI is a pathological disorder that occurs after blood flow is restored to ischemic tissue. It can occur after myocardial ischemia, profound hypovolemia, acute kidney injury, and after organ transplantation. If this injury is prolonged, it can lead to allograft dysfunction after organ transplantation [26]. It has been postulated that the injury of IRI induces metabolic derangements, leading to ATP depletion and the release of reactive oxygen species. This induces cell death and the release of endogenous activators of the innate immune system. Possible ligands include HA and HMGB1. HA is a glycosaminoglycan component of the extracellular matrix, and its release has been associated with kidney IRI and acute allograft rejection [27, 28]. As stated above, HA signals via TLRs 2/4, but also CD44. Experimental models have shown that the absence of these receptors can abrogate inflammation induced by kidney IRI [29, 30]. HMGB1 is another endogenous activator that has been implicated in various models of IRI [31]. HMGB1 is a nuclear protein that aids gene transcription and is released during cell death. This protein can signal via the receptor of advanced glycation end-products (RAGE), in addition to several TLRs (e.g., TLRs 2, 4, and 9). HMGB1 has been primarily implicated in liver IRI, since the level of this protein increases during liver IRI and inhibiting HMGB1 reduces the degree of liver injury and inflammation during IRI [32]. Consistent with these findings, mice that are deficient in TLR4 are also protected from the injury of liver IRI [33]. Moreover, there is evidence that inhibition of HMGB1 delays the onset of acute cardiac allograft rejection in mice [34].

The role of TLRs has also been implicated in cardiac IRI and during ischemic brain injury. In experimental murine models, absence of either TLR 2 or 4 reduces myocardial necrosis induced by coronary ischemia and subsequent reperfusion [35, 36]. Interestingly, TLRs have been implicated in the pathogenesis of atherosclerosis as crossing TLR-deficient mice (e.g., TLR 2 or 4) with mice that are genetically prone to atherosclerosis (e.g., apoE$^{-/-}$ or LDL receptor$^{-/-}$) abrogates the development of atherosclerosis [37]. Furthermore, signaling via MyD88 may also be important for flow-mediated vascular adaptation [38].

PRRs and alloimmunity

As noted above, PRRs were first recognized for their ability to induce inflammatory responses in innate immune cells. With recognition of the ability of TLR-ligands to promote maturation of DCs, it became clear that these were immune adjuvants that linked innate and adaptive responses by enabling DCs to optimally activate naive T cells in response to peptides, proteins, or alloantigens [15]. However, expression of TLRs is not limited to the innate immune system, as they can be found on T cells, B cells, endothelium, and many epithelial cells as well. Thus, studies of the role of TLRs (and perhaps other PRRs) on the response to allografts, unless done in cell-specific knockouts, must be interpreted in the light of their widespread distribution, and effects attributed to individual cell types only with great caution.

Experimental studies

TLRs were first found to be critical for acute transplant rejection in a minor mismatched skin transplant model [39]. In agreement with prior literature in nontransplant models, this study found that impaired TLR signaling, specifically absence of MyD88, led to impaired DC maturation and migration after skin transplantation [39]. This was associated with an impaired ability to prime graft-specific T cells. Hence, this study provided evidence that innate activation via MyD88 signaling primed adaptive alloimmune T cell responses. A subsequent study found that in more immunogenic experimental murine transplant models (skin and vascularized organs) in which donor and recipient MHC mismatch existed, MyD88 signaling was dispensable for acute allograft rejection [40]. However, MyD88 signaling did promote Th1 anti-donor cellular immune responses. Another study found that skin transplants that were deficient in all TLR signaling, specifically deficient in both MyD88 and TRIF, exhibited a modest but significant delay in time to allograft rejection in wild-type recipients compared with wild-type allografts [41].

Although TLR signaling via MyD88 is not critical for acute skin allograft rejection in highly immunogenic donor–recipient strain combinations [40], several investigators have found that TLR activation has very important implications for transplant tolerance induction. Two research groups found that recipients that were deficient in MyD88 exhibited indefinite skin allograft survival mediated by costimulatory blockade [42, 43]. Typically, wild-type recipients are resistant to such therapy and only exhibit a small delay in time to allograft rejection. In one study, absence of MyD88 impaired inflammatory responses in DCs after transplantation [42]. This was associated with an impaired ability of T cell priming in these recipients compared with wild-type recipients both after treatment with costimulatory blockade and without immune modulation. This defective priming of effector T cells allowed these cells to be more easily immune suppressed by regulatory T cells. A recent study mechanistically evaluated which inflammatory cytokines prevented the efficacy of costimulatory blockade to extend skin allograft survival [44]. This study found that cooperation between IL-6 and TNF-α impaired the ability of costimulatory blockade to delay the onset of acute allograft rejection. Furthermore, it demonstrated that recipients that were deficient in IRAK-M, a negative regulator of TLR activation, resisted the allograft-prolonging properties of costimulatory-based regimens [44].

Complementary experimental studies found that administration of systemic TLR activators abrogated the induction of transplantation tolerance [45–47]. Either lipopolysaccharide (which activates TLR4), CpG (which activates TLR9), or poly I:C (a synthetic TLR3 activator) impaired the ability of costimulatory blockade to extend allograft survival, an effect that was dependent upon type I interferons or IL-12 depending upon the model. In sum, all the above studies indicate that TLR responses are involved in the allograft response, and that inflammatory mediators that are induced by TLR activation in the context of organ transplantation can impair tolerance induction.

Clinical studies

The first study to document an association with TLRs and acute allograft rejection in clinical organ transplantation was in lung allograft recipients. The lungs are unique as an allograft as they can be exposed to inhaled toxins, including those that activate TLRs (e.g., LPS, a TLR4 stimulator). Using a genetic approach, the study demonstrated that recipients that were heterozygous for a single nucleotide polymorphism in the TLR4 receptor, which impairs signaling via TLR4, exhibited reduced frequency of biopsy-proven acute rejection compared with wild-type recipients 3 years after transplantation [48, 49]. Interestingly, there was a trend towards less chronic rejection (bronchiolitis obliterans) in the mutant TLR4 recipient group. However, the presence of the TLR4 mutation within the donor allograft had no impact on the frequency of acute allograft rejection. Similar findings have been found in kidney transplant recipients, with a longer duration of follow up (95 months) [50]. A recent study found a role for TLR4 signaling within the donor allograft in the setting of human kidney transplantation [51]. This study found that this effect was greater for deceased rather than living related donors and that this phenotype was associated with increased HMGB1 levels within deceased donors rather than living related. A possible explanation for these findings is that increased IRI that occurs with cadaveric organ harvest induces more HMGB1 release than living-related donor transplants, with subsequent increased activation of the innate immune system after implantation. Regarding other organs, a clinical study in cardiac transplantation associated increased TLR4 gene expression with allograft endothelial dysfunction, a vascular defect that may be involved in chronic allograft vasculopathy [52]. However, mechanistic studies, either experimental or clinical, examining the importance of TLRs in the development of chronic rejection are still lacking.

Other innate pathways in organ transplantation

Cellular mediators of the innate system, including neutrophils, NK cells, and macrophages, have been found to play a role in alloimmunity, although none of them are critical for transplant rejection responses, unless a specific pathway has been deleted; for example, NK cell-dependent rejection of vascularized allografts in CD28-deficient mice. However, the role of these cells may be complex. For example, it has been shown that NK cells can promote transplant tolerance by killing donor antigen-presenting cells located in donor tissues [53].

The innate immune system also has a soluble component, the complement system, which is evolutionarily very old and which also links to adaptive responses. It consists of three pathways: classic, alternative, and lectin. All of these pathways converge on C3, leading to the assembly of the membrane attack complex, which induces pore formation in the invading pathogen. Furthermore, the production of C5a initiates inflammatory responses. The complement system also has regulatory components, including decay-accelerating factor (DAF), which leads to the dissociation of the C3/C5 complex. Regarding the importance of complement in transplant rejection, one study found in an experimental renal allograft model that local production of C3 within the allograft was critical for T cell priming and subsequent allograft rejection [54]. Another study found that the DAF regulatory protein influenced the antigen-presenting cell–T cell interaction to enhance alloimmunity and transplant rejection [55].

Interaction between TLRs and immune suppressants used in organ transplantation

Clinically, it would be attractive if currently used immune suppressants were found to inhibit the innate immune response. There have been some studies that have examined the impact of certain immune suppressants, or pathways targeted by these medications, on TLR immune responses. For example, one study found that calcineurin acted as a negative regulator of certain TLR signaling pathways, in particular TLRs 2 and 4, and the adaptors MyD88 and TRIF [56]. The results of this study imply that calcineurin inhibitors, such as cyclosporine and tacrolimus, used in clinical organ transplantation would enhance TLR 2 and 4 signaling. Furthermore, another experimental study found evidence that cyclosporine induced nephrotoxicity via activating TLRs [57]. Thus, these experimental studies suggest that this class of medication might further activate the innate immune system after solid organ transplantation and may have unanticipated detrimental effects, an issue that should be evaluated clinically.

Regarding other types of immune suppressant, an experimental study found evidence that the mTOR inhibitor, sirolimus, inhibited TLR4-induced IL-6 production and reduced colon cancer development [58]. However, it is not known if this class of medication alters TLR signaling in solid organ transplantation. Glucocorticoids are pleiotropic immune suppressants that the majority of organ transplant recipients receive in the early phase after implantation. A clinical study of patients with autoimmunity found that TLR signaling within DCs, specifically the production of proinflammatory cytokines, such as IL-12 and TNF-α, was impaired by glucocorticoids, despite the fact that this medication increased TLR 2, 3, and 4 expression [59]. In conclusion, currently employed immune suppressant regimens may alter TLR signaling in organ transplant recipients, but clinical studies need to be conducted to examine this directly.

Possible future experimental strategies

Given that experimental evidence indicates that certain inflammatory mediators, such as IL-6 and TNF-α, may impair transplant tolerance induction [44], one plausible future strategy would be to incorporate inhibitors of these cytokines in future clinical protocols aimed at inducing transplantation tolerance. Clinical agents that inhibit IL-6 or TNF-α exist and are used in certain autoimmune disorders. However, caution will be needed in such future trials, as inhibiting innate signaling pathways may also impair host defense to pathogens in solid organ transplant recipients, a group of patients who are already susceptible to infection due the administration of generalized immune suppressants. Alternatively, inhibiting TLR signaling pathways or other innate immune pathways (e.g., components of the complement system) in donor allografts, in particular cadaveric organs, may reduce the injury induced by IRI and such an approach awaits the outcomes of future clinical studies.

Conclusion

Both recent and clinical studies have shed important insights into the role of the innate immune system in organ transplantation. Despite these advances, important questions remain to be answered. Specifically, experimental studies should investigate TLR responses in chronic vasculopathy. Clinical studies should examine how currently used immune suppressants interact with the innate immune system. Furthermore, strategies should be developed to incorporate modification of innate immune signaling either within the donor or the recipient as adjunctive therapy in experimental protocols aimed at inducing clinical transplantation tolerance. However, caution will be required in these approaches, as altering innate immune signaling may predispose to infection.

References

1 Roach JC, Glusman G, Rowen L *et al*. The evolution of vertebrate Toll-like receptors. *Proc Natl Acad Sci U S A* 2005; 102(27):9577–9582. DOI: 10.1073/pnas.0502272102.

2 Siamon G. Elie Metchnikoff: father of natural immunity. *Eur J Immunol* 2008;38(12):3257–3264.

3 Suttles J, Stout RD. Macrophage CD40 signaling: a pivotal regulator of disease protection and pathogenesis. *Sem Immunol* 2009;21:257–264.

4 Mellman I, Steinman RM. Dendritic cells: specialized and regulated antigen processing machines. *Cell* 2001;106:255–258.

5 Ramaiah SK, Jaeschke H. Role of neutrophils in the pathogenesis of acute inflammatory liver injury. *Toxicol Pathol* 2007;35(6):757–766.

6 Menendez A, Brett Finlay B. Defensins in the immunology of bacterial infections. *Curr Opin Immunol* 2007;19(4):385–391.

7 Janeway CA, Jr. Approaching the asymptote? Evolution and revolution in immunology. *Cold Spring Harb Symp Quant Biol* 1989;54(Pt 1):1–13.

8 Lemaitre B, Nicolas E, Michaut L *et al*. The dorsoventral regulatory gene cassette spätzle/Toll/cactus controls the potent antifungal response in *Drosophila* adults. *Cell* 1996;86(6):973–983.

9 Medzhitov R, Preston-Hurlburt P, Janeway CA, Jr. A human homologue of the *Drosophila* Toll protein signals activation of adaptive immunity. *Nature* 1997;388(6640):394–397.

10 Beutler BA. TLRs and innate immunity. *Blood* 2009;113(7):1399–1407.

11 Poltorak A, He X, Smirnova I *et al*. Defective LPS signaling in C3H/HeJ and C57BL/10ScCr mice: mutations in Tlr4 gene. *Science* 1998;282(5396):2085–2088.

12 Shirali A, Goldstein D. Tracking the Toll of kidney disease. *J Am Soc Nephrol* 2008;19(8):1444–1450.

13 Akira S, Takeda K. Toll-like receptor signalling. *Nat Rev Immunol* 2004;4(7):499–511.

14 Kawai T, Akira S. Toll-like receptor and RIG-1-like receptor signaling. *Ann N Y Acad Sci* 2008;1143:1–20.

15 Goldstein DR. Toll like receptors and the link between innate and acquire alloimmunity. *Curr Opin Immunol* 2004;16(5):538–544.

16 Iwasaki A, Medzhitov R. Toll-like receptor control of the adaptive immune responses. *Nat Immunol* 2004;5(10):987–995.

17 Tesar BM, Jiang D, Liang J *et al*. The role of hyaluronan degradation products as innate alloimmune agonists. *Am J Transplant* 2006;6(11):2622–2635.

18 Termeer C, Benedix F, Sleeman J *et al*. Oligosaccharides of hyaluronan activate dendritic cells via Toll-like receptor 4. *J Exp Med* 2002;195(1):99–111.

19 Fritz JH, Ferrero RL, Philpott DJ, Girardin SE. Nod-like proteins in immunity, inflammation and disease. *Nat Immunol* 2006;7(12):1250–1257.

20 Stetson DB, Medzhitov R. Antiviral defense: interferons and beyond. *J Exp Med* 2006;203(8):1837–1841.

21 Stetson DB, Medzhitov R. Recognition of cytosolic DNA activates an IRF3-dependent innate immune response. *Immunity* 2006;24(1):93–103.

22 O'Neill LAJ, Bowie AG. The family of five: TIR-domain-containing adaptors in Toll-like receptor signaling. *Nat Rev Immunol* 2007;7:353–364.

23 Hoebe K, Janssen EM, Kim SO *et al*. Upregulation of costimulatory molecules induced by lipopolysaccharide and double-stranded RNA occurs by Trif-dependent and Trif-independent pathways. *Nat Immunol* 2003; 4(12):1223–1229.

24 Shen H, Tesar BM, Walker WE, Goldstein DR. Dual signaling of MyD88 and TRIF is critical for maximal TLR4-induced dendritic cell maturation. *J Immunol* 2008;181(3):1849–1858.

25 Obhrai J, Goldstein DR. The role of Toll-like receptors in solid organ transplantation. [Editorial]. *Transplantation* 2006;81(4):497–502.

26 Land WG. The role of postischemic reperfusion injury and other nonantigen-dependent inflammatory pathways in transplantation. *Transplantation* 2005; 79(5):505–514.

27 Hällgren R, Gerdin B, Tufverson T. Hyaluronic acid accumulation and redistribution in rejecting rat kidney graft. *J Exp Med* 1990;171:2063–2076.

28 Wells A, Larsson E, Hanas E *et al*. Increased hyaluronan in acutely rejecting human kidney grafts. *Transplantation* 1993;55(6):1346–1349.

29 Rouschop KMA, Roelofs JJTH, Claessen N *et al*. Protection against renal ischemia reperfusion injury by CD44 disruption. *J Am Soc Nephrol* 2005;16(7): 2034–2043.

30 Leemans JC, Stokman G, Claessen N *et al*. Renal-associated TLR2 mediates ischemia/reperfusion injury in the kidney. *J Clin Invest* 2005;115(10):2894–903.

31 Erlandsson Harris H, Andersson U. Mini-review: The nuclear protein HMGB1 as a proinflammatory mediator. *Eur J Immunol* 2004;34(6):1503–1512.

32 Tsung A, Sahai R, Tanaka H *et al*. The nuclear factor HMGB1 mediates hepatic injury after murine liver ischemia–reperfusion. *J Exp Med* 2005;201(7): 1135–1143.

33 Izuishi K, Tsung A, Jeyabalan G *et al*. Cutting Edge: High-mobility group box 1 preconditioning protects against liver ischemia–reperfusion injury. *J Immunol* 2006;176(12):7154–7158.

34 Huang Y, Yin H, Han J *et al*. Extracellular Hmgb1 functions as an innate immune-mediator implicated in murine cardiac allograft acute rejection. *Am J Transplant* 2007;7(4):799–808.

35 Shishido T, Nozaki N, Yamaguchi S *et al*. Toll-like receptor-2 modulates ventricular remodeling after myocardial infarction. *Circuation* 2003;108(23): 2905–2910.

36 Oyama J-i, Blais C, Jr, Liu X *et al.* Reduced myocardial ischemia-reperfusion injury in Toll-like receptor 4-deficient mice. *Circulation* 2004;109(6):784–789.

37 Michelsen KS, Wong MH, Shah PK *et al.* Lack of Toll-like receptor 4 or myeloid differentiation factor 88 reduces atherosclerosis and alters plaque phenotype in mice deficient in apolipoprotein E. *Proc Natl Acad Sci U S A* 2004;101(29):10679–10684.

38 Tang PCY, Qin L, Zielonka J *et al.* MyD88-dependent, superoxide-initiated inflammation is necessary for flow-mediated inward remodeling of conduit arteries. *J Exp Med* 2008;205(13):3159–3171.

39 Goldstein DR, Tesar BM, Akira S, Lakkis FG. Critical role of the Toll-like receptor signal adaptor protein MyD88 in acute allograft rejection. *J Clin Invest* 2003;111(10):1571–1578.

40 Tesar BM, Zhang J, Li Q, Goldstein DR. TH1 immune responses to fully MHC mismatched allografts are diminished in the absence of MyD88, a Toll like receptor signal adaptor protein. *Am J Transplant* 2004;4(9):1429–1439.

41 McKay D, Shigeoka A, Rubinstein M *et al.* Simultaneous deletion of MyD88 and Trif delays major histocompatibility and minor antigen mismatch allograft rejection. *Eur J Immunol* 2006;36(8): 1994–2002.

42 Walker WE, Nasr IW, Camirand G *et al.* Absence of innate MyD88 signaling promotes inducible allograft acceptance. *J Immunol* 2006;177(8):5307–5316.

43 Chen L, Wang T, Zhou P *et al.* TLR engagement prevents transplantation tolerance. *Am J Transplant* 2006;6(10):2282–2291.

44 Shen H, Goldstein DR. IL-6 and TNF-α synergistically inhibit allograft acceptance. *J Am Soc Nephrol* 2009;20(5):1032–1040.

45 Thornley TB, Brehm MA, Markees TG *et al.* TLR agonists abrogate costimulation blockade-induced prolongation of skin allografts. *J Immunol* 2006; 176(3):1561–1570.

46 Chen L, Wang T, Zhou P *et al.* TLR engagement prevents transplantation tolerance. *Am J Transplant* 2006;6:2282–2291.

47 Porrett PM, Yuan X, LaRosa DF *et al.* Mechanisms underlying blockade of allograft acceptance by TLR ligands. *J Immunol* 2008;181(3):1692–1699.

48 Palmer SM, Burch LH, Davis RD *et al.* The role of innate immunity in acute allograft rejection after lung transplantation. *Am J Respir Crit Care Med* 2003;168(6):628–632.

49 Palmer SM, Burch LH, Trindade AJ *et al.* Innate immunity influences long-term outcomes after human lung transplant. *Am J Respir Crit Care Med* 2005;171(7):780–785.

50 Ducloux D, Deschamps M, Yannaraki M *et al.* Relevance of Toll-like receptor-4 polymorphisms in renal transplantation. *Kidney Int* 2005;67(6):2454–2461.

51 Krüger B, Krick S, Dhillon N *et al.* Donor Toll-like receptor 4 contributes to ischemia and reperfusion injury following human kidney transplantation. *Proc Natl Acad Sci U S A* 2009;106(9):3390–3395.

52 Methe H, Zimmer E, Grimm C *et al.* Evidence for a role of Toll-like receptor 4 in development of chronic allograft rejection after cardiac transplantation. *Transplantation* 78(9):1324–1331.

53 Yu G, Xu X, Vu MD *et al.* NK cells promote transplant tolerance by killing donor antigen-presenting cells. *J Exp Med* 2006;203(8):1851–1858.

54 Pratt JR, Basheer SA, Sacks SH. Local synthesis of complement component C3 regulates acute renal transplant rejection. *Nat Med* 2002;8:582–587.

55 Pavlov V, Raedler H, Yuan S *et al.* Donor deficiency of decay-accelerating factor accelerates murine T cell-mediated cardiac allograft rejection. *J Immunol*; 181(7):4580–9458.

56 Kang YJ, Kusler B, Otsuka M *et al.* Calcineurin negatively regulates TLR-mediated activation pathways. *J Immunol* 2007;179(7):4598–4607.

57 Lim SW, Li C, Ahn KO *et al.* Cyclosporine-induced renal injury induces Toll-like receptor and maturation of dendritic cells. *Transplantation* 2005;80(5): 691–699.

58 Sun Q, Liu Q, Zheng Y, Cao X. Rapamycin suppresses TLR4-triggered IL-6 and PGE$_2$ production of colon cancer cells by inhibiting TLR4 expression and NF-κB activation. *Mol Immunol* 2008;10:2929–2936.

59 Rozkova D, Horvath R, Bartunkova J, Spisek R. Glucocorticoids severely impair differentiation and antigen presenting function of dendritic cells despite upregulation of Toll-like receptors. *Clin Immunol* 2006;3:260–271.

CHAPTER 6

Regulation of the Alloimmune Response

Kathryn J. Wood[1] and Terry B. Strom[2]

[1]Transplantation Research Immunology Group, Nuffield Department of Surgical Sciences, University of Oxford, John Radcliffe Hospital, Oxford, UK

[2]Harvard Medical School, Beth Israel Deaconess Medical Center, Transplant Institute, Boston, MA, USA

Introduction and basic definitions

Transplantation of an organ, tissue, or cells from an allogeneic donor triggers a dialogue between the innate and adaptive immune systems that results in a cascade of mechanisms that not only initiate, but also direct the destruction of the transplant if they are allowed to run their full course. At the same time, but at a slower pace, mechanisms that can regulate or control these same immune responses are established. Unfortunately, in the case of transplantation, without active intervention the natural mechanisms of immune regulation are established too slowly and are not powerful enough to prevent rejection. Nevertheless, these fail-safe mechanisms that are built into every immune response are essential to ensure that each immune response an individual makes is appropriate to the context in which it is triggered. Immune responses that are too weak will not, in the case of an infection, clear the infectious agents, thereby threatening the survival of the host. In contrast, immune responses that are too vigorous have the potential to cause damage to the host's own tissues, again potentially compromising the host's wellbeing. The immune system, therefore, strives to make an appropriate, measured response that is sufficient to eliminate the antigen that triggered it, but not so vigorous that long-lasting tissue damage is caused. In the case of transplantation, the immune response that elicits rejection or destruction of allogeneic transplanted cells or tissues is arguably at the more vigorous end of the spectrum. Importantly, experimental data are demonstrating that the natural mechanisms of control/regulation that are triggered during an alloimmune response can be harnessed to control the response and prevent rejection, especially when immunotherapy that supports immune regulation is used.

Cellular and molecular regulation of the alloimmune response: regulation of T cell and B cell responses

T cells play a pivotal role in the destructive arm of the adaptive immune response that can lead to rejection, but they also participate in the regulatory/suppressor arms of the response.

Anergy

Anergy is a term used to describe the functional inactivation of lymphocytes, resulting in the cells becoming refractory or unresponsiveness to further stimulation. T cell activation is a product of signals delivered from the T cell receptor (TCR) following binding or ligation of a relevant peptide–MHC (pMHC) complex and from ligand–receptor pairs

Immunotherapy in Transplantation: Principles and Practice, First Edition. Edited by Bruce Kaplan, Gilbert J. Burckart and Fadi G. Lakkis.
© 2012 Blackwell Publishing Ltd. Published 2012 by Blackwell Publishing Ltd.

on the T cell and antigen-presenting cell that are collectively known as costimulatory pathways. These costimulatory pathways include those that augment T cell reactivity, such as the CD28–CD86 interaction and many other more recently characterized pathways, as well as counterparts that have the potential to limit or control T cell activation, such as the CD152 (CTLA-4)–CD80 interaction.

In vitro, antigen recognition (i.e., TCR ligation by the relevant pMHC complex) in the absence of costimulation was shown to induce T cell anergy [1]. The absence of cositmulation, through CD28, at the time of antigen recognition, was demonstrated to be critical for the induction of T cell anergy in these in vitro systems. In vivo, induction of T cell anergy has also been shown to be dependent on CTLA-4 ligation [2]. The costimulatory molecule programmed death 1 (PD-1) is highly expressed on anergic T cells and in some tissues, and its interaction with its ligand, another member of the B7 family, has also been shown to be involved in the induction of T cell anergy in some settings [3]. Hence, in vitro and in vivo, T cell anergy can result from ligation of TCRs in the absence of the correct additional costimulatory signals, resulting in the control of T cell activation and attenuation of the ability of T cells to respond [4].

Cell death
Central deletion of alloantigen reactive T cells

Intrathymic modulation of the immunological repertoire underpins the concept of central immunological tolerance. T cell precursors arise in the bone marrow and migrate to the thymus. Upon entry into the thymus, these progenitor cells begin to rearrange their TCR genes and undergo a program of selection. $CD4^+CD8^+$ thymocytes expressing a complete $\alpha\beta$TCR then undergo positive and negative selection before emigration into the periphery as mature single positive T cells expressing either CD4 or CD8. Only those cells with TCRs of sufficiently high affinity to self-pMHC complexes receive survival signals in the thymus as part of a process termed positive selection. The remaining T cells that have too low an affinity for self-pMHC complexes become apoptotic and are deleted [5]. In addition, those cells with TCRs that have too high

an affinity for self-pMHC are also deleted in a process known as negative selection [6]. In this way, T cells capable of recognizing self-MHC molecules bound to foreign peptides, often referred to as self-restricted T cells, that have the potential of being useful to the host immune system are maintained, while ensuring that the majority of dangerous self- or auto-reactive T cells are deleted (i.e. eliminated from the emerging T cell repertoire).

The process of negative selection in the thymus is incomplete; meaning that some potentially harmful T cells may escape negative selection. The immune system, therefore, has developed a fail-safe mechanism that can control the activity of these unwanted T cells. Thus, in addition to positive selection of T cells that are potentially useful in combating infections, the process of thymic selection also results in the selection of a population of thymus-derived or naturally occurring Tregs [7–9]. T cells with regulatory activity are thought to have an intermediate rather than a high affinity for self-pMHC complexes and express the transcription factor Foxp3 [10]. Following selection, Tregs migrate to the periphery alongside other T cells, where they control any potentially harmful self-reactive T cells that have escaped deletion in the thymus [10].

The phenomenon of central tolerance (i.e., deletion of unwanted T cells) has been exploited experimentally for the induction of transplantation tolerance. For example, central deletion of alloreactive T cells has been achieved via direct delivery of alloantigen into the thymus via intrathymic injection (e.g., [11, 12]). The establishment of allogeneic mixed bone marrow chimeras in the mouse has also been shown to result in deletion of donor-reactive thymocytes as a result of the presence of donor-derived leukocytes in the thymus [13]. These studies provide proof of principle that mechanisms of central tolerance through deletion of antigen reactive T cells may be harnessed to facilitate operational transplantation tolerance.

Peripheral deletion of alloantigen-reactive T cells: activation-induced cell death or immune exhaustion

Apoptosis of antigen-reactive T cells via activation-induced cell death (AICD) is another means by which T cell reactivity can be controlled as a consequence of deletion of antigen-reactive T cells. AICD is a process in which T cells undergo cell death in the periphery, following restimulation through TCRs and the engagement of specific receptors, including CD95 (FAS), or upon exposure to reactive oxygen species [14]. A number of different molecules, including CD95, tumour necrosis factor receptor 1 (TNFR1), and tumour necrosis factor-related apoptosis-inducing ligand receptor (TRAILR) in the case of CD8$^+$ T cells activated in the absence of CD4$^+$ T cell help can play a role in AICD depending on the circumstances triggering a complex series of signaling events which ultimately lead to caspase activation, DNA fragmentation, cytoskeletal degradation, and cell death. For example, ligation of CD95 by CD95L induces the formation of the CD95 death-inducing signaling complex (CD95 DISC) in which caspase 8 and caspase 10 are activated. These caspases either directly activate caspase 3, caspase 6, and caspase 7 or cleave the B cell lymphoma-2 (bcl-2) family protein BID into truncated BID (tBID). tBID mediates the release of cytochrome C from the mitochondria, which in turn triggers the formation of the apoptosome. This leads to the activation of caspase 9, which subsequently cleaves and activates the downstream effector capsases [15].

Immunoregulation/suppression
Regulatory T cells

T-cell-mediated immunoregulation or suppression is one of the key mechanisms responsible for maintaining specific immunological unresponsiveness or tolerance in vivo and for controlling T cell homeostasis. This mechanism can be used to control not only immune responses to self-antigens, thereby preventing autoimmune disease, but also responses to non-self molecules that are introduced into the host [16]. It is interesting to note that the existence of leukocytes able to suppress alloantigen-specific immune responses was first described by Billingham *et al.* over 50 years ago [17]. Thus, the concept of suppression or active regulation of the immune response in the setting of transplantation is by no means a new idea. What is new is the ability to

characterize the cell populations responsible for this phenomenon in detail at both a cellular and a molecular level.

CD25$^+$CD4$^+$foxp3$^+$Tregs are one of the key populations responsible for immunoregulation in vivo. As mentioned above, thymus-derived or naturally occurring CD25$^+$CD4$^+$foxp3$^+$Treg (nTreg) is generated as a distinct population in the thymus. nTregs are an actively dividing, differentiated population that is maintained by self-renewal [18]. Importantly for therapeutic strategies, CD25$^+$CD4$^+$foxp3$^+$Tregs that are phenotypically and functionally similar can also be generated under certain conditions after antigen exposure in vivo and ex vivo (e.g., [19–22]). Such populations of Tregs are known as induced or adaptive Tregs. In many of these situations the resulting Treg population present in the periphery is a mixture of nTregs and induced Tregs, some of which may have been the result of conversion [23].

It is likely that the ability of extracellular signals to drive the stable expression of foxp3, and differentiation of CD4$^+$ cells towards a Treg phenotype following antigen exposure, may vary between individuals depending on recipient factors such as age, sex, genetic background, and epigenetic modification [10, 24, 25]. In mice, Foxp3 has been shown to regulate T cell commitment and function in a dose-dependent manner, suggesting that a sustained minimum level of expression would be required to retain functionality. This is supported by the observation that expression of Foxp3 in mature Tregs is required to maintain the transcriptional program established during their commitment [26]. Moreover, epigenetic modification of the foxp3 locus in mice is required for stable expression, and thus stable functional activity of Tregs [10, 27].

Alloantigen-induced Tregs have been shown to be able to prevent acute as well as delayed graft rejection. Importantly, following transplantation, the immune system is constantly exposed to donor alloantigens while graft function is maintained. This may enable the generation of antigen-induced Tregs and the stabilization of foxp3 expression allowing the functional activity of Tregs to be sustained in vivo. In mouse models, our own laboratory has demonstrated that Tregs induced in response to alloantigen in vivo can prevent the rejection of heart allografts in naive mice with an intact immune repertoire [28], as well as in more subtle adoptive transfer models using immunodeficient hosts [29, 30]. We have also demonstrated recently that these same populations of alloantigen-induced Tregs can prevent the development of transplant arteriosclerosis in mouse [31] as well as in a humanized mouse model [32].

The ability and effectiveness of Tregs to control an immune response in vivo is linked, in part, to the conditions that prevail at the time they are generated and/or function, such as the presence or absence of inflammation [33], the number and potency of Tregs relative to that of potential effector cells, naive as well as memory [34–36], and their ability to migrate and function in the relevant microenvironment in vivo [37, 38]. Interestingly, immunosuppressive drugs may also influence the generation and function of Tregs, an important factor to consider in the setting of transplantation [39].

The draining lymphoid tissue is the primary, initial site of interaction between Tregs and naive T cells following transplantation [38, 40, 41]. However, there are also data demonstrating that, as the length of time after transplantation increases, Tregs are also present within the allograft itself [37]. In the setting of clinical transplantation, in both liver and kidney transplant recipients, evidence has been obtained that T cells with the phenotypic characteristics of regulatory cells are present in both the peripheral blood and the graft [42–44].

The mechanisms by which Tregs prevent T cell priming either in the draining lymphoid tissue or within the graft are multifactorial. Tregs have the potential to influence antigen-presenting cells as well as T cell function. Following reactivation in vivo, Tregs produce IFNγ rapidly and transiently [45]. Production of IFNγ in a defined microenvironment in vivo will induce expression of new immunomodulatory molecules, including indoleamine 2,3-dioxygenase (IDO), with the potential to modify cell function and inhibit alloimmune responses. The role of IFNγ in transplantation and other settings is paradoxical [46]. On the one hand, allograft rejection is a process frequently associated with a dominant Th1 IFNγ response, whereas the absence of intra-graft IFNγ often correlates with long-term graft survival [47, 48]. This association of IFNγ and rejection is partially explained by the fact that IFNγ can induce macrophage activation, mononuclear infiltration, edema, and tissue necrosis. On the other hand, IFNγ does appear to be essential for acute cellular rejection, as both IFNγ-deficient and wild-type mice reject cardiac allografts with similar kinetics [49] and at least one study has demonstrated that IFNγ$^{-/-}$ recipients reject skin allografts more rapidly than their wild-type littermates [50]. Moreover, although the classical view of IFNγ is that it favors Th1 cell development, it is becoming apparent that IFNγ can also play an important regulatory role. For example, IFNγ can limit the number of Th1 effector cells via inducible nitric oxide synthase (iNOS) [45], can inhibit the proliferation of IL-4-producing Th2 cells [51], and can suppress the development of the recently identified Th17 effector cell subset now known to play an important role in many autoimmune models [52, 53]. In addition, IFNγ also plays an important role in the maintenance of T cell homeostasis by inducing apoptosis-dependent activation-induced cell death to limit T cell expansion following antigen encounter [54] (see "Peripheral deletion of alloantigen-reactive T cells" section).

Expression of cell-surface molecules has also been linked to the mechanism of immunoregulation by Tregs. CD152 (CTLA-4) has powerful immunomodulatory effects and can act as a negative regulator of T cell activation [55]. CD152 is expressed by Tregs and is critical for their function in vivo (e.g., [30, 56–60]. The mechanism by which CD152 functions on Tregs is not completely understood. Engagement of CD80/86 on dendritic cells (DCs) can induce IDO expression [61] and is a potent activator of LFA-1 clustering and adhesion [62]. CTLA-4 can modulate T cell motility and the threshold for T cell activation [63]. In vivo, Tregs have been shown to have prolonged interactions with DCs in the draining lymph nodes that preceded the inhibition of T cell activation [41].

Reactivation of Tregs in vivo also upregulates expression of a receptor for hyaluronic-acid-mediated migration [64], which, like CD44, can bind to the extracellular matrix protein hyaluronic acid and α-mannosidase, and impact the ability to migrate and interact with other leukocytes [65].

The coordinated expression of CD39/CD73 on Tregs and the adenosine A2A receptor on activated T effector cells generates immunosuppressive loops that play an important role in the inhibitory function of Tregs [66]. CD39 and CD73 are members of a larger family of ectoenzymes that degrade nucleotides and include molecules with roles in lymphocyte activation and migration. CD39 is expressed on different cellular lineages in addition to Tregs, such as B lymphocytes and Langerhans cells, and its biochemical activity is the rate-limiting component of the ectoenzymatic chain that metabolizes extracellular nucleoside di- and tri-phosphates, ultimately to the respective nucleosides, such as adenosine. Thus, CD39 has the potential to modulate immune cell–cell contacts by catalyzing local changes in extracellular nucleotides. Adenosine generated from the hydrolysis of nucleotides exerts substantive inhibitory effects, thereby contributing as one of the mechanisms that Tregs use to regulate immune responses [67].

Regulatory activity has also been identified within the CD8$^+$ T cell population, including amongst CD8$^+$CD28$^-$ T cells. In transplantation, alloantigen-specific CD8$^+$CD28$^-$ Tregs were found to function by inducing tolerogenic DCs which were characterized by reduced expression of costimulatory molecules and upregulation of immunoglobulin-like transcript 3 and 4 (ILT3 and ILT4) [68]. CD8$^{-/-}$CD28$^{-/-}$ double knockout mice have an increased severity of experimental autoimmune encephalomyelitis, and this can be reversed by the adoptive transfer of CD8$^+$CD28$^-$ T cells but not by CD8$^+$CD28$^+$ T cells [69]. Interestingly, naive, freshly isolated human CD8$^+$CD28$^-$ T cells do not exhibit regulatory activity; but, upon priming, these cells become regulatory and also upregulate molecular markers such as glucocorticoid-induced TNF-receptor-family-related protein (GITR), Foxp3, CTLA-4, CD62L, and CD25, molecules that are typically associated with subsets of CD4$^+$ Tregs [70].

Regulatory B cells

B cells with the capacity to suppress the development of autoimmune diseases in mice were first described in the 1980s. Regulatory B cells (Bregs) express high levels of CD1d, CD21, CD24, and IgM and moderate levels of CD19, although some heterogeneity has been described that different subsets may exist [71]. Human Bregs have several properties in common with their mouse counterparts, including an immature phenotype, and comprise a small subset of the total B cell pool. One of the characteristics of B cells with regulatory activity is their ability to secrete IL-10. CD40 stimulation appears to be required to stimulate IL-10 production and has been reported to be necessary for activation of Bregs, enabling them to manifest their functional activity and suppress Th1 differentiation. It has been suggested that there is a link between Bregs and T cells, with Bregs acting as potent generators of Tregs. Interestingly, in renal transplant recipients who have a functioning graft in the absence of immuno-suppression, a B cell signature has been found to be associated with the operationally tolerant state [72, 73]. Clearly more work is required to determine the role of Bregs in the regulation of alloimmune responses.

Dendritic cells

DCs are central to the activation/priming of an immune response, but paradoxically they can also promote the development of tolerance [74–77]. One of the keys to both functions of DCs is their state of maturity. Initially, immature myeloid DCs that express low levels of MHC class II and costimulatory molecules at the cell surface were identified as the dominant form of DCs that had the capacity to induce T cell tolerance. In contrast, mature myeloid DCs that express much higher levels of both MHC and costimulatory molecules were found to prime T cell responses most efficiently. However, subsequently, mature DCs have also been shown to have the capacity induce tolerance; therefore, the relationship between the state of maturity of a DC and its tolerogenic potential is now less clear.

Immature DCs can promote tolerance to solid organ allografts and bone marrow grafts. For example, a single injection of immature donor-derived DCs 7 days before transplantation of an MHC-mismatched heart allograft extends [78] or prolongs survival indefinitely [79] in a donor-specific manner. The potential tolerogenic effects of immature DCs can be potentiated by the coadministration of immune-modulating agents, such as costimulation blockade [80]. "Alternatively activated" or "regulatory" DCs, that have low costimulatory ability, were also found to protect MHC-mismatched skin grafts from rejection [81] and mice from lethal acute graft-versus-host disease and when administered 7 days before transplantation [82].

Reports showing that mature DCs can induce tolerance despite expressing high levels of MHC and costimulatory molecules include in vitro data with human cells demonstrating that maturation of human monocyte-derived DCs with tumor necrosis factor-α and prostaglandin E2 triggered cross-priming and proliferation of CD8$^+$ T cells with tolerogenic properties [83] and that mature, but not immature, DCs can prime CD4$^+$ T cells that inhibit allogeneic mixed leukocyte reactions [84]. In vivo, bone-marrow-derived DCs matured with TNF-α, but not lipopolysaccharide or antibody to CD40, protected mice from CD4$^+$ T-cell-mediated experimental autoimmune encephalomyelitis, despite the expression of high levels of MHC class II and costimulatory molecules [85].

Plasmacytoid DCs have also been found to have a role in tolerance induction. Plasmacytoid DCs were originally defined by their capacity to secrete large amounts of type I interferons in response to viruses and to play an essential role in protecting individuals against inflammatory responses to harmless antigens. Plasmacytoid DCs have now also been shown to be able to induce Tregs in vitro that produce significant amounts of interleukin IL-10, low IFNγ, and no IL-4, IL-5, or transforming growth factor beta (TGFβ) [86].

Donor-derived preplasmacytoid DCs infused 7 days before transplant were found to be capable of prolonging subsequent heart allograft survival (from 9 to 22 days) in the absence of immunosuppressive therapy [87], but this effect was markedly enhanced by anti-CD154 monoclonal antibody (mAb) administration [88]. In mice, preplasmacytoid DCs appear to be the principal cell type that facilitates hematopoietic stem cell engraftment and induction of donor-specific skin graft tolerance in allogeneic recipients [86].

Taking the data using different populations of DCs together, it seems that both myeloid and plasmacytoid DCs can promote tolerance, and that maturation by itself is not the distinguishing feature that separates their immunogenic from their tolerogenic function. Indeed, maturation is more of a continuum than an "on–off" switch, and a "semi-mature" state, in which DCs are phenotypically mature but remain poor producers or proinflammatory cytokines, appears to be linked to tolerogenic function. The combination of DCs administered with costimulatory blockade may be the most promising approach identified thus far.

Myeloid-derived suppressor cells

Myeloid-derived suppressor cells (MDSCs) have been associated with many suppressive functions, antigen specific and nonspecific, including regulation of innate immunity, T cell activation, and tumor immunity. MDSCs are a heterogeneous population of progenitor cells that can accumulate in tissues during an inflammatory immune response. The expansion and activation of MDSCs is regulated by factors produced by other cells in the same microenvironment, including stromal cells, activated T cells, and the tumor cells themselves when a tumor is present.

A number of MDSC subsets have been described in both mice and humans [89]. Despite the heterogeneity described in the literature, each subset expresses common phenotypic markers: Gr1 and CD11b in mice and CD33, CD11b, CD34, and low MHC class II in humans. Activated MDSCs suppress proliferation and cytokine production by T, B, and NK cells in vitro through mechanisms that include the enzymes inducible nitric oxide synthase 1 that induces nitric oxide production and arginase 1 that depletes arginine. Both pathways invoke several mechanisms that inhibit cell function. MDSCs also appear to be able to be modify T cell differentiation pathways, and it has been reported that they promote Treg differentiation [89].

In experimental models, MDSCs have been shown to play a role in the induction of tolerance to alloantigens. Transplantation tolerance could not be induced in mice that did not express MHC class II on circulating leukocytes, a finding consistent with a requirement for recipient MHC class II + cells for the induction of tolerance to alloantigens [90]. Direct evidence of a tolerogenic role for CD11b$^+$CD115$^+$Gr1$^+$ monocytes for heart allografts in mice [91] and iNOS-expressing MDSCs in kidney allografts in rats has subsequently been reported [92].

Ignorance

The simplest mechanism that facilitates the maintenance of peripheral tolerance is T cell ignorance of self-antigen. In this setting, autoreactive T cells escape negative selection within the thymus and enter the periphery, but such T cells are either barred access to sites that express their cognate peptide or they never see enough peptide to enable them to overcome activation thresholds [93]. In transplantation it is hard to envisage how this mechanism could operate to regulate the alloimmune response effectively.

Relevance to immunotherapy

In parallel with development of new small-molecule immunosuppressive drugs, biological therapies, including polyclonal anti-lymphocyte antibodies, Ig fusion proteins, chimeric mouse–human and humanized monoclonal antibodies, are administered with increasing frequency, to transplant recipients as part of a multifaceted treatment regimen. Biologics may be required to induce dominant Treg-dependent tolerance because of the precise molecular targeting afforded by this technology. This review of biologic agents and regimens in use or under development will emphasize the pertinence to attempts to tilt the balance of immunity toward dominant-type immunoregulation-dependent tolerance. Most regimens now in use effectively suppress rejection but do not enhance immunoregulation, as they exert potent effects upon both cytopathic and cytoprotective immune responses.

Conventional polyclonal rabbit (Thymoglobulin) or horse (ATGAM) thymocyte/lymphocyte antibodies

These are in widespread used as a potent means to produce immunosuppression as a consequence of lymphopenia. To make these products, rabbits or horses are immunized with human lymphocytes to produce cytotoxic antibodies directed against antigens expressed on human lymphocytes. The lots are processed to deplete unwanted antibodies and achieve some consistency on the composition of the cytotoxic antibodies.

Treatment with these products creates lymphopenia whose magnitude and duration are proportional to the amount of drug and the number of injections administered. Lymphopenia is responsible for the increased occurrence of opportunistic infections and the virally driven lymphoproliferative syndrome observed in treated patients. Homoeostatic proliferation of lymphocytes follows cessation of treatment as the lymphocyte pool recovers size and leads to the development of memory cells. Memory lymphocytes, including those capable of cross-reaction with allogeneic tissues, are not as readily depleted by cytotoxic antibodies, nor are they as responsive to immunoregulations as are resting or recently activated lymphocytes. Hence, profound lymphodepletion creates a barrier to dominant-type, immunoregulation-dependent transplant tolerance [94]. In-vitro models suggest sparing of Tregs by Thymoglobulin [95]. While the intense immunosuppression provided by antilymphocyte antibodies prevents rejection in the rejection-prone early transplant period, active treatment can promote through homeostatic proliferation the expansion of memory cells and does not per se aid dominant-type transplant tolerance. Lymphodepletive therapies can be used as an immunosuppressive prolog to create tolerance through use of other treatment modalities, such as creation of robust persistent mixed lineage hematopoietic chimerism in rodents [96].

Chimeric and humanized monoclonal antibodies

Mouse or other foreign xenoantibodies are often neutralized rapidly by human anti-xeno antibodies. To avoid a neutralizing immune response, mouse–human and humanized chimeric mAbs have been designed and produced to create mAbs that possess humanized immunogenicity. Moreover, the use of humanized or chimeric antibodies leads to enhanced longevity of the antibody in the circulation. Chimeric antibodies are produced by a gene fusion strategy: codons for the entire antigen-binding region (Fv), comprising both the immunoglobulin heavy- and light-chain variable regions ($V_L + V_H$), from an existing murine mAb are joined to codons for human Fc sequences. This simple approach has been extended and refined to create hyperchimeric or humanized antibodies [97]. In this strategy, as little of the xenogeneic rodent variable region sequences as possible is introduced while retaining antigen specificity and affinity of the parental rodent antibody. A variety of monoclonal chimeric and humanized immunosuppressive antibodies are of interest.

Anti-CD52 (alemtuzumab) mAb

This has been used as an induction agent [98]. As CD52 is expressed upon all lymphocytes, albeit at different levels, anti-CD52 also creates long-lived lymphopenia. Thus, the concerns that accompany profound lymphopenia (i.e., homeostatic proliferation of the lymphocyte pool, opportunistic infection, and cancer) are of concern in anti-CD52-treated patients. The precise role of this agent as a transplant therapeutic and potential for use in the creation of tolerance remains to be resolved, and its role in the creation of tolerance induction is subject to the same considerations and concerns as polyclonal antilymphocyte preparations.

Chimeric (basiliximab) and humanized (dacluzimab) anti-CD25 (IL-2R) mAbs

These are approved for clinical use as induction agents. CD25, the molecular target, is the alpha chain of the trimolecular interleukin 2 receptor (IL-2R). CD25 is not expressed upon conventional resting T cells, B cells, or other mononuclear leukocytes. It is robustly expressed upon Tregs, and recently activated T cells, B cells, or other activated mononuclear leukocytes. Hence, anti-CD25 mAbs target recently activated donor-reactive conventional lymphocytes, not the vast majority of the lymphocytes pool. They do, however, also target CD25^{hi} Tregs. The desired loss of both donor-reactive effector and the inevitable associated undesirable loss of regulatory cells potentially make these agents ill-suited for the creation of transplant tolerance.

Anti-CD20 mAb (rituximab)

This is expressed by mature B cells, but not by antibody-producing plasma cells. Surprisingly, anti-CD20 mAb treatment has proven efficacious in the treatment of several T-cell-dependent autoimmune diseases [99]. Some hypothesize that elimination of CD20$^+$ antigen-presenting cells by rituximab provides the basis for these interesting effects. Nonetheless, it seems unlikely that anti-CD20 mAbs, certainly as a monotherapy, offer a potent tool to create transplant tolerance.

Humanized anti-CD3 mAbs

Two parallel strategies have been used to impair the capacity of anti-CD3 antibodies to polymerize on the cell surface after binding CD3 by the Waldmann and the Bluestone laboratories [100]. Polymerization of CD3 activates the signaling pathway downstream of the TCR, thereby leading to transient T cell activation and a virulent cytokine release syndrome. These designer anti-CD3 mAbs retain T cell stimulatory capacity, albeit greatly impaired as a consequence of the failure of these designer antibodies to readily polymerize targeted CD3 molecules on the cell surface. Interestingly, these antibodies stimulate T cells to express the TGFβ, a potent, quintessential immunosuppressive cytokine, an effect crucial to immune tolerizing effects achieved in autoimmune models [100]. Both of the humanized "non-stimulatory" anti-CD3 mAbs have been used with success in inducing remissions in humans with new onset type 1 diabetes, but neither has been introduced into clinical transplantation [100]. The doses of anti-CD3 used to obtain drug-free remissions of type 1 diabetes trials caused the cytokine release syndrome, and lower doses failed to confer benefit in patients with new onset type 1 diabetes. While anti-CD3 mAbs can tilt the balance of immunity toward tolerance, adjunctive agents may be required to enable using safe non-toxic doses in attempts to create tolerance.

Anti-p40 mAb (usekinumab)

The IL-12 and IL-23R bimolecular complexes share a p40 subunit [101]. Both IL-12 and IL-23 deliver important cues to naive CD4 T cells, instructing them to become Th1 cells or stabilizing their commitment to the Th17 phenotype. Hence, targeting the p40 common chain of the IL-12 and IL-23 receptor complexes serves to target both Th1 and Th17 cells. While targeting the p40 subunit has not been extensively studied in transplant models, this strategy has proven useful in autoimmunity. It seems dubious that monotherapy with anti-p40 would be efficacious in creating transplant tolerance; however, this agent might well prove a useful component of a multi-agent regimen given the specificity of anti-p40 for a cytokine receptor crucial for commitment of CD4$^+$ T cells to the Th1 and Th17 phenotypes.

Ig-based fusion proteins

In some cases, cell-surface proteins are targeted by Ig fusion proteins. The usual function of these cell-surface-targeted Ig-based fusion proteins is to serve as site-specific pharmacological antagonists or (less commonly) agonists. In accordance with these goals, cytokines, cytokine receptors, or the ectodomain of cell-surface receptor proteins have generally been utilized as the targeting domain of the nonlytic, Fc$^{-/-}$-based fusion proteins. A variety of IgG heavy-chain-based fusion proteins have been created in which a peptide homing sequence, replacing the V$_H$ region, has been genetically fused to the hinge, CH2, and CH3 regions of FcΥ. The Fc domain of IgG serves as an effector domain and imparts several crucial attributes to the fusion protein. IgG proteins possess an exceptional circulating half-life following parenteral administration. The sequences responsible for this extraordinary longevity reside in the Fc region; therefore, FcΥ sequences impart a prolonged half-life to the peptide sequence chosen as the targeting device (homing domain) for the fusion protein. In the event that the desired therapeutic effect requires lysis of the target cell, the FcΥ region of an appropriate IgG isotype is chosen.

Belatacept

Belatacept, a second-generation CTLA-4-related.Ig fusion protein has been created using a mutated ectodomain of the CTLA-4 T cell surface protein. T cell surface CTLA-4 and CD28 both bind to the B7 (CD80 and CD86) costimulatory proteins expressed upon antigen-presenting cells. Ligation with CTLA4 transmits an immunoregulatory signal, while CD28 transmits a positive immunostimulatory signal. Belatacept is designed to better insure that T cell costimulatory signals triggered by interaction of T cell CD28 surface proteins with the CD80 and CD86 surface proteins upon antigen-presenting cells are blunted. In clinical practice, belatacept has proven to be an interesting and effective therapeutic agent, but use in regimens now being tested does not create transplant tolerance in clinical transplantation. The possibility is that incorporation into a multi-agent regimen may prove useful to the creation of transplant tolerance [102].

LFA-3.Ig (alefacept)

This is created by a gene fusion strategy in which the extracellular domain of LFA-3 is fused to IgG to target CD2. LFA-3.Ig binds to and polymerizes cell-surface CD2. This interaction leads to selective elimination of memory T cells. Combined treatment with CTLA-4.Ig and alefacept, in the absence of calcineurin inhibitors, corticosteroids, or lymphodepleting agents, prevents early acute rejection, enabling prolonged engraftment of renal transplants in the nonhuman primate transplant model [103]. This is a notable achievement. While tolerance was not produced, this regimen may serve as a platform to achieve elimination of memory cells, a major barrier to tolerance induction.

IL-2-based therapies

Both recently activated effector T cells and Tregs bear the high-affinity trimolecular IL-2R complex. A variety of cell types, including resting NK and NKT cells, bear the bimolecular intermediate-affinity IL-2R complex. Repeated stimulation of recently activated effector T cells, but not Tregs, by IL-2 triggers activation-induced cell death [39]. Activation of Tregs by IL-2 induces expression and activation of the STAT5 transcription factor. Creation and maintenance of the Treg phenotype requires stimulation by transforming growth factor beta and IL-2-triggered STAT5 activation. Indeed, Tregs, but not effector T cells, expand with IL-2 administration [104]. Hence, IL-2 selectively programs antigen-activated effector or conventional

T cells for apoptosis while maintaining the viability and function of Tregs.

The therapeutic potential for IL-2 therapy is limited by the short half-life of IL-2 in the circulation and by the wide range of cell types that bear the high- or intermediate-IL-2R complexes. In order to selectively target high-affinity-bearing T cells and not NK or NKT cells, cells that can produce massive amounts of cytokines following IL-2 stimulation, it is necessary to avoid circulating IL-2 levels that will activate the intermediate-affinity (10^9) receptor. The high-affinity receptor is saturated with IL-2 concentrations of 10^{12}. The ability to maintain low-dose, high-affinity saturating IL-2 concentrations that do rise to the levels that activate the intermediate-affinity IL-2R require constant, not peak and valley, pharmacokinetics. Because the half-life of circulating IL-2 is so short (minutes), it is impossible to administer IL-2 into the bloodstream and maintain the proper blood levels long term unless indwelling lines are used. Several strategies have been used to overcome these obstacles, the simplest of which is to inject IL-2 subcutaneously or intramuscularly. Administration in these sites creates a slow-release system that has been used to promote a tolerant state in preclinical models.

IL-2: anti-IL-2 complexes

IgG is the protein with longest known circulating half-life [104]. Hence, IL-2:anti-IL-2 complexes exhibit a far longer half-life than IL-2. Anti-IL-2 antibodies that do not bind to IL-2 epitopes crucial for receptor binding do not necessarily neutralize IL-2 activity. Thus, non-neutralizing, anti-IL-2 antibodies can be complexed with IL-2 and the mixture infused to provide a long-lived tolerance-promoting drug. Through fusion of IL-2 with downstream IgG heavy-chain Fc sequences, the resultant fusion protein possesses unimpaired IL-2 action and receptor site affinity plus properties contributed by the Fc sequences. These properties include a greatly prolonged circulating half-life and the ability to kill IL-2.Ig-coated cells via activation of Fc receptor bearing mononuclear leukocytes. IL-2 promotes activation-induced cell death of activated conventional T cells but serves to maintain the survival and functional integrity of Tregs [105].

IL-15 receptor blocking therapies

IL-15 is a potent T cell growth factor produced primarily by non-T cells that drives proliferation of effector T cells and release of proinflammatory cytokines by a variety of activated mononuclear leukocytes. The IL-15 receptor is expressed upon activated but resting T cells and other mononuclear leukocytes. The capacity of IL-2 to produce activation-induced cell death in effector T cells is totally blocked by IL-15 [106].

Mutant antagonist type IL-15.Ig

Introducing subtle mutations in fourth helix of IL-15 has created a high-affinity IL-15R-specific antagonist [107]. The antagonist binds to the alpha and beta chains, but not the common gamma chain, of the IL-15R. As binding to the common gamma chain activates the JAK STAT pathway, the mutant IL-15 is a high-affinity IL-15R antagonist. Through fusion of the mutant IL-15 with downstream IgG heavy-chain Fc sequences, the resultant fusion protein possesses unimpaired IL-15 receptor blocking action plus the prolonged half-life and cell lytic properties contributed by the Fc sequences. Blockade of the IL-15R serves to prevent IL-15 from overriding the ability of IL-2 to promote activation-induced cell death of activated conventional CD4[+] T cells [106]. In addition, the stimulatory effects of IL-15 upon CD8 and NKT cells and the ability of IL-15 to trigger expression of proinflammatory cytokines by non-lymphocyte mononuclear leukocytes are blocked.

Power mix

This regimen consists of: (i) an agonist (wild-type) IL-2.Ig fusion protein to enhance activation-induced cell death of effector, but not regulatory, T cells [106] and to provide IL-2-mediated nonredundant function in the differentiation of (Foxp3[+]) regulatory T cells [108]; (ii) a high-affinity IL-15Rα antagonist, mutant IL-15.Ig fusion protein (mutIL-15 Ig) [107, 109] to block proliferation and promote passive cell death of activated effector T cells by aborting proliferative and antiapoptotic IL-15 signals [105, 106, 110] and to block the ability of IL-15 to induce expression of proinflammatory cytokines by activated mononuclear inflammatory cells [111]; and (iii) rapamycin to blunt the proliferative response of activated T cells to T cell growth factors without inhibiting the activation-induced cell death signal imparted by IL-2 [112]. Moreover, the agonist IL-2-related and antagonist IL-15-related proteins were designed as IgG2a-derived Fc fusion proteins to ensure a prolonged circulating half-life and a potential means to kill activated effector, but not regulatory, IL-2R$^+$ and IL-15R$^+$ target cells via the activation of complement and FcR$^+$ leukocytes [111]. Hence, the IgG2a-based complement-dependent and antibody-dependent cell-cytotoxicity-activating Ig-related fusion proteins are potentially cytotoxic proteins that target certain vulnerable activated IL-2R$^+$/IL-15R$^-$, not IL-2R$^-$/IL-15R$^-$ resting, mononuclear leukocytes [105, 107].

In short, power mix is intended to tilt the balance of anti-donor immunity toward tolerance by (i) inciting IL-2-triggered apoptosis of activated cytopathic, but not regulatory, T cells, (ii) blocking the stimulatory effects of IL-15 upon T cells, B cells, and non-lymphocytic mononuclear cells, and (iii) inhibiting IL-15-triggered release of proinflammatory cytokines. This strategy has proven highly effective in restoring euglycemia and self-tolerance in the mouse type 1 diabetes model [113], and creation of tolerance in stringent murine transplant models and long-term drug-free survival of nonhuman primate islet allografts. In the mouse, indefinite drug-free survival of allogeneic islets placed into frankly diabetic autoimmune hosts was achieved despite the combined onslaught of auto- and allo-immune T cells. Drug-free survival of cynomolgus islet allografts was obtained for up to 1 year (manuscript in preparation).

Taming adverse inflammation as a means to promote tolerance

The texture of the inflammatory milieu in which T cells recognize antigen determines whether T cells adopt and maintain a cytoprotective or cytopathic phenotype. A microenvironment dominated by IL-12, a monokine, or IL-4 cells prompts naive CD4$^+$ T cells to commit to the Th1 or Th2 effector phenotypes. While a microenvironment dominated by the presence of transforming growth factor

alpha promotes commitment of naive T cells to the Treg phenotype, the addition of proinflammatory cytokines such as IL-6, IL-21, TNF-α, and IL-1 beta to TGFβ prevents or breaks commitment to the Treg phenotype and instead promotes acquisition of the powerfully proinflammatory Th17 phenotype. Organ transplants undergo ischemia reperfusion injury. Cell transplants such as islet transplant undergo anoxic and hypoxic injury as these cells are stripped from their blood supply and require neo-vacularization post-transplantation. As a direct consequence, organ and tissue transplantation are inevitably associated with intragraft expression of the proinflammatory, cytodestructive cytokines listed above that both promote delayed graft function and inhibit acquisition of regulatory phenotype. These proinflammatory, cytodestructive cytokines create injury of the transplant, releasing allo- and tissue-antigens in the context of a milieu that favors commitment of donor reactive T cells to cytopathic phenotypes while precluding commitment to cytoprotective phenotypes. It seems reasonable to assume that treatments that favorably shift the balance of intragraft inflammation from dominance by proinflammatory cytokines toward dominance by anti-inflammatory and cytoprotective cytokines such as TGFβ and interleukin 1 receptor antagonist during the peri-transplant period would tilt the allograft response toward tolerance. Currently, corticosteroids are the only anti-inflammatory agents regularly used as part of the treatment regimen for recipients. Corticosteroids inhibit expression of both pro- and anti-inflammatory cytokines and, therefore, do not selectively support cytoprotective immunity. Available for clinical trial in transplantation are inhibitors of the IL-1 beta, TNF-α, and IL-6 pathways. These agents might prove useful as adjunctive therapies given in the peri-transplant period. Another approach is the therapeutic use of select serpin family acute-phase reactants such as α1-antitrypsin or perhaps C1 esterase inhibitor. Under normal conditions these proteins are present in the circulation. Expression of A1AT by the liver is robustly enhanced in response to inflammation.

Individuals born with defects in the A1AT or C1 esterase inhibitor genes are subject to premature death. Replacement therapy with these serpin proteins purified from human blood is routine and safe. Overall, these proteins act to curtail expression of pro- but not anti-inflammatory cytokines, thrombosis, and complement activation. Not surprisingly, A1AT and C1 esterase inhibitor protect from ischemia reperfusion injury. Useful, indeed, are the immune tolerizing therapeutic effects of A1AT treatment that have been documented in mouse islet allograft [114] and the spontaneous autoimmune NOD diabetes models [113]. While A1AT does not directly alter T cell activation conducted in the absence of mononuclear T cells, A1AT through its effect on innate immunity promotes cytoprotection and immune tolerance by providing an environment in which T cells are activated in a milieu dominated by immuno-regulatory cytokines but not proinflammatory cytokines. In this regard, it is not surprising that A1AT therapy provides potent cytoprotection to islets transplanted into syngeneic hosts, thereby reducing the mass of islets required to render a diabetic host normoglycemic long term in autologous and syngeneic monkey and mouse models.

The use of biomarkers to identify recipients tolerant to their transplants

Some recipients are tolerant to their transplants, but conventional measures, such as a smooth rejection-free course, do not accurately identify these patients. The incidence among recipients of liver transplants with a rejection-free course for at least several years is approximately 20%, as deduced by efforts to wean such patients off maintenance immunosuppression. Far more accurate detection of tolerance patients can be undertaken through application of gene profiling techniques of circulating blood cells in appropriate candidates. Serial studies suggest that the immune response to transplants is subject to change over time after the inflammatory milieu present in the peri-transplant period has long disappeared, and reductions in the doses of conventional medications, particularly calcineurin inhibitors and corti-costeroids, that given in full doses can impair function of regulatory cells as drastically as that of

effector cells. While the incidence of renal transplant recipients with tolerance is almost certainly far less common than with liver transplant recipients, an almost curious B cell signature has been detected in patients who have successfully ceased taking immunosuppressive drugs. A small subset of recipients receiving maintenance immuno-suppression has been identified. Perhaps these patients will prove appropriate for planned cessation of immunosuppressives. This effort should be undertaken using biomarker evaluations for detection of incipient rejection during the weaning phase and continued thereafter [72, 73, 115].

Dose minimization and tolerance

In order to induce tolerance it will be necessary to tilt the balance of anti-donor immunity from a tissue-destructive to tissue-protective mode. In theory there are at least means of accomplishing this goal. The most obvious, but perhaps more difficult, strategy is to permanently delete donor-reactive tissue-destructive T cells. While this can readily be executed through establishment of mixed donor and recipient mixed chimerism in rodent models, this goal has not been reproducibly accomplished in nonhuman primates or in humans. Intense treatment strategies using radiation, lymphodepletive biologic therapy, and conventional small drugs that often create robust multi-lineage hematopoietic chimerism in mice while failing to create robust mixed chimerism were sufficient to enable four of five treated recipients with renal failure secondary to multiple myeloma to maintain long-term, drug-free engraftment of renal transplants.

Maybe we should not hurry to create tolerance

To sum up the foregoing, it is difficult to create tolerance in humans. In the immediate post-transplant period, application of the most interesting strategies for creation of tolerance, in our estimation, entails a multidrug regimen. Regulatory agency requirements and rivalry between pharmaceutical companies complicate plans for clinical execution. As the intense proinflammatory consequences of the organ or tissue harvest, preservation, and transplant procedures must complicate successful creation of an environment conducive to the enduring functional dominance of Tregs over effector T cells, a scenario is required for dominant-type tolerance. We submit that it might prove more productive in the short term to apply potentially tolerizing therapies after inflammation has subsided and the intensity of tolerant unfriendly regimens has been minimized. It seems likely that the prudent use of biomarkers can guide this effort [115].

Abbreviations

Breg	regulatory B cell
IL-2	interleukin 2
IL-2R	interleukin 2 receptor
mAb	monoclonal antibody
MDSC	myeloid-derived suppressor cell
PD1	programmed death 1
Treg	regulatory T cell

References

1 Jenkins MK, Pardoll DM, Mizuguchi J et al. T-cell unresponsiveness in vivo and in vitro: fine specificity of induction and molecular characterization of the unresponsive state. *Immunol Rev* 1987;95:113–135.

2 Perez V, van Parijs L, Biuckians A et al. Induction of peripheral T cell tolerance in vivo requires CTLA-4 engagement. *Immunity* 1997;6(4):411–417.

3 Tsushima F, Yao S, Shin T et al. Interaction between B7-H1 and PD-1 determines initiation and reversal of T-cell anergy. *Blood* 2007;110(1):180–185.

4 Francisco LM, Sage PT, Sharpe AH. The PD-1 pathway in tolerance and autoimmunity. *Immunol Rev* 2010;236(1):219–242.

5 Benoist C, Mathis D. Positive selection of the T cell repertoire: where and when does it occur? *Cell* 1989;58:1027–1033.

6 Kappler JW, Roehm N, Marrack P. T cell tolerance by clonal elimination in the thymus. *Cell* 1987;49:273–280.

7 Sakaguchi S, Sakaguchi N, Asano M et al. Immunologic self tolerance maintained by activated T cells expressing IL-2 receptor alpha chains (CD25). Breakdown of a single mechanism of self tolerance causes various autoimmune diseases. *J Immunol* 1995;155:1151–1164.

8 Suri-Payer E, Amar AZ, Thornton AM, Shevach EM. CD4$^+$CD25$^+$ T cells inhibit both the induction and effector function of autoreactive T cells and represent a unique lineage of immunoregulatory cells. *J Immunol* 1998;160(3):1212–1218.

9 Ohkura N, Sakaguchi S. Regulatory T cells: roles of T cell receptor for their development and function. *Semin Immunopathol* 2010;32(2):95–106.

10 Josefowicz SZ, Rudensky A. Control of regulatory T cell lineage commitment and maintenance. *Immunity* 2009;30(5):616–625.

11 Posselt A, Barker C, Friedman A et al. Intrathymic inoculation of islets at birth prevents autoimmune diabetes and pancreatic insulitis in the BB rat. *Transplant Proc* 1993;25:301–302.

12 Jones N, Fluck N, Mellor A et al. Deletion of alloantigen-reactive thymocytes as a mechanism of adult transplantation tolerance induction following intrathymic antigen administration. *Eur J Immunol* 1997;27:1591–1600.

13 Manilay J, Pearson D, Sergio J et al. Intrathymic deletion of alloreactive T cells in mixed bone marrow chimeras prepared with a nonmyeloablative conditioning regime. *Transplantation* 1998;66:96–102.

14 Krammer PH, Arnold R, Lavrik IN. Life and death in peripheral T cells. *Nat Rev* 2007;7(7):532–542.

15 Strasser A, Jost PJ, Nagata S. The many roles of FAS receptor signaling in the immune system. *Immunity* 2009;30(2):180–192.

16 Wood KJ, Sakaguchi S. Regulatory T cells in transplantation tolerance. *Nat Immunol Rev* 2003;3:199–210.

17 Billingham RE, Brent L, Medawar PB. Actively acquired tolerance of foreign cells. *Nature* 1953;172:603–606.

18 Rubtsov YP, Niec RE, Josefowicz S et al. Stability of the regulatory T cell lineage in vivo. *Science* 2010;329(5999):1667–1671.

19 Oliveira V, Sawitzki B, Chapman S et al. Anti-CD4-mediated selection of Treg in vitro – in vitro suppression does not predict in vivo capacity to prevent graft rejection. *Eur J Immunol* 2008;38(6):1677–1688.

20 Feng G, Gao W, Strom TB et al. Exogenous IFN-γ ex vivo shapes the alloreactive T-cell repertoire by inhibition of Th17 responses and generation of functional Foxp3$^+$ regulatory T cells. *Eur J Immunol* 2008;38(9):2512–2527.

21 Zheng SG, Wang JJ, Wang P et al. IL-2 is essential for TGF-β to convert naive CD4$^+$CD25$^-$ cells to CD25$^+$Foxp3$^+$ regulatory T cells and for expansion of these cells. *J Immunol* 2007;178:2018–2027.

22 Battaglia M, Stabilini A, Roncarolo M-G. Rapamycin selectively expands CD4$^+$CD25$^+$FoxP3$^+$ regulatory T cells. *Blood* 2005;105(12):4743–8.

23 Francis RS, Feng G, Tha-In T *et al*. Induction of transplantation tolerance converts potential effector T cells into graft-protective regulatory T cells. *Eur J Immunol* 2011;41(3):726–738.

24 Long E, Wood KJ. Understanding FOXP3: progress towards achieving transplantation tolerance. *Transplantation* 2007;84:459–461.

25 Zheng Y, Rudensky AY. Foxp3 in control of the regulatory T cell lineage. *Nat Immunol* 2007;8(5):457–462.

26 Williams L, Rudensky A. Maintenance of the Foxp3-dependent developmental program in mature regulatory T cells requires continued expression of Foxp3. *Nat Immunol* 2007;8:277–284.

27 Floess S, Freyer J, Siewert C *et al*. Epigenetic control of the foxp3 locus in regulatory T cells. *PLoS Biol* 2007;5:169–178

28 Bushell A, Morris P, Wood K. Transplantation tolerance induced by antigen pretreatment and depleting anti-CD4 antibody depends on CD4+ T cell regulation during the induction phase of the response. *Eur J Immunol* 1995;25:2643–2649.

29 Hara M, Kingsley C, Niimi M *et al*. IL-10 is required for regulatory T cells to mediate tolerance to alloantigens in vivo. *J Immunol* 2001;166:3789–3796.

30 Kingsley CI, Karim M, Bushell AR, Wood KJ. CD25+CD4+ regulatory T cells prevent graft rejection: CTLA-4- and IL-10-dependent immunoregulation of alloresponses. *J Immunol* 2002;168(3):1080–1086.

31 Warnecke G, Bushell A, Nadig S, Wood KJ. Regulation of transplant arteriosclerosis by CD25+CD4+ T cells generated to alloantigen in vivo. *Transplantation* 2007;83:1459–1465.

32 Issa F, Hester J, Goto R *et al*. Ex vivo-expanded human regulatory T cells prevent the rejection of skin allografts in a humanised mouse model. *Transplantation* 2010;90:1321–1327.

33 Weaver C, Harrington L, Mangan P *et al*. Th17: an effector CD4 T cell lineage with regulatory T cell ties. *Immunity* 2006;24:677–688.

34 Wells A, Li X, Li Y *et al*. Requirement for T cell apoptosis in the induction of peripheral transplantation tolerance. *Nat Med* 1999;5:1303–1307.

35 Adams A, Williams MA, Jones T *et al*. Heterologous immunity provides a potent barrier to transplantation tolerance. *J Clin Invest* 2003;111:1887–1895.

36 Yang J, Brook MO, Carvalho-Gaspar M *et al*. Allograft rejection mediated by memory T cells is resistant to regulation. *Proc Natl Acad Sci U S A* 2008;104: 19954–19959.

37 Carvalho-Gaspar M, Jones ND, Luo S *et al*. Location and time-dependent control of rejection by regulatory T cells culminates in a failure to generate memory T cells. *J Immunol* 2008;180(10):6640–6648.

38 Fan Z, Spencer JA, Lu Y *et al*. In vivo tracking of "color-coded" effector, natural and induced regulatory T cells in the allograft response. *Nat Med* 2010;16(6): 718–722.

39 Li X, Strom T, Turka L, Wells A. T cell death and transplantation tolerance. *Immunity* 2001;14:407–416.

40 Graca L, Cobbold SP, Waldmann H. Identification of regulatory T cells in tolerated allografts. *J Exp Med* 2002;195(12):1641–1646.

41 Tang Q, Adams J, Tooley A *et al*. Visualizing regulatory T cell control of autoimmune responses in nonobese diabetic mice. *Nat Immunol* 2006;7:83–92.

42 Li Y, Koshiba T, Yoshizawa A *et al*. Analyses of peripheral blood mononuclear cells in operational tolerance after pediatric living donor liver transplantation. *Am J Transplant* 2004;4(12):2118–2125.

43 Li Y, Zhao X, Cheng D *et al*. The presence of Foxp3 expressing T cells within grafts of tolerant human liver transplant recipients. *Transplantation* 2008;86(12): 1837–1843. DOI: 10.097/TP.0b013e31818febc4.

44 Martinez-Llordella M, Puig-Pey I, Orlando G *et al*. Multiparameter immune profiling of operational tolerance in liver transplantation. *Am J Transplant* 2007;7(2):309–319.

45 Sawitzki B, Kingsley CI, Oliveira V *et al*. Interferon gamma production by alloantigen reactive CD25+CD4+ regulatory T cells is important for their regulatory function in vivo. *J Exp Med* 2005;201:1925–1935.

46 Wood KJ, Sawitzki B. Interferon γ: a crucial role in the function of induced regulatory T cells in vivo. *Trends Immunol* 2006;27:183–187.

47 Konieczny B, Dai Z, Elwood E *et al*. IFN-γ is critical for long-term allograft survival indcued by blocking the CD28 and CD40 ligand T cell costimulation pathways. *J Immunol* 1998;160:2059–2064.

48 Yu X-Z, Albert MH, Martin PJ, Anasetti C. CD28 ligation induces transplantation tolerance by IFN-γ-dependent depletion of T cells that recognize alloantigens. *J Clin Invest* 2004;113(11):1624–1630.

49 Saleem S, Konieczny B, Lowry R *et al*. Acute rejection of vascularized heart allografts in the absence of IFNγ. *Transplantation* 1996;62:1908–1911.

50 Markees TG, Phillips NE, Gordon EJ *et al*. Long term survival of skin allografts induced by donor splenocytes and anti-CD154 antibody in thymectomised mice requires CD4+ T cells, interferon-γ and CTLA-4. *J Clin Invest* 1998;101:2446–2455.

51 Gajewski TF, Fitch FW. Anti-proliferative effect of IFN-gamma in immune regulation. I. IFN-gamma inhibits

the proliferation of Th2 but not Th1 murine helper T lymphocyte clones. *J Immunol* 1988;140(12): 4245–4252.

52 Bettelli E, Carrier Y, Gao W *et al.* Reciprocal developmental pathways for the generation of pathogenic effector TH17 and regulatory T cells. *Nature* 2006; 441:235–238.

53 Heidt S, San D, Chadha R, Wood KJ. The impact of Th17 cells on transplant rejection and the induction of tolerance. *Curr Opin Organ Transplant* 2010;15(4): 456–461. DOI: 10.1097/MOT.0b013e32833b9bfb.

54 Tewari K, Nakayama Y, Suresh M. Role of direct effects of IFN-γ on T cells in the regulation of CD8 T cell homeostasis. *J Immunol* 2007;179(4):2115–2125.

55 Thompson C, Allison J. The emerging role of CTLA-4 as an immune attenuator. *Immunity* 1997;7:445–450.

56 Walunas T, Bluestone J. CTLA-4 regulates tolerance induction and T cell differentiation in vivo. *J Immunol* 1998;160:3855–3860.

57 Walunas T, Lenschow D, Bakker C *et al.* CTLA-4 can function as a negative regulator of T cell activation. *Immunity* 1994;1:405–413.

58 Waterhouse P, Penninger J, Timms E *et al.* Lymphoproliferative disorders with early lethality in mice deficient in CTLA-4. *Science* 1995;270:985–988.

59 Read S, Malmström V, Powrie F. Cytotoxic T lymphocyte associated antigen 4 plays an essential role in the function of CD25⁺CD4⁺ regulatory cells that control intestinal inflammation. *J Exp Med* 2000;192:295–302.

60 Read S, Greenwald R, Izcue A *et al.* Blockade of CTLA-4 on CD4⁺CD25⁺ regulatory T cells abrogates their function in vivo. *J Immunol* 2006;177:4376–4383.

61 Fallarino F, Grohmann U, Hwang KW *et al.* Modulation of tryptophan catabolism by regulatory T cells. *Nat Immunol* 2003;4:1206–1212.

62 Schneider H, Valk E, da Rocha S *et al.* CTLA-4 upregulation of lymphocyte function-associated antigen 1 adhesion and clustering as an alternative basis for co-receptor function. *Proc Natl Acad Sci U S A* 2005; 102:12861–12866.

63 Schneider H, Downey J, Smith A *et al.* Reversal of the TCR stop signal by CTLA-4. *Science* 2006;313(5795): 1972–1975.

64 Sawitzki B, Bushell A, Steger U *et al.* Identification of gene markers for the prediction of allograft rejection or permanent acceptance. *Am J Transplant* 2007;7(5): 1091–1102.

65 Long ET, Baker S, Oliveira V *et al.* Alpha-1,2-Mannosidase and hence *N*-glycosylation are required for regulatory t cell migration and allograft tolerance in mice. *PLoS One* 2010;5(1):e8894.

66 Deaglio S, Dwyer KM, Gao W *et al.* Adenosine generation catalyzed by CD39 and CD73 expressed on regulatory T cells mediates immune suppression. *J Exp Med* 2007;204:1257–1265.

67 Junger WG. Immune cell regulation by autocrine purinergic signalling. *Nat Rev* 2011;11(3):201–212.

68 Chang C, Ciubotariu R, Manavalan J *et al.* Tolerization of dendritic cells by TS cells: the crucial role of inhibitory receptors ILT3 and ILT4. *Nat Immunol* 2002;2: 237–243.

69 Najafian N, Chitnis T, Salama AD *et al.* Regulatory functions of CD8⁺CD28⁻ T cells in an autoimmune disease model. *J Clin Invest* 2003;112(7):1037–1048.

70 Scotto L, Naiyer AJ, Galluzzo S *et al.* Overlap between molecular markers expressed by naturally occurring CD4⁺CD25⁺ regulatory T cells and antigen specific CD4⁺CD25⁺ and CD8⁺CD28⁻ T suppressor cells. *Hum Immunol* 2004;65(11):1297–1306.

71 Mauri C, Blair PA. Regulatory B cells in autoimmunity: developments and controversies. *Nat Rev Rheumatol* 2010;6(11):636–643.

72 Sagoo P, Perucha E, Sawitzki B *et al.* Development of a cross-platform biomarker signature to detect renal transplant tolerance in humans. *J Clin Invest* 2010;120(6):1848–1861.

73 Newell KA, Asare A, Kirk AD *et al.* Identification of a B cell signature associated with renal transplant tolerance in humans. *J Clin Invest* 2010;120(6): 1836–1847.

74 Morelli AE, Thomson AW. Dendritic cells: regulators of alloimmunity and opportunities for tolerance induction. *Immunol Rev* 2003;196:125–146.

75 Barratt-Boyes SM, Thomson AW. Dendritic cells: tools and targets for transplant tolerance. *Am J Transplant* 2005;5(12):2807–2813.

76 Van Kooten C, Lombardi G, Gelderman KA *et al.* Dendritic cells as a tool to induce transplantation tolerance: obstacles and opportunities. *Transplantation* 2011;91(1):2–7. DOI: 10.1097/TP.0b013e31820263b3.

77 Morelli AE, Thomson AW. Tolerogenic dendritic cells and the quest for transplant tolerance. *Nat Rev* 2007;7(8):610–621.

78 Fu F, Li Y, Qian S *et al.* Costimulatory molecule-deficient dendritic cell progenitors (MHC class II⁺, CD80ᵈⁱᵐ, CD86⁻) prolong cardiac allograft survival in nonimmunosupressed recipients. *Transplantation* 1996;62:659–665.

79 Lutz M, Suri R, Niimi M *et al.* Immature dendritic cells generated with low doses of GM-CSF in the absence of IL-4 are maturation resistant and prolong allograft survival in vivo. *Eur J Immunol* 2000;30:1813–1822.

80 Lu L, Li W, Fu F *et al*. Blockade of the CD40–CD40 ligand pathway potentiates the capacity of donor-derived dendritic cell progenitors to induce long-term cardiac allograft survival. *Transplantation* 1997;64: 1808–1815.

81 Roelen D, Schuurhuis D, van den Boogaardt D *et al*. Prolongation of skin graft survival by modulation of the alloimmune response with alternatively activated dendritic cells. *Transplantation* 2003;76:1608–1615.

82 Sato K, Yamashita N, Yamashita N *et al*. Regulatory Dendritic cells protect mice from murine acute graft-versus-host disease and leukemia relapse. *Immunity* 2003;18:367–379.

83 Albert ML, Jegathesan M, Darnell RB. Dendritic cell maturation is required for cross-tolerisation of CD8⁺ T cells. *Nat Immunol* 2001;2:1010–1017.

84 Verhasselt V, Vosters O, Beuneu C *et al*. Induction of FOXP3-expressing regulatory CD4pos T cells by human mature autologous dendritic cells. *Eur J Immunol* 2004;34:762–772.

85 Menges M, Rößner S, Voigtländer C *et al*. Repetitive injections of dendritic cells matured with tumor necrosis factor induce antigen-specific protection of mice from autoimmunity. *J Exp Med* 2001;195:15–22.

86 Gilliet M, Liu Y-J. Generation of human CD8 T regulatory cells by CD40 ligand-activated plasmacytoid dendritic cells. *J Exp Med* 2002;195(6):695–704.

87 Abe M, Wang Z, de Creus A, Thomson AW. plasmacytoid dendritic cell precursors induce allogeneic T-cell hyporesponsiveness and prolong heart graft survival. *Am J Transplant* 2005;5(8):1808–1819.

88 Bjorck P, Coates PTH, Wang Z *et al*. Promotion of long-term heart allograft survival by combination of mobilized donor plasmacytoid dendritic cells and anti-CD154 monoclonal antibody. *J Heart Lung Transplant* 2005;24(8):1118–1120.

89 Boros P, Ochando JC, Chen S-H, Bromberg JS. Myeloid-derived suppressor cells: natural regulators for transplant tolerance. *Hum Immunol* 2010;71(11): 1061–1066.

90 Yamada A, Chandraker A, Laufer TM *et al*. Cutting Edge: Recipient MHC class II expression is required to achieve long-term survival of murine cardiac allografts after costimulatory blockade. *J Immunol* 2001; 167(10):5522–5526.

91 Garcia MR, Ledgerwood L, Yang Y *et al*. Monocytic suppressive cells mediate cardiovascular transplantation tolerance in mice. *J Clin Invest* 2010;120(7): 2486–2496.

92 Dugast A-S, Haudebourg T, Coulon F *et al*. Myeloid-derived suppressor cells accumulate in kidney allograft

tolerance and specifically suppress effector T cell expansion. *J Immunol* 2008;180(12):7898–7906.

93 Walker LSK, Abbas AK. The enemy within: keeping self-reactive T cells at bay in the periphery. *Nat Rev* 2002;2(1):11–19.

94 Wu Z, Bensinger SJ, Zhang J *et al*. Homeostatic proliferation is a barrier to transplantation tolerance. *Nat Med* 2004;10(1):87–92.

95 Lopez M, Clarkson MR, Albin M *et al*. A novel mechanism of action for anti-thymocyte globulin: induction of CD4+CD25⁺Foxp3⁺ regulatory T cells. *J Am Soc Nephrol* 2006;17(10):2844–2853.

96 Cosimi AB, Sachs DH. Mixed chimerism and transplantation tolerance. *Transplantation* 2004;77(6): 943–946.

97 Jones PT, Dear PH, Foote J *et al*. Replacing the complementarity-determining regions in a human antibody with those from a mouse. *Nature* 1986; 321(6069):522–525.

98 Hale G, Xia MQ, Tighe HP *et al*. The CAMPATH-1 antigen (CDw52). *Tissue Antigens* 1990;35(3):118–127.

99 Edwards JC, Szczepanski L, Szechinski J *et al*. Efficacy of B-cell-targeted therapy with rituximab in patients with rheumatoid arthritis. *N Engl J Med* 2004; 350(25):2572–2581.

100 Chatenoud L. Immune therapy for type 1 diabetes mellitus – what is unique about anti-CD3 antibodies? *Nat Rev Endocrinol* 2010;6(3):149–157.

101 Luo J, Wu SJ, Lacy ER *et al*. Structural basis for the dual recognition of IL-12 and IL-23 by ustekinumab. *J Mol Biol* 2010;402(5):797–812.

102 Ferguson R, Grinyo J, Vincenti F *et al*. Immunosuppression with belatacept-based, corticosteroid-avoiding regimens in de novo kidney transplant recipients. *Am J Transplant* 2011;11(1):66–76.

103 Weaver TA, Charafeddine AH, Agarwal A *et al*. Alefacept promotes co-stimulation blockade based allograft survival in nonhuman primates. *Nat Med* 2009;15(7):746–749.

104 Webster KE, Walters S, Kohler RE *et al*. In vivo expansion of T reg cells with IL-2–mAb complexes: induction of resistance to EAE and long-term acceptance of islet allografts without immunosuppression. *J Exp Med* 2009;206(4):751–760.

105 Zheng XX, Sanchez-Fueyo A, Sho M *et al*. Favorably tipping the balance between cytopathic and regulatory T cells to create transplantation tolerance. *Immunity* 2003;19(4):503–514.

106 Li XC, Demirci G, Ferrari-Lacraz S *et al*. IL-15 and IL-2: a matter of life and death for T cells in vivo. *Nat Med* 2001;7(1):114–118.

107 Kim YS, Maslinski W, Zheng XX *et al.* Targeting the IL-15 receptor with an antagonist IL-15 mutant/Fc gamma2a protein blocks delayed-type hypersensitivity. *J Immunol* 1998;160(12):5742–5748.

108 Fontenot JD, Rasmussen JP, Gavin MA, Rudensky AY. A function for interleukin 2 in Foxp3-expressing regulatory T cells. *Nat Immunol* 2005;6(11):1142–1151.

109 Ferrari-Lacraz S, Zanelli E, Neuberg M *et al.* Targeting IL-15 receptor-bearing cells with an antagonist mutant IL-15/Fc protein prevents disease development and progression in murine collagen-induced arthritis. *J Immunol* 2004;173(9):5818–5826.

110 Waldmann TA, Dubois S, Tagaya Y. Contrasting roles of IL-2 and IL-15 in the life and death of lymphocytes: implications for immunotherapy. *Immunity* 2001;14(2):105–110.

111 Zheng XX, Maslinski W, Ferrari-Lacraz S, Strom TB. Cytokines in the treatment and prevention of autoimmune responses-a role of IL-15. *Adv Exp Med Biol* 2003;520:87–95.

112 Charrad RS, Li Y, Delpech B *et al.* Ligation of the CD44 adhesion molecule reverses blockage of differentiation in human acute myeloid leukemia. *Nat Med* 1999;5(6):669–676.

113 Koulmanda M, Bhasin M, Hoffman L *et al.* Curative and beta cell regenerative effects of α1-antitrypsin treatment in autoimmune diabetic NOD mice. *Proc Natl Acad Sci U S A* 2008;105(42):16242–16247.

114 Lewis EC, Mizrahi M, Toledano M *et al.* α1-Antitrypsin monotherapy induces immune tolerance during islet allograft transplantation in mice. *Proc Natl Acad Sci U S A* 2008;105(42):16236–16241.

115 Sanchez-Fueyo A, Strom TB. Immunologic basis of graft rejection and tolerance following transplantation of liver or other solid organs. *Gastroenterology* 2011;140(1):51–64.

PART 2
Transplantation Clinical Pharmacology

CHAPTER 7

Pharmacokinetics

Venkateswaran C. Pillai[1] and Raman Venkataramanan[1,2]

[1]School of Pharmacy, University of Pittsburgh, Pittsburgh, PA, USA

[2]Thomas Starzl Transplantation Institute, Magee-Womens Research Institute, Department of Pathology, McGowan Institute for Regenerative Medicine, Pittsburgh, PA, USA

Introduction

Pharmacokinetics deals with the time course of drug concentration in the body. Pharmacokinetics describes the various rate processes involved in absorption, distribution, metabolism, and excretion (ADME) of a drug.

- Absorption is defined as the process by which a drug moves from the site of application to the site of measurement. This absorption process can be passive (simple diffusion against a concentration gradient) or active (involving a transporter).
- Distribution is a reversible process of movement of drugs from and to the site of measurement. Distribution of the drug is influenced by the permeability of the drug to various tissues, the blood flow to the various tissues/organs, and binding of drugs to plasma proteins (typically albumin or alpha 1 acid glycoprotein) and tissue proteins.
- Metabolism is a process where one chemical is converted to another chemical through an enzymatic pathway. Metabolism typically takes place in the liver, but certain drugs can undergo metabolism in the gut wall as well. Organs such as brain, lung, and kidney also contain drug-metabolizing enzymes and may contribute to regional concentration of drug and metabolite and, hence, to efficacy or toxicity, but they do not contribute very much to the overall systemic exposure of the drug.

- Excretion is the irreversible loss of drug from the body as the unchanged parent drug through the urine, bile, lung, or sweat.

Elimination is the sum of metabolism and excretion and represents the total irreversible loss of the drug from the body. In certain cases, the term disposition is used to refer to the combination of distribution and elimination. For a detailed description of the pharmacokinetic concepts, readers are referred to several textbooks in this area [1–10]. Table 7.1 lists some general guidelines in conducting pharmacokinetic studies.

Value of pharmacokinetic information

Pharmacokinetic parameters are useful in understanding the behavior of a drug in the body, in predicting the drug concentration–time profile in the body, in estimating the availability of a drug from a formulation, in determining the effect of changes in drug formulations, changes in physiological factors, and changes in pathological factors on systemic drug exposure, in evaluating drug–drug interactions, in adjusting the dosing regimen of drugs in certain disease states, in correlating the drug exposure to drug response, and in individualizing the dosing regimen of a drug in a patient.

Immunotherapy in Transplantation: Principles and Practice, First Edition. Edited by Bruce Kaplan, Gilbert J. Burckart and Fadi G. Lakkis.
© 2012 Blackwell Publishing Ltd. Published 2012 by Blackwell Publishing Ltd.

Table 7.1 General guidelines for pharmacokinetic studies.

It is important to analyze the dosage form for drug content in a pharmacokinetic study to know the exact dose used.

The same iv line must not be used to administer drug and withdraw blood samples for a pharmacokinetic study.

It is important to collect blood samples for at least three half-lives of the drug in order to obtain proper pharmacokinetic parameters.

It is important to know exactly when a blood sample is collected in a pharmacokinetic study.

It is critical to make sure samples are handled/processed properly (such as a avoiding hemolysis, temperature effects on blood cell partitioning, temperature effect on stability of the drug) when drug concentrations are to be measured in biological fluids.

A specific and sensitive assay method must be used to measure drug concentrations and to calculate pharmacokinetic parameters.

Whenever possible, the major metabolites must also be measured.

To characterize a rate constant from a straight line, at least three data points must be used.

To characterize the absorption and disposition, at least three data point in the absorptive phase and three data points in the disposition phase must be obtained.

Parameters (CL and Vd) calculated after extravascular administration will not always be equal to those calculated from IV data due to the less than complete bioavailability of the drug after extravascular administration.

In order to obtain all the pharmacokinetic parameters, drug must be given intravenously, whenever possible.

It is not possible to obtain an absolute bioavailability estimate for a drug without obtaining data from iv drug administration.

Routes of administration and drug concentration–time profile

Vascular administration

Most of the biological processes obey a first-order process, which implies that the rate of the process is a function of drug concentration. At high concentrations the rate of decline in drug concentration will be high, and as the concentration of drug decreases the rate of decline will become slower. This gives a curvilinear appearance for the drug concentration versus time profile in a regular Cartesian scale (Figure 7.1a).

Figure 7.1a illustrates the blood concentration versus time profile for a drug administered intravascularly as a bolus injection. A drug that is administered intravascularly (intravenous or intra-arterial) undergoes a process of distribution and elimination, which are governed by the physico-chemical characteristics of the drug and its physico-chemical and biochemical interactions within the body. If a drug is given intravenously as a bolus injection, the highest concentration C_0 is achieved immediately at the end of drug administration (typically referred to as time zero), and the drug concentration subsequently decreases with time. A drug that distributes instantaneously to various parts of the body is referred to as a drug that exhibits a one-compartment behavior. A drug that does not instantaneously distribute in the entire body is referred to as a drug that exhibits multicompartmental behavior (Figure 7.1a). Such drugs distribute immediately into certain parts of the body (referred to as the central compartment), but take more time to distribute into other parts of the body (referred to as the peripheral or tissue compartment).

When the concentrations are log or ln transformed, the curve becomes linear if the drug undergoes a one-compartment behavior. For a drug that exhibits multicompartment behavior, one observes an initial curvilinear portion, which

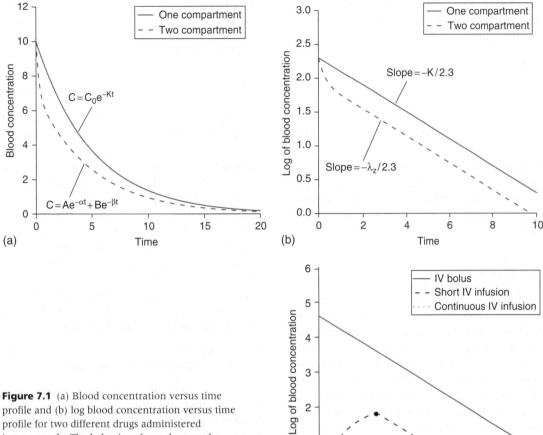

Figure 7.1 (a) Blood concentration versus time profile and (b) log blood concentration versus time profile for two different drugs administered intravenously. The behavior of one drug can be characterized by a one-compartment model and the other by a two-compartment model. (c) The log blood concentration versus time profile for a drug administered as an iv bolus, iv short infusion, and iv continuous infusion.

is followed by a linear decline once a distribution equilibrium is reached, on log or ln transformation (Figure 7.1b). If a drug is administered as an infusion, the initial concentration will be zero and the concentration will increase with time and eventually reach a steady state, where the concentration stays relatively constant with time as long as the drug is continuously administered at the same infusion rate (Figure 7.1c). In the case of a drug that is administered as continuous infusion, on stopping the infusion of the drug concentration will decline similar to what is observed with an iv

bolus or a short infusion. Immunosuppressive drugs like mycophenolate mofetil are given as a short infusion (a few hours), while cyclosporine and tacrolimus are given as a short infusion or as a continuous infusion (24 h infusion) to steady state.

The slope of the terminal linear portion (disposition phase) of a log or ln concentration versus time plot is determined by the disposition rate constant (K or λ_z). This is a rate constant that is normally expressed in units of 1/time. This is the rate constant associated with the elimination or disposition of the drug from the body. This is calculated from concentration data points in the terminal linear portion of the log (or ln) concentration versus time plots using linear regression analysis

Slope of the terminal portion (log scale) =

$$-\frac{K}{2.3} \quad \text{or} \quad -\frac{\lambda_z}{2.3} \tag{7.1}$$

$$K \text{ or } \lambda_z = \frac{\ln C_1 - \ln C_2}{t_2 - t_1} \text{ (h}^{-1}) \tag{7.2}$$

The apparent half-life $T_{1/2}$ normally represented in minutes or hours, is the time that it takes for an amount or concentration to decrease to one half of the amount or concentration. Mathematically this is given as

$$T_{1/2} = \frac{0.693}{K \text{ or } \lambda_z} \text{ (h)} \tag{7.3}$$

It typically takes five or six half-lives to eliminate most of the administered drug from the body. It also takes five or six half-lives to reach a steady state once a new dosing regimen is initiated or when a dosing regimen is changed. It is important to collect blood samples for at least three half-lives in order to reasonably estimate the $T_{1/2}$ in pharmacokinetic studies.

In a typical pharmacokinetic study, drug concentrations are measured at several time points during a dosing interval. The area under the blood or plasma concentration versus time curve, AUC (amount × time/volume unit), is a measure of the overall drug exposure in a patient. Area under the curve is calculated by the trapezoidal rule or using an empiric equation. In using the trapezoidal rule, the blood or plasma concentration versus time profile is considered to be made up of several trapezoids and the AUC for each trapezoid is calculated as given in Equation (7.4) and summed up to the last measured concentration. The AUC from the last measured concentration to time infinity (when all the drug is lost from the body) is calculated as C_{last}/K, where C_{last} is the last measured concentration.

$$\text{AUC}_{0-\text{infinity}} = \sum \left[\left(\frac{C_n + C_{n+1}}{2} \right)(T_{n+1} - t_n) \right] + \frac{C_{last}}{\lambda_z} ((\mu g / mL)h) \tag{7.4}$$

where C_n and C_{n+1} correspond to the concentrations measured at times n and $n+1$, where n ranges from zero to the last number of samples collected. AUC can also be calculated as follows:

$$\text{AUC} = \sum_{i=1}^{n} (c_i / \lambda_i) \tag{7.5}$$

where i can range from 1 to n and c_i is the intercept on the y-axis and λ_i is the corresponding slope of the straight line. Area under the curve is normally expressed in concentration × time (($\mu g/mL$)h). The higher the AUC, the higher the drug exposure is in a given patient; and the smaller the AUC, the smaller is the drug exposure in a given patient.

From the AUC one can calculate the total body clearance CL (volume/time) of a drug. This is defined as the volume of blood or plasma that is completely cleared of the drug per unit time. Clearance is also a proportionality constant that relates the rate of loss of drug from the body to the concentration of drug in blood or plasma.

Rate of drug loss from the body
$$= \text{CL} \times \text{Concentration in blood or plasma} \tag{7.6}$$

Clearance is normally calculated as the total amount of drug cleared from the body/AUC. When the drug is given by a vascular route, the amount cleared will be equal to the dose of the drug administered and the clearance is given as follows:

$$\text{CL} = \frac{\text{Dose}}{\text{AUC}} \text{ (mL / h)} \tag{7.7}$$

The extent to which a drug is distributed in the body is normally determined by the apparent volume of distribution Vd (volume units). This relates the concentration of the drug at the site of measurement (plasma or blood) to the total amount of drug in the body. This is calculated as follows after an iv bolus dose for a drug that exhibits a one-compartment behavior:

$$\text{Vd} = \frac{\text{Dose}}{\text{Cp}^0} \text{ (mL)} \tag{7.8}$$

where Cp^0 is the concentration at time zero, when a drug is administered as an iv bolus. The concentration at time zero is typically not measured and is a value that is obtained from the y-axis intercept of the extrapolated log concentration versus time line. Vd can also be obtained from equation below:

$$Vd = \frac{CL}{K} \quad (mL) \tag{7.9}$$

If a drug exhibits a multicompartment behavior, the distribution of the drug is described by several volume terms and they are measured as follows:

$$Vc = \frac{Dose}{Cp^0} \quad (mL) \tag{7.10}$$

where the term Vc describes the volume of the central compartment into which the drug distributes instantaneously and a product of Vc and concentration of the drug in blood or plasma gives us an estimate of the amount of the drug in this central compartment. Another volume of distribution term Vd_β or Vd_{area} is defined as follows:

$$Vd_\beta \text{ or } Vd_{area} = \frac{Dose}{AUC \times K} \text{ in one compartment } (mL) \tag{7.11}$$

$$= \frac{Dose}{AUC \times \lambda_z} \text{ in multicompartment} (mL) \tag{7.12}$$

$$= \frac{CL}{K} \quad \text{or} \quad \frac{CL}{\lambda_z} \quad (mL) \tag{7.13}$$

where Vd_β is the volume of distribution term that relates the blood or plasma concentration to the amount of drug in the body during the terminal disposition phase (post distributive phase). The true distribution of a drug is given by another term, Vdss:
for iv bolus

$$Vdss = CL\left(\frac{AUMC}{AUC}\right) \quad (mL) \tag{7.14}$$

for iv bolus

$$Vdss = Dose\left(\frac{AUMC}{AUC^2}\right) \quad (mL) \tag{7.15}$$

for iv infusion

$$Vdss = \left[Dose\left(\frac{AUMC}{AUC^2}\right)\right] - \left[\left(\frac{t_i \times Dose}{2 \times AUC}\right)\right] \quad (mL) \tag{7.16}$$

where t_i is the infusion time and AUMC is the area under the first moment curve and is given by

$$AUMC = \sum\left[\left(\frac{C_n + C_{n+1}}{2}\right)(T_{n+1} - t_n)\right]\left(\frac{T_{n+1} + t_n}{2}\right) + \left(\frac{T_{last}C_{last}}{\lambda_z}\right) + \left(\frac{C_{last}}{\lambda_z^2}\right)(mg / mL)h^2 \tag{7.17}$$

$$Vss = R_0 T - \frac{CL \times AUC_{0-T}}{Css} \quad (mL) \tag{7.18}$$

where R_0 is the rate of infusion Vdss is volume of distribution at steady state and can give an estimate of the amount of drug in the body at steady state. Vdss gives a measure of drug distribution and is independent of drug elimination parameters, while Vd_β is influenced by changes in drug elimination.

In addition, one can also calculate the mean residence time (MRT) for a drug administered as an iv bolus, which is the average time that the absorbed molecules reside in the body and is given as

$$MRT = \frac{AUMC}{AUC} \quad (h) \tag{7.19}$$

$$MRT = \frac{1}{\lambda_z} \quad (h) \tag{7.20}$$

It is mathematically equal to the time when 63 % of the iv dose is eliminated from the body.

When the drug is given as an iv infusion the MRT is given as

$$MRT_{iv} = \frac{t_i}{2} + \frac{1}{\lambda_z} \quad (h) \tag{7.21}$$

where t_i is the time of infusion.

Time course of drug concentration

The blood concentration versus time profile of a drug administered intravenously as a bolus is mathematically given as follows for one and two compartment drugs:

$$C = C_0 e^{-Kt} \quad \text{(one – compartment iv bolus)} \, (\mu g / mL) \tag{7.22}$$

$$C = A e^{-\alpha t} + B e^{-\beta t} \tag{7.23}$$
$$\text{(two – compartment iv bolus)} (\mu g / mL)$$

where α and β are the distribution and disposition rate constants and A an B are the y-axis intercepts of the two straight lines.

When the drug is given as a continuous iv infusion the following equation describes the time course of the drug.

$$C = \frac{R_0}{KV}(1 - e^{-Kt}) \ (\mu g / mL) \tag{7.24}$$

$$C = \frac{R_0}{\text{Clearance}}(1 - e^{-Kt}) \ (\mu g / mL) \tag{7.25}$$

where R_0 is the infusion rate. When the infusion is continued after reaching steady state the equation simplifies as follows:

$$C = \frac{R_0}{\text{Clearance}} \ (\mu g / mL) \tag{7.26}$$

Extravascular administration

A drug that is administered extravasculary (such as oral, subcutaneous, intramuscular, intraperitoneal) undergoes a process of absorption, distribution, and elimination, which in addition also depends on the formulation factors and its interactions within the body. If a drug is given extravascularly, the initial concentration at time zero will be zero; the concentration will reach a maximum and then the drug concentrations will fall with time. In addition to the disposition rate constant, half-life, and AUC, several other specific parameters are associated with extravascular administration of a drug.

The rate of absorption of a drug from the extravascular route is a function of the rate constant of absorption k_a (units of 1/time) and the amount available for absorption. The k_a is calculated from the blood or plasma concentration versus time profile using a method referred to as feathering or residual analysis. Changes only in the absorption rate constant, such as due to formulation changes, can change the time course of the drug in the body but will not change the AUC.

The amount available for absorption is a product of fraction of the dose absorbed and the dose of drug given. With extravascular administration, the fraction of the dose absorbed from the site of administration may not always be one. This is especially true for drugs administrated orally.

The time to maximum concentration (t_{max} or t_{peak}) is the time when the concentration of a drug is at its highest within a dosing interval. At this time point,

the rate at which the drug comes into the body equals the rate at which drug is removed from the body. t_{max} is typically a value observed from the drug concentration versus time profile. This parameter is influenced by the rate constants associated with the absorption (k_a) and elimination (K or λ_z) of the drug from the body and is independent of the dose or the fraction of the dose absorbed or the volume of distribution of the drug:

$$t_{max} \ \text{or} \ t_{peak} = \frac{\ln(k_a / K)}{k_a - K} \ (h) \tag{7.27}$$

The concentration maximum C_{max} is the highest concentration observed during a dosing interval (that is, concentration at t_{max} or t_{peak}). This is typically a value observed from the drug concentration versus time profile. This parameter is influenced by the dose, volume of distribution, the fraction of the drug that is bioavailable F, absorption rate constant, and disposition rate constant:

$$C_{max} = \left(\frac{F \times \text{Dose}}{\text{Vd}}\right) e^{-kt_{max}} \ (\mu g / mL) \tag{7.28}$$

When a drug is given by extravascular route, it is not always possible to know the total amount cleared, as one will not know the total amount of drug that is bioavailable. Therefore, in order to get the clearance value one needs to know the fraction bioavailable:

$$\text{CL} = \frac{F \times \text{Dose}}{\text{AUC}} \ (mL / h) \tag{7.29}$$

So when administered dose is divided by the observed AUC one gets the apparent oral clearance estimate (CL/F):

$$\frac{\text{CL}}{F} = \frac{\text{Dose}_{oral}}{\text{AUC}_{oral}} \ (mL / h) \tag{7.30}$$

In a similar manner, we can only calculate the apparent volume of distribution Vd/F after extravascular administration of a drug. This is calculated from the intercept of the extrapolated terminal disposition phase of the log concentration versus time data after extravascular drug administration. Since the actual dose absorbed is not known after extravascular administration, the parameter estimated is Vd/F:

$$\frac{\text{Vd}}{F} = \frac{\text{Dose}}{\text{AUC} \times \lambda_z} \text{ (mL)} \tag{7.31}$$

$$\frac{\text{Vdss}}{F} = \text{CL}\left(\frac{\text{AUMC}}{\text{AUC}}\right) \text{ (mL)} \tag{7.32}$$

The MRT for a drug administered extravascularly is given as follows:

$$\text{MRT}_{\text{extravascular}} = \frac{1}{k_a} + \frac{1}{\lambda_z} \text{ (h)} \tag{7.33}$$

The mean absorption time (MAT) can be obtained from iv and oral data as follows:

$$\text{MAT} = \text{MRT}_{\text{extravascular}} - \text{MRT}_{\text{iv}} \text{ (h)} \tag{7.34}$$

In addition, one very important parameter for a drug that is administered extravascularly is the bioavailability. Bioavailability is a measure of rate and extent to which a drug is absorbed from a dosage form and becomes available to the systemic circulation or at the site of action. While the rate of absorption can be inferred from t_{max} and C_{max}, the extent of absorption is inferred from the AUC:

$$\text{Absolute bioavailability} = \frac{\text{AUC}_{\text{extravascular}}}{\text{AUC}_{\text{iv}}} \tag{7.35}$$

$$\text{Relative bioavailability} = \frac{\text{AUC}_{\text{extravascular}}}{\text{AUC}_{\text{non-iv}}} \tag{7.36}$$

The blood or plasma concentration of a drug administered extravascularly is shown in Figure 7.2a and b and is given as follows:

$$C = \frac{k_a F \times \text{Dose}}{\text{Vd}(k_a - K)}(e^{-kt} - e^{-k_a t}) \text{ (µg / mL)} \tag{7.37}$$

Multiple dosing of drugs

The pharmacokinetic properties of a drug ultimately determine the appropriate dose and the dosing frequency for that drug. In practice, drugs are administered on a chronic basis. Typically, a given dose is repeated every dosing interval T. The gen-

eral rule of thumb is to administer the drug once every half-life. However, from a practical point of view, a drug with a short half-life may have to be given much less frequently than its half-life and a drug with a half-life that is greater than 24 h may have to be given more often (at least once every day). Drugs such as tacrolimus cyclosporine and mycophenolic acid have a $T_{1/2}$ of 8–12 h and are given typically twice a day. Drugs such as sirolimus with a half-life greater than 24 h are given once a day. Monoclonal antibodies with a half-life in days are given once a week or much less frequently.

$$\text{Maximum amount at steady state} = \frac{\text{Dose}}{1 - e^{-KT}} \text{ (µg)} \tag{7.38}$$

Minimum amount of drug in the body at steady

$$\text{state} = \frac{\text{Dose}}{1 - e^{-KT}} e^{-KT}$$

In other words, the amount of drug in the body at any time during steady state can be calculated from the amount of the drug in the body after a single dose using the multiple dose function $1/(1 - e^{-KT})$, assuming that the pharmacokinetics of the drug are not altered on chronic dosing.

When a drug is taken repeatedly it may accumulate in the body. Accumulation represents build up of the drug in the body when it is given on a multiple dose basis. It is calculated as follows:

$$\text{Accumulation ratio} = \frac{\text{Css}_{\text{max}}}{\text{C}_{1\text{max}}} \tag{7.39}$$

$$= \frac{\text{Css}_{\text{min}}}{\text{C}_{1\text{min}}} \tag{7.40}$$

$$= \frac{1}{1 - e^{-KT}} \tag{7.41}$$

where Css_{max} and $\text{C}_{1\text{max}}$ correspond to the maximum concentration at steady state and maximum concentration after the first dose; Css_{min} and $\text{C}_{1\text{min}}$ correspond to the minimum concentration at steady state and minimum concentration after the first dose. Accumulation depends on the half-life of the drug and the frequency of drug dosing. If a drug is given more often than once every five half-lives it will accumulate in the body. The more often a

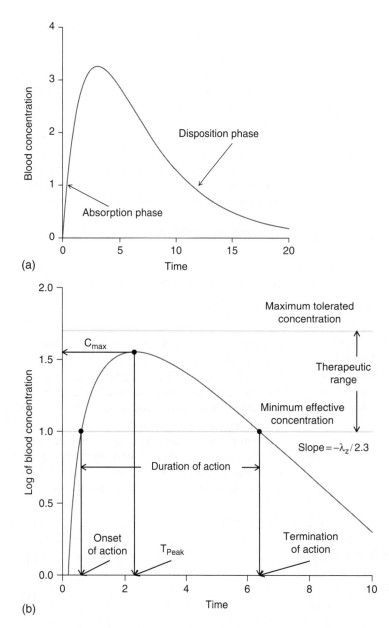

(a)

(b)

Figure 7.2 (a) Blood concentration versus time profile and (b) log blood concentration versus time profile for a drug administered by an extravascular route.

drug is given in reference to its half-life, the more of that drug will accumulate in the body.

Repeated administration of a drug leads to steady state when the dose lost during a dosing interval equals the dose administered (for iv dose) or dose absorbed (for extravascular dose). The concentration–time profile of a drug at steady state will be similar from one dosing interval to the next, assuming the drug does not alter its own pharmacokinetics.

Another parameter, fluctuation, represents the change in drug concentration over a dosing interval. Fluctuation is calculated as follows:

$$\text{Fluctuation} = \frac{C_{1\text{max}}}{C_{1\text{min}}} \tag{7.42}$$

$$= \frac{\text{Css}_{\text{max}}}{\text{Css}_{\text{min}}} \qquad (7.43)$$

Fluctuation depends on the half life and frequency of dosing of a drug. The more often a drug is given in reference to its half-life, the less the drug concentrations will fluctuate in the body.

Another parameter of interest is the average concentration of the drug at steady state $C_{\text{ss average}}$:

$$C_{\text{ss average}} = \frac{F \times \text{Dose}}{\text{CL} \times T} \; (\mu g / mL) \qquad (7.44)$$

$$= \frac{\text{AUC}}{T} \; (\mu g / mL) \qquad (7.45)$$

Average steady-state concentration is not an arithmetic mean of the maximum and minimum concentrations, but falls within the maximum and the minimum concentrations. Average steady-state concentration is a parameter that when multiplied by the dosing interval T gives one the AUC for the drug.

The blood concentration versus time course after multiple iv doses of a drug is described as follows:

$$(Cn)t = \frac{C_0(1-e^{-nKT})}{1-e^{-KT}} e^{-Kt} \; \mu g / mL \qquad (7.46)$$

where n is the dose number, t is the time after dose, and T is the dosing interval.

In the case of extravascular administration, the following equation describes the concentration versus time profile:

$$(Cn)t = \left[\frac{k_a F \times \text{Dose}}{V(k_a - K)} \right] \left(\frac{1-e^{-nKT}}{1-e^{-KT}} e^{-Kt} \right)$$
$$- \left(\frac{1-e^{-nk_aT}}{1-e^{-k_aT}} e^{-k_at} \right) (\mu g / mL) \qquad (7.47)$$

Pharmacokinetic parameters for a drug can be calculated after single dose or after multiple doses. If a drug is given more frequently than its half life, it will not be possible to get a good estimate of the $T_{1/2}$ of the drug during multiple dosing.

The AUC at steady state during one dosing interval is mathematically equal to AUC from time zero to infinity after a single dose:

$$\text{AUC}_{0-T} \text{SS} = \text{AUC}_{0-\text{infinity}} \text{ after single dose} \qquad (7.48)$$

Therefore, clearance of the drug can be calculated from AUC at steady state as follows:

$$\text{CL} = \frac{\text{Dose at steady state}}{\text{AUC at steady state}} \; (mL / min) \qquad (7.49)$$

If the pharmacokinetic study is conducted under non-steady-state conditions, it is important to exclude the AUC of the drug that comes from the previous dose and to include AUC for the study dose that spills into the next dose in order to get the correct AUC, using reverse superposition principles.

Loading dose

Since it takes five half-lives to reach steady state, it will take several days to reach desired concentrations for drugs with a long $T_{1/2}$. In such cases one can reach the desired steady concentrations faster using a loading dose:

$$\text{Loading dose} = \frac{\text{Maintenance dose}}{1-e^{-KT}} \; (mg) \qquad (7.50)$$

This indicates that for a dosing interval that is equal to the $T_{1/2}$ of a drug the loading dose should be twice the maintenance dose. In order to obtain steady state faster, a loading dose is useful for a drug like sirolimus, which has a long $T_{1/2}$.

Metabolite kinetics

Measurement of metabolites provides additional information on the disposition characteristics of a drug.

$$\frac{\text{AUC(m)}}{\text{AUC(p)}} = \frac{\text{CLm}}{\text{CL(m)}} \qquad (7.51)$$

where AUC(m) is the AUC for the metabolite, AUC(p) is the AUC for the parent drug, CLm is the formation clearance of the metabolite, and CL(m) is the elimination clearance of the metabolite. For example, knowing the AUC and clearance of mycophenolic acid and AUC of the mycophenolic acid glucuronide (MPAG) one can infer about the elimination clearance of MPAG in a patient using the above equation.

Table 7.2 Analytical methods/biological fluids used for measurement of immunosuppressive drugs.

Cyclosporine	Immunoassays, HPLC, HPLC–MS-MS	Blood
Tacrolimus	Immunoassay, HPLC–MS-MS	Blood
Sirolimus	Immunoassay, HPLC, HPLC–MS-MS	Blood
Mycophenolic acid	Immunoassay, HPLC, HPLC–MS-MS	Plasma
Leflunomide	HPLC, HPLC–MS-MS	Plasma

HPLC: high-performance liquid chromatography;
MS-MS: tandem mass spectrometry.

Factors that influence pharmacokinetic parameters estimated

Variation with biological fluid in which the drug concentration is measured

Pharmacokinetic parameters are normally calculated based on the drug concentrations measured in blood or plasma or serum (Table 7.2). Given that blood and plasma concentrations are normally different, the pharmacokinetic parameters obtained will vary with the biological fluid used in measuring the drug concentrations. The clearance parameters calculated for cyclosporine and tacrolimus are higher based on plasma concentrations than those calculated based on blood concentrations, as the blood-to-plasma ratio for these drugs is greater than one, indicating red blood cell uptake of these drugs. Since it is the blood that takes the drug through the organs of elimination, it is informative to calculate the blood clearance of the drug even if drug concentrations are measured in plasma using the following equation:

$$\text{Blood clearance} = \text{Plasma clearance} \times \left[\frac{\text{concentration in plasma}}{\text{concentration in blood}} \right]$$

(7.52)

Variation with assay methodology used

The pharmacokinetic parameters estimated are only as good as the measured concentrations of the drug in the biological fluids. It is important to utilize a sensitive and specific assay method (HPLC, HPLC–MS-MS) for measuring the concentration of the drugs in the biological fluids (Table 7.2). In the past, nonspecific immunoassays (radioimmunoassay, enzyme immunoassays) have been used to measure drug concentrations. Such assays measured not only the parent drug, but also some of the metabolites that tended to cross-react with the antibodies used. Pharmacokinetic parameters (CL, Vd) calculated using nonspecific immunoassays tend to be smaller than what is obtained using specific assay methods. With nonspecific assays the half-life estimated may either be longer than or similar to what is obtained based on drug concentrations measured using specific assay methods.

It is important to interpret the pharmacokinetic parameters in reference to the assay methods used.

Factors that affect the pharmacokinetics of a drug

Absorption

The rate and extent of absorption of drugs can be altered by several factors. These can broadly be classified into formulation factors, physicochemical factors, and physiologic factors. Formulation factors include disintegration and dissolution of the drug from the dosage form. Physicochemical factors include particle size, solubility, dissolution, and complexation. Physiologic factors include gastric pH, gastric motility, intestinal motility, surface area, fluid volume, food–drug interactions, drug–drug interactions, intestinal metabolism, and intestinal uptake and efflux through transporters.

According to the Biopharmaceutical Drug Classification System [11], drugs can be broadly classified based on their aqueous solubility and permeability into four classes. Class 1 consists of drugs that are highly soluble and highly permeable. These drugs are normally well absorbed if there is no chemical degradation, no complexation, and no significant first pass hepatic metabolism. For such drugs, dissolution from the solid dosage form is normally the rate-limiting step in the overall blood concentration profile. Class 2 consists of drugs that are poorly soluble but highly permeable. These drugs are normally rapidly absorbed if in solution in an absorbable form. Most of the immunosuppressive drugs, such as cyclosporine, tacrolimus, sirolimus, and mycophenolic acid, fall into this category. All of these drugs are fairly rapidly absorbed, as illustrated by the small t peak (1–4 h). Improved and consistent absorption of cyclosporine from the microemulsion compared with olive oil formulation also speaks to the importance of the availability of the drug for absorption from the dosage form. Dissolution will be the rate-limiting step for absorption of class 2 drugs from a solid dosage form. When generic formulations are manufactured it is important to keep this in mind. Class 3 consists of drugs that are highly soluble but poorly permeable. For these drugs, intestinal permeability will limit the absorption of the drugs. Class 4 consists of drugs that are poorly soluble and poorly permeable, and such drugs are not likely to be useful systemically.

A few years ago a modified version of the Biopharmaceutics Classification System (BCS) classification system was proposed [12]. This system, known as the Biopharmaceutics Drug Disposition Classification System (BDDCS), may be useful in predicting overall drug disposition that includes drug elimination process, involvement of efflux and absorptive transporters on oral drug absorption and food interactions. In this system the major route of elimination serves as the permeability criteria. Class 1 drugs are highly soluble and highly metabolized. Class 2 drugs are poorly soluble but highly metabolized, Class 3 drugs are highly soluble but poorly metabolized. Class 4 drugs are poorly soluble and poorly metabolized. Immunosuppressive drugs such as cyclosporine, tacrolimus and sirolimus belong to class 2 and are predicted to have predominate efflux drug transporter involvement, which has been experimentally shown.

The overall systemic availability of a drug can be predicted by the following equation:

$$F = f_a f_g f_h \qquad (7.53)$$

where f_a is the fraction of the drug that is not lost in the feces as unabsorbed drug, f_g is the fraction of the drug that is not lost in the gut and escapes gut metabolism, and f_h is the fraction of the drug that escapes hepatic metabolism [13].

f_a can be less than one if the drug is not completely absorbed, or is complexed in the gut, or degraded in the gut. f_g can be less than one if the drug is metabolized or effluxed in the gut. f_h can be less than one if the drug is metabolized in the liver. For a drug that is completely permeable and is absorbed completely, is not complexed with gut content or degraded in the gut, is not metabolized or effluxed in the gut, and is not metabolized in the liver, F will be equal to or close to one. Immunosuppressive drugs such as cyclosporine, tacrolimus and sirolimus are relatively well permeable, are not complexed or degraded in the gut, but are metabolized and effluxed in the gut wall and metabolized in the liver. The poor oral bioavailability of these drugs (15–30 %) is primarily related to the metabolism and efflux in the gut wall and minimally due to hepatic first-pass metabolism.

Distribution

The distribution of a drug in the body is influenced by various factors. The apparent volume of distribution of the drug is influenced by blood or plasma volume, total body water, drug binding to plasma proteins, and drug binding to tissue proteins. These parameters are related as follows:

$$V_{ss} = V_p + V_t(f_u / f_t) \qquad (7.54)$$

where V_p is the volume of plasma, V_t is the difference of the volume of total body water and plasma volume, f_u is the fraction of the drug unbound in plasma and f_t is the fraction of the drug unbound in tissues. Drugs such as tacrolimus, cyclosporine, and sirolimus have a large volume of distribution, indicating uptake and binding to different tissue proteins. Monoclonal antibodies typically have a small volume of distribution and are predominantly in the vascular space.

Metabolism

The total body clearance of the drug can be due to metabolic and nonmetabolic clearance. For a drug that is only cleared by metabolism, the total body clearance will be equal to its metabolic clearance. For a drug that is only metabolized by the liver, the hepatic clearance will be the metabolic clearance. The hepatic clearance CL_h of the drug can be influenced by the hepatic blood flow Q, the intrinsic ability of the liver to metabolize a drug CL_{int}, and the fraction of the drug that is unbound in plasma f_u as follows:

$$CL_h = \frac{Qf_u CL_{int}}{Q + f_u \times CL_{int}} \ (mL/min) \qquad (7.55)$$

The highest clearance of a drug by the liver will correspond to the hepatic blood flow. The highest ability of the organ to clear a drug will depend on the blood flow rate to that organ.

For drugs with low intrinisic clearance (limited ability of the liver to metabolize the drug – low-clearance drug), the equation simplifies to

$$CL_h = f_u \times CL_{int} \ (mL/min) \qquad (7.56)$$

This implies that, for low-clearance drugs, changes in f_u and CL_{int} will change the hepatic clearance and changes in hepatic blood flow (within physiological limits) will have limited to no effect on the hepatic clearance.

For drugs with high intrinsic clearance (high capacity of the liver to metabolize the drug – high-clearance drugs), the equation simplifies to

$$CL_h \approx Q \ (mL/min) \qquad (7.57)$$

This implies that, for high-clearance drugs, changes in Q will change the clearance, and changes in f_u and CL_{int} will have limited to no effect on the hepatic clearance.

In general, hepatic blood flow can be altered by physiological, pathological, and pharmacological factors. The intrinsic clearance can be altered by physiological, pathological, and pharmacological factors as well. Certain drugs, such as rifampin, phenobarbital, phenytoin, and carbamazepine, can induce enzymes (increase in intrinsic clearance) and certain drugs, such as azole antifungal agents, erythromycin, and ritonavir, can inhibit enzymes (decrease in intrinsic clearance). Several drug–drug interactions have been reported with cyclosporine, tacrolimus, and sirolimus, which are substrates for cytochrome P450 3A enzyme system in the liver and small intestine. In addition, herb–drug interactions involving increase in intrinsic clearance have also been reported with St. John's wort and cyclosporine and tacrolimus.

Such interactions can lead to loss of transplanted graft due to lower systemic concentrations of the immunosuppressive drugs.

The unbound fraction of a drug can also be altered by physiological, pathological, and pharmacological factors. Subsequent to a liver transplant surgery, the concentration of albumin will increase in liver transplant patients, leading to more binding of drug and a lowering of unbound fraction, as has been documented for mycophenolic acid [14]. Since mycophenolic acid is a low-clearance drug, this leads to a decrease in overall total body clearance of the mycophenolic acid with time after transplantation.

The clearance of a drug can also be influenced by age, gender, diet, other drugs, and environmental and genetic factors. It is well known that the clearance of cyclosporine, tacrolimus, sirolimus, and mycophenolic acid are higher in pediatric patients than in adults. Pediatric patients require a higher dose on a milligram/kilogram basis in order to have similar exposure to the adult patients.

For a drug that is metabolized in the liver, the fraction of a drug that is likely to be bioavailable can be predicted using

$$F = 1 - E \qquad (7.58)$$

where E is the extraction ratio of the drug in the liver. Since

$$E = \frac{CL}{Q} \qquad (7.59)$$

$$F = 1 - \frac{CL}{Q} \qquad (7.60)$$

$$F = 1 - \frac{Dose_{iv}}{AUC_{iv} \times Q} \qquad (7.61)$$

Therefore, knowing the iv dose and AUC and assuming a physiologic liver blood flow of 1.5 L/min, one can predict the theoretical availability of a drug that is administered orally. Deviation from the prediction can imply incomplete drug absorption, degradation of drug in the gut, gut-wall metabolism, or gut-wall efflux in cases of overprediction, and saturable hepatic metabolism in the case of underprediction by Equation (7.61).

Further modifying the above equation, one can relate F to blood flow, intrinsic clearance, and f_u as follows:

$$F = \frac{Q}{Q + f_u \times CL_{int}} \quad (7.62)$$

When CL_{int} is very low (a low-clearance drug), then F will approach one. When CL_{int} is very high, then

$$F \approx \frac{Q}{f_u \times CL_{int}} \quad (7.63)$$

In such cases, as Q increases, so F will also increase, as the drug spends less time in the liver, where it is eliminated. As f_u and CL_{int} increase, F decreases, as drug is cleared more readily. While changes in intrinsic clearance will have limited to no effect on the kinetics of a high-clearance drug given intravenously, after oral administration the changes in intrinsic clearance will alter the kinetics of high-clearance drugs as well.

Excretion

Kidney is the primary organ of drug elimination. Renal clearance CL_r of the drug can simply be obtained using the expression

$$CL_r = \frac{\text{Cumulative amount excreted in the urine}}{AUC} \quad (7.64)$$

$$CL_r = \frac{\text{Amount excreted over a time period}}{\text{Plasma concentration of drug at midpoint of urine collection}} \quad (7.65)$$

This expression can be used independent of whether a drug is given intravascularly or extravascularly.

A drug can be excreted through glomerular filtration and/or active secretion and may undergo tubular reabsorption. The renal clearance of such compounds can be given as

$$CL_r = (CL_{filt} + CL_{sec})(1 - F_{reabs}) \quad (7.66)$$

where CL_{filt} is the filtration clearance, CL_{sec} is the secretion clearance, and F_{reabs} is the fraction that is reabsorbed in the tubules.

Certain drugs can be excreted in the bile. If the drug is excreted unchanged or a metabolite of the drug that can be converted to the drug in the gut is eliminated in the bile, the drug can undergo a process of enterohepatic recirculation. This process increases the drug exposure in a patient. Mycophenolic acid, an immunosuppressive drug, undergoes conjugation and the conjugate is secreted in the bile and is cleaved and reabsorbed back into systemic circulation.

Individualization of drug dosing

Pharmacokinetic parameters reported for a drug are only a mean or average in a population of patients studied. Individualization of the dosing regimen of a drug will involve evaluation of the pharmacokinetics of a drug in a particular patient and adjusting the dose based on the observed parameters in order to obtain a desired drug exposure (Table 7.3). Typically, if the clearance of the drug in a patient is much higher than expected in that patient population, an increase in dose is a logical approach. If the $T_{1/2}$ in a patient is much smaller than expected in that patient population, then an increase in frequency of dosing may be considered. Such approaches are used in immunosuppressive drug dosing in certain patients. Pediatric patients not

Table 7.3 Steps in individualizing dosing regimen of drugs in patients.

Selection of a dose and dosing regimen

Administration of a drug to patients

Collection of biological fluids

Analysis of drug/metabolite concentrations

Pharmacokinetic calculations – noncompartmental and population pharmacokinetics

Interpretation of the data with patient covariates

Recommendation for dosage change

Follow up to evaluate performance

only require a higher dose than adults do, but also may need more frequent dosing due to the shorter $T_{1/2}$ compared with adult patients.

In routine clinical care of the patients it may not be possible to obtain several blood samples in order to obtain the AUC. In such cases, limited sampling strategies and mini AUC evaluations have been proposed. More commonly, drug exposure is inferred from measurement of the trough concentrations (lowest concentration in a dosing interval, typically just prior to start of the subsequent dose). In order to use trough concentrations as a surrogate marker of drug exposure it is important to document the relationship between AUC and trough concentrations. For immunosuppressive drugs such as tacrolimus and sirolimus, this relationship has been documented in several patient populations [15].

In summary, this chapter has provided some background information on generating and interpreting pharmacokinetic parameters for a drug. Understanding the limitations and assumptions surrounding the various parameters measured will help in properly utilizing these parameters in optimizing the drug therapy in a patient population.

References

1 Jambhekar SS, Breen PJ. *Basic Pharmacokinetics*. London: Pharmaceutical Press; 2010.

2 Ritchel WA, Kearns G. *Handbook of Basic Pharmacokinetics*, 6th edn. Washington, DC: APhA; 2008.

3 Bauer L. *Applied Clinical Pharmacokinetics*, 2nd edn. McGraw-Hill; 2008.

4 Gabrielson J, Winter D. *Pharmacokinetics and Pharmacodynamics Data Analysis, Concepts and Applications*, 4th edn. Boca Raton, FL: CRC Press; 2007.

5 Bonate PL, Howard DR. Pharmacokinetics in Drug Development, vols. 1–3. Arlington, VA: AAPS Press; 2004.

6 Hedaya MA. *Basic Pharmacokinetics*. Baco Raton, FL: CRC Press; 2007.

7 Krishna R. *Applications of Pharmacokinetics Principles in Drug Development*. New York: Kluwer Academic/Plenum; 2004.

8 Evans WE, Schentag J, Jusko WJ. *Applied Pharmacokinetics*. Vancouver, WA: Applied Therapeutics; 1992.

9 Rowland M, Tozer TN. *Clinical Pharmacokinetics. Concepts and Applications*, 4th edn. Philadelphia, PA: Williams and Wilkins Media; 2011

10 Gibaldi M, Perrier D. *Pharmacokinetics*, 2nd edn. New York: Marcel Dekker; 1982.

11 Amidon GL, Lennernäs H, Shah VP, Crison JR. A theoretical basis for a biopharmaceutics drug classification: the correlation of in vitro drug product dissolution and in vivo bioavailability. *Pharm Res* 1995;12:413–420.

12 Wu C, Benet LZ. Predicting drug disposition via application of BCS: transporter/absorption/elimination interplay and development of a biopharmaceuitcs drug disposition classification system. *Pharm Res* 2005;22:11–23.

13 Wu CY, Benet LZ, Hebert MF *et al*. Differentiation of absorption and first pass gut metabolism in humans: studies with cyclosporine. *Clin Pharmacol Ther* 1995; 58:492–497.

14 Pisupati J, Jain A, Burckart G *et al*. Intraindividual and interindividual variations in the pharmacokinetics of mycophenolic acid in liver transplant patients. *J Clin Pharmacol* 2005;45:34–41.

15 Schubert M, Venkataramanan R, Holt DW *et al*. Pharmacokinetics of sirolimus and tacrolimus in pediatric transplant patients. *Am J Transplant* 2004; 4(5):767–773.

CHAPTER 8

Therapeutic Drug Monitoring for Immunosuppressive Agents

Michael C. Milone and Leslie M.J. Shaw

Hospital of the University of Pennsylvania, Philadelphia, PA, USA

Introduction

Optimal immunosuppressive drug (ISD) therapy is critical to the success of solid organ and bone marrow transplantation. These drugs are also used in the treatment of autoimmune disorders. Their safe and effective use poses serious challenges due to highly variable pharmacokinetic behavior and the narrow therapeutic index of many of these agents. Therapeutic drug monitoring (TDM), often used synonymously with blood concentration monitoring, therefore plays an important role during ISD therapy.

An important prerequisite to successful TDM is the ability to measure the drug of interest. Using modern technologies that are available within most analytical chemistry laboratories, the measurement of most drugs, including ISDs and their metabolites, is readily achieved. Unfortunately, many of these analytical techniques, such as liquid chromatography with mass spectrometry detection (LC–MS) are highly complex, requiring analysts with specialized expertise and expensive equipment that is not available in most hospital laboratories. Immunoassay techniques for commonly used ISDs that can be run on high-throughput automated chemistry analyzers has made methods for measuring these drugs available to most moderate- to high-complexity clinical laboratories [1]. Although these routine immunoassay techniques are well validated

for their clinical applications, there are important differences between the various analytical techniques that can have a profound impact on the care of individual patients. Thus, the analytical performance of the methods used to measure drugs, including the ISDs, must be understood for the safe and effective use of TDM for these agents.

The complexity of the concentration monitoring process is one of the greatest challenges to the practice of TDM. Many individuals are involved in the TDM process. Each must perform his or her role correctly in order for TDM to be useful (see Figure 8.1). This complexity combined with the resource-intensive nature of monitoring limits the application of TDM to only a small number of drugs [2]. The decision to use TDM for a particular agent is generally based upon criteria as outlined in Table 8.1. For the most part, ISDs meet these general criteria, and some form of TDM is accepted as standard practice. Despite the widespread application of TDM to ISDs, the clinical utility of monitoring remains controversial for some drugs, such as mycophenolate mofetil (MMF) [3, 4]. This controversy stems, in part, from the challenges inherent in the complex TDM process; however, individualized drug therapy also requires more than just an understanding of a drug's pharmacokinetic behavior. The relationship between drug exposure and important clinical outcomes of toxicity or efficacy (the pharmacodynamic response) also varies

Immunotherapy in Transplantation: Principles and Practice, First Edition. Edited by Bruce Kaplan, Gilbert J. Burckart and Fadi G. Lakkis.
© 2012 Blackwell Publishing Ltd. Published 2012 by Blackwell Publishing Ltd.

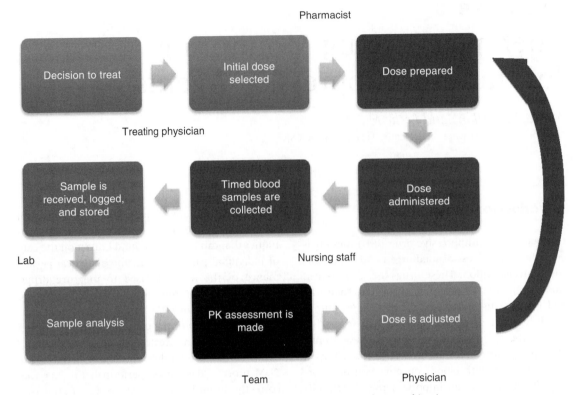

Pharmacist

Treating physician

Lab

Nursing staff

Team

Physician

Figure 8.1 The complicated feedback loop of monitored drug therapy. PK = pharmacokinetics.

Table 8.1 General criteria that support the need for drug concentration monitoring and applied pharmacokinetics (PK).

Concentration–response relationship exists for the drug
Narrow therapeutic index
Unable to adequately predict drug concentrations due to significant inter-individual variability in pharmacokinetic behavior
Treatment failure or toxicity is serious
Failure or toxicity is not immediately obvious

greatly for the commonly used ISDs [5]. Unfortunately, measured drug concentrations tell us nothing about the pharmacodynamic aspects of drug therapy in an individual patient.

In the broadest sense, TDM encompasses an array of testing modalities beyond traditional drug concentration monitoring. Serum creatinine and the white blood count are often used to monitor ISDs such as tacrolimus (TRL) and MMF respectively for toxicity. Monitoring for over-immunosuppression that may lead to opportunistic infection or under-immunosuppression that fails to prevent transplant rejection still poses significant clinical challenges. Both are recognized only after complications arise. Some transplant centers routinely perform biopsies of the transplanted organ in an effort to detect rejection early. This procedure, although somewhat effective, is invasive. It also only detects under-immunosuppression after it has already occurred. Thus, there is a significant need for improved assays that can be used to detect inappropriate immunosuppression before the onset of infection or rejection. Laboratory assays that provide information on the immunomodulatory pharmacodynamic effects of ISDs have been reported over the past several years [6], including one that is commercially available as an Food and Drug Administration-cleared test [7]; however, their role in clinical practice remains unclear.

Even with a highly informative pharmacodynamic and pharmacokinetic assessment of immuno-suppression, traditional TDM still requires that patients receive the drug prior to making an assessment with the associated risks. Pharmacogenomic testing offers the possibility of predicting the PK and pharmacodynamics (PD) effects of drugs prior to their administration (see Chapter 10). Unfortunately, even the most successful pharmacogenomic testing cannot fully characterize the PK and PD variability of any drug, as there are a multitude of nongenetic factors that contribute to PK and PD variability.

TDM in the future will likely encompass a combination of all three monitoring modalities. Integration of these modalities will not be simple; however, they are beginning to be applied clinically to some drugs, such as warfarin. While still early in their development, these combined monitoring approaches offer the possibility of truly individualized approaches to ISD therapy.

General principles of TDM

Concentration monitoring is employed for two primary clinical purposes. A drug concentration can be a useful diagnostic test during the evaluation of a patient experiencing signs and symptoms of reduced efficacy or toxicity. TDM data are also used in the prospective control of a drug's concentration in order to minimize the pharmacokinetic variability. The interpretation of a drug concentration depends upon the clinical context under which it is performed. This section will discuss some of the important pharmacokinetic and analytical concepts before delving into specific drugs. The reader is referred to texts on TDM for detailed discussions of these and other aspects of drug concentration monitoring [8–11].

Therapeutic range

A "therapeutic" range is always provided with a drug concentration to assist in its interpretation.

Generally defined as the range of drug concentrations associated with maximal efficacy and minimal toxicity, there is currently no standard defining an acceptable level of toxicity or efficacy, nor are there consistent procedures used to establish a therapeutic range. The 5th and 95th percentiles of a drug's concentration in stable patients without evidence of toxicity are sometimes used to define the boundaries of the range. In other situations, the range is defined through pharmacodynamic studies that have determined the relationship between a drug's concentration and toxicity and/or efficacy endpoints. The boundaries of the range are then set according to acceptable levels of both endpoints. Since the development of the range is probabilistic in nature, a concentration that is within the "therapeutic range" for a given drug does not exclude the possibility that signs and symptoms of toxicity experienced by an individual patient are related to the monitored drug. A concentration outside of the range also does not indicate that a patient will experience toxicity or reduced efficacy; however, the likelihood of either is certainly lower. Another limitation of these target therapeutic range studies is that the majority of them are retrospective in nature, although there are a few formal studies that have used a prospective study design based on retrospective data reviews and included a control empiric dosing arm (see section below on mycophenolic acid (MPA)).

It is important to recognize that the therapeutic range is not necessarily valid outside of the population used to establish it. This is particularly critical for ISDs, as most patients that are treated with these drugs receive additional immunosuppressive agents. A change in dosing of one drug may have a profound impact on the pharmacodynamic relationship of another. The nature of the transplanted organ (e.g., cadaveric versus living-related donor kidneys), age, and co-morbid illness can all have important influences on the pharmacodynamic response. The importance of these factors should not be ignored. Thus, the therapeutic range is a modest guide at best for monitoring therapy, and physicians must not overrely on it in treating patients with these drugs.

Testing error

Interpretation of concentration data is also challenged by the practicalities of collecting the data. Error is inherent in all measurement. Random error, the cumulative result of numerous immeasurable and uncontrollable variations that affect the testing process (e.g., electromagnetic field fluctuations), leads to analytical imprecision. While the causes of random error are immeasurable, the overall imprecision of an analytical method can be quantified, and the selection of analytical method is often based upon a determination of an acceptable level of method imprecision. In contrast to random errors, systematic errors are those errors that have a measurable and often consistent effect on the testing process. In some cases, these errors are sometimes quite insidious, such as calibration errors in liquid chromatography with tandem mass spectrometry detection (LC–MS/MS) methods, lot-to-lot variations in immunoassay reagents, or analytical interference [12]. Interferences may occur in all methods; however, they are particularly problematic for immunoassay platforms due to metabolite cross-reactivity and human anti-mouse antibodies (HAMAs) [13]. The increasing use of murine monoclonal antibodies as immuno-modulatory agents has the potential to increase the likelihood of HAMA development.

A major source of systematic error contributing to differences in results across laboratories is the lack of standardized reference materials (SRMs) for ISDs. In their absence, there is often great difficulty in ensuring that the calibration of an analytical method is similar from one laboratory to another, even those using the same method. All laboratories performing TDM in the USA must participate in external proficiency testing that is aimed towards avoiding gross inconsistencies and bias in measurement across clinical laboratories. Nevertheless, the potential for significant differences across laboratories is still significant due to both random and systematic errors. Proficiency testing data for TRL shows that concentrations within a clinically relevant range for this widely used ISD can vary by more than 100 % across laboratories even using the same analytical method [1].

Beyond the analytical phase of testing, there are many other places where error can creep into the testing process. Incorrect dosing and/or timing of drug administration can affect the ensuing concentrations. Although most of the ISDs have good stability in blood specimens, improper collection and/or handling (e.g., significant delays in processing or inappropriate storage conditions for MPA) can adversely affect the measured drug concentrations. Without adequate attention to these factors, TDM data can be rendered useless and perhaps even detrimental to the care of patients.

Applied pharmacokinetics

In most cases, the area under the concentration curve (AUC) is the best measure of exposure to a drug. Accurate estimation of AUC requires the measurement of 10 or more concentrations over an 8 or 12 h dose interval [14]. Since this intensive blood sampling cannot be easily done in most out-patient treatment settings, clinicians must often rely upon a single (e.g., pre-dose trough concentration) or limited number of drug concentrations to estimate the AUC. The concentration(s) chosen for monitoring may not be the best correlated with the AUC. Rather, concentrations such as the C_0 (concentration at the start of the dose interval, which is also often referred to as trough or pre-dose concentration) are chosen simply because it is most convenient or practical in the outpatient setting.

Since knowledge of the AUC is often desired, two approaches are commonly employed to predict the AUC from a limited set of concentration data. These methods are typically referred to as limited sampling or abbreviated sampling strategies to distinguish them from the more intense sampling used to calculate an AUC. The less-complex approach uses multivariate regression analysis to identify a limited set of concentrations that predict the AUC with a "reasonable" degree of uncertainty [15–17]. In practice, while this limited sampling approach is relatively straightforward to develop using statistical methods such as stepwise linear regression, they have limited tolerance for errors in the timing of specimen collection. The results of these approaches are also highly dependent upon the population used to develop the regression equations, and equations should not be transferred to other patient populations without validation. Despite these challenges, once these limited sampling methods are developed, they are relatively easy to implement in the clinic with tools as simple as a calculator.

Bayesian forecasting approaches are a bit more complicated to implement, but have several advantages over the simpler regression-based approaches [17, 18]. Based upon the application of Bayes' theorem, these methods can take into account past as well as current concentration data available for a patient. Thus, they offer the ability to limit intra-patient in addition to inter-patient variability. They also can incorporate information from population pharmacokinetic studies, such as important clinical factors (e.g., weight, age, or creatinine) that affect the pharmacokinetic behavior of a drug. The details of these statistical methods are well beyond the scope of this chapter.

While the literature is filled with various limited sampling strategies (LSSs) to predict AUC, there are relatively few prospective clinical studies demonstrating increased efficacy or reduced toxicity associated with most of these strategies. Owing to the increased complexity of limited sampling approaches, especially the Bayesian approaches, these strategies are also not generally available to most physicians caring for patients. The increasing use of computers in clinical practice continues to reduce barriers to these more-complex monitoring approaches. Electronic medical records also make the aggregation of the required clinical and laboratory data relatively simple. It is likely, therefore, that these LSSs will expand in the decades to come.

Notwithstanding the current limitations to using concentration data to guide drug therapy, concentration monitoring is still advocated for most immunosuppressive agents. Recommendations for monitoring are largely supported by both retrospective and prospective studies demonstrating a relationship between concentration data and pharmacodynamic endpoints. In a few cases, the risks and benefits of TDM have been evaluated through prospective, double-blinded, randomized clinical trials; however, these latter studies are fairly expensive to conduct, and they are generally restricted to kidney transplant recipients due to the large numbers of patients needed to achieve adequate statistical power. There is also limited incentive to study TDM, as it generates a logistical barrier to using a drug even if the benefits of TDM might outweigh the risks and increased costs associated with its use. Although cost is not generally considered in the decision to monitor, cost considerations are becoming increasingly important in the evaluation of any therapeutic agent or diagnostic test. TDM has the potential to improve the cost of transplant care by reducing complications of under- and over-immunosuppression that can be expensive to treat, especially graft failure that may require a second transplant. Cost should, therefore, be an outcome measure in all trials evaluating TDM for ISDs.

Monitoring of individual immunosuppressive agents

Cyclosporine A (CsA)
Rationale for monitoring CsA

Introduced in the 1980s, CsA revolutionized the care of transplant patients through its potent inhibition of acute cellular transplant rejection. Early studies with intravenous CsA demonstrated modest pharmacokinetics (PK) variability across healthy individuals; however, clinical use of the drug required an oral formulation to make it practical. The original formulation of CsA (Sandimmune) was an oral solution of CsA dissolved in oil due to the highly lipophilic nature of the drug. This solution was then mixed with a liquid such as juice prior to consumption. Slow and erratic absorption with poor bioavailability led to significant intra- and inter-individual variability in CsA exposure. The wide pharmacokinetic variability combined with the narrow therapeutic index necessitated the use of therapeutic drug monitoring during the early trials. Improved bioavailability of the CsA was obtained through reformulation into an oil-based micro-emulsion (Neoral) that was approved in 1995 [19]. The microemulsion formulation shows superior dose linearity with greater exposure due to the improved absorption compared with Sandimmune.

Despite these improvements in formulation, significant pharmacokinetic variability remains, with the dose-adjusted AUC of microemulsion-formulated cyclosporine demonstrating a >20% coefficient of variation (CV) across individuals [20].

In addition to the wide variability in absorption, the variability in CsA metabolism and elimination is also important. CsA is subject to numerous drug and food interactions. Grapefruit and red wine, as well as herbal medicines such as St. John's wort, exhibit significant interactions with CsA through their common metabolism by the CYP3A enzymatic system and membrane transport by P-glycoprotein (also known as MDR1). Commonly co-administered ISDs, such as corticosteroids and sirolimus, also exert clinically relevant affects on CsA PK.

The documented pharmacokinetic variability combined with the narrow therapeutic index of this drug provides a rationale for the use of therapeutic drug monitoring. Monitoring has been endorsed by experts in the field of transplant medicine and is a standard of care across the vast majority of transplant centers.

Over the past decade, a number of generic formulations of CsA have also been introduced on the US market. While these newer formulations have demonstrated bioequivalence to Neoral, most of these bioequivalence studies were performed in healthy subjects. The transferability of this data to transplant recipients is unclear, further supporting the use of therapeutic monitoring for this drug.

Measurement of CsA concentrations

The gold standard method for measurement of CsA is LC–MS/MS. This method demonstrates the greatest specificity for the compound along with a high degree of reproducibility. High-pressure liquid chromatography with ultraviolet detection (HPLC–UV) is also a highly specific analysis method, although not as specific as mass spectrometry-based methods. While chromatographic methods are the best currently available for CsA measurement, the equipment necessary for these methods is both expensive and complicated to operate, requiring specialized technical expertise. Thus, these methods are not generally available in most hospital laboratories outside of major academic medical

centers. Most transplant centers, therefore, use an immunoassay method for CsA concentration monitoring. In 2010, only approximately 10% of clinical laboratories in the USA were using a liquid chromatography-based method. The remainder use one of seven different commercially available immunoassay platforms [1].

Owing to the significant binding of CsA to cyclophilin proteins within red blood cells (RBCs), the concentrations of CsA in plasma or serum are generally quite low compared with total blood concentrations. Plasma and serum concentrations are also dependent upon the RBC mass or hematocrit of the specimen, which can be quite variable in transplant patients. Thus, methods for CsA predominantly use whole blood with an initial RBC lysis and drug extraction step prior to analysis. Immunoassay methods that employ a quick sample lysis without the need for a centrifugation prior to analysis have been developed, allowing some methods to be automated (e.g., CEDIA® CsA assay). Traditionally, LC–MS/MS methods were significantly more labor intensive owing to the need for organic solvent extraction prior to analysis. A number of methods have been developed for CsA that employ a simple, single RBC lysis and protein precipitation step followed by a sample cleanup using a C18 extraction pre-column in line with the liquid chromatography separation column. Although still a complex method, these developments have made LC–MS/MS much simpler and cheaper to perform.

Initial immunoassays developed in the 1980s to monitor cyclosporine were plagued by a number of problems including poor assay specificity, lack of assay standardization, and significant analytical variability. Complex matrix effects were also common and problematic. More specific assays were developed through the incorporation of monoclonal antibodies with greater specificity for CsA compared with its metabolites. An evaluation of immunoassay bias and accuracy of a number of commercially available immunoassay platforms by Werner Steimer demonstrated that significant and nonconstant bias is frequently observed between platforms when compared against the more specific HPLC method [21]. The most commonly used TDx monoclonal immunoassay method for cyclosporine showed an average bias of 57 % compared with HPLC. In some individual patients, the differences between the immunoassay and HPLC methods exceeded 100 %. Some of the observed differences are likely explained by the variable specificity of the platform antibodies to CsA metabolites compared with the parent drug. While the hydroxylated metabolites AM1 and AM9 and the demethylated metabolite AM4N lack significant immunosuppressive activity, they show anywhere from 2 % to as much as 20 % cross-reactivity, depending upon the immunoassay platform evaluated. Variability in metabolite production and elimination can, therefore, contribute substantially to the immunoassay-measured CsA concentration.

The nonconstant metabolite bias inherent in immunoassays in addition to any analytical error poses hurdles to applying concentration-monitoring data in the clinic. The differences across immunoassay platforms make it imperative to pay close attention to the methods used in any study when evaluating the use of TDM for CsA.

Clinical utilization and impact of monitoring CsA

The relationship between CsA exposure and clinically important endpoints such as nephrotoxicity and organ rejection was investigated early owing to the highly variable pharmacokinetic behavior of this drug. In one of the earliest studies of CsA PK, Lindholm and Kahan reported on a population of 160 consecutive kidney transplant patients treated with once daily intravenous or oral CsA [22]. Although transplant rejection (40 %) and graft loss (23 %) were significantly higher in this study compared with the incidence observed with current induction and maintenance immunosuppressive regimens, patients with higher CsA concentrations had significantly lower rates of graft rejection and higher rates of graft survival at 1 year. Subsequent studies have supported the pharmacodynamic relationship between CsA exposure and clinically relevant endpoints [23–28]. These studies have also confirmed the wide variability in pharmacokinetic behavior of this drug, particularly during the early part of the dose interval. Thus, concentration

monitoring of CsA is generally considered a standard of care across transplant centers.

Although $AUC_{0-12\,h}$ provides the best measure of drug exposure, the impracticality of making these AUC measurements, particularly in the outpatient setting, has led to the use of other surrogate measures of exposure. Since most of the variability in CsA PK occurs during the initial 4 h following dosing, AUC over this early post-dose period (e.g., $AUC_{0-4\,h}$) has been explored as a surrogate for the full dose interval $AUC_{0-12\,h}$; however, even these abbreviated sampling approaches pose real challenges to collection in the clinic [28]. C_0 (trough or pre-dose concentration), therefore, remains the most commonly used single, timed concentration for CsA monitoring. Unfortunately, the correlation between C_0 and $AUC_{0-12\,h}$ is relatively poor. Reported r^2 values for the relationship between C_0 and AUC_{0-12h} or AUC_{0-4h} generally fall within the 0.4–0.6 range. C_0 also appears to be a poor predictor of CsA efficacy or toxicity [23–28]. In a prospective study by Grant et al. that compared the PK of Neoral and Sandimmune formulations of CsA, AUC_{0-6h} demonstrated a significant correlation with graft rejection, with patients in the lowest quartile of AUC exposure showing a more than twofold increased incidence of rejection than those in the highest exposure quartile. No significant relationship between C_0 and efficacy or toxicity endpoints in either formulation group could be demonstrated [25].

No single, timed concentration is likely to provide as much information regarding CsA exposure as an AUC. Nevertheless, multiple studies support the 1 or 2 h post-dose concentration, close to the C_{max} for microemulsion-formulated CsA, as a significantly better surrogate for the 12 h dose interval AUC compared with C_0 with reported r^2 values generally >0.8 [23–27, 29–31]. Based upon this improved correlation, the 2 h post-dose concentration C_2 has been advocated as a single concentration monitoring alternative to C_0. Knight and Morris systematically reviewed the literature for studies directly comparing C_2 and C_0 monitoring in both de novo and stable kidney, liver, heart, and lung transplant recipients [32]. Although most retrospective studies demonstrate a relationship between C_2 and clinically relevant endpoints such as rejection and nephrotoxicity, the benefits of C_2 monitoring on clinically relevant endpoints in prospective clinical studies is more limited. Dosing differences for CsA have been observed for C_2 compared with C_0 monitored therapy. Of the 10 randomized, controlled studies comparing C_2 with C_0 monitoring, only a single study demonstrated a significant improvement in rejection and nephrotoxicity with C_2 monitoring; however, Knight and Morris point out that this study (presented only in abstract form) in Chinese kidney transplant recipients lacks a number of important details, such as the C_0 target range used or how well patients achieved the targeted ranges [33]. Thus, there is insufficient evidence currently to support C_2 monitoring as superior to C_0, despite the improved correlation with AUC. This may, in part, relate to the generally small study sizes available and the numerous other challenges to successful ISD therapy (e.g., compliance) that impact upon the clinically important endpoints.

Tacrolimus (TRL)

Rationale for monitoring

TRL, also frequently referred to by its investigational name FK506, was introduced into clinical practice in 1994 as an alternative to CsA. Although more easily formulated than CsA, TRL, like CsA, also suffers from highly variable absorption, metabolism, and elimination. The bioavailability of TRL varies from as low as 5 % to as high as 95 % in some individuals (mean ~25 %). Clearance varies by >25 %, with some studies showing as much as a 50 % CV. Much of the variability in absorption and elimination may be explained by genetic differences among individuals in the cytochrome P450 enzymes and the P-glycoprotein drug transporter (see Chapter 10). TRL PK is also affected by age, gender, several drug interactions, and liver function. Not surprising given the tremendous pharmacokinetic variability, there is little observed correlation between dose and pre-dose trough concentrations of TRL (see Figure 8.2, unpublished data).

Although PK is variable, TRL exposure correlates with the important clinical endpoints of rejection

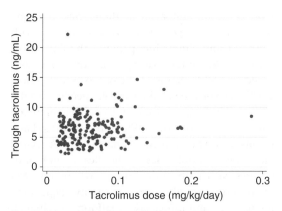

Figure 8.2 Tacrolimus trough concentrations correlate poorly with the weight-normalized tacrolimus dose.

and toxicity. Laskow *et al.* were the first to document a clear pharmacokinetic–pharmacodynamic relationship for TRL in a prospective, concentration-controlled exposure escalation trial [34]. In that study, 120 kidney transplant patients were prospectively randomized to three different levels of TRL exposure with low (5–15 ng/mL), intermediate (16–25 ng/mL), or high (26–40 ng/mL) target blood trough concentrations adjusted over 42 days. More rejection events occurred in the low target exposure group and more toxicity, including severe, life-threatening toxicity, was observed in the high target exposure group; however, serum creatinine and estimated glomerular filtration rate were not significantly different among the three target groups. Logistic regression analysis of trough concentrations in relation to both rejection and toxicity endpoints demonstrated a significant relationship. These findings were further supported by several subsequent studies. In a study by Venkataramanan *et al.*, 111 liver transplant recipients were prospectively evaluated over 12 weeks following transplantation [35]. A strong concentration–response relationship was demonstrated between nephrotoxicity and trough TRL concentrations in that study, with the risk of toxicity <10 % at concentrations under 5 ng/mL rising to >80 % at concentrations of over 20 ng/mL.

TRL dosing is presumed to benefit from concentration-monitored therapy due to the narrow therapeutic index of this drug and the overall variable pharmacokinetic behavior. The package insert currently recommends concentration-monitored therapy. In addition, several consensus conferences, most notably the Lake Louis conference in 1995, have supported this recommendation [36]. TDM for TRL is currently considered the standard of care in all centers using the drug.

Measurement of drug concentrations

Immunoassays predominate across the USA owing to their ease of use. Approximately 10 % of laboratories use a mass spectrometry-based reference method of analysis, generally considered the gold standard. Although HPLC-based methods have been reported, the poor UV absorption of TRL greatly limits the sensitivity of these assays and their utility.

Similar to CsA, TRL concentrations in the serum or plasma are quite low owing to high binding to immunophilin proteins, predominantly the FK506 binding protein 12, within all cells, including RBCs. Like CsA, plasma and serum concentrations are affected by the hematocrit. As a result, whole blood has become the principal sample used for TRL concentration monitoring, with extraction accomplished through cell lysis and protein denaturation steps that are similar or identical to those used for CsA analysis. In addition, LC–MS/MS methods have also been published. These methods increasingly utilize online C18 pre-column extraction, with some methods capable of analyzing multiple immunosuppressive agents simultaneously, including CsA, TRL, and rapamycin, by taking advantage of the tremendous specificity of mass spectrometry-based methods.

Immunoassays for TRL, like CsA, are also subject to interference by metabolites. Immunoassay results are generally consistent with LC–MS/MS results. Most studies report an average bias of 10–15 %; however, bias may depend upon the population studied. The bias can also be quite higher in some individuals. Accumulation of certain metabolites in patients with poor liver function is particularly problematic. The 15-O-desmethyl- and 31-O-desmethyl-tacrolimus metabolites exhibit close to 90–100 % cross-reactivity with the antibodies used in many immunoassays. Unlike

CsA, where the major metabolites appear to have little or no immunosuppressive activity, the predominant TRL metabolites also have a broad range of activity from 100 % (31-O-desmethyl-tacrolimus) to 0 % (15-O-desmethyl-tacrolimus) compared with the parent drug, further compounding the problems of cross-reactivity [37]. Fortunately, the fraction of total immunoreactivity that is contributed by these metabolites is small for most patients, so that monitoring of the parent drug appears adequate for routine monitoring.

Beyond the specificity issues, immunoassays for TRL are also increasingly challenged by the reduced concentrations presented with calcineurin-sparing immunosuppressive regimens. In our center, which is fairly representative of most centers in the USA, the target concentration range for renal transplant recipients beyond 3 months is 4–8 ng/mL. A study by Soldin et al. demonstrated that the CV of the most widely used immunoassay was greater than 12–15 % below 10 ng/mL, and the precision further declined with decreasing concentration [38].

Many of these assay deficiencies may be improved with new immunoassay designs, sample processing methods, and/or improved antibodies. Despite the fact that LC–MS/MS methods demonstrate extremely high analytical specificity, even these methods are subject to variability across laboratories due to differences in specimen processing and analysis. Interpretation of blood TRL concentrations must, therefore, be made only with a thorough understanding of the testing methods used by the laboratory performing the test.

In addition to whole-blood measurements, attempts have also been made to measure TRL directly in tissue using biopsy material from the transplanted organ. A study by Capron et al. measured TRL in liver biopsy material by LC–MS/MS [39]. These investigators reported a limit of detection (LOD) and a lower limit of quantitation (LLOQ) of 1 pg/mg and 5 pg/mg respectively compared with transplanted liver tissue concentrations, which ranged from 5 to 387 pg/mg. Although this analysis required a dedicated biopsy specimen for analysis with at least 1 mg of tissue dry weight, this study clearly demonstrated the feasibility of measuring

TRL within the transplanted organ. These investigators further demonstrated that the tissue concentration of TRL correlated better with rejection severity by histologic assessment in comparison with blood concentrations, raising the possibility that transplanted tissue might be a superior specimen for analysis; however, further study is clearly required to determine the safety and efficacy of this significantly more invasive monitoring approach.

Clinical utilization and impact of monitoring

Although TRL TDM is widely used, there is limited data from concentration-controlled studies to support its use. The study by Laskow *et al.* represents the only prospective trial that evaluated the ability of concentration-controlled therapy to achieve desired exposure levels [34]. Unfortunately, owing to ethical concerns with study design, a control arm managed without TDM was not included for comparison to demonstrate a benefit to monitored therapy. Nevertheless, monitoring of trough (predose) TRL concentration C_0 is, by far, the most commonly applied TDM approach. This is undoubtedly due to the ease of collecting this specimen over other timed specimens or the multiple samples required over a dose interval for AUC estimation. However, the strength of the correlation between C_0 and exposure as assessed in a full dose interval AUC has been the subject of much debate. The correlation between trough TRL and AUC is variable, with r^2 values ranging from 0.97 to 0.34 [40–45]. Despite the data supporting a relationship between TRL exposure as assessed by AUC and the clinically relevant endpoints of toxicity and efficacy, the correlation between blood TRL C_0 and clinically relevant outcomes is still somewhat controversial.

Alternative single time-point concentrations and LSSs have been explored to enhance the accuracy of estimating the TRL AUC while retaining a sample collection scheme that is reasonable to apply to the outpatient clinic setting. Ting *et al.* provide the most recent critical analysis of LLSs for TRL AUC estimation [15]. Of the seven published approaches available in 2006, all utilized multiple linear regression to derive relationships between either single or multiple timed TRL concentrations within the initial 6 h period following TRL dosing and TRL AUC. Only a single published study, by Dansirikul *et al.*, used prospectively collected data and provided validation of the derived LSS equation in a separate group of patients [46]. A few additional studies have been published beyond those reviewed by Ting *et al.* with similar results and limitations to the previously published studies [47–49]. These approaches may provide some utility in the evaluation of challenging patients; however, the improvement over traditional C_0 monitoring remains unknown. The transferability of LSS derived in one patient population to another, given the variability in transplant type, concomitant drug therapy, and genetic factors (e.g., CYP3A5 genetic differences among racial groups) that influence TRL PK, presents an additional major challenge to using any LSS. Caution must, therefore, be exercised with their use.

Notwithstanding the lack of randomized controlled trial evidence to support the use of TDM to optimize TRL therapy, the substantial evidence showing a correlation between blood TRL concentrations and toxicity has led to monitoring as standard of care. C_0 monitoring remains the primary approach even in light of the known limitations; however, AUC measurements should be considered for some patients, particularly those with clinical findings of rejection and/or toxicity that are inconsistent with the apparent level of immunosuppression.

Mycophenolic acid (MPA)
Rationale for monitoring

Mycophenolate mofetil (MMF, CellCept), the morpholinoester prodrug of MPA, was originally introduced in the USA in 1995. This drug has since become the predominant anti-metabolite ISD used in the transplant setting. Although monitoring is not currently recommended in the package insert, the variability in exposure to MPA across individuals taking a fixed dose of the drug soon became clear. MPA pharmacokinetic behavior is affected by several factors, including impaired renal and hepatic function, food intake, plasma albumin concentration, and co-administered drugs. Significant intra-individual variability in PK has also been observed. The greatest variability in MPA PK is noted in the initial 2 months following transplantation, when adequate immunosuppression is critical to graft function and survival. It has also become apparent from longer term PK studies that exposure to MPA increases over time due to reduced clearance of the drug.

A relationship between MPA exposure and the clinically relevant pharmacodynamic endpoint of transplant rejection has also been demonstrated. The randomized concentration-controlled trial (RCCT) [50], designed to evaluate the impact of MPA TDM on outcome, randomized 154 adult patients following kidney transplant into three groups with different MPA AUC targets. All patients in this study were receiving concomitant CsA and prednisone therapy as maintenance immunosuppression. Although patients within the three groups achieved average AUC target levels that were higher than originally proposed, a pharmacokinetic/pharmacodynamic analysis of this study demonstrated that the median MPA AUC over the 6 month time course of the study was inversely related to incidence of acute rejection. No relationship was apparent between MPA dose and efficacy. Three studies evaluated prospectively the utility of TDM using either (1) a Bayesian forecasting approach for AUC determination [51], (2) an abbreviated sampling AUC estimation approach [52], or (3) the pre-dose trough concentration [53] to adjust MMF dosing. Each of these three studies utilized a no TDM empiric dosing control arm. A full discussion of the details of these studies is beyond the scope of this chapter. The APOMYGRE study confirmed the earlier findings in the RCCT study that, in renal transplant patients whose immunosuppression regimen was MMF and CsA based, the control of MPA AUC to achieve target values of 45 (mg h)/L led to a lower rate of early acute rejection compared with the empiric dosed patients. On the other hand, the fixed-dose concentration-controlled (FDCC) and Opticept studies (each included a majority of patients on TRL therapy) did not demonstrate a significantly lower rate of rejection in concentration-controlled patients compared with empirically dosed patients [52, 53] in a setting where the rejection rates at 1 year were <10 % across the study arms, a value substantially below the anticipated rate of rejection based on earlier studies (~20 %) that likely led to underpowered studies. Nevertheless, for both of these studies a statistically significant relationship between AUC and risk for rejection (FDCC) or trough concentration and risk for rejection (Opticept) were shown. An important conclusion reached by the FDCC investigators was the recommendation for a higher starting dose of 3 g/day in patients receiving TRL would assure faster achievement of the target AUC of 45 (mg h)/L. The Opticept investigators discovered that at the extremes of weight there was a substantially higher AUC (low weight subgroup) or lower AUC (high weight group) compared with the range of AUC values achieved in patients whose weights were between the two extremes [54]. A number of additional studies in other transplant groups have shown similar pharmacodynamic relationships between MPA exposure and efficacy. The association between MPA AUC and adverse events such as suppression of hematopoiesis, GI toxicity, or infectious complications is less clear; however, several studies have supported a relationship between some of these endpoints and pharmacokinetic measures [55, 56].

Based upon the marked PK variability observed with MPA and the pharmacodynamic relationship of PK parameters to rejection outcome, several scientific societies and consensus conferences have advocated the use of concentration monitoring for patients undergoing treatment with MMF or enteric-coated MPA (EC-MPA) [57].

Measurement of drug concentrations
MPA is routinely measured in serum or plasma. Currently, HPLC–UV and mass spectrometry-based methods are the principle methods used for MPA monitoring. An immunoassay is also available outside the USA from Dade Behring (EMIT Mycophenolic Acid®), which can be run on automated clinical chemistry analyzers. The agreement between the EMIT immunoassay and the gold-standard LC–MS/MS method or HPLC is generally good. Not surprisingly, the immunoassay consistently overestimates the MPA concentration. Metabolites are likely a contributing factor in the immunoassay overestimation. A recently introduced automated receptor (human IMPDH)-based assay

provides results comparable to either validated HPLC–UV or LC-MS/MS methods [58]. Although the glucuronide metabolites of MPA are generally inactive as immunosuppressants, the acyl-glucuronide metabolite may play a role in toxicity related to MPA; however, this latter metabolite is generally quite low in comparison with the parent drug and the primary glucuronide metabolite. Methods have been developed to measure both metabolites of MPA using LC–MS/MS. Analyses of a subset of study data from the FDCC study have shown no predictive value for plasma concentrations of the acyl-glucuronide, but suggest that local gastrointestinal concentrations are the likely best correlate for gastrointestinal toxic effects of MMF [59]. Thus, the parent drug is the only moiety routinely measured.

MPA binding to albumin is also an important factor that restricts MPA clearance, with 99 % of MPA typically bound. Similar to the problems encountered with drugs like phenytoin and valproate, total MPA levels, while generally reflective of active drug concentrations, can occasionally be deceptive when conditions occur that displace drug from binding to albumin (e.g., uremia) [60] or with extremely low albumin concentrations. Under these conditions, measurement of free MPA concentrations may be a better correlate of clinical efficacy and toxicity than total MPA concentrations. Equilibrium dialysis followed by HPLC or LC–MS measurement of the protein-free dialysate represents the gold standard for free MPA measurements. However, since free drug concentrations measured by validated filtration methods have been shown to provide equivalent results compared with equilibrium dialysis, but are much more practical to perform [61], this is the preferred technique for MPA free measurement. Under most circumstances, MPA-free fraction is relatively constant in relationship to total concentration, and measurement of free MPA is regarded as a measure of interest in the research setting, but not in routine clinical practice.

Clinical utilization and impact of monitoring

C_0 measurements or AUC estimations based upon an LSS are the primary method used for monitor-

ing MMF therapy. Although a relationship between AUC and outcome exists, the clinical utility of concentration monitoring, particularly C_0 monitoring for MMF, has been questioned. Over the past decade, several studies were conducted to evaluate the clinical utility of prospective concentration-controlled MMF therapy. While these studies were anticipated to fully clarify the utility of monitored MMF therapy, the outcomes from these studies are conflicting and have done little to settle the controversies surrounding this area of therapeutic drug monitoring.

The data supporting the use of C_0 monitoring is the weakest. Although this time point is the most convenient for monitoring in the outpatient setting, C_0 shows a very poor relationship to AUC. This is likely due to the complex pharmacokinetic profile exhibited by MPA. MPA undergoes a significant enterohepatic circulation (EHC) leading to a complex concentration–time curve during a dose interval. There are typically two MPA concentration peaks over an MMF dose interval, with the intensity and timing of the secondary peak in concentration varying greatly from 4 to 10h following dose administration. Food intake and concomitant ISD use are important factors that can impact upon the EHC of MPA. In particular, CsA, in contrast to TRL, inhibits EHC. Thus, the ability of a single concentration such as the C_0 to predict the AUC over an entire dose interval is limited. The poor correlation coefficients that typically range from an r^2 of 0.23 to 0.66 support this; however, the correlation coefficients are better for patients on TRL compared with CsA as the concomitant ISD [53].

Sirolimus (rapamycin) and everolimus (Zortress)
Rationale for monitoring

Sirolimus, a cyclic 31-membered ring macrolide antibiotic, first isolated from *Streptomyces hygroscopicus*, a fungus isolated from soil samples collected at the Vai Atari region of Rapa Nui (Easter Island), exerts immunosuppressive activity by selective inhibition of mammalian target of rapamycin (*mTOR*). Sirolimus was introduced in the USA in 1999 as an ISD that, when administered together with CsA, reduced the incidence of acute rejection in renal transplant recipients [62]. Following this, in 2003 sirolimus was approved by the US Food and Drug Administration for a second indication, namely substitution for, and reduction of, the nephrotoxic burden of calcineurin inhibitors, CsA or TRL. Approved use of sirolimus is restricted to renal transplant patients >13 years old [63]. Like CsA and TRL, sirolimus absorption, metabolism, and clearance are highly variable and subject to clinically important drug–drug interactions. Oral bioavailability is low, with an average of 13.6 % (10.3–16.9 %, 95 % CI), elimination half-life is prolonged, 59.2 ± 18.5 h (mean ± SD), and trough concentrations vary widely within and between patients (%CV 45 % and 38 % respectively) [64]. Concomitant administration of CsA, diltiazem, ketocanazole, erythromycin, verapamil, or food cause increased sirolimus concentration, whereas rifamycin causes decreased sirolimus concentration [65, 66] As already discussed for CsA and TRL, processing of sirolimus via oxidative metabolism via CYP3A4/5 is the major metabolic clearance pathway, and the P-glycoprotein countertransport system is the major transport system governing gastrointestinal absorption and distribution into and out of tissues. These two processes are the sites for drug–drug interaction effects via competition for binding sites between sirolimus and interacting drug. Good correlation between trough sirolimus concentration and the 24 h dose-interval AUC was observed ($r = 0.96$) [64], thus supporting the use of this parameter for sirolimus exposure measurement. As with any therapeutic drug monitoring test, a key to ultimate reliability of trough sirolimus concentration, in addition to use of a qualified bioanalytical method, is systematically accurate timing of trough samples in relationship to the medication administration time.

As observed for CsA and TRL, distribution of sirolimus in whole blood is primarily into blood cells. In an investigation of sirolimus distribution in blood of stable renal transplant patients the blood to plasma concentration ratio (mean ± SD) is 36.5 ± 17.9 [64].

The extensive variability of sirolimus clearance from patient to patient explains the unpredictability of blood concentration per unit of drug dose.

Investigations of the relationship between steady-state trough sirolimus concentration and clinical effects (acute rejection and side effects) led to the recommendation of therapeutic drug monitoring for all patients taking sirolimus [63]. Close monitoring of blood sirolimus concentration is especially important at the initiation of therapy in conjunction with a loading dose, when there is a change in the dosage form of the drug, when there is significant change in liver function, or when concomitant CsA dosage is tapered or withdrawn. Kahan *et al.* provided the first retrospective analysis of sirolimus blood concentration versus clinical outcome data in a cohort of 150 renal transplant patients who received concomitant CsA [67]. Sirolimus was measured in whole blood samples using a well-validated HPLC–UV methodology [68]. According to their analyses, there was a significant association between trough sirolimus concentrations <5 ng/mL and the incidence of acute rejection. Trough concentrations were reported to be significantly higher in subjects at the time of experiencing the following side effects: thrombocytopenia (<100 000 mm^3), leukopenia (<4000 mm^3), and hypertriglyceridemia (>400 mg/ dL), leading to a provisional recommendation of 15 ng/mL as the upper end of the therapeutic range. Statistical analyses of sirolimus concentration versus acute rejection in five clinical studies during the clinical development of the drug in renal transplant patients receiving concomitant CsA led to the definition of 5 ng/mL as the lower end of the therapeutic range [69].

Measurement of drug concentrations

In the USA, the majority of laboratories use an immunoassay for sirolimus measurement. The microparticle enzyme immunoassay (MEIA) had been the most widely used immunoassay until its discontinuation by Abbott Laboratories in early 2010. The MEIA method was replaced by the Abbott Architect chemiluminescence immunoassay, and the latter is now the most commonly used immunoassay in clinical laboratories. LC–MS/MS is used in 25 % of US laboratories according to the 2010 College of American Pathologists Proficiency Testing survey for sirolimus TDM [1] and 57 % of participants in the Analytical Services International proficiency testing scheme use this more selective technology [70]. According to study data developed in our laboratory, sirolimus concentration values using the Architect average 20 % (20 ± 14 %) higher than LC–MS/MS in transplant patient blood samples. Since there are substantial sample-to-sample differences in the high bias, the results from one assay method cannot be converted to the other by a simple proportionality factor. Metabolites of sirolimus are the likely contributor to the immuno-assay bias. Hydroxy-, dihydroxy-, dimethyl- and didemethyl-sirolimus metabolites have been detected in human blood samples from patients on sirolimus, CsA, and corticosteroid therapy, and their aggregate concentration was reported to be greater than that of the parent drug [71]. The currently available therapeutic range guideline is based on parent drug sirolimus measurement by HPLC methodology. Since the more commonly used immunoassays like the Architect produce a result with a high but variable bias, and since contemporary immunosuppression regimens differ from those used at the time the therapeutic range data were developed, further studies are needed to develop new therapeutic range information to guide the use of this procedure in contemporary practice.

Clinical utilization and impact of monitoring

Although sirolimus TDM is considered a standard of practice for transplant patients prescribed this immunosuppressant, and is recommended by the manufacturer, there is only retrospective concentration versus clinical outcome data for the combination of sirolimus, CsA, and corticosteroid therapy. The study of Kahan *et al.* [67] and report of Zimmerman [69] provide good retrospective evidence that <5 ng/mL is associated with significantly increased risk for acute rejection using HPLC-based methodology. However, owing to the widespread use of immunoassays with varying metabolite bias, use of different regimens (e.g., sirolimus in combination with TRL), and lack of prospective studies of using therapeutic drug monitoring of sirolimus in contemporary practice, further investigations are warranted. A

memorandum was circulated by Wyeth (now Pfizer) to prescribers at the time of the introduction of the new Architect immunoassay stating that "switching between platforms, whether between immunoassay platforms or between immunoassay and HPLC, can produce differing results that may be clinically significant" [72]. This information and emphasis onthe differences in concentrations measured by different methods is an important statement of caution when interpreting sirolimus concentration data.

Everolimus (Zortress)
Rationale for monitoring

In April 2010, everolimus, a more water-soluble analog of sirolimus was approved for use in CsA-sparing regimens, including the requirement for adjusting everolimus doses using target trough blood concentrations in renal transplant patients. The target ranges were established from earlier studies [73–76] and used prospectively to demonstrate equivalent acute rejection rates compared with the combination of traditional full dose/blood exposure levels of CsA and empiric dose MMF [77]. Using LC–MS/MS methodology in all of these studies, a trough everolimus concentration of <3 ng/mL was identified as the low threshold concentration below which risk for acute rejection is increased significantly in regimens that include everolimus, CsA, and corticosteroid.

The mechanism of action and pharmacodynamic effects of everolimus are comparable to those for sirolimus. Wide variability of metabolism and clearance for everolimus as for CsA, TRL, and sirolimus is governed by CYP3A5/5 and P-glycoprotein, and the observed drug–drug interactions are comparable to that observed for sirolimus. The within- and between-patient variability of dose-interval AUC was 27 % and 31 % respectively in a study in 731 renal transplant patients studied over a 6 month period post-transplantation [78]. There was no detectable influence of sex, age (16–66 years), or weight (42–132 kg) on AUC, but everolimus exposure was significantly lower by an average of 20 % in blacks. In a study of 659 AUC profiles the correlation between trough concentration and overall exposure (AUC) there was a significant linear correlation with a coefficient (*r* value) of 0.89 and corresponding coefficient of determination (*r²* value) of 0.79. Similar degrees of correlation between everolimus trough concentration and thrombocytopenia, leukopenia, hypertriglyceridemia, or hypercholesterolemia were observed in an investigation of 54 stable renal transplant patients (18–68 years) [79].

Measurement of drug concentrations

The bioanalytical method used for measurement of everolimus concentration in the pharmacokinetic assessments and prospective therapeutic drug monitoring protocols of many clinical investigations is a validated HPLC–tandem mass spectrometry method [73, 77]. Use of this bioanalytical methodology provides for sensitive and selective measurement of everolimus, and this attribute is important for reliable measurement of blood concentrations at the low end of the recommended target concentration range (3 ng/mL) in currently utilized immunosuppression protocols [77, 80] In the future we can anticipate the availability of immunoassays for everolimus and it will be essential to understand the comparison between these methods and any biases between them.

Conclusion

Monitored drug therapy has undergone a tremendous change over the past quarter of a century with the increasing availability of bench-top LC–MS/MS and immunoassay techniques in many clinical laboratories. The possibility of accurately and specifically measuring almost any drug in any biological fluid is a reality. While TDM has become a standard of care for most ISDs, TDM practices will continue to evolve with the field of transplantation. New ISDs, such as the protein kinase C inhibitor sotrastaurin, exhibit PK variability comparable to that seen with currently used ISDs and may benefit from monitoring therapy [81]. Although TDM of biologic drugs such as belatacept have not been reported in clinical trials to date, potentially useful

pharmacodynamic assays that can be performed on blood specimens have been described [82]. Many of the novel ISDs in clinical development may also impact the PK and/or PD of existing drugs, such as the interaction between sotrastaurin and TRL, requiring changes in the way that we monitor existing drugs. We are also likely to see a number of pharmacodynamic and pharmacogenetic assays for ISDs in the next decade. Integrating these newer assays with traditional PK monitoring schemes offers the potential for increasingly personalized therapy for these complex patients. With the paucity of new drugs in the pipeline, improving our ability to use existing drugs will likely be critical to the success of transplantation well into the foreseeable future.

Abbreviations

AUC	area under the concentration–time curve
AUC$_{0-12h}$	AUC from time = 0 h to time = 12 h
AUC$_{0-4h}$	AUC from time = 0 h to time = 4 h
AUC$_{0-6h}$	AUC from time = 0 h to time = 6 h
C$_0$	concentration at time = 0 h (often termed pre-dose or trough concentration)
CsA	cyclosporine A
CV	coefficient of variation
CYP3A	cytochrome P450 3A
EC-MPA	enteric-coated mycophenolic acid
EHC	enterohepatic circulation
EMIT	enzyme-multiplied immunoassay technique
HAMA	human anti-mouse antibody
HPLC	high-pressure liquid chromatography
HPLC–UV	high-pressure liquid chromatography with ultraviolet detection
IMPDH	inosine monophosphate dehydrogenase
ISDs	immunosuppressive drugs
LC–MS/MS	liquid chromatography with tandem mass spectrometry detection
LLOQ	lower limit of quantitation
LOD	limit of detection
LSS	limited sampling strategy

MDR1 multidrug resistance gene 1 (also known as P-glycoprotein)
MEIA microparticle enzyme immunoassay
MMF mycophenolate mofetil
MPA mycophenolic acid
PD Pharmacodynamics
PK Pharmacokinetics
SRM standardized reference material
TDM therapeutic drug monitoring
TRL Tacrolimus

References

1 2010 Immunosuppressive Drug Proficiency Testing Survey Results. College of American Pathologists; 2010.

2 Schumacher GE, Barr JT. Therapeutic drug monitoring: is it cost-effective? *Expert Rev Pharmacoecon Outcomes Res* 2002;2(6):619–624.

3 Van Gelder T. Mycophenolate blood level monitoring: recent progress. *Am J Transplant* 2009;9(7):1495–1499.

4 Barraclough KA, Staatz CE, Isbel NM, Johnson DW. Therapeutic monitoring of mycophenolate in transplantation: is it justified? *Curr Drug Metab* 2009;10(2):179–187.

5 Yatscoff RW, Aspeslet LJ, Gallant HL. Pharmacodynamic monitoring of immunosuppressive drugs. *Clin Chem* 1998;44(2):428–432.

6 Oellerich M, Barten M, Armstrong V. Biomarkers: the link between therapeutic drug monitoring and pharmacodynamics. *Ther Drug Monit* 2006;28(1):35–38.

7 Kowalski R, Post D, Schneider M *et al.* Immune cell function testing: an adjunct to therapeutic drug monitoring in transplant patient management. *Clin Transplant* 2003;17(2):77–88.

8 Burton ME. *Applied Pharmacokinetics & Pharmacodynamics: Principles of Therapeutic Drug Monitoring*, 4th edn. Baltimore: Lippincott Williams & Wilkins; 2006.

9 Hammett-Stabler CA, Dasgupta A (eds.). *Therapeutic Drug Monitoring Data: A Concise Guide*, 3rd edn. Washington, DC: AACC Press; 2007.

10 Rowland M, Tozer TN. *Clinical Pharmacokinetics, Concepts and Applications*. Philadelphia: Lea & Febiger; 1980.

11 Schumacher GE. *Therapeutic Drug Monitoring*. Norwalk, CT: Appleton & Lange; 1995.

12 Tietz NW, Burtis CA, Ashwood ER, Bruns DE. *Tietz Textbook of Clinical Chemistry and Molecular Diagnostics*, 4th edn. St. Louis, MO.: Elsevier Saunders; 2006.

13 Kricka LJ. Human anti-animal antibody interferences in immunological assays. *Clin Chem* 1999;45(7):942–956.

14 Gibaldi M, Perrier D. *Pharmacokinetics. Drugs and the Pharmaceutical Sciences*, 2nd edn. New York: Dekker; 1982, pp. 445–449.

15 Ting L, Villeneuve E, Ensom M. Beyond cyclosporine: a systematic review of limited sampling strategies for other immunosuppressants. *Ther Drug Monit* 2006;28(3):419–430.

16 Bruchet NK, Ensom MHH. Limited sampling strategies for mycophenolic acid in solid organ transplantation: a systematic review. *Expert Opin Drug Metab Toxicol* 2009;5(9):1079–1097.

17 Marquet P. Clinical application of population pharmacokinetic methods developed for immunosuppressive drugs. *Ther Drug Monit* 2005;27(6):727–732.

18 Jelliffe RW, Schumitzky A, Bayard D *et al.* Model-based, goal-oriented, individualised drug therapy. Linkage of population modelling, new "multiple model" dosage design, Bayesian feedback and individualised target goals. *Clin Pharmacokinet* 1998;34(1):57–77.

19 Dunn CJ, Wagstaff AJ, Perry CM *et al.* Cyclosporin: an updated review of the pharmacokinetic properties, clinical efficacy and tolerability of a microemulsion-based formulation (neoral)1 in organ transplantation. *Drugs* 2001;61(13):1957–2016.

20 Keown P, Landsberg D, Halloran P *et al.* A randomized, prospective multicenter pharmacoepidemiologic study of cyclosporine microemulsion in stable renal graft recipients. Report of the Canadian Neoral Renal Transplantation Study Group. *Transplantation* 1996;62(12):1744–1752.

21 Steimer W. Performance and specificity of monoclonal immunoassays for cyclosporine monitoring: how specific is specific? *Clin Chem* 1999;45(3):371–381.

22 Lindholm A, Kahan BD. Influence of cyclosporine pharmacokinetics, trough concentrations, and AUC monitoring on outcome after kidney transplantation. *Clin Pharmacol Ther* 1993;54(2):205–218.

23 Clase CM, Mahalati K, Kiberd BA *et al.* Adequate early cyclosporin exposure is critical to prevent renal allograft rejection: patients monitored by absorption profiling. *Am J Transplant* 2002;2(8):789–795.

24 Cantarovich M, Barkun JS, Tchervenkov JI *et al.* Comparison of neoral dose monitoring with cyclosporine through levels versus 2-hr postdose levels in

stable liver transplant patients. *Transplantation* 1998; 66(12):1621–1627.

25 Grant D, Kneteman N, Tchervenkov J *et al.* Peak cyclosporine levels (Cmax) correlate with freedom from liver graft rejection: results of a prospective, randomized comparison of neoral and sandimmune for liver transplantation (NOF-8). *Transplantation* 1999; 67(8):1133–1137.

26 Barakat O, Peaston R, Rai R *et al.* Clinical benefit of monitoring cyclosporine C2 and C4 in long-term liver transplant recipients. *Transplant Proc* 2002;34(5): 1535–1537.

27 International Neoral Renal Transplantation Study Group. Cyclosporine microemulsion (Neoral) absorption profiling and sparse-sample predictors during the first 3 months after renal transplantation. *Am J Transplant* 2002;2(2):148–156.

28 Mahalati K, Belitsky P, West K *et al.* Approaching the therapeutic window for cyclosporine in kidney transplantation: a prospective study. *J Am Soc Nephrol* 2001;12(4):828–833.

29 Cantarovich M, Barkun J, Besner JG *et al.* Cyclosporine peak levels provide a better correlation with the area-under-the-curve than trough levels in liver transplant patients treated with Neoral. *Transplant Proc* 1998; 30(4):1462–1463.

30 Cantarovich M, Besner JG, Barkun JS *et al.* Two-hour cyclosporine level determination is the appropriate tool to monitor Neoral therapy. *Clin Transplant* 1998; 12(3):243–249.

31 Jaksch P, Kocher A, Neuhauser P *et al.* Monitoring C2 level predicts exposure in maintenance lung transplant patients receiving the microemulsion formulation of cyclosporine (Neoral). *J Heart Lung Transplant* 2005;24(8):1076–1080.

32 Knight SR, Morris PJ. The clinical benefits of cyclosporine C2-level monitoring: a systematic review. *Transplantation* 2007;83(12):1525–1535.

33 Wang X, Xu D (eds.). Using Neoral C2 monitoring as the predictor in de novo renal transplant patients: a prospective study. *XIXth International Congress of the Transplantation Society*; 2002, Aug 25–30, Miami, FL.

34 Laskow DA, Vincenti F, Neylan JF *et al.* An open-label, concentration-ranging trial of FK506 in primary kidney transplantation: a report of the United States Multicenter FK506 Kidney Transplant Group. *Transplantation* 1996;62(7):900–905.

35 Venkataramanan R, Shaw LM, Sarkozi L *et al.* Clinical utility of monitoring tacrolimus blood concentrations in liver transplant patients. *J Clin Pharmacol* 2001; 41(5):542–551.

36 Soldin SJ, Shaw LM, Yatscoff RW (eds.). *Proceedings of the International Consensus Conference on Immunosuppressive Drugs*, Lake Louise, Alberta, Canada, May 5–7, 1995. *Ther Drug Monit 1995*;17(6):559–703.

37 Murthy JN, Davis DL, Yatscoff RW, Soldin SJ. Tacrolimus metabolite cross-reactivity in different tacrolimus assays. *Clin Biochem* 1998;31(8):613–617.

38 Soldin SJ, Steele BW, Witte DL *et al.* Lack of specificity of cyclosporine immunoassays. Results of a College of American Pathologists Study. *Arch Pathol Lab Med* 2003;127(1):19–22.

39 Capron A, Lerut J, Verbaandert C *et al.* Validation of a liquid chromatography-mass spectrometric assay for tacrolimus in liver biopsies after hepatic transplantation: correlation with histopathologic staging of rejection. *Ther Drug Monit* 2007;29(3):340–348.

40 Jorgensen K, Povlsen J, Madsen S *et al.* C2 (2-h) levels are not superior to trough levels as estimates of the area under the curve in tacrolimus-treated renal-transplant patients. *Nephrol Dial Transplant* 2002;17(8):1487–1490.

41 Jorgensen KA, Povlsen JV, Poulsen JH. Optimal time for determination of blood tacrolimus level. *Transplant Proc* 2001;33(7–8):3164–3165.

42 Braun F, Peters B, Schutz E *et al.* Therapeutic drug monitoring of tacrolimus early after liver transplantation. *Transplant Proc* 2002;34(5):1538–1539.

43 Wong KM, Shek CC, Chau KF, Li CS. Abbreviated tacrolimus area-under-the-curve monitoring for renal transplant recipients. *Am J Kidney Dis* 2000;35(4): 660–666.

44 Cantarovich M, Fridell J, Barkun J *et al.* Optimal time points for the prediction of the area-under-the-curve in liver transplant patients receiving tacrolimus. *Transplant Proc* 1998;30(4):1460–1461.

45 Ku YM, Min DI. An abbreviated area-under-the-curve monitoring for tacrolimus in patients with liver transplants. *Ther Drug Monit* 1998;20(2):219–223.

46 Dansirikul C, Staatz CE, Duffull SB *et al.* Sampling times for monitoring tacrolimus in stable adult liver transplant recipients. *Ther Drug Monit* 2004;26(6): 593–599.

47 Armendáriz Y, Pou L, Cantarell C *et al.* Evaluation of a limited sampling strategy to estimate area under the curve of tacrolimus in adult renal transplant patients. *Ther Drug Monit* 2005;27(4):431–434.

48 Delaloye JR, Kassir N, Lapeyraque AL *et al.* Limited sampling strategies for monitoring tacrolimus in pediatric liver transplant recipients. *Ther Drug Monit* 2011;33(4):380–386.

49 Miura M, Satoh S, Niioka T *et al.* Limited sampling strategy for simultaneous estimation of the area under

the concentration-time curve of tacrolimus and mycophenolic acid in adult renal transplant recipients. *Ther Drug Monit* 2008;30(1):52–59.

50 Hale MD, Nicholls AJ, Bullingham RE *et al*. The pharmacokinetic-pharmacodynamic relationship for mycophenolate mofetil in renal transplantation. *Clin Pharmacol Ther* 1998;64(6):672–683.

51 Le Meur Y, Buchler M, Thierry A *et al*. Individualized mycophenolate mofetil dosing based on drug exposure significantly improves patient outcomes after renal transplantation. *Am J Transplant* 2007;7(11): 2496–2503.

52 Van Gelder T, Silva HT, de Fijter JW *et al*. Comparing mycophenolate mofetil regimens for de novo renal transplant recipients: the fixed-dose concentration-controlled trial. *Transplantation* 2008;86(8):1043–1051.

53 Gaston RS, Kaplan B, Shah T *et al*. Fixed- or controlled-dose mycophenolate mofetil with standard- or reduced-dose calcineurin inhibitors: the Opticept trial. *Am J Transplant* 2009;9(7):1607–1619.

54 Kaplan B, Gaston RS, Meier-Kriesche HU *et al*. Mycophenolic acid exposure in high- and low-weight renal transplant patients after dosing with mycophenolate mofetil in the Opticept trial. *Ther Drug Monit* 2010;32(2):224–227.

55 Mourad M, Malaise J, Chaib Eddour D *et al*. *Correlation of mycophenolic acid pharmacokinetic parameters with side effects in kidney transplant patients treated with mycophenolate mofetil. Clin Chem* 2001;47(1):88–94.

56 Weber LT, Shipkova M, Armstrong VW *et al*. The pharmacokinetic–pharmacodynamic relationship for total and free mycophenolic acid in pediatric renal transplant recipients: a report of the German Study Group on Mycophenolate Mofetil Therapy. *J Am Soc Nephrol* 2002;13(3):759–768.

57 Van Gelder T, Le Meur Y, Shaw LM *et al*. Therapeutic drug monitoring of mycophenolate mofetil in transplantation. *Ther Drug Monit* 2006;28(2):145–154.

58 Brandhorst G, Marquet P, Shaw LM *et al*. Multicenter evaluation of a new inosine monophosphate dehydrogenase inhibition assay for quantification of total mycophenolic acid in plasma. *Ther Drug Monit* 2008; 30(4):428–433.

59 Heller T, van Gelder T, Budde K *et al*. Plasma concentrations of mycophenolic acid acyl glucuronide are not associated with diarrhea in renal transplant recipients. *Am J Transplant* 2007;7(7):1822–1831.

60 Kaplan B, Meier-Kriesche HU, Vaghela M *et al*. Withdrawal of mycophenolate mofetil in stable renal transplant recipients. *Transplantation* 2000;69(8): 1726–1728.

61 Sophianopoulos JA, Durham SJ, Sophianopoulos AJ *et al*. Ultrafiltration is theoretically equivalent to equilibrium dialysis but much simpler to carry out. *Arch Biochem Biophys* 1978;187(1):132–137.

62 Miller JL. Sirolimus approved with renal transplant indication. *Am J Health Syst Pharm* 1999;56(21): 2177–2178.

63 Pfizer. Rapammune (sirolimus) Oral Solution and Tablets. Package Insert; 2010.

64 Kahan BD, Camardo JS. Rapamycin: clinical results and future opportunities. *Transplantation* 2001; 72(7):1181–1193.

65 Zimmerman JJ, Ferron GM, Lim HK, Parker V. The effect of a high-fat meal on the oral bioavailability of the immunosuppressant sirolimus (rapamycin). *J Clin Pharmacol* 1999;39(11):1155–1161.

66 Kaplan B, Meier-Kriesche HU, Napoli KL, Kahan BD. The effects of relative timing of sirolimus and cyclosporine microemulsion formulation coadministration on the pharmacokinetics of each agent. *Clin Pharmacol Ther* 1998;63(1):48–53.

67 Kahan BD, Napoli KL, Kelly PA *et al*. Therapeutic drug monitoring of sirolimus: correlations with efficacy and toxicity. *Clin Transplant* 2000;14(2):97–109.

68 Napoli KL, Kahan BD. Routine clinical monitoring of sirolimus (rapamycin) whole-blood concentrations by HPLC with ultraviolet detection. *Clin Chem* 1996; 42(12):1943–1948.

69 Zimmerman JJ. Exposure–response relationships and drug interactions of sirolimus. *AAPS J* 2004;6(4):e28.

70 Analytical Services International Sirolimus Proficiency Survery Results [October 1, 2010]; available from: http://www.bioanalytics.co.uk.

71 Streit F, Christians U, Schiebel HM *et al*. Sensitive and specific quantification of sirolimus (rapamycin) and its metabolites in blood of kidney graft recipients by HPLC/electrospray-mass spectrometry. *Clin Chem* 1996;42(9):1417–1425.

72 Wyeth. Dear Health Care Provider Letter [updated December 17, 2009]; available from: http://www.fda.gov/downloads/Safety/MedWatch/SafetyInformation/SafetyAlertsforHumanMedicalProducts/UCM197064.pdf.

73 Chan L, Greenstein S, Hardy MA *et al*. Multicenter, randomized study of the use of everolimus with tacrolimus after renal transplantation demonstrates its effectiveness. *Transplantation* 2008;85(6): 821–826.

74 Kovarik JM, Tedesco H, Pascual J *et al*. Everolimus therapeutic concentration range defined from a prospective trial with reduced-exposure cyclosporine in de

novo kidney transplantation. *Ther Drug Monit* 2004; 26(5):499–505.

75 Nashan B, Curtis J, Ponticelli C *et al*. Everolimus and reduced-exposure cyclosporine in de novo renal-transplant recipients: a three-year phase II, randomized, multicenter, open-label study. *Transplantation* 2004;78(9):1332–1340.

76 Pascual J. Concentration-controlled everolimus (Certican): combination with reduced dose calcineurin inhibitors. *Transplantation* 2005;79(9 Suppl):S76–S79.

77 Tedesco Silva H, Jr, Cibrik D, Johnston T *et al*. Everolimus plus reduced-exposure CsA versus mycophenolic acid plus standard-exposure CsA in renal-transplant recipients. *Am J Transplant* 2010;10(6):1401–1413.

78 Kovarik JM, Kaplan B, Silva HT *et al*. Pharmacokinetics of an everolimus–cyclosporine immunosuppressive regimen over the first 6 months after kidney transplantation. *Am J Transplant* 2003;3(5):606–613.

79 Budde K, Neumayer HH, Lehne G *et al*. Tolerability and steady-state pharmacokinetics of everolimus in maintenance renal transplant patients. *Nephrol Dial Transplant* 2004;19(10):2606–2614.

80 Korecka M, Solari SG, Shaw LM. Sensitive, high throughput HPLC–MS/MS method with on-line sample clean-up for everolimus measurement. *Ther Drug Monit* 2006;28(4):484–490.

81 Kovarik JM, Steiger JU, Grinyo JM *et al*. Pharmacokinetics of sotrastaurin combined with tacrolimus or mycophenolic acid in de novo kidney transplant recipients. *Transplantation* 2011;91(3): 317–322.

82 Latek R, Fleener C, Lamian V *et al*. Assessment of belatacept-mediated costimulation blockade through evaluation of CD80/86-receptor saturation. *Transplantation* 2009;87(6):926–933.

CHAPTER 9

Pharmacometrics: Concepts and Applications to Drug Development

Mallika Lala[1] and Jogarao V.S. Gobburu[2]

[1]Division of Pharmacometrics, Office of Clinical Pharmacology, Center for Drug Evaluation and Research, US Food and Drug Administration, Silver Spring, MD, USA

[2]University of Maryland School of Pharmacy, Baltimore, MD, USA

What is pharmacometrics?

Introduction

Pharmacometrics is the science of quantitaive clinical pharmacology that influences decision-making throughouht the drug development and regulatory review process. It is an amalgamation of several research areas, including, among others, pharmacokinetics (PK), pharmacodynamics (PD), pathophysiology, and statistics. Pharmacometrics is comprised of an array of techniques that are primarily based on modeling and simulation of data, which include, but are not limited to, population pharmacokinetic analysis, exposure–response (E–R, or PK–PD) determination for drug efficacy and safety, clinical trial simulations, and disease progression modeling.

Several organizations have discussed the increasing importance of modeling and simulation for enhancing drug development [1–4]. The pharmaceutical industry has conducted surveys to evaluate the role of pharmacometric analysis in their drug development process. A study at Parke-Davis [5] found that, in almost half (5 of 12) of the cases reviewed, the population analysis provided information that influenced the direction of individual development programs and may have facilitated review and approval. A similar study at Hoffmann La Roche [6] found that a modeling and simulation-guided approach contributed toward making clinical drug development more rational and efficient, by better dose selection for clinical trials and time savings up to several months.

The following sections of this chapter describe the general applications of pharmacometrics during drug development and regulatory review, as well as different concepts and methods employed. Case studies, which bring out the role that pharmacometric analyses have played in various aspects of drug development, and a future perspective on the field, are also provided.

Quantitative disease–drug–trial models

Disease–drug–trial models may be considered mathematical expressions of the time course of biomarkers, clinical outcomes, placebo effects, drug effects, and trial execution characteristics [7]. Accrual of information from across drug development programs enables efficient future planning, for which quantified disease, drug, and trial information can serve as a helpful guide.

Disease models quantify the relevant biological system in the absence of drug (see detailed discussion in "Disease models" section). Drug models characterize the E–R relationship for both efficacy and safety of drugs. Among other decisions, such models drive the determination of optimal dosing regimens. Using drug models early on can reduce unexpected safety/efficacy outcomes during the

Immunotherapy in Transplantation: Principles and Practice, First Edition. Edited by Bruce Kaplan, Gilbert J. Burckart and Fadi G. Lakkis.

late clinical phase [8, 9]. Trial models attempt to account for patient characteristics and behaviors such as eligibility criteria, baseline variables and their correlation, protocol adherence [10], and dropout rates, which may significantly influence outcomes in clinical trials. Trial models have great potential contribution towards more efficient and successful future clinical trials.

Applications

Pharmacometrics can be applied at all stages of the drug lifecycle, right from the preclinical phase through clinical development, and regulatory review, as well as post-marketing. Potential applications range from molecule screening and identification of biomarkers and surrogates, to dosing regimen and trial design selection and optimization, to prognostic factor and benefit–risk evaluation. These methods have the unique ability to leverage all prior and current information, providing a rational, scientifically sound framework to maximize knowledge and efficiency of drug development programs. The many and varied applications of pharmacometrics are illustrated in Figure 9.1.

Clinical trial design

It has been observed over time that registration trials fail to demonstrate effectiveness or safety, often due to ignorance of prior knowledge, both drug-specific and nonspecific (placebo effect or natural disease progression) and/or employment of one-size-fits-all dosing strategies [1, 11]. Disease–drug–trial models and clinical trial simulations are useful tools that can help reduce such trial failures. Potential benefits include upfront comparison of candidate study designs, dose and safety outcomes selection, sample size and power determination, and evaluation of drug interactions and co-morbidities [12]. The resources needed to perform the pharmacometric analyses are negligible compared with the costs of unsuccessful trials.

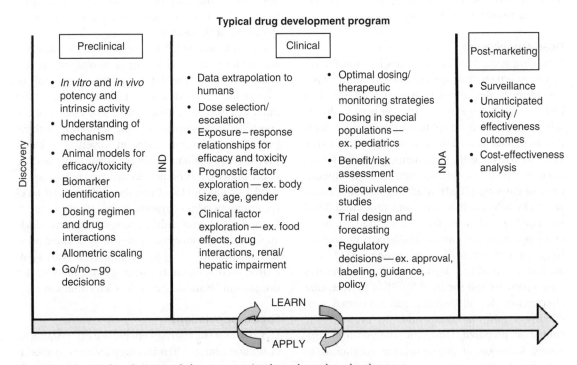

Figure 9.1 Potential applications of pharmacometrics throughout drug development.

For instance, nesiritide, developed for the treatment of acute congestive heart failure, was initially not approved because the dosing regimen used in the first registration trial was suboptimal. Modeling led to suggestion of a new, optimal dosing regimen, and results of simulated trials based on this regimen matched well with those of the second registration trial that led to eventual approval of the drug [13]. In retrospect it appears as though an early dose optimization could have saved 3 years of drug development time and one failed clinical trial.

Another instance is for a drug to treat type 2 diabetes mellitus [14]. A semi-mechanistic model to describe the time course of fasting plasma glucose (FPG) and hemoglobin A1c (HbA1c) was developed and extensive simulations were performed to evaluate two different trial designs: genotype-stratified and biomarker enrichment designs. The biomarker-enrichment design with a bid dosing regimen was proposed for future trials with an understanding that the trial results would be used to derive an optimal dosing strategy, such as genotype-based dosing. An important resulting drug development decision was the need to develop a sustained-release formulation of the drug.

Dose optimization

Exploring several dosing strategies in clinical trials is often impractical, costly, and in some cases unethical. Under such circumstances, simulations can be used to explore all competing dosing schemes and select an optimal strategy. If no single dosing scheme is able to achieve target drug exposures in the majority of patients, there may be a need for dose individualization and therapeutic drug monitoring (TDM). Modeling and simulation can help forecast this need and provide a TDM strategy [1]. This was observed in the case of an oral suspension product for prophylaxis of invasive fungal infections in high-risk patients [15]. E–R analysis revealed very high variability in exposures across patients and the need for TDM to maximize effectiveness for all patients, and supported conducting a post-marketing study to evaluate the benefit of proposed TDM. The analysis also supported inclusion of administration conditions to optimize drug absorption, emphasizing the impor-

tance of adequate plasma concentrations, in the drug label.

Usually, only dosing regimens "directly" studied in clinical trials are proposed in drug labels. However, a drug model may effectively be used to explore the suitability of intermediate doses that are not directly studied, but which could potentially offer similar effectiveness as the dosing regimens studied [16, 17]. But extrapolating outside the dose range studied may not be feasible. The ability of a well-developed E–R relationship to support approval of a dosing regimen not directly studied in clinical trials is, in fact, one of the strongest merits of modeling and simulation. Unfortunately, this tool is not being fully exploited currently.

Covariate/prognostic factor determination

Apart from dose-ranging studies, the clinical pharmacology characterization of a new drug involves a number of bridging studies to identify influential covariates or prognostic factors such as body size, age, gender, food intake, co-morbidities, co-medications, and others. While effectiveness and safety data may not be collected in bridging studies, they could be simulated from a previously developed drug model.

For instance, Sular is a once-a-day controlled-release formulation of the drug nisoldipine, which is approved in the USA for the treatment of hypertension. Food was found to increase the bioavailability (Cmax increases up to 245%) of the controlled–release product. The influence of these higher drug concentrations on lowering of blood pressure was evaluated using simulation of the drug effect under fed condition from a previously developed E–R model [18]. Even though the Sular label recommends administration on an empty stomach for optimal bioavailability, these simulations alleviated the safety concern of a large drop in blood pressure, should the drug be administered with food. Hence, there is no safety warning in the label for the drug to not be administered in a fed condition.

Special populations

Pharmacometric analyses enable the understanding of unique clinical pharmacology features in special populations, such as pediatrics, geriatrics, renal/

hepatic impairment, and others. A case in point is docetaxel, where the E–R relationship in patients with cancer was successful in identifying a subpopulation, patients with liver impairment, to be more prone to grade 4 neutropenia [19]. This important finding improved the safety profile of the drug and was the basis of the dosing recommendation for patients with hepatic insufficiency in the label. The drug development program of docetaxel exemplifies the value added by prospective modeling and simulation while planning clinical trials.

The US Food and Drug Administration (FDA) offers a 6 month extension on the marketing exclusivity for a new drug, should the sponsor fulfill the requirement of a written request to characterize the E–R relationship of the drug in pediatrics. Hence, one of the most sought out special populations to study for labeling changes is pediatrics. A well-defined E–R relationship of a drug in adults, be it for a biomarker, surrogate, or clinical endpoint, can facilitate development of the same drug for use in pediatrics. Modeling and simulation is a powerful tool that can be used to provide plausible trial design, rational dosing recommendations, and useful labeling information in pediatrics when sufficient understanding of adult and pediatric pharmacology is available [20].

For instance, a pediatric population analysis [21], and further modeling and simulation [22], provided the labeled dosing recommendations for the anti-arrhythmic agent sotalol in pediatrics aged 1 month to 12 years. The E–R analysis found drug effects in pediatrics to be consistent with adults. In this case, dosing for patients <2 years of age was selected specifically based on modeling, and not studied directly in trials.

Regulatory considerations

The US FDA routinely utilizes pharmacometric methods as an aid in making regulatory decisions during the investigational new drug (IND), biologics license application (BLA), and new drug application (NDA) review processes. The role of pharmacometric analyses in various regulatory decisions are summarized in Table 9.1.

A survey of 42 NDAs submitted between 2000 and 2004, which included a pharmacometric

Table 9.1 Summary of the types of regulatory decisions influenced by pharmacometric analyses [1].

Regulatory decision	Role of pharmacometric analyses
Trial design guidance	• Selection of dose or exposure range for registration trials • Derivation of optimal sampling schemes (PK and PD)

Approval	• Development of approval criteria
	• Evaluation of:
	  ○ evidence of effectiveness
	  ○ benefit–risk
	  ○ targeted safety studies (e.g., QT evaluation)
	  ○ clinical implications of failed bioequivalence studies

Labeling	• Recommendation of dosing strategy:
	  ○ dose and regimen
	  ○ individualized doses, where required
	  ○ therapeutic drug monitoring, where required
	  ○ dosing in special populations (e.g., pediatrics)
	  ○ drug interactions
	• Evidence for warnings and precautions

Policy	• Evaluation of:
	  ○ alternative primary analysis methods
	  ○ competing recommendations for guidances
	  ○ bioequivalence criteria

component, revealed that pharmacometric analyses were pivotal in regulatory decision making in more than half of the cases. Of the 14 reviews where such analyses were key to approval related decisions, five identified the need for additional trials and six identified reduction in the burden of conducting additional trials [1].

The proceedings of an advisory committee meeting for cardio-renal drug products are noteworthy [23]. The meeting devoted 50 % of the total time to discuss the role of E–R in cardio-renal drug development. The advisory committee concluded that model-dependent analysis to learn about the shape of the E–R curve and more innovative designs to potentially allow both frequentist and Bayesian types of data analysis were needed.

Table 9.2 Comparison of systems biology, semi-mechanistic and empirical approaches to disease models [7].

Approach \ Feature	Data source	Validation	Complexity and resources	Application
Systems biology models	*Wide range*: underlying biology, interrelationships with related systems, multiple detailed experiments, etc.	Extremely challenging	*High*: diverse expertise involved	• target identification • dose selection • trial design optimization • risk projection based on biomarker data
Semi-mechanistic models	*Limited range*: one or more experiments; related systems not considered	Relatively simple	*Low*: lesser expertise involved	• go/no-go decisions • dose selection • trial design optimization
Empirical models	*Limited range*: one or more experiments; may not accommodate design variations and related systems not considered			

The FDA issues guidance to industry to facilitate a smoother drug development and approval process. The guidance to industry on population pharmacokinetics [16] emphasizes the role of modeling and simulation in designing and analyzing trials. The FDA Modernization Act (FDAMA) [17] has a section for "extrapolation from existing studies" which emphasizes the ability to use knowledge from previous clinical trials for approval of the same drug product for pediatric use, or for establishing equivalence of alternative formulations, provided the original trial yielded well-defined E–R relationships. The FDA has also implemented end-of-phase-IIA (EOP2A) meetings with sponsors [24] and published the Critical Path Initiative [25], which again emphasize the usefulness of pharmacometrics in enhancing drug development. The premise for all these regulatory initiatives is that, with efficient planning, sponsors can economize valuable drug development time and resources, which is in the public health interest, as well as reap full advantage of the resulting incentives.

Disease models

A disease model is a mathematical representation of a given biological (or pathological) system in the absence of drug that attempts to quantify the time course of the disease [7]. There are three major sub-models that capture the relevant aspects of disease modeling, namely the relationship between biomarkers and clinical outcomes, the natural disease progression, and the placebo effect. In addition, there are three general approaches to building any disease model: systems biology, semi-mechanistic, and empirical modeling. The main features of the three approaches are summarized in Table 9.2.

Biomarkers and clinical outcomes

In several cases, particularly when clinical endpoints occur after prolonged periods of time, biomarkers are used as outcomes in clinical trials rather than the actual clinical endpoints. Characterization of the relationship between biomarkers and clinical outcomes for both efficacy and safety for a particular disease condition is thus a very important aspect of disease modeling, and can help develop surrogate endpoints. Such models can then aid in trial design optimization and risk projection based on biomarker data. Systems biology models, although complex, are very useful for this purpose [26]. They are based on an understanding of the underlying biological system, much like physiologically based models. They represent the system at the molecular level, with an ability to account for pathological disturbances. The model parameters are estimated from multiple, detailed in-vitro and ex-vivo experiments [7].

On the other hand, semi-mechanistic and empirical models are predominantly data driven and tend to disregard details of related diseases [27]. Semi-mechanistic models sufficiently simplify the biological system to be able to describe the available data well, and could be the first step toward a systems biology model. Empirical disease models are essentially mathematical expressions used to interpolate between observed data, and seldom relate to the underlying biology. Even so, such models are useful, depending on the problem at hand. Empirical models are simple and frequently all that are available, and are often invaluable in making go/no-go decisions and designing pivotal trials. The empirical parametric hazard model [28] that describes the relationship between the change in tumor size and survival is one such example.

It may be correct to say that every model will include some empirical component. For instance, in the case of diabetes, a detailed systems biology model with more than 50 parameters [29] and a semi-mechanistic model [30] have been proposed. While the systems biology model takes into account glucose and HbA1c data, as well as other related information such as blood pressure, cardiac output, family history, cholesterol, and smoking status, the semi-mechanistic model focuses on just the glucose and HbA1c information. Similarly, the outputs of the systems biology model include risks of retinopathy, nephropathy, and neuropathy, while the semi-mechanistic model is restricted to prediction of changes in glucose and HbA1c. Having said that, the systems biology model will still need to establish a relationship between change in blood pressure and/or glucose and a binary event such as myocardial infarction, thus incorporating an empirical component [7].

Natural disease progression

The natural disease progression aspect of disease modeling aims at describing the time course of changes observed in the clinical outcome. Drug therapy may alter natural progression of the disease, and such models can then provide insights into the management of several diseases [31]. For this purpose, empirical models have been used most commonly. The natural progression of

Alzheimer's disease as measured by the Alzheimer's disease assessment scale–cognitive score (ADAS–COG) and that of Parkinson's disease using the total unified Parkinson disease rating scale (UPDRS) have been described using empirical models [32–34]. However, mechanistic models, which are more generalizable, are also being studied. A mechanistic disease progression model for arthritis in rats has been proposed [35].

Placebo effect

The effect in a placebo group refers to the psychosocially induced biochemical changes in a patient's brain and body that in turn may affect both the natural course of a disease and the response to therapy [36]. Thus, even though the placebo effect is not directly related to the disease, it can significantly impact outcomes. This is particularly true for disease conditions that are measured symptomatically, such as pain and depression. Therefore, modeling the magnitude and time course of the placebo effect has value in discerning true drug effects and also aids in estimating sample size during trial design. Recently, a Bayesian model that describes the time course of the Hamilton depression rating scale (HAMD-17) clinical score in the placebo arms of antidepressant trials, combined with a dropout mechanism, has been developed [37]. This model provides new insights on the validity of the results of several longitudinal registration trials currently used for new drug products. A placebo model for Crohn's disease trials [38] is also available.

Population analysis

Conceptual framework

A population model typically comprises structural and statistical model components. Structural models are deterministic in nature and account for population or "fixed effects" (primary model parameters), but do not account for variability. The typical value of systemic clearance (CL) for a 70 kg individual and the mean potency (EC50) of a drug are examples of fixed effects. A population model suite would include four structural models: PK model, PD model, covariate (or prognostic factor) model, and disease progression model.

Statistical models are stochastic in nature and account for the variability or "random effects" seen at both the individual and the observational levels. A population model suite would include three statistical models: between-subject variability (BSV) model, between-occasion variability (BOV) model, and within-subject variability (WSV) model. Random-effects models usually assume that the between-subject and between-occasion errors η are normally distributed with mean zero and variance Ω^2, and that the within-subject or residual errors ε are normally distributed with mean zero and variance σ^2. BSV signifies deviations among different subjects and BOV signifies deviations among different occasions. WSV signifies deviation between predicted and observed values for each subject, and may be the result of measurement error or even model misspecification.

Nonlinear mixed-effects models are called so because they attempt to account for both fixed and random effects together. The "mixed effects" concept is depicted in Plate 9.1. Consider a one-compartment PK model where the drug is given as an intravenous bolus and the volume of distribution V is identical in every individual (no BSV for V). Then, the concentration in the ith subject at the jth time point (C_{ij}) can be described using the equations

$$C_{ij} = \frac{\text{Dose}}{V} e^{-(CL_i/V)t} + \varepsilon_{ij} \qquad (9.1)$$

$$CL_i = CL_{POP} + \eta_{CL,i} \qquad (9.2)$$

where CL_i is the estimated clearance of the ith subject, CL_{POP} is the estimated population mean clearance, $\eta_{CL,i}$ is the difference between the population mean and individual clearances, and ε_{ij} is the residual error of the jth sample of the ith subject.

Analysis methods

A primary goal of population analysis is to estimate the mean value of relevant parameters (such as CL, V, and EC50) in the population of interest, the variances in these parameters, and the residual variability of observations. Another goal is to explain the observed BSV using patient covariates such as body size, age, genotype, and so on. In addition, estimating individual PK parameters (such as CL_i and V_i) is required to impute concentrations for performing E–R analysis and any other simulations at a later stage.

The known methods for performing a population analysis are: naive pooled, naive averaged, two-stage (TS), and nonlinear mixed-effects (NM) or one-stage analysis. The main features of these analysis methods are summarized in Table 9.3.

In naive pooled analysis, individual observations from all subjects are pooled (as though all data

Table 9.3 Main features of the common population analysis methods.

Method \ Feature	Covariate exploration	Uncertainty at observational level	Uncertainty at subject level	Relative complexity and time involved
Naive pooled	*Indirect*: a model with known relevant covariates can be imposed	*Ignored*: mean estimates will be unduly closer to outliers (extreme observations).	*Ignored*: all subjects are weighted equally, regardless of number of observations per subject	*Low*
Naive averaged	*Indirect*: subjects can be divided into groups based on relevant covariates			
Two-stage	*Convenient*: a covariate model can be estimated in stage 2	*Accounted*: models will not be unduly influenced by extreme observations.	*Accounted*: subjects with more data are also weighted more.	*High*: special training is required.
One-stage	*Convenient*: a covariate model can be included in the optimization step			

came from a single, giant subject) to obtain average PK parameters. A minor variation of this method is the naive averaged analysis, which involves determination of the mean of the data at each time point. Both these methods provide only the central tendency of the model parameters and no random effects are estimated. These methods are used more often for preclinical data and are appealing because of their simplicity. However, since BSV is not estimated and cannot be accounted for using covariates, the potential applications of naive pooled or naive averaged analyses are very limited.

In TS analysis, the first stage involves estimation of the average parameters for each subject from their individual observations, while the second stage involves the estimation of the population mean and variance of the parameters, after adjusting for covariates, if necessary. Estimates of both the central tendency and the inter-individual variability can be obtained reasonably well. The TS method requires collection of rich data to have sufficient samples per subject (greater than the number of model parameters to be estimated), which is the usual requirement with experimental data. One concern is this method assumes that the individual parameters, estimated in stage 1, are known without any uncertainty. More serious drawbacks include the inability to model sparse data and concentration (or dose)-dependent nonlinear processes. The conventional PK noncompartmental analysis (NCA) is a type of TS population analysis approach.

In NM analysis, data from all subjects are simultaneously modeled to yield estimates of both population mean parameters and variance. Since both stages of the TS method are performed in one step, the NM technique is also known as the "one-stage" method. Individual parameters are calculated post hoc, subsequent to this one-stage optimization. NM modeling is perhaps the most powerful technique for analyzing both rich and sparse data, and does not share the drawbacks of the other methods discussed earlier. One of the main advantages of the NM method is its ability to conduct meta-analyses, which enables incorporating all data across a drug development program. The primary disadvantage of this method is that

sophisticated software are required for the analysis, which mandates special training for its use, while learning resources are limited. In addition, these analyses can be highly time consuming.

Model qualification

All models are required to be qualified and credible for their wider adoption. Validation implies a procedure of utmost robustness. However, the fact that the true model and its parameters are not known discourages the use of the term "validation" for population PK–PD models. Hence, qualification may be a better suited term.

The purpose for which the model is being developed should be clearly specified as a prerequisite before undertaking any model building. Based on the purpose of the model, qualification methods can test either the descriptive capacity or the extrapolation capacity of a given model. Developing an acceptable descriptive model is critical for making labeling recommendations. However, drug labels, usually, do not extrapolate results beyond the range of data observed.

Adequate description of the data at hand will ensure that the proposed model and its parameters are qualified to make reliable inferences, within the range of the data studied. This can be assessed using the routine diagnostic tests, such as goodness-of-fit plots (independent variable versus observed and individual/population model predictions), summary statistics, and precision of the parameter estimates. A model and its parameters may be deemed "qualified" to perform the particular task(s) if they satisfy certain prespecified criteria. Application of a predictive check to a model and its parameters along with Monte Carlo simulations [39,40] is an effective method used for qualification of population models.

Physiological interpretation of model parameters is one of the most important aspects of model qualification. A model and its parameters may be deemed "credible" to perform a particular task if the conceptual foundation on which the model was proposed is satisfactory to a panel of experts. It is important to note that there is no formal means to assess whether a model can be used for extrapolation. Hence, the credibility of the model (i.e., whether the model was derived from sound mechanistic principles, which appear reasonable to subject matter experts) is important. Thus, a model (and its parameters) may be considered qualified to predict beyond the range of the data used for building the model if the descriptive capacity of the model is acceptable and the model is credible.

Types of data and trial designs

Data
Pharmacometrics data (referring to PK/PD measurements) that may be collected during clinical trials, in general, are of two types: rich data and sparse data. Typically, rich data, which refers to several (10–20) samples from each subject, are collected under controlled conditions in trials conducted in a small number of patients over a short duration of time. Data from each subject can be analyzed independent of the others, in most cases, and then summarized. Such data are the best for building structural models. Dose-escalation studies, bioequivalence studies, and bridging (for prognostic factor effects) studies are examples of trials where rich data are collected.

On the other hand, late-phase clinical trials that are conducted in a large number of patients and for relatively longer durations typically collect sparse data. A few (one to five) samples are taken from each individual owing to practical limitations, which makes it challenging to analyze the data from each subject separately. Sparse data are most suited to build statistical models. Pivotal or registration safety–efficacy trials are examples of studies that tend to collect sparse data.

Trial designs
Broadly, three of the most commonly used trial designs that employ population analyses are parallel, cross-over, and titration. In a parallel study design, subjects are randomized to one of several treatment options; for instance, control, dose1, dose2, or dose3. Such a design supports the estimation of population E–R characteristics well, but not that of individual characteristics. In a cross-over design, each subject receives all the treatment

options. This is the most powerful study design for estimating the individual E–R relationships. However, such trials are longer in duration and may experience carry-over effects from previous treatments. The titration design is one where patients are usually initiated at a low dose, which is then gradually increased either until no additional benefit is observed or until dose-limiting toxicity occurs. This design resembles clinical practice most closely and individual E–R determination is possible. However, it may so happen that patients who are less sensitive to the drug need higher doses, making it (falsely) appear as though the response decreases after a certain dose. In several cases, particularly for the cross-over and titration designs, sophisticated data analysis, such as mixed-effects modeling, is required.

Further, based on the assignment of randomized groups in the trial, there are different designs possible. Subjects may be randomized to receive a particular dose or concentration of the test drug or to a particular effect elicited by the drug. Accordingly, such trials are referred to as a randomized dose-controlled trial (RDCT), a randomized concentration-controlled trial (RCCT), or a randomized effect-controlled trial (RECT). An active control group is used where a placebo control is considered unethical.

In an RDCT, the different doses of the drug to be tested are randomly administered to the subjects. Data are then collected throughout the trial and analyzed using an appropriate method. Such trials are the most commonly seen design owing to the relatively simple execution and analysis involved.

In an RCCT, a set of target drug concentration levels are selected based on the E–R relationship established from previous studies. Subjects are then randomized to one of these prespecified target concentrations [41]. Such a design obviates a dose-titration period during which the dose that ensures achieving concentrations within the selected target range (e.g., $5 \pm 0.5 \mu g/L$) is identified. A variation of the RCCT design is when doses are prespecified based on a certain demographic variable. For instance, body-weight-adjusted doses are routinely administered in pediatric studies. Similarly, in an RECT, subjects are randomly assigned to a prespecified target effect level. Again, the target effects are chosen based on prior knowledge of the drug's E–R, and the dose is titrated accordingly.

RCCT and RECT designs have similar requirements, such as prior E–R relationship, to select the appropriate target concentration or effect ranges, an efficient and sensitive analytical assay method with a short turn-around time, and sufficient strengths of the formulation to allow for any required dose adjustments. Candidate drugs for such trial designs are those where the PK has a large unexplained variability (RCCT) and those where the PD has a large unexplained variability (RECT). In addition, when the measured effect (desired/undesired) is symptomatic (for instance, effects such as pain or nausea that are "felt" by patients) the RECT could be applicable. When the symptoms are not obvious, the RCCT may be a better choice. Unfortunately, very few drug development programs utilize RCCT or RECT designs, perhaps due to their complicated execution and data analysis, relative to the RDCT design, as well as the cost of implementing TDM if the drug is approved [42, 43]. Notably, trials for immunosuppressant drugs used in transplantation generally employ the RCCT design.

Case studies

Pharmacometric analyses have been employed at various stages of the drug development process. Several case studies where such analyses have had pragmatic value in decision making are discussed. Cases include drugs used as immunotherapy during transplantation, as well as other drugs. Table 9.4 summarizes all cases presented, while a few selected cases have been discussed in detail.

Tacrolimus: liver, kidney, heart transplantation
Background
Tacrolimus is an immunosuppressive agent indicated for the prophylaxis of organ rejection in allogeneic liver, kidney, or heart transplants. A large amount of variability has been observed in the PK

and PD of this drug. Pharmacometric methods have been employed throughout the drug development stages of tacrolimus, to select rational dosing regimens and optimize therapy [46].

Key questions
The key questions are:
1. What is a safe and effective dosing regimen for first-time-in-man clinical studies?
2. What is a rational target therapeutic concentration range for tacrolimus?
3. What is an optimal initial dose of tacrolimus for late-phase clinical trials?
4. What is an optimal TDM strategy for managing patients on tacrolimus therapy?

Role of pharmacometrics
The starting dose of tacrolimus (0.15 mg/(kg day) IV) used in early-phase clinical trials was extrapolated from a synthesis of safe doses in two animal models (rat and dog). The target concentration range for monitoring the drug therapy during these trials was also based on the same animal models, augmented with in vitro PD modeling using the IC_{50} values from mixed lymphocyte reactions. Collectively, all the animal models studied were also highly predictive of the systemic toxicities observed with tacrolimus in humans. A pilot compassionate-use early clinical study in patients with refractory liver rejection suggested that the 0.15 mg/kg starting dose was clinically effective, but toxic in some patients, and doses had to be individualized to the patient. A reduced starting dose (0.05 mg/(kg day) IV) was predicted by simulations before onset of the pivotal trial, and the need for this dose reduction was dramatically confirmed during the US and European multicenter registration trials. In addition, an artificial intelligent modeling system (AIMS) was developed to efficiently guide dosing and monitoring of patients on tacrolimus. The AIMS-based TDM led to clinical and pharmacoeconomic benefits in a subsequent prospective pilot clinical study.

Impact
Preclinical models proved to be a reliable guide for identifying a safe and effective dose and a therapeutic concentration range for tacrolimus.

Table 9.4 Summary of case studies, where pharmacometric analysis had an impact on decision making, during different stages of drug development.

Drug	Stage	Key questions	Decision impacted	Comments
5c8, mAb [44]	☒ Pre-clinical ☐ Early clinical ☐ Late clinical ☐ EOP2A ☐ Post-marketing	☒ Molecule screening ☒ Trial/experimental design ☒ Dose selection ☐ Covariate determination ☐ Evidence of effectiveness ☐ Benefit/risk evaluation	☒ Go/no-go ☒ Dose optimization ☐ Improved trial design ☐ Approval ☐ Labeling ☐ Special population – dose selection	*Perceived impact of model developed:* • optimized sample collection in experiments • anticipated E–R in humans • quantified other antigen-provoked responses • projected utility of 5c8 in treatment of antibody-mediated autoimmune disease
rPSGL-Ig [45]	☒ Pre-clinical ☒ Early clinical ☒ Late clinical ☐ EOP2A ☐ Post-marketing	☒ Molecule screening ☐ Trial/experimental design ☒ Dose selection ☐ Covariate determination ☐ Evidence of effectiveness ☐ Benefit/risk evaluation	☒ Go/no-go ☒ Dose optimization ☐ Improved trial design ☐ Approval ☐ Labeling ☐ Special population – dose selection	• developed allometric models across animal species to predict PK and dose range for first-time-in-man clinical trial
Tacrolimus [46]	☒ Pre-clinical ☒ Early clinical ☒ Late clinical ☐ EOP2A ☐ Post-marketing	☐ Molecule screening ☒ Trial/experimental design ☒ Dose selection ☐ Covariate determination ☒ Evidence of effectiveness ☐ Benefit/risk evaluation	☐ Go/no-go ☒ Dose optimization ☒ Improved trial design ☒ Approval ☐ Labeling ☐ Special population – dose selection	• derived early-phase trials starting dose using two animal models • derived target conc. range for RCCT trials and TDM using animal and in-vitro PD models • derived final starting dose for pivotal trial using simulations • improved TDM strategy and cost-efficiency
Rivoglitazone [47]	☐ Pre-clinical ☒ Early clinical ☐ Late clinical ☐ EOP2A ☐ Post-marketing	☐ Molecule screening ☒ Trial/experimental design ☒ Dose selection ☐ Covariate determination ☐ Evidence of effectiveness ☒ Benefit/risk evaluation	☐ Go/no-go ☒ Dose optimization ☒ Improved trial design ☐ Approval ☐ Labeling ☐ Special population – dose selection	• developed a "best-in-class" compound using modeling and simulation • selected biomarker/endpoint, dose, sampling, washout, eligibility and discontinuation criteria, and forecasted trials for late clinical phase • built disease model from related drug information
Mycophenolate mofetil [48, 49]	☐ Pre-clinical ☒ Early clinical ☐ Late clinical ☐ EOP2A ☐ Post-marketing	☐ Molecule screening ☒ Trial/experimental design ☒ Dose selection ☐ Covariate determination ☐ Evidence of effectiveness ☐ Benefit/risk evaluation	☐ Go/no-go ☒ Dose optimization ☐ Improved trial design ☐ Approval ☐ Labeling ☐ Special population – dose selection	• derived dosing regimen for a late-phase clinical trial (RCCT) using E-R model based on a pilot study

Drug	Phase (☒ checked)	Application (☒ checked)	Impact (☒ checked)	Outcomes
Degarelix [50, 51]	Pre-clinical ☐ Early clinical ☐ Late clinical ☒ EOP2A ☐ Post-marketing ☐	Molecule screening ☐ Trial/experimental design ☐ Dose selection ☒ Covariate determination ☐ Evidence of effectiveness ☒ Benefit/risk evaluation ☐	Go/no-go ☐ Dose optimization ☒ Improved trial design ☐ Approval ☒ Labeling ☐ Special population – dose selection ☐	• explored alternative dosing strategies based on five phase 1/2 studies • selected final dosing regimen for registration trial that eventually led to drug approval
Piperacillin/Tazobactam [52]	Pre-clinical ☐ Early clinical ☐ Late clinical ☒ EOP2A ☐ Post-marketing ☐	Molecule screening ☐ Trial/experimental design ☐ Dose selection ☒ Covariate determination ☐ Evidence of effectiveness ☐ Benefit/risk evaluation ☒	Go/no-go ☐ Dose optimization ☐ Improved trial design ☐ Approval ☐ Labeling ☒ Special population – dose selection ☒	• recommended two-step weight-based PIP/TAZ pediatric dosing regimen in drug label for patients aged ≥2 months • verified no new safety concerns than those in adults
Busulfan [1, 53]	Pre-clinical ☐ Early clinical ☐ Late clinical ☒ EOP2A ☐ Post-marketing ☐	Molecule screening ☐ Trial/experimental design ☐ Dose selection ☒ Covariate determination ☐ Evidence of effectiveness ☐ Benefit/risk evaluation ☐	Go/no-go ☐ Dose optimization ☐ Improved trial design ☐ Approval ☐ Labeling ☒ Special population – dose selection ☒	• recommended two-step weight-based pediatric dosing regimen in drug label • proposed TDM strategy in label to enhance therapeutic targeting
Everolimus/cyclosporine [15]	Pre-clinical ☐ Early clinical ☐ Late clinical ☒ EOP2A ☐ Post-marketing ☐	Molecule screening ☐ Trial/experimental design ☐ Dose selection ☒ Covariate determination ☐ Evidence of effectiveness ☐ Benefit/risk evaluation ☒	Go/no-go ☐ Dose optimization ☒ Improved trial design ☐ Approval ☒ Labeling ☐ Special population – dose selection ☒	• projected likely outcomes of altered dosing schemes • proposed new dosing regimen that reduced renal toxicity while maintaining efficacy thus improving benefit/risk profile than seen in registration trial • cardio-renal advisory committee recommended new regimen to be evaluated in future trial
Apomorphine [1]	Pre-clinical ☐ Early clinical ☒ Late clinical ☒ EOP2A ☐ Post-marketing ☐	Molecule screening ☐ Trial/experimental design ☒ Dose selection ☒ Covariate determination ☒ Evidence of effectiveness ☐ Benefit/risk evaluation ☐	Go/no-go ☐ Dose optimization ☐ Improved trial design ☐ Approval ☐ Labeling ☒ Special population – dose selection ☒	• demonstrated a 50 % increase in exposure in renal impairment • derived maximum recommended dose and titration strategy and dose adjustment in renal impairment in drug label
Zoledronic acid [1]	Pre-clinical ☐ Early clinical ☐ Late clinical ☒ EOP2A ☐ Post-marketing ☒	Molecule screening ☐ Trial/experimental design ☐ Dose selection ☒ Covariate determination ☒ Evidence of effectiveness ☒ Benefit/risk evaluation ☐	Go/no-go ☐ Dose optimization ☐ Improved trial design ☐ Approval ☐ Labeling ☒ Special population – dose selection ☒	• suggested a correlation between risk of renal deterioration and drug exposure • recommended dose adjustments in mild and moderate renal impairment patients in drug label

(Continued)

Table 9.4 Summary of case studies, where pharmacometric analysis had an impact on decision making, during different stages of drug development (*Continued*).

Drug	Stage	Key questions	Decision impacted	Comments
Oxcarbeazepine [1, 54]	☐ Pre-clinical ☐ Early clinical ☒ Late clinical ☐ EOP2A ☐ Post-marketing	☐ Molecule screening ☐ Trial/experimental design ☒ Dose selection ☐ Covariate determination ☒ Evidence of effectiveness ☐ Benefit/risk evaluation	☐ Go/no-go ☐ Dose optimization ☐ Improved trial design ☒ Approval ☒ Labeling ☒ Special population – dose selection	• found no important differences in placebo and drug effects between adults and pediatrics • supported evidence for approving drug as monotherpay in pediatric patients with partial seizures • derived dosing instructions in drug label • saved additional controlled trials
Micafungin [15]	☐ Pre-clinical ☐ Early clinical ☒ Late clinical ☐ EOP2A ☐ Post-marketing	☐ Molecule screening ☐ Trial/experimental design ☒ Dose selection ☐ Covariate determination ☐ Evidence of effectiveness ☒ Benefit/risk evaluation	☐ Go/no-go ☒ Dose optimization ☐ Improved trial design ☒ Approval ☒ Labeling ☐ Special population – dose selection	• derived dosing recommendation and supported approval of drug for esophageal candidiasis • provided evidence for label to indicate greater potential for liver toxicity at approved dose
Varenicline [15]	☐ Pre-clinical ☐ Early clinical ☒ Late clinical ☐ EOP2A ☐ Post-marketing	☐ Molecule screening ☐ Trial/experimental design ☒ Dose selection ☒ Covariate determination ☐ Evidence of effectiveness ☐ Benefit/risk evaluation	☐ Go/no-go ☒ Dose optimization ☐ Improved trial design ☐ Approval ☒ Labeling ☐ Special population – dose selection	• showed much higher drug exposures in renal impairment • found baseline smoking status and age to be prognostic of abstinence from smoking • found marginal dose increase to increase effectiveness but also significantly increase toxicity (nausea) • recommended lowering dose in case of intolerance to adverse effects in drug label
Drug to treat a life-threatening rheumatologic disorder [1]	☐ Pre-clinical ☐ Early clinical ☒ Late clinical ☐ EOP2A ☐ Post-marketing	☐ Molecule screening ☒ Trial/experimental design ☒ Dose selection ☐ Covariate determination ☒ Evidence of effectiveness ☐ Benefit/risk evaluation	☐ Go/no-go ☐ Dose optimization ☒ Improved trial design ☐ Approval ☐ Labeling ☐ Special population – dose selection	• showed that biomarker was predictive of clinical outcome but a 65 % reduction would achieve significance, after two failed registration trials • recommended exploring doses that achieve greater reduction in the biomarker or maximal tolerated dose for future trials
Drug to treat a debilitating neurological disorder [15]	☐ Pre-clinical ☐ Early clinical ☒ Late clinical ☐ EOP2A ☐ Post-marketing	☐ Molecule screening ☐ Trial/experimental design ☐ Dose selection ☐ Covariate determination ☒ Evidence of effectiveness ☐ Benefit/risk evaluation	☐ Go/no-go ☐ Dose optimization ☐ Improved trial design ☒ Approval ☐ Labeling ☐ Special population – dose selection	• showed that reduction in symptoms was related with drug dose while withdrawal effects were significant and consistent, after one failed and one successful registration trial • supported evidence of effectiveness for drug approval • saved additional clinical trial

Case	Development phase	Activity	Impact	Outcomes
Drug to treat a mild, moderate, or severe life-threatening disease [15]	☐ Pre-clinical ☐ Early clinical ☒ Late clinical ☐ EOP2A ☐ Post-marketing	☐ Molecule screening ☒ Trial/experimental design ☐ Dose selection ☐ Covariate determination ☒ Evidence of effectiveness ☐ Benefit/risk evaluation	☐ Go/no-go ☐ Dose optimization ☒ Improved trial design ☐ Approval ☐ Labeling ☐ Special population – dose selection	• identified nonresponder subgroup: patients with mild disease • showed consistent effectiveness in patients with moderate and severe disease • elucidated inconsistent results from previous trials • recommended future study in only moderate and severe disease patients
New class of antivirals [14]	☐ Pre-clinical ☐ Early clinical ☐ Late clinical ☒ EOP2A ☐ Post-marketing	☐ Molecule screening ☒ Trial/experimental design ☒ Dose selection ☐ Covariate determination ☐ Evidence of effectiveness ☐ Benefit/risk evaluation	☐ Go/no-go ☒ Dose optimization ☒ Improved trial design ☐ Approval ☐ Labeling ☐ Special population – dose selection	• distinguished QD and BID dosing regimens using a mechanistic viral-dynamic model that previous models could not achieve • allowed assessment of impact of variability, dosing regimen, patient compliance, and dropout on trial outcomes • proposed a lower dose BID regimen for future trials
Drug to treat insomnia [14]	☐ Pre-clinical ☐ Early clinical ☐ Late clinical ☒ EOP2A ☐ Post-marketing	☐ Molecule screening ☒ Trial/experimental design ☒ Dose selection ☐ Covariate determination ☐ Evidence of effectiveness ☐ Benefit/risk evaluation	☐ Go/no-go ☐ Dose optimization ☒ Improved trial design ☐ Approval ☐ Labeling ☐ Special population – dose selection	• recommended healthy subject studies for selecting doses for sleep onset but not for sleep maintenance evaluation • recommended patient trial durations of more than 30 days for reliable identification of doses and persistent sleep maintenance
Pro-drug to treat a life-threatening disease [14]	☐ Pre-clinical ☐ Early clinical ☐ Late clinical ☒ EOP2A ☐ Post-marketing	☐ Molecule screening ☒ Trial/experimental design ☒ Dose selection ☒ Covariate determination ☐ Evidence of effectiveness ☐ Benefit/risk evaluation	☐ Go/no-go ☒ Dose optimization ☒ Improved trial design ☐ Approval ☐ Labeling ☐ Special population – dose selection	• revealed body weight to be prognostic for toxicity and effectiveness and that per kilogram dosing of both test and reference drugs would allow more appropriate investigation of noninferiority indirectly, also derived optimal dosing of reference drug for wider application across other development programs

Implementation of the AIMS improved the TDM strategy by three- to four-fold reduction in number of blood samples drawn and a reduction in length of hospitalization after liver transplantation. Thus, modeling and simulation enabled more efficient trial design and data analysis of the RCCTs conducted during development of tacrolimus and improved the cost effectiveness of therapy.

Degarelix: prostate cancer
Background
Degarelix is indicated for the treatment of advanced prostate cancer patients. During its clinical development, the primary endpoint used in trials was suppression of testosterone levels (<0.5 ng/mL) from day 28 of treatment initiation through 1 year of therapy in 90 % patients. The dosing goals were to achieve this challenging endpoint. The sponsor conducted five early- and late-phase dose-finding clinical studies but was unable to derive an optimal dosing regimen. An EOP2A meeting was arranged between the FDA and the sponsor to discuss a better drug development plan for degarelix.

Key question
What is a rational dosing regimen that would maximize the effectiveness of degarelix in advanced prostate cancer patients?

Role of pharmacometrics
Population analysis was conducted to develop an E–R model for degarelix based on the five dose-finding studies conducted by the sponsor [50, 51]. The FDA suggested alternative dosing strategies and clarified the regulatory expectations of the NDA. For initial suppression of testosterone levels by day 28, a higher loading dose requirement was explored. A lower maintenance dose was derived to sustain the testosterone suppression through 1 year of drug therapy. Using a mechanistic E–R model and extensive clinical trial simulations, an optimal dosing regimen was derived. All pharmacometric analyses were conducted by the sponsor, under the guidance of the FDA. The model-based regimen was used in a registration trial that resulted in positive outcomes and led to approval of degarelix for this indication.

Impact
Degarelix was approved for use in advanced prostate cancer based on a registration trial that employed a modeling and simulation-derived dosing regimen, which several prior clinical studies failed to derive. Trials in prostate cancer patients are challenging and costly and early interaction between the sponsor and the FDA enabled more cost-efficient drug development and a smoother review process.

Busulfan: bone marrow transplantation
Background
Busulfex, an intravenous formulation of the drug busulfan, is used in combination with cyclophosphamide as an immunosuppressive conditioning regimen for bone marrow ablation prior to hematopoietic stem cell transplantation. The drug was initially approved for use in adults with chronic myelogenous leukemia. The dose-limiting toxicity associated with busulfan is potentially fatal hepatic venoocclusive disease (HVOD). Clinical studies suggested that a therapeutic window of 900–1500 μmol/(L min) in adults was appropriate to balance safety (occurrence of HVOD and leukemic relapse) and efficacy (successful engraftment). The FDA issued a written request to the sponsor to determine the PK of busulfan in pediatrics (aged 4–17 years) and the optimal dosing regimen for this population that would achieve target exposures.

Key question
What is the appropriate dosing strategy for busulfex in pediatric patients?

Role of pharmacometrics
A population PK study was conducted to characterize the PK of intravenous busulfan in pediatrics and provide dosing recommendations [53]. Clinical studies indicated that the therapeutic window was similar for pediatric and adult patients. However, this was confounded by the increased variability in the PK of oral busulfan seen in pediatric patients compared with adults. Hence, a target therapeutic window with a lower, more conservative threshold for toxicity, than in adults, was used for pediatric

patients (900–1350 μmol/(L min)). Body weight, body surface area, age, and gender were explored for their impact on pediatric dosing. Simulations suggested that the mg/kg- and mg/m²-based dosing regimens were similar in their efficiency. Exposures obtained by different dosing regimens, with one to seven dosing steps including various combinations of weights and doses, were evaluated. All the dosing regimens explored had, at best, 60% patients achieving target exposures after the first dose. Notably, the model revealed that the unexplained BSV (25%) was larger than the WSV (6%), indicating that BSV is the key determinant of therapeutic success. This finding, coupled with the narrow therapeutic window for busulfan, supported implementation of therapeutic drug monitoring for optimizing drug therapy.

Impact

Based on the modeling and simulation, and practical considerations, a two-step dosing regimen was proposed from this study: 1.1 mg/kg for patients weighing ≤12 kg and 0.8 mg/kg (adult dose) for patients weighing >12 kg. In addition, considering that about 40% patients may not achieve target exposures after the first dose, even with the optimized regimen, a TDM strategy was proposed to enhance therapeutic targeting. These dosing recommendations, which had not been directly tested in clinical trials, were incorporated into the drug label.

Perspective

Learn–apply paradigm

The strongest merit of model-based drug development lies in its ability to incorporate the entire base of relevant prior knowledge into decision-focused recommendations for the future. A learn–apply paradigm is being proposed as an effective means to leverage pharmacometric methods and enhance drug development [55]. Accordingly, learning refers to transforming information (such as clinical trial data) into knowledge, while applying refers to utilizing this knowledge to make informed decisions (such as confirmation of effectiveness, dose

selection, etc.). This is an extension to the learn-and-confirm philosophy in modeling that has been promoted by Lewis Sheiner [56].

Currently, pharmacometric models are typically developed at the end of phase 3. A more prudent way to economize time and costs to develop models is by maintaining a progressive model-building philosophy. The essence of progressive model building is to continuously update the current model as new knowledge is accrued. The advantages are at least twofold: the ability to "carry-forward" knowledge all along the development of a given drug product and the ability to divide a big problem into several small components that are easier to solve. For instance, in the case of developing a "best-in-class" compound, model-based drug development can use the wealth of knowledge from predecessor drugs with a similar mechanism of action [47]. Right from the phase 1 stage, efficacy and safety drug models can be developed based on preclinical data of the new drug, as well as clinical experience with predecessors. As the clinical development advances, the models can be continually updated, and thus the characteristics of the new drug would become increasingly well defined. However, implementation of such a paradigm calls for more open collaboration of scientists from all disciplines and an institutional commitment to use the "current" model while designing the next trial.

Future considerations

The late-phase attrition rates in drug development are alarmingly high at both the registration trial and the regulatory review stages, and it is believed that timely application of pharmacometric methods can enhance future development plans and reduce these attrition rates [1–7, 11, 57].

Quantitative disease–drug–trial model suites can serve as a valuable tool for improving future drug development and should be increasingly employed to design trials using clinical trial simulations. The FDA has set a target to design 50% of all pediatric trials using simulations by 2015 and 100% by 2020. Upon development of and experience with a particular disease–drug–trial model suite, a standardized template can be created for the trial design, data analysis, and review for all drugs under that indication. Consortia on specific topics are perhaps effective means for developing such model suites.

Early-on interaction between the FDA and drug sponsors may help in more efficient planning. The EOP2A meetings are a good platform to facilitate this goal via more rational dose selection and trial design and reduction in number of cycles involved in the NDA review [24].

However, modeling and simulation must not be viewed as a substitute for clinical trials altogether, nor seen as a tool to salvage failed trials, which were poorly designed, for regulatory approval. The aim is simply to employ these techniques into a continuous learn–apply paradigm, capitalize on prior knowledge, improve trial design, and support evidence for approval and labeling of drugs.

Increased collaboration between the industry, academia, and the FDA is essential for the growth and wider application of pharmacometrics. In addition, increased interaction across the board between experts, such as clinicians, pharmacometricians, and statisticians, is a must for better appreciation of this field. Finally, training in this area is currently not offered by many academic institutions, and this may be an important step forward in the future.

Abbreviations

ADAS-COG	Alzheimer's disease assessment scale – cognitive score
BOV	between-occasion variability
BSV	between-subject variability
BLA	biologic license application
CL	clearance
Cmax	maximum plasma drug concentration
EOP2A	end-of-phase-IIA
ER	exposure–response
FDA	Food and Drug Administration
FDAMA	Food and Drug Administration Modernization Act
FPG	fasting plasma glucose
HAMD-17	Hamilton depression rating scale
HbA1c	hemoglobin A1c
HVOD	hepatic veno-occlusive disease
IC$_{50}$	half maximal inhibitory concentration of drug
IND	investigational new drug
IV	intravenous
NCA	noncompartmental analysis
NDA	new drug application
NM	nonlinear mixed-effects
PD	pharmacodynamics
PK	pharmacokinetics
RCCT	randomized concentration-controlled trial
RDCT	randomized dose-controlled trial
RECT	randomized effect-controlled trial
TDM	therapeutic drug monitoring
TS	two-stage
UPDRS	unified Parkinson disease rating scale
V	volume of distribution
WSV	within-subject variability

References

1 Bhattaram VA, Booth BP, Ramchandani RP *et al.* Impact of pharmacometrics on drug approval and labeling decisions: a survey of 42 new drug applications. *AAPS J* 2005;7(3):E503–E512.

2 Lalonde RL, Kowalski KG, Hutmacher MM *et al.* Model-based drug development. *Clin Pharmacol Ther* 2007; 82(1):21–32.

3 Meibohm B, Derendorf H. Pharmacokinetic/pharmacodynamic studies in drug product development. *J Pharm Sci* 2002;91(1):18–31.

4 Zhang L, Sinha V, Forgue ST *et al.* Model-based drug development: the road to quantitative pharmacology. *J Pharmacokinet Pharmacodyn* 2006;33(3):369–393.

5 Olson SC, Bockbrader H, Boyd RA *et al.* Impact of population pharmacokinetic-pharmacodynamic analyses on the drug development process: experience at Parke-Davis. *Clin Pharmacokinet* 2000;38(5):449–459.

6 Reigner BG, Williams PE, Patel IH *et al.* An evaluation of the integration of pharmacokinetic and pharmacodynamic principles in clinical drug development. Experience within Hoffmann La Roche. *Clin Pharmacokinet* 1997;33(2):142–152.

7 Gobburu JV, Lesko LJ. Quantitative disease, drug, and trial models. *Annu Rev Pharmacol Toxicol* 2009;49: 291–301.

8 Garnett CE, Beasley N, Bhattaram VA *et al.* Concentration–QT relationships play a key role in the

evaluation of proarrhythmic risk during regulatory review. *J Clin Pharmacol* 2008;48(1):13–18.

9 Sheiner LB, Steimer JL. Pharmacokinetic/pharmacodynamic modeling in drug development. *Annu Rev Pharmacol Toxicol* 2000;40:67–95.

10 Girard P, Blaschke TF, Kastrissios H, Sheiner LB. A Markov mixed effect regression model for drug compliance. *Stat Med* 1998;17(20):2313–2333.

11 Gordian M, Singh N, Zemmel R, Elias T. Why products fail in phase III. *In Vivo* 2006;4:1–9.

12 Bonate PL. Clinical trial simulation in drug development. *Pharm Res* 2000;17(3):252–256.

13 Publication Committee for the VMAC Investigators. Intravenous nesiritide vs nitroglycerin for treatment of decompensated congestive heart failure: a randomized controlled trial. *J Am Med Assoc* 2002;287(12): 1531–1540.

14 Wang Y, Bhattaram AV, Jadhav PR *et al*. Leveraging prior quantitative knowledge to guide drug development decisions and regulatory science recommendations: impact of FDA pharmacometrics during 2004–2006. *J Clin Pharmacol* 2008;48(2):146–156.

15 Bhattaram VA, Bonapace C, Chilukuri DM *et al*. Impact of pharmacometric reviews on new drug approval and labeling decisions – a survey of 31 new drug applications submitted between 2005 and 2006. *Clin Pharmacol Ther* 2007;81(2):213–221.

16 US FDA. Exposure–Response Guidance to Industry; 2003. Available from: http://www.fda.gov/downloads/Drugs/GuidanceComplianceRegulatoryInformation/Guidances/ucm072109.pdf (accessed 12 June 2010).

17 US FDA. Food and Drug Administration Modernization Act (FDAMA) of 1997; 2011. Available from: http://www.fda.gov/RegulatoryInformation/Legislation/FederalFoodDrugandCosmeticActFDCAct/SignificantAmendmentstotheFDCAct/FDAMA/default.htm.

18 Schaefer HG, Heinig R, Ahr G *et al*. Pharmacokinetic–pharmacodynamic modelling as a tool to evaluate the clinical relevance of a drug–food interaction for a nisoldipine controlled-release dosage form. *Eur J Clin Pharmacol* 1997;51(6):473–480.

19 Bruno R, Hille D, Riva A *et al*. Population pharmacokinetics/pharmacodynamics of docetaxel in phase II studies in patients with cancer. *J Clin Oncol* 1998:16(1): 187–196.

20 Jadhav PR, Zhang J, Gobburu JV. Leveraging prior quantitative knowledge in guiding pediatric drug development: a case study. *Pharm Stat* 2009;8(3):216–224.

21 Shi J, Ludden TM, Melikian AP *et al*. Population pharmacokinetics and pharmacodynamics of sotalol in pediatric patients with supraventricular or ventricular tachyarrhythmia. *J Pharmacokinet Pharmacodyn* 2001; 28(6):555–575.

22 US FDA. Sotalol Review; 2001. Available from: http://www.accessdata.fda.gov/drugsatfda_docs/nda/2001/19-865S010_Betapace_biopharmr.pdf (accessed 12 June 2010).

23 Gobburu JVS, Lipicky RJ.Dose–response characterization in current drug development: do we have a problem? Presented at the FDA's Cardio-renal Advisory Committee Meeting 2000. Available from: http://www.fda.gov/ohrms/dockets/ac/00/backgrd/3656b2a.pdf.

24 US FDA. Advisory Committee for Pharmaceutical Science, Clinical Pharmacology Subcommittee; 2003. Available from: http://www.fda.gov/ohrms/dockets/ac/03/slides/3998s1.htm.

25 US FDA. Critical Path Initiative; 2004. Available from: http://www.fda.gov/oc/initiatives/criticalpath/whitepaper.html.

26 Michelson S. The impact of systems biology and biosimulation on drug discovery and development. *Mol Biosyst* 2006;2(6–7):288–291.

27 Mitsis GD, Marmarelis VZ. Nonlinear modeling of glucose metabolism: comparison of parametric vs. nonparametric methods. *Conf Proc IEEE Eng Med Biol Soc* 2007;2007:5968–5971.

28 Wang Y, Sung C, Dartois C *et al*. Elucidation of relationship between tumor size and survival in non-small-cell lung cancer patients can aid early decision making in clinical drug development. *Clin Pharmacol Ther* 2009;86(2):167–174.

29 Eddy DM, Schlessinger L. Archimedes: a trial-validated model of diabetes. *Diabetes Care* 2003;26(11):3093–3101.

30 Jauslin PM, Silber HE, Frey N *et al*. An integrated glucose–insulin model to describe oral glucose tolerance test data in type 2 diabetics. *J Clin Pharmacol* 2007;47(10):1244–1255.

31 Chan PL, Holford NH. Drug treatment effects on disease progression. *Annu Rev Pharmacol Toxicol* 2001;41:625–659.

32 Holford NH, Peace KE. Methodologic aspects of a population pharmacodynamic model for cognitive effects in Alzheimer patients treated with tacrine. *Proc Natl Acad Sci U S A* 1992;89(23):11466–11470.

33 Holford NH, Chan PL, Nutt JG *et al*. Disease progression and pharmacodynamics in Parkinson disease – evidence for functional protection with levodopa and other treatments. *J Pharmacokinet Pharmacodyn* 2006;33(3):281–311.

34 Bhattaram VA, Siddiqui O, Kapcala LP, Gobburu JVS. Endpoints and analyses to discern disease-modifying

drug effects in early Parkinson's disease. *AAPS J* 2009;11(3):456–464.

35 Earp JC, Dubois DC, Molano DS *et al*. Modeling corticosteroid effects in a rat model of rheumatoid arthritis I: mechanistic disease progression model for the time course of collagen-induced arthritis in Lewis rats. *J Pharmacol Exp Ther* 2008;326(2):532–545.

36 Benedetti F. Mechanisms of placebo and placebo-related effects across diseases and treatments. *Annu Rev Pharmacol Toxicol* 2008;48:33–60.

37 Gomeni R, Lavergne A, Merlo-Pich E. Modelling placebo response in depression trials using a longitudinal model with informative dropout. *Eur J Pharm Sci* 2009;36(1):4–10.

38 Su C, Lichtenstein GR, Krok K *et al*. A meta-analysis of the placebo rates of remission and response in clinical trials of active Crohn's disease. *Gastroenterology* 2004;126(5):1257–1269.

39 Jadhav PR, Gobburu JV. A new equivalence based metric for predictive check to qualify mixed-effects models. *AAPS J* 2005;7(3):E523–E531.

40 Post TM, Freijer JI, Ploeger BA, Danhof M. Extensions to the visual predictive check to facilitate model performance evaluation. *J Pharmacokinet Pharmacodyn* 2008;35(2):185–202.

41 Sanathanan LP, Peck CC. The randomized concentration-controlled trial: an evaluation of its sample size efficiency. *Control Clin Trials* 1991;12(6):780–794.

42 Endrenyi L, Zha J. Comparative efficiencies of randomized concentration- and dose-controlled clinical trials. *Clin Pharmacol Ther* 1994;56(3):331–338.

43 Ebling WF, Levy G. Population pharmacodynamics: strategies for concentration-and effect-controlled clinical trials. *Ann Pharmacother* 1996;30(1):12–19.

44 Gobburu JV, Tenhoor C, Rogge MC *et al*. Pharmacokinetics/dynamics of 5c8, a monoclonal antibody to CD154 (CD40 ligand) suppression of an immune response in monkeys. *J Pharmacol Exp Ther* 1998;286(2):925–930.

45 Khor SP, McCarthy K, DuPont M *et al*. Pharmacokinetics, pharmacodynamics, allometry, and dose selection of rPSGL-Ig for phase I trial. *J Pharmacol Exp Ther* 2000;293(2):618–624.

46 Lieberman R, McMichael J. Role of pharmacokinetic–pharmacodynamic principles in rational and cost-effective drug development. *Ther Drug Monit* 1996; 18(4):423–428.

47 Rohatagi S, Carrothers TJ, Jin J *et al*. Model-based development of a PPARγ agonist, rivoglitazone, to aid dose selection and optimize clinical trial designs. *J Clin Pharmacol* 2008;48(12):1420–1429.

48 Bullingham RE, Nicholls A, Hale M. Pharmacokinetics of mycophenolate mofetil (RS61443): a short review. *Transplant Proc* 1996;28(2):925–929.

49 Hale MD, Nicholls AJ, Bullingham RE *et al*. The pharmacokinetic–pharmacodynamic relationship for mycophenolate mofetil in renal transplantation. *Clin Pharmacol Ther* 1998;64(6):672–683.

50 Jadhav PR, Agersø H, Tornøe CW, Gobburu JV. Semi-mechanistic pharmacodynamic modeling for degarelix, a novel gonadotropin releasing hormone (GnRH) blocker. *J Pharmacokinet Pharmacodyn* 2006;33(5):609–634.

51 Tornøe CW, Agersø H, Senderovitz T *et al*. Population pharmacokinetic/pharmacodynamic (PK/PD) modelling of the hypothalamic–pituitary–gonadal axis following treatment with GnRH analogues. *Br J Clin Pharmacol* 2007;63(6):648–664.

52 Tornøe CW, Tworzyanski JJ, Imoisili MA *et al*. Optimising piperacillin/tazobactam dosing in paediatrics. *Int J Antimicrob Agents* 2007;30(4):320–324.

53 Booth BP, Rahman A, Dagher R *et al*. Population pharmacokinetic-based dosing of intravenous busulfan in pediatric patients. *J Clin Pharmacol* 2007;47(1):101–111.

54 US FDA. Oxcarbazepine Review; 2003. Available from: http://www.accessdata.fda.gov/drugsatfda_docs/nda/2003/021014_S003_TRILEPTAL%20TABLETS_BIOPHARMR.pdf (accessed 12 June 2010).

55 Gobburu J. Learn–apply paradigm: re-confirming the goals of drug development; 2011. Available from: http://www.fda.gov/downloads/Drugs/NewsEvents/UCM209136.pdf.

56 Sheiner LB. Learning versus confirming in clinical drug development. *Clin Pharmacol Ther* 1997;61(3):275–291.

57 Kola I, Landis J. Can the pharmaceutical industry reduce attrition rates? *Nat Rev Drug Discov* 2004;3(8):711–715.

CHAPTER 10

Pharmacogenomics and Organ Transplantation*

Gilbert J. Burckart[1] and Richard M. Watanabe[2]

[1]Office of Clinical Pharmacology, Center for Drug Evaluation and Research, US Food and Drug Administration, Silver Spring, MD, USA

[2]Division of Biostatistics, Preventive Medicine and Physiology & Biophysics, Keck School of Medicine, University of Southern California, Los Angeles, CA, USA

Introduction

Pharmacogenomics (PGx) studies in solid organ transplantation have been conducted for the last two decades. During the 1990s, genetic studies focused on immunogenetic markers such as single nucleotide polymorphisms in tumor necrosis factor (TNF), interleukin-10 (IL-10), interleukin-6 (IL-6) and interferon-gamma. Studies from 2002 to today have examined drug-specific pharmacogenomic single-nucleotide polymorpisms (SNPs). During both periods, most studies have reported the association of a single SNP with an outcome measure following organ transplantation, such as biopsy-proven acute rejection (BPAR). More recently, genome-wide association (GWA) studies of organ transplantation have begun to appear in the literature.

The definition of PGx used in this chapter is broad, and encompasses the effect of genetics on drug disposition, drug effect, and adverse drug effects. The definition of the US Food and Drug Administration for PGx is the study of variations of DNA and RNA characteristics as related to drug response [1]. The potential for PGx to impact on transplant outcome is notable: drug therapy

interactions with the immune and inflammatory systems are complex; the immunosuppressive drugs presently used are highly metabolized, have major toxicities, and have multiple drug interactions; and drug therapy outcomes are likely to be influenced by the complex donor–recipient tissue interaction. Therefore, the long-term impact of PGx on organ transplant outcomes should be large, and should represent multiple opportunities for therapeutic intervention [2].

However, the hurdles to the clinical use of pharmacogenomic information are substantial and come from multiple sources. Perhaps the largest obstacle to overcome is establishing the phenotype of the transplant patient for use in any pharmacogenomic study of organ transplant patients. This variability starts with the patient and the donor–recipient interaction, includes the center-to-center effect in transplant patient management, and encompasses both major and minor differences in drug treatment protocols between centers. If this variability in transplant patient phenotype can be made manageable, remaining obstacles include test availability, test reimbursement, and acceptance by clinicians and health care provider institutions.

The objectives of this chapter are to discuss the use of candidate gene and GWA studies in organ transplant patients, to discuss the obstacles to the acceptance of PGx into transplant clinical practice,

---

*Disclaimer: all of the materials presented in this chapter are the opinions of the authors, and are in no way meant to represent the position of the US Food and Drug Administration.

Immunotherapy in Transplantation: Principles and Practice, First Edition. Edited by Bruce Kaplan, Gilbert J. Burckart and Fadi G. Lakkis.
© 2012 Blackwell Publishing Ltd. Published 2012 by Blackwell Publishing Ltd.

and to summarize the opportunities for PGx to contribute to the care of the organ transplant patient.

Genetic studies in organ transplantation

A critical component of any genetic association study, whether a candidate gene, GWA, or GWA meta-analysis, is independent replication in other samples. Independent replication has been held as the standard by which any initial association can be considered "true" in the face of small effect sizes and multiple testing issues. Replication has been relatively easy for genetic studies of complex human diseases, given that large epidemiologic studies of many diseases have been ongoing for years and typically entail similar ascertainment schemes and measurement of endophenotypes. Furthermore, clinical definitions of many human diseases, while perhaps not optimal for genetic studies, are nonetheless standardized, making classification of cases and controls relatively straightforward. The same cannot be said for clinical drug trials, where ascertainment, treatment regimen, drug combination and dosage, monitoring, drug compliance, and a multitude of other factors may significantly differ across studies. This is particularly true in organ transplantation. Thus, identifying an independent study with similar, if not the same, study design is extremely difficult, complicating the ability to perform independent replication. This raises the question of whether some level of standardization in study design is needed to facilitate pharmacogenomic studies.

Variability in patient management from one center to another and clinical trial design is a major problem in PGx studies in organ transplantation. One recent study pointed out the differences in the center-to-center occurrence of acute rejection [3]. Therefore, independent replication of a PGx finding from a single transplant center study to another transplant center is extremely difficult. Other sources of variability in transplant PGx studies includes subsetting of the patient population due to differences in race or ethnicity [4], accuracy of genotyping due to variations in methodology and lack of use of control samples, and the large number of demographic factors used to describe the transplant population.

Another consideration is that PGx studies are not performed in isolation from other testing on patients. Therefore, PGx tests must be integrated with other available patient information from physical exam, laboratory tests, and histology if a biopsy was performed. While PGx can add additional information, it is unlikely in the future that PGx will entirely take the place of other tests that are routinely performed on transplant patients today. The two common instances where this suggestion is made are with therapeutic drug concentration monitoring and with biopsies of the transplanted organ. While PGx may be able to suggest drug selection or initial dosing with some drugs, it will not be able to replace measuring drug concentrations in blood or plasma when it is available for a transplant drug [5]. Therapeutic drug monitoring and PGx should be complementary. Similarly, while experience with Allomap® peripheral blood testing for gene expression has had some success because of its negative predictive value for cardiac transplant rejection [6], the poor positive predictive value of such a test is unlikely to eliminate the need for cardiac biopsies in the near future.

The following discussion will be broken into candidate gene studies and GWA studies. GWA studies in organ transplantation to date have been limited to cells [7] and harvested organs [8]. GWA studies are much more mature in areas like diabetes mellitus (DM) than in organ transplantation, so many of the examples provided are in DM. However, many of the same considerations for a complex disease process like DM would be expected to apply for organ transplantation.

Candidate gene studies

Studies in organ transplantation started examining the effects of SNPs on transplant outcome in the mid 1990s. These initial studies examined SNPs in genes relating to the regulation of immune function such as TNF, IL-10, gamma interferon, IL-6, and transforming growth factor beta. The outcome measure for most of these gene association studies was not clinical outcome, but rather a biomarker for the clinical efficacy of the drug regimen.

A representative biomarker of a clinical outcome is also defined as a surrogate marker, and the most common biomarker for pharmacogenomic SNP association studies in organ transplantation is BPAR. Almost 30 years after the first drug approval based on changes in the incidence of BPAR, we now realize that BPAR is a heterogeneous process and that BPAR is not a good surrogate marker for long-term outcome after organ transplantation. While BPAR is still considered important as a drug-preventable adverse outcome in transplant patients, its use as a primary outcome measure in gene association studies is questionable. The choice of an adequate biomarker, including genomic biomarkers, for transplant outcome remains a considerable problem for drug development in organ transplantation [9].

The inability to reproduce the association between a gene polymorphism and BPAR may represent a center effect [3]. Even for transplant centers that use the same major immunosuppressive therapy, the details of patient management are frequently different between centers. The next most frequent biomarker for PGx association studies in organ transplantation is the plasma or blood drug concentration in relation to drug dose.

Some of the immunosuppressant drugs used in transplantation have assays readily available for the clinical measurement of plasma or blood concentrations. Tacrolimus, sirolimus, cyclosporine, and mycophenolic acid (MPA) have assays available for therapeutic drug monitoring. The ability of PGx gene polymorphisms to predict the pharmacokinetics and the pharmacodynamics of a drug has been discussed previously [5]. At the present time, drug concentration monitoring represents the best method for individualizing drug dosing and managing drug interactions in an individual transplant patient. The dilemma is that routine drug concentration monitoring is only available for the four agents mentioned, and does not include corticosteroids, biological agents, and many other drugs administered to a transplant patient. Also, the relationship between the drug concentrations, gene polymorphisms, and transplant outcome is not predictable in individual patients. Consequently, immunosuppressive drug concentrations often serve only as a marker of drug compliance or a gross measure for dose adjustment.

Recent gene polymorphism association studies have focused on the prediction of drug concentrations, and serve to emphasize the role of metabolic enzymes and transporters in transplant drug disposition [10]. Numerous studies have now been published on the association of SNPs of *CYP3A5* with tacrolimus drug concentration per dose. As expected, the patients who express the cytochrome P450 3A5 enzyme require a higher dose to achieve the same blood concentrations as the patients with genotypes considered to be nonexpressors of the enzyme. However, careful examination of individual patients reveals considerable overlap between the expressors and nonexpressors of CYP3A5 [11]. Similarly, *ABCB1*, which encodes for the membrane transporter P-glycoprotein, has had a number of reports examining the effect of *ABCB1* SNPs on tacrolimus blood concentrations in transplant patients. Even with *ABCB1* haplotyping and restriction of the patient population to CYP3A5 nonexpressors, the association is not one that can be used for the clinical prediction of tacrolimus dosing in individual transplant patients [12].

A more complicated candidate gene association analysis would be necessary with a drug such as MPA. MPA disposition and effect are mediated through a number of polymorphic genes. The polymorphisms that may affect plasma drug concentrations of MPA are those of *ABCB1* and *MRP2* [13], which may affect drug absorption or enterohepatic recirculation, of the organic anion transport protein affecting MPA uptake into hepatocytes, and of the uridine glycosyltransferases (UGTs), which affect phase 2 metabolism [2]. The immunosuppressant effect of MPA is manifest through polymorphic enzymes inosine monophosphate dehydrogenase (IMPDH)-1 and IMPDH-2 [14, 15]. Finally, MPA-induced adverse effects such as gastrointestinal intolerance and leukopenia have been associated with these same SNPs [16, 17]. Most of these studies have examined polymorphisms in a single gene, and no clinical application has come from any of these reports. Some composite measure of the impact of these gene polymorphisms on MPA therapeutic or toxic effect would have to be made for this information to be useful in the clinical management of transplant patients.

Interpretation of GWA results

Over a decade ago, Risch and Merikangas formally demonstrated that genetic association was statistically more powerful than genetic linkage studies and introduced the notion of GWA as a means to rapidly identify susceptibility variants underlying complex human diseases [18]. However, such a scale of genomic analysis was not possible even in the most sophisticated laboratories at that time. The era of GWA and large-scale human genomic research was made possible by the integration of a series of landmark achievements: advances in genomic technology [19], the sequencing of the human genome [20, 21], and the cataloging of human variation across the genome [22]. The success of GWA is evidenced by the Catalog of Genome-wide Association Studies (http://www.genome.gov/26525384), which at the time of writing has logged 3044 SNPs associated with a variety of human conditions from 625 publications. While GWA studies have mostly been completed in a variety of common human diseases, PGx-based GWA studies have just now started to appear in the literature [23–26].

One of the advantages of GWA studies is the ability to interrogate a large proportion of the human genome for common genetic variants that may be associated with a phenotype of interest in an unbiased fashion. Coverage of the human genome is extended well beyond genotyped markers through imputation, which leverages haplotype information from other sources (typically the HapMap [22, 27]) to infer genotypes for markers that were not included in the original genotyping [28, 29]. The "unbiased" aspect of GWA studies refers to the fact that no a priori assumptions are made with regard to the location or identity of potential genetic loci, nor are any specific biologic considerations made. Thus, GWA represents an anonymous

survey of the genome for variation that may underlie a given phenotype.

The findings from GWA studies are commonly described in terms of "genes," when in fact association signals from such studies only identify loci. This distinction is important, given that many times the SNPs identified from GWA studies do not fall within coding regions of any gene. In fact, it has been rare for a signal from a GWA study to be a nonsynonymous coding variant. An example is rs13266634 (C→T), which is associated with type 2 DM and results in an arginine to tryptophan conversion at codon 325 in solute carrier family 30 (zinc transporter), member 8 (*SLC30A8*) [30–33].

In most cases, association signals fall within intronic regions of genes, immediate 5'- or 3'-UTR regions of genes, or between known genes, with the last category being the most common in GWA studies. The convention in the field has been to report the gene that is physically closest to the association signal in cases where GWA signals fall between genes. The sometimes ambiguous nature of GWA results is partly a consequence of one of the strengths of GWA studies, namely leveraging linkage disequilibrium (LD) across the human genome.

The LD pattern allows investigators to capture information from the "functional" variant using a proxy SNP. However, in some cases, LD extends over long distances and can encompass multiple genes, which confounds interpretation of GWA results. One could argue that examination of the biologic function of genes within a given LD block could allow for inference of "the" susceptibility gene. However, in many cases there are multiple "logical" candidate genes within a region. A good example again comes from the type 2 DM literature. GWA studies identified rs1111875 as being associated with type 2 diabetes [30–33], and hematopoietically expressed homeobox (*HHEX*) has been typically used to identify this locus even though rs1111875 is ~7.5 kb downstream from *HHEX*. HHEX has plausible biology related to type 2 DM; however, there is an extended block of LD in this region of the genome in individuals of northern European ancestry. There are two additional genes within this block of LD that have plausible biology related to type 2 diabetes: kinesin family member 11 (*KIF11*) and insulin-degrading enzyme (*IDE*). Recent functional studies suggest *HHEX* is indeed the type 2 DM susceptibility locus [34], illustrating how additional fine-mapping, functional, and/or sequencing studies will be required to identify "the" gene.

There are additional weaknesses with regard to the GWA approach. First, the SNPs typically genotyped and imputed for such studies are common variants. Thus, rare variants with high penetrance will not be detected using this approach. Second, other structural variations in the genome, such as copy number or insertion/deletion polymorphisms [35, 36], have been shown to have biologic consequences [37, 38] and should be considered in any comprehensive genomic analysis of disease or other phenotype. Such variation can be in LD with common SNPs and, therefore, captured in GWA studies; however, common SNPs are relatively poor proxies for structural variation, and by some estimates upwards to 30 % of copy number variants are not adequately tagged by common SNPs [39]. Thus, targeted genome-wide analysis of such structural variation is required to understand their potential contribution to the phenotype of interest.

The statistical properties of GWA studies, mainly the penalty for multiple testing, result in only the relatively "low hanging fruit" to be followed up for replication and validation. The fact that a specific locus is not identified by GWA analysis does not necessary mean that the locus does not contribute to the phenotype. Once again, results from the type 2 DM literature highlight this issue. The first of the type 2 DM case–control GWA studies initially identified 10 susceptibility loci for the disease [30–33, 40]. Ever larger case–control samples, the largest consisting of 42 542 cases and 98 912 controls, have identified additional susceptibility loci [41–44]. However, independent studies of type 2 DM-related quantitative traits, specifically fasting and 2 h glucose, identified loci associated with variation in these traits, which, when subsequently assessed in type 2 DM case–control samples, showed evidence for association with disease [45–48]. Thus, not all disease susceptibility loci can be identified through case–control samples, and other disease-related phenotypes should be considered. The combined effort of examining both type 2 DM

and type 2 DM-related quantitative traits has resulted in the identification of 38 susceptibility loci to date and provides an important lesson for PGx studies.

GWA considerations for PGx

The successful application of GWA studies to complex human disease has generated several misconceptions. Among them, the low genetic effect sizes observed in complex diseases has generated debate regarding the public health relevance of genetic variation and whether gene variants are even biologically or clinically relevant [49–51]. It is important to remember that the effect size of a genetic association result should not be equated to biologic or clinical relevance of the locus. There are two specific examples from the type 2 DM literature that are relevant for PGx, although other examples exist related to the general biology of type 2 DM. The E23K variant (rs5219) in potassium inwardly-rectifying channel, subfamily J, member 11 (*KCNJ11*) is a type 2 DM susceptibility locus [52, 53]. KCNJ11 is an ATP-sensitive K-channel that plays a critical role in insulin secretion by pancreatic β-cells and is the target of the sulfonylurea class of DM medications, highlighting the biologic and clinical importance of this gene. Furthermore, a series of studies by Gloyn and coworkers has shown that mutations in *KCNJ11* are associated with neonatal diabetes [54, 55] and neonatal diabetes accompanied by developmental delay and epilepsy (DEND) syndrome [54, 56–58]. The mutations associated with neonatal diabetes and DEND syndrome are KCNJ11-activating mutations, meaning the K-channel remains open, preventing depolarization of the pancreatic β-cell membrane and subsequent insulin release. Patients with this condition lack circulating insulin due to the continued activity of the K-channel are typically misdiagnosed by clinicians as having type 1 DM, and typically started on traditional insulin therapy. Pearson *et al.* demonstrated that most patients with *KCNJ11* mutations can be successfully taken off insulin therapy and treated using sulfonylureas [55], with similar success achieved with DEND syndrome patients [59–61]. Such clinical translation is not limited to rare mutations in *KCNJ11*. The common E23K variant has been associated with risk of sulfonylurea-induced hypoglycemia [62] and secondary failure to sulfonylurea therapy [63], allowing clinicians to adjust sulfonylurea therapy appropriately for those individuals with carrying this variants.

Therefore, patients who are at risk for the development of DM may be identifiable. In transplantation, identifying patients at risk for developing an adverse effect, such as DM, would be critical for minimizing major drug adverse effects. Similar to *KCNJ11*, peroxisome proliferator-activated receptor-γ (*PPARG*) is another example of a type 2 DM susceptibility locus [64, 65] with very high biologic and clinical significance. Thiazolidinediones are insulin sensitizing agents that act as agonists for PPARG and used to treat type 2 DM. Studies also show that treating at-risk individuals with thiazolidinediones may also be effective in significantly reducing, or possibly preventing, development of future type 2 DM [66–71]. Studies have shown that 30–40 % of patients treated with a thiazolidinedione do not respond to the drug with an improvement in insulin sensitivity. Pharmacogenomic studies of *PPARG* are limited, but it as been shown that the common Pro12Ala (rs1801282) type 2 DM susceptibility variant is not associated with response to thiazolidinedione therapy [72–74]. There is evidence that variation elsewhere in *PPARG* is associated with response to troglitazone therapy [75], but troglitazone was removed from the market owing to hepatotoxicity. It is unknown if variants that were associated with troglitazone response are associated with response to pioglitazone or rosiglitazone, the two other thiazolidinediones that are currently available. Currently, no PGx studies have been reported that identify DM susceptibility as a means of preventing new onset DM after transplantation.

Another misconception generated by GWA studies is that, for any complex human phenotype, genetic effect sizes are small; therefore, sample sizes for genetic association studies must be extremely large or meet genome-wide significance levels for associations to be valid. The genome-wide significance level of $p < 5 \times 10^{-8}$ was determined under the assumption that SNPs across the entire human genome would be tested for association with an outcome of interest and that the effect size would be small [76], making the prior probability of a true association very small. This builds upon the original "common gene, common disease" hypothesis that posits that multiple genes of small effect contribute to risk for a common disease. Thus, the genome-wide significance cut-off represents a value that is modestly smaller than a Bonferroni-corrected $p = 0.05$. Correction for multiple testing is important to minimize type 1 error rates; however, assuming that parameters derived for common diseases apply to all gene association studies is not appropriate. Nelson *et al.* have nicely shown that adverse drug responses tend to have very large effect sizes, such that a genome-wide analysis could be performed with a modest number of cases matched to a large set of clinically matched or population controls [77]. Taking one specific example from their study, they show that neutropenia occurs in ~20 % of patients treated with irinotecan. *GCT1A1*28* is a risk allele for this adverse reaction that has a frequency of ~32 % in the population and a genetic effect of 28 as determined by the genetic relative risk for the homozygous genotypes. Nelson *et al.* estimated that a total of 58 cases and 200 clinically matched or population controls would be required to have 80 % power to detect association at a significance level of $p = 10^{-7}$ given these parameters [77]. The analysis by Nelson and colleagues suggests that GWA studies for adverse drug events are very feasible with modest sample sizes. Furthermore, similar genome-wide studies are also likely to be feasible for other drug-related phenotypes, such as drug response, where effect sizes are likely to fall between those observed for common disease variation and drug adverse events. Nelson and colleagues have created the Population Reference Sample (POPRES) to provide population-based reference material for use in PGx [78]; the samples are available through dbGAP (http://www.ncbi.nlm.nih.gov/sites/entrez?Db=gap).

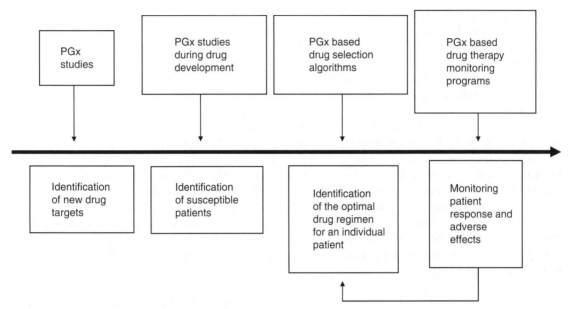

Figure 10.1 Depiction of the continuum of contributions that pharmacogenomics (PGx) could make to drug development and patient care in organ transplantation. Genome-wide association (GWA) studies are most likely to be used in the identification of new drug targets and in the identification of patients who will respond or will develop an adverse effect.

Pharmacogenomic applications in clinical transplant patient care

The application of PGx to care of the organ transplant patient may occur in several ways. PGx can (1) serve as the basis for an algorithm for drug selection, (2) serve as a biomarker for drug efficacy and outcome after transplantation, (3) help to identify patients at risk for adverse drug effects, and (4) help to identify new drug targets for drug development in organ transplantation. Figure 10.1 demonstrates how PGx studies can contribute to the continuum of drug development and optimal drug use in patients.

Individualizing the drug therapy regimen has now become a realistic goal for transplantation. Sufficient numbers of new immunomodulating agents, both small molecules and biological agents, are available to provide drug selection potential. Larger numbers of transplant researchers and clinicians are now involved in "transplantomics," and personalizing care for the transplant patient is one

of their goals [79]. The PGx basis for drug selection could be the recipient and/or donor genotype for the initial drug regimen, and PGx could be used to monitor and adjust therapy after transplantation. The development of simple drug-selection algorithms has previously been discussed [80].

Having the PGx test (whether it be RNA, protein, or metabolite expression) be the biomarker for drug efficacy is one of the most promising of the PGx applications to transplant patient care. These tests in peripheral blood and urine will be able to predict acute rejection significantly before clinical recognition or a biopsy. Transplantation has no lack of previously identified biomarkers, but fully qualifying these biomarkers for clinical use has been a major problem [9]. The actual incorporation of these testing methods into clinical practice is a problem that will be discussed in the next section.

Adverse drug effects remain a major problem in organ transplantation. DM, renal failure, and hypertension are all problems that have been associated with the calcineurin antagonists. Genetic predisposition to these adverse effects is likely, based upon a racial predilection to develop some adverse effects like DM, as discussed previously. If we could identify patients at risk for a particular adverse drug effect using PGx, then we may be able to adjust the drug therapy so as to avoid this problem [81].

PGx may hold the key to drug development efforts which could finally make a major improvement in long-term graft and patient survival. Understanding the pathogenesis of chronic allograft dysfunction through PGx may not only provide biomarkers for patient management, but may also identify novel targets for drug development. In February 2011, the US Food and Drug Administration published their draft guidance for industry on using PGx in early phase clinical studies [82].

PGx acceptance in clinical practice

The final acceptance of PGx into clinical practice in organ transplantion will require an acceptance by a complex group of participants. The clinician may ultimately decide the applicability of the test to the care of the individual transplant patient. The institution (hospital, health maintenance organization) may have to decide on whether to make the test available, therefore limiting the ability of the clinician to use the test. The test provider will have to be able to provide sufficient numbers of tests for the institution to make the test available. And the government may have to approve the test in order for the test to be paid for by third parties. The three factors which relate to the sustainability of medical innovations are legitimacy, organizational factors, and intermediary functions [83, 84].

Legitimacy relates to a number of factors. Foremost is that the innovation, or the PGx test in this case, has to be validated and accepted. Clinicians have to accept the test as being legitimate before they will take the time to learn to use the test. The test has to be cost effective for it to be accepted. Finally, the test is more likely to be adopted if there is public policy behind it.

In May 2008, a US Department of Health and Human Services report was published on "Realizing the Potential of Pharmacogenomics: Opportunities and Challenges" [85]. Also called the Secretary's Advisory Committee on Genetics, Health, and Society or SACGHS report on PGx, the report was strongly supportive of the development of PGx so that it meets a public health need. The recommendations of the committee were wide ranging, from public health education to the development of guidances by the US Food and Drug Administration. Therefore, public policy does support the incorporation of PGx into clinical practice.

The organizational factors supporting medical innovation relate to the experience of the organization in dealing with new techniques, and prestige associated with the use of a particular new test. If PGx testing is to be used clinically in transplantation, it will be initiated by one of major transplant centers, much as occurred when the calcineurin antagonists were new drugs for transplantation.

Finally, the intermediary functions describe the ability of the company making the PGx test to work with organizations to properly perform the test accurately and in a timely manner. This ability is very much dependent upon a large staff which can work with a broad range of institutions, so will likely be carried out by a major diagnostics or pharmaceutical company.

An alternative scenario is for the co-development of a PGx test and a new drug for transplantation. If the PGx test is developed to select the patient population most likely to respond to the new transplant drug, or selects patients based on an adverse effect profile, then the drug and the PGx test can be considered for concurrent approval by the US Food and Drug Administration. Figure 10.2 demonstrates the concept of the co-development of a PGx test and a drug concurrently.

Conclusion

PGx remains one of the bright spots on the horizon for organ transplantation. PGx can potentially provide a test for drug individualization for transplant patients, can help to guide the therapy of transplant patients, can help to avoid critical

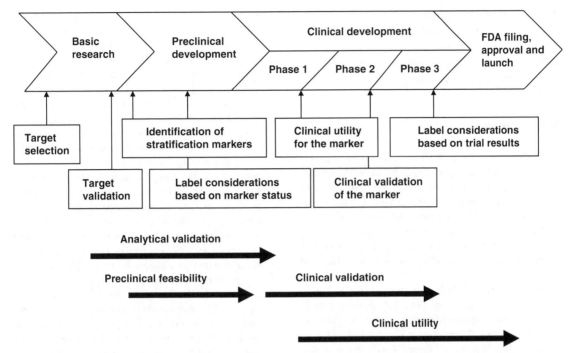

Figure 10.2 This figure depicts how co-development of a drug and a pharmacogenomics (PGx) test can be performed concurrently within a drug development program. The large arrow has all of the components of a drug development program, and below the arrow are the steps taken for test development, validation, and clinical testing. From a public FDA presentation by Felix W. Frueh: http://www.fda.gov/downloads/Drugs/ScienceResearch/ResearchAreas/Pharmacogenetics/ucm085626.pdf.

adverse drug effects, and can find new targets for drug development that can change long-term transplant outcome for the first time in 30 years. However, none of these goals will be obtained easily. New consortia must be formed and funding must be found for the required studies.

GWA studies are now making substantial contributions to complex diseases such as DM, and will increasingly be used in organ transplantation. As new targets are identified and new biomarkers discovered, the goal of applying this information to transplant patient care will eventually be realized. Governmental support exists for the incorporation of PGx into patient care systems, and guidances from the US Food and Drug Administration are available to guide the use of PGx in drug development programs for organ transplantation. The early availability of a microarray-derived peripheral blood test for cardiac rejection and the establish-ment of a yearly "transplantomics" meeting demonstrate the potential and the willingness of transplant clinicians and researchers to embrace PGx. The required pieces for establishing the legitimacy of PGx testing in organ transplantation are in place. While considerable work remains, there is little doubt that PGx will help to transform organ transplantation from a protocol-driven to a patient-individualized care process.

Abbreviations

BPAR	biopsy-proven acute rejection
DEND	developmental delay and epilepsy
DM	diabetes mellitus
GWA	genome-wide association
IL-6	interleukin-6
IL-10	interleukin-10

LD   linkage disequilibrium
MPA   mycophenolic acid
PGx   pharmacogenomics
SNPs   single nucleotide polymorphisms
TNF   tumor necrosis factor

References

1 US Food and Drug Administration. Guidance for industry: E15 definitions for genomic biomarkers, pharmacogenomics, pharmacogenetics, genomic data and sample coding categories; 2008. Access at: http://www.fda.gov/downloads/Drugs/GuidanceCompliance RegulatoryInformation/Guidances/UCM073162.pdf.

2 Burckart GJ. Pharmacogenomics: the key to improved drug therapy in transplant patients. *Clin Lab Med* 2008;28:411–422.

3 Israni A, Leduc R, Holmes J *et al*. Single-nucleotide polymorphisms, acute rejection, and severity of tubulitis in kidney transplantation, accounting for center-to-center variation. *Transplantation* 2010;90:1401–1408.

4 Girnita DM, Webber SA, Ferrell R *et al*. Disparate distribution of 16 candidate single nucleotide polymorphisms among racial and ethnic groups of pediatric heart transplant patients. *Transplantation* 2006;82: 1774–1780.

5 Burckart GJ, Liu XI. Pharmacogenetics in transplant patients: can it predict pharmacokinetics and pharmacodynamics? *Ther Drug Monit* 2006;28:23–30.

6 Deng MC, Eisen HJ, Mehra MR *et al*. Noninvasive discrimination of rejection in cardiac allograft recipients using gene expression profiling. *Am J Transplant* 2006;6: 150–160.

7 Grigoryev YA, Kurian SM, Nakorchevskiy AA *et al*. Genome-wide analysis of immune activation in human T and B cells reveals distinct classes of alternatively spliced genes. *PLoS One* 2009;4:e7906.

8 Wilflingseder J, Kainz A, Muhlberger I *et al*. Impaired metabolism in donor kidney grafts after steroid pretreatment. *Transpl Int* 2010;23:796–804.

9 Burckart GJ, Amur S, Goodsaid FM *et al*. (2008) Qualification of biomarkers for drug development in organ transplantation. *Am J Transplant*;8:267–270.

10 Burckart GJ, Amur S. Update on the clinical pharmacogenomics of organ transplantation. *Pharmacogenomics* 2010;11:227–236.

11 Zheng H, Zeevi A, Schuetz E *et al*. Tacrolimus dosing in adult lung transplant patients is related to cytochrome P4503A5 gene polymorphism. *J Clin Pharmacol* 2004;44:135–140.

12 Wang J, Zeevi A, McCurry K *et al*. Impact of ABCB1 (MDR1) haplotypes on tacrolimus dosing in adult lung transplant patients who are CYP3A5 *3/*3 nonexpressors. *Transpl Immunol* 2006;15:235–240.

13 Wang J, Figurski M, Shaw LM, Burckart GJ. The impact of P-glycoprotein and Mrp2 on mycophenolic acid levels in mice. *Transpl Immunol* 2008;19:192–196.

14 Wang J, Zeevi A, Webber S *et al*. A novel variant L263F in human inosine 5′-monophosphate dehydrogenase 2 is associated with diminished enzyme activity. *Pharmacogenet Genomics* 2007;17:283–290.

15 Wang J, Yang JW, Zeevi A *et al*. IMPDH1 gene polymorphisms and association with acute rejection in renal transplant patients. *Clin Pharmacol Ther* 2008;83:711–717.

16 Ohmann EL, Burckart GJ, Chen Y *et al*. Inosine 5′-monophosphate dehydrogenase 1 haplotypes and association with mycophenolate mofetil gastrointestinal intolerance in pediatric heart transplant patients. *Pediatr Transplant* 2010;14:891–895.

17 Ohmann EL, Burckart GJ, Chen Y *et al*. Impact of inosine 5′-monophosphate dehyrogenase 1,2 and multidrug resistance protein 2 genetic polymorphisms on mycophenolate mofetil related adverse events in pediatric heart transplant patients. *J Heart Lung Transplant* 2008;27:S181.

18 Risch N, Merikangas K. The future of genetic studies of complex human diseases. *Science* 1996;273:1516–1517.

19 Fan JB, Oliphant A, Shen R *et al*. Highly parallel SNP genotyping. *Cold Spring Harb Symp Quant Biol* 2003; 68:69–78.

20 International Human Genome Mapping Consortium. A physical map of the human genome. *Nature* 2001; 409:934–941.

21 The Genome Sequencing Consortium. Initial sequencing and analysis of the human genome. *Nature* 2001; 409:860–921.

22 The International HapMap Consortium. A haplotype map of the human genome. *Nature* 2005;437:1299–1320.

23 Ising M, Lucae S, Binder EB *et al*. A genomewide association study points to multiple loci that predict antidepressant drug treatment outcome in depression. *Arch Gen Psychiatry* 2009;66:966–975.

24 Perlis RH, Smoller JW, Ferreira MA *et al*. A genomewide association study of response to lithium for prevention of recurrence in bipolar disorder. *Am J Psychiatry* 2009;166:718–725.

25 Aberg K, Adkins DE, Bukszar J *et al*. Genomewide association study of movement-related adverse antipsychotic effects. *Biol Psychiatry* 2010;67:279–282.

26 Garriock HA, Kraft JB, Shyn SI *et al*. A genomewide association study of citalopram response in major depressive disorder. *Biol Psychiatry* 2010;67:133–138.

27 The International HapMap Consortium. The international HapMap project. *Nature* 2003;426:789–796.

28 Ellinghaus D, Schreiber S, Franke A, Nothnagel M. Current software for genotype imputation. *Hum Genomics* 2009;3:371–380.

29 Nothnagel M, Ellinghaus D, Schreiber S *et al.* A comprehensive evaluation of SNP genotype imputation. *Hum Genet* 2009;125:163–171.

30 Sladek R, Rocheleau G, Rung J *et al.* A genome-wide association study identified novel risk loci for type 2 diabetes. *Nature* 2007;445:881–885.

31 Diabetes Genetics Initiative of Broad Institute of Harvard and MIT, Lund University, and Novartis Institutes of BioMedical Research, Saxena R, Voight BF, Lyssenko V, Burtt NP, de Bakker PI *et al.* Genome-wide association analysis identifies loci for type 2 diabetes and triglyceride levels. *Science* 2007;316:1331–1336.

32 Scott LJ, Mohlke KL, Bonnycastle LL *et al.* A genome-wide association study of type 2 diabetes in Finns detects multiple susceptibility variants. *Science* 2007; 316:1341–1345.

33 Zeggini E, Weedon MN, Lindgren CM *et al.* Replication of genome-wide association signals in U.K. samples reveals risk loci for type 2 diabetes. *Science* 2007; 316:1336–1341.

34 Ragvin A, Moro E, Fredman D *et al.* Long-range gene regulation links genomic type 2 diabetes and obesity risk regions to *HHEX*, *SOX₄*, and *IRX₃*. *Proc Natl Acad Sci U S A* 2010;107:775–780.

35 Feuk L, Carson AR, Scherer SW. Structural variation in the human genome. *Nat Rev Genet* 2006;7:85–97.

36 Freeman JL, Perry GH, Feuk L *et al.* Copy number variation: new insights in genome diversity. *Genome Res* 2006;16:949–961.

37 Parmeggiani F, Costagliola C, Gemmati D *et al.* Predictive role of coagulation-balance gene polymorphisms in the efficacy of photodynamic therapy with verteporfin for classic choroidal neovascularization secondary to age-related macular degeneration. *Pharmacogenet Genomics* 2007;17:1039–1046.

38 Hebbring SJ, Moyer AM, Weinshilboum RM. Sulfotransferase gene copy number variation: pharmacogenetics and function. *Cytogenet Genome Res* 2008; 123:205–210.

39 Cooper GM, Zerr T, Kidd JM *et al.* Systematic assessment of copy number variant detection via genome-wide SNP genotyping. *Nat Genet* 2008;40:1199–1203.

40 Steinthorsdottir V, Thorleifsson G, Reynisdottir I *et al.* A variant in CDKAL1 influences insulin response and risk of type 2 diabetes. *Nat Genet* 2007;39:770–775.

41 Zeggini E, Scott LJ, Saxena R *et al.* Meta-analysis of genome-wide association data and large-scale replication identifies additional susceptibility loci for type 2 diabetes. *Nat Genet* 2008;40:638–645.

42 Yasuda K, Miyake K, Horikawa Y *et al.* Variants in *KCNQ1* are associated with susceptibility to type 2 diabetes mellitus. *Nat Genet* 2008;40:1092–1097.

43 Unoki H, Takahashi A, Kawaguchi T *et al.* SNPs in *KCNQ1* are associated with susceptibility to type 2 diabetes in East Asian and European populations. *Nat Genet* 2008;40:1098–1102.

44 Voight BF, Scott LJ, Steinthorsdottir V *et al.* Twelve type 2 diabetes susceptibility loci identified through large-scale association analysis. *Nat Genet* 2010;42: 579–589.

45 Bouatia-Naji N, Bonnefond A, Cavalcanti-Proenca C *et al.* A variant near *MTNR1B* is associated with increased fasting plasma glucose levels and type 2 diabetes risk. *Nat Genet* 2009;41:89–94.

46 Prokopenko I, Langenberg C, Florez JC *et al.* Variants in *MTNR1B* influence fasting glucose levels. *Nat Genet* 2009;41:77–81.

47 Saxena R, Hivert MF, Langenberg C *et al.* Genetic variation in *GIPR* influences the glucose and insulin responses to an oral glucose challenge. *Nat Genet* 2010;42:142–148.

48 Dupuis J, Langenberg C, Prokopenko I *et al.* New genetic loci implicated in fasting glucose homeostasis and their impact on type 2 diabetes risk. *Nat Genet* 2010;42:105–116. [Erratum: *Nat Genet* 2010; 42(5):464.]

49 Goldstein DB. Common genetic variation and human traits. *New Engl J Med* 2009;360:1696–1698.

50 Hirschhorn JN. Genomewide association studies – illuminating biologic pathways. *New Engl J Med* 2009;360:1699–1701.

51 Kraft P, Hunter DJ. Genetic risk prediction – are we there yet? *New Engl J Med* 2009;360:1701–1703.

52 Barroso I, Luan J, Middelberg RP *et al.* Candidate gene association study in type 2 diabetes indicates a role for genes involved in beta-cell function as well as insulin action. *Plos Biol* 2003;1:E20. [Erratum: *PLoS Biol* 2003;1(3):445.]

53 Gloyn AL, Weedon MN, Owen KR *et al.* Large-scale association studies of variants in genes encoding the pancreatic β-cell K_{ATP} channel subunits Kir6.2 (*KCNJ11*) and SUR1 (*ABCC8*) confirm that the *KCNJ11* E23K variant is associated with type 2 diabetes. *Diabetes* 2003;52:568–572.

54 Gloyn AL, Pearson ER, Antcliff JF *et al.* Activating mutations in the gene encoding the ATP-sensitive potassium-channel subunit Kir6.2 and permanent neonatal diabetes. *New Engl J Med* 2004;350:1838–1849. [Erratum: *N Engl J Med* 2004;351(14):1470.]

55 Pearson ER, Flechtner I, Njolstad PR *et al.* Switching from insulin to oral sulfonylureas in patients with diabetes due to Kir6.2 mutations. *New Engl J Med* 2006;355:467–477.

56 Proks P, Antcliff JF, Lippiat J *et al.* Molecular basis of Kir6.2 mutations associated with neonatal diabetes or neonatal diabetes plus neurological features. *Proc Natl Acad Sci U S A* 2004;101:17539–17544.

57 Proks P, Girard C, Haider S *et al.* A gating mutation at the internal mouth of the Kir6.2 pore is associated with DEND syndrome. *EMBO Rep* 2005;6:470–475.

58 Gloyn AL, Diatloff-Zito C, Edghill EL *et al. KCNJ11* activating mutations are associated with developmental delay, epilepsy and neonatal diabetes syndrome and other neurological features. *Eur J Hum Genet* 2006;14:824–830.

59 Slingerland AS, Nuboer R, Hadders-Algra M *et al.* Improved motor development and good long-term glycaemic control with sulfonylurea treatment in a patient with the syndrome of intermediate developmental delay, early-onset generalised epilepsy and neonatal diabetes associated with the V59M mutation in the *KCNJ11* gene. *Diabetologia* 2006;49:2559–2563.

60 Stanik J, Gasperikova D, Paskova M *et al.* Prevalence of permanent neonatal diabetes in Slovakia and successful replacement of insulin with sulfonylurea therapy in *KCNJ11* and *ABCC8* mutation carriers. *J Clin Endocrinol Metab* 2007;92:1276–1282.

61 Slingerland AS, Hurkx W, Noordam K *et al.* Sulphonylurea therapy improves cognition in a patient with the V59M *KCNJ11* mutation. *Diabet Med* 2008;25:277–281.

62 Holstein A, Hahn M, Stumvoll M, Kovacs P. The E23K variant of *KCNJ11* and the risk for severe sulfonylurea-induced hypoglycemia in patients with type 2 diabetes. *Horm Metab Res* 2009;41:387–390.

63 Sesti G, Laratta E, Cardellini M *et al.* The E23K variant of *KCNJ11* encoding the pancreatic β-cell adenosine 5'-triphosphate-sensitive potassium channel subunit Kir6.2 is associated with an increased risk of secondary failure to sulfonylurea in patients with type 2 diabetes. *J Clin Endocrinol Metab* 2006;91:2334–2339.

64 Deeb SS, Fajas L, Nemoto M *et al.* A Pro12Ala substitution in PPARγ2 associated with decreased receptor activity, lower body mass index and improved insulin sensitivity. *Nat Genet* 1998;20:284–287.

65 Altshuler D, Hirschhorn JN, Klannemark M *et al.* The common PPARγ Pro12Ala polymorphism is associated with decreased risk of type 2 diabetes. *Nat Genet* 2000;26:76–80.

66 Nolan JJ, Ludvik B, Beerdsen P *et al.* Improvement in glucose tolerance and insulin resistance in obese subjects treated with troglitazone. *New Engl J Med* 1994;331:1188–1193.

67 Antonucci T, Whitcomb R, McLain R *et al.* Impaired glucose tolerance is normalized by treatment with the thiazolidinedione troglitazone. *Diab Care* 1997;20:188–193. [Erratum: *Diab Care* 1998;21(4):678.]

68 Buchanan TA, Xiang AH, Peters RK *et al.* Preservation of pancreatic β-cell function and prevention of type 2 diabetes by pharmacological treatment of insulin resistance in high-risk hispanic women. *Diabetes* 2002;51:2796–2803.

69 The Diabetes Prevention Program Research Group. Prevention of type 2 diabetes with troglitazone in the Diabetes Prevention Program. *Diabetes* 2005;54:1150–1156.

70 Xiang AH, Peters RK, Kjos SL *et al.* Effect of pioglitazone on pancreatic β-cell function and diabetes risk in Hispanic women with prior gestational diabetes. *Diabetes* 2006;55:517–522.

71 The DREAM (Diabetes REduction Assessment with ramipril and rosiglitazone Medication) Trial Investigators. Effect of rosiglitazone on the frequency of diabetes in patients with impaired glucose tolerance or impaired fasting glucose: a randomised controlled trial. *Lancet* 2006;368:1096–1105.

72 Bluher M, Lubben G, Paschke R. Analysis of the relationship between the Pro12Ala variant in the PPAR-γ2 gene and the response rate to therapy with pioglitazone in patients with type 2 diabetes. *Diab Care* 2003;26:825–831.

73 Snitker S, Watanabe RM, Ani I *et al.* Changes in insulin sensitivity in response to troglitazone do not differ between subjects with and without the common, functional Pro12Ala peroxisome proliferator-activated receptor-γ2 gene variant: results from the Troglitazone in Prevention of Diabetes (TRIPOD) study. *Diab Care* 2004;27:1365–1368.

74 Florez JC, Jablonski KA, Sun MW *et al.* Effects of the type 2 diabetes-associated *PPARG* P12A polymorphism on progression to diabetes and response to troglitazone. *J Clin Endocrinol Metab* 2007;92:1502–1509.

75 Wolford JK, Yeatts KA, Dhanjal SK *et al.* Sequence variation in *PPARG* may underlie differential response to troglitazone. *Diabetes* 2005;54:3319–3325.

76 Pe'er I, Yelensky R, Altshuler D, Daly MJ. Estimation of the multiple testing burden for genomewide association studies of nearly all common variants. *Genet Epidemiol* 2008;32:381–385.

77 Nelson MR, Bacanu SA, Mosteller M *et al.* Genome-wide approaches to identify pharmacogenetic contributions to adverse drug reactions. *Pharmacogenomics J* 2009;9:23–33.

78 Nelson MR, Bryc K, King KS *et al.* The Population Reference Sample, POPRES: a resource for population, disease, and pharmacological genetics research. *Am J Hum Genet* 2008;83:347–358.

79 Sarwal MM, Benjamin J, Butte AJ *et al.* Transplantomics and biomarkers in organ transplantation: a report from the first international conference. *Transplantation* 2011;91:379–382.

80 Burckart GJ, Hutchinson IV, Zeevi A. Pharmacogenomics and lung transplantation: clinical implications. *Pharmacogenomics J* 2006;6:301–310.

81 Bai JP, Lesko LJ, Burckart GJ. Understanding the genetic basis for adverse drug effects: the calcineurin inhibitors. *Pharmacotherapy* 2010;30:195–209.

82 US Food and Drug Administration. Guidance for industry: clinical pharmacogenomics: premarketing evaluation in early phase clinical studies; 2011. Access at: http://www.fda.gov/downloads/Drugs/GuidanceComplianceRegulatoryInformation/Guidances/UCM243702.pdf.

83 Racine DP. Reliable effectiveness: a theory on sustaining and replicating worthwhile innovations. *Adm Policy Ment Health* 2006;33:356–387.

84 Burckart GJ, Frueh FW, Lesko LJ. Progress in the direct application of pharmacogenomics to patient care: sustaining innovation. *J Appl Pharmacol* 2007;15:1–6.

85 US Department of Health and Human Services. Realizing the potential of pharmacogenomics: opportunities and challenges; 2008. Access at: http://oba.od.nih.gov/oba/SACGHS/reports/SACGHS_PGx_report.pdf.

CHAPTER 11

Study Design/Process of Development: Clinical Studies

Richard D. Mamelok
Mamelok Consulting, Palo Alto, CA, USA

Introduction

The clinical trials that comprise the late development of a new drug range from the first administration of a new drug to humans through relatively large trials designed to investigate the efficacy and safety of the drug in the population of patients for whom the drug is intended. Taken individually, each trial should be considered as an experiment seeking to answer well-defined questions. The data generated from each trial, evaluated collectively, should provide a comprehensive picture of the drug's pharmacokinetics, pharmacodynamics, the relationship of dose and/or exposure of drug to selective clinical outcomes, the balance of benefits and risks of the drug, and, when appropriate, a comparison with established therapeutic approaches.

Somewhat arbitrary phases of clinical drug development have been defined, each with a specific goal. Phase I explores dose tolerability and pharmacokinetics and determines which doses will be explored initially for clinical efficacy. Phase II investigates, in a preliminary way, the efficacy and safety of a new drug, establishing the doses that are most likely to produce the optimal risk–benefit ratio. Results from Phase II establish the hypothesis that will be rigorously tested in Phase III. The results of Phase III form the primary basis of the approval by regulatory agencies and either confirm or refute a hypothesis generated from earlier development. These phases proceed in sequence as the main questions posed in each phase are answered. However, other trials are usually conducted concurrently with late Phase II and Phase III, investigating such things as the effects of renal and hepatic function on pharmacokinetics, drug–drug interaction, the effect of food on pharmacokinetics, and the effects of a drug on cardiac conduction and repolarization.

This chapter will initially discuss the phases of drug development in people in somewhat general terms. This will be followed by more specific discussion and considerations related to transplant patients, particularly with regard to endpoints.

Phase I: initial studies in humans

The first study in humans is almost always a single-dose study in subjects who are closely supervised during the dosing and for some time after. Subjects are monitored for pharmacologic effects with an emphasis on toxicity. Intensive pharmacokinetic sampling is performed. Pharmacodynamic testing of an effect on specific molecular targets or physiologic function may also be monitored. The development of subjective symptoms should be sought by nondirective questioning such as "How do you feel?" rather than by soliciting for the occurrence of a specific symptom. Depending on the molecular

Immunotherapy in Transplantation: Principles and Practice, First Edition. Edited by Bruce Kaplan, Gilbert J. Burckart and Fadi G. Lakkis.
© 2012 Blackwell Publishing Ltd. Published 2012 by Blackwell Publishing Ltd.

targets and expected toxicities and risk, the first dosing may be done in healthy volunteers or in transplant patients.

In general, patients are preferred because they may differ significantly from healthy people in their pharmacokinetics and sensitivity to effects. However, especially in the setting of the early post-transplant period, patients are on multiple drugs and are medically unstable and thus it is difficult in the small number of subjects in the first dose tolerability study to isolate the drug's effects. Thus, if the pharmacologic profile allows, the first trial is often done in healthy volunteers and then, based on the findings, repeated in patients possibly with a modified dosing scheme. Stable transplant patients are sometimes entered into the first trial in humans, but the confounding factor of concurrent therapy is not eliminated in that setting. Nevertheless, for a drug intended for use in the immediate post-transplant period, eventually the drug will have to be tested in the target population.

The general design of the first study in humans is one that progresses through a series of ascending single doses administered to different cohorts. Often a cohort consists of a randomized, blinded study in which six subjects receive drug and two receive placebo. While it is not uncommon to dose all subjects in a cohort simultaneously, when a novel drug with high potential for having widespread systemic effects that might occur in a rapidly advancing cascade is being tested it is advisable that dosing within a cohort be staggered. Six subjects per full cohort are often studied because the power to detect adverse events increases most rapidly as the size of the cohort increases to six. A sample size of six yields 80% power to observe an event that would occur in the population being studied at an incidence of 25% [1]. Thus, in Phase I studies, only the most common drug-induced adverse effects are likely to be observed. Of course, the power would increase further if cohorts were even larger, but a compromise is made between power and the efficiency of determining the doses that should be carried forward for further testing. At the conclusion of the study, the results in the placebo patients can be pooled, increasing the chance of correctly evaluating treatment-emergent events as caused by the actual drug.

One of the most difficult decisions made in drug development is choosing the first dose to test in humans. The studies in animal models that precede clinical trials in humans establish key information on which to base this decision, but there is always uncertainty because animals may metabolize and eliminate the drug differently than humans or may have different sensitivity to the drug's pharmacologic effects. Furthermore, idiosyncratic reactions cannot be predicted reliably from animal-based toxicology. Drugs that are based on human or humanized proteins will have drastically different pharmacokinetics in animals than in humans, and the duration of exposure in animals is severely limited because of the production of antibodies against the humanized protein. Also, there will be differences in and uncertainty about receptor homology, the distribution and density of receptors, receptor specificity, and binding constants. Clearly, one needs to choose a dose that is highly unlikely to cause any harm, and this is also a dose that is unlikely to produce any observable pharmacologic effect. The first study in humans continues until one of several outcomes is observed: a dose is found which is not well tolerated; there is little or no incremental exposure based on pharmacokinetic measurements with increasing dose; or a dose is reached that is so high that either administering more would not be feasible, such as too high a volume for injection or too much drug to be conveniently administered orally, or the dose would not be economically feasible to manufacture.

There are several methods of choosing the first dose. One of the simplest and long-standing approaches has been to choose some fraction of the maximum dose that was devoid of effects in animals observed in studies lasting about 4–13 weeks [2]. The range of the fraction chosen is wide, such that if toxicity studies revealed unusual toxicities or severe effects, then a smaller fraction would be used. More recently, and more commonly used today, methods that are still evolving employ some sort of modeling that seeks to predict the likely exposures in humans based on data from several animal species. This type of approach includes "interspecies scaling" and has several variations [3, 4]. Sometimes dosing is based either on body mass equivalence, which assumes that the equivalent dose is proportional to body mass, or on surface area equivalence, which assumes that the equivalent dose is proportional to body surface area. A somewhat more sophisticated approach employs allometric models, which assume that a relevant measure of toxicity, such as the lowest dose to produce an observed adverse effect, is a power function of mass, with empirically determined coefficients and exponents [3]. Such scaling leads to predictions of doses that are likely to produce effects in humans similar to those observed in animals, as well as predictions of pharmacokinetic attributes such as clearance and volume of distribution. Once the data from several species are fitted statistically to an acceptable model, it is assumed that human data will also adhere to the model's predictions. While these approaches were initially developed for small molecules, they have also been applied to proteins such as monoclonal antibodies, clotting factors, and cell-surface proteins [5–7].

Recently, the US Food and Drug Administration and the European Committee for Medicinal Products for Human Use have issued guidelines for first dosing in humans [8, 9]. While the details of these documents differ, the overall goal is similar and seeks to define the "minimal anticipated biological effect level" (or MABEL) and the "maximum recommended starting dose" (or MSRD). In animal studies, the highest dose level that does not produce a significant increase in adverse effects in comparison with the control group is determined and is referred to the NOAEL (no observable adverse effect level). Based on the NOAEL, the dose response in animals for effects of interest and an appropriate scaling factor are determined empirically, the "human equivalent dose" (or HED) is determined for each species for the NOAEL and the MABEL. The HED may also be determined from pharmacokinetic–pharmacodynamic modeling that may be able to incorporate multiple variables that determine pharmacologic and toxic effects. In the absence of a reason to do otherwise, the animal species used to determine the HED to be used in the first human trial should be the most sensitive species. However, this choice may be modified if there are known differences between species in absorption, distribution of the drug in tissues, metabolism, and

elimination, or if a particular species is known to be most predictive for a particular class of molecules. When a molecule has a known molecular target, knowledge of which animal species expresses the most relevant receptors needs to be considered. Once the appropriate HED is chosen, then a safety factor is chosen, such as 1/10 of the HED of the NOAEL or a smaller fraction of the MABEL (e.g., 1/1000). The safety factor may be smaller if a drug has a steep dose–response curve, has demonstrated severe toxicities, has a toxicity that cannot be clinically monitored or predicted from less severe expressions of the dose limiting toxicity, has a nonreversible toxicity, has nonlinear pharmacokinetics, is the first drug of its class ever to be tested, or has a novel molecular target. Finally, a judgment regarding the overall utility and predictability of the animal models used in preclinical work has to be made. If there is a large amount of uncertainty in a model's predictiveness, then a small fraction for scaling should be used. Extra caution must also be taken when the drug's target is connected to multiple signaling pathways or targets that are expressed in many tissues. While MABEL will always be larger than NOAEL by definition, if they are widely disparate, the NOAEL should be used.

There are several approaches to increasing the dose as the first study in humans proceeds. A balance has to be chosen between minimizing risk by not having increments that are too large and determining the maximally tolerated dose efficiently. The scheme for progressively increasing the dose in the first human trial is primarily based on the presumed steepness of the dose–response curve and the severity of the anticipated toxic effects. The steeper the curve and the more severe a potential toxicity could be, the smaller the interval between doses will be. Doses can be increased linearly, logarithmically, by a modified Fibonacci series, or by some combination or modification of these. Sometimes the first trials in humans allow some flexibility, so that the increment to the next dose can be made smaller once a level that produced a drug-related effect has been reached. Often, a committee made up of investigators and the commercial sponsor of a trial meet when a given cohort has completed dosing to decide, within guidelines specified in the protocol, what the next dose level should be.

In addition to getting a first sense of dose tolerability, the other information obtained in Phase I is pharmacokinetic data in humans, most importantly clearance and half-life. Clearance allows one to estimate the exposure (area under the curve or AUC) of the drug when dosed to steady state. Half-life determines how long it takes to get to steady state, which is approximately reached in four to five half-lives. Also, when a drug is dosed intermittently, as most drugs taken by transplant patients are and as essentially any drug targeted to outpatients is, half-life allows one to estimate the range of concentrations in blood or plasma that will be found over the course of a given dosing interval.* This knowledge, along with knowledge of the actual concentrations that are obtained with a given dose, allows one to choose an appropriate dose for multiple dosing and an appropriate dosing interval. If the relationship of pharmacologic and/ or toxic effects and concentration of drug has been estimated from preclinical studies, one can make an even better estimate of the appropriate dose to eventually take forward into more advanced testing. Other considerations in moving to further testing include whether the dosing regimen that is likely to be effective can be delivered by an acceptable formulation.

In conducting the pharmacokinetic sampling in Phase I, it is important to sample most frequently around when the presumed maximum concentration is reached. Otherwise, large errors can be made in estimating this concentration, and thus in the calculation of AUC. If the drug is given intravenously, then frequent sampling during the infusion is done. It is very important to obtain a sample as soon as the infusion ends as well. In order to get an accurate determination of half-life it is important to sample for at least two, and preferably more, half-lives. For the first trial one has to make an educated guess as to when the maximum concentration will

be reached and how long the half-life is likely to be. Since these guesses are not always correct, it is not uncommon to perform a number of pharmacokinetic studies subsequent to the initial dose tolerability studies.

If the main route of administration anticipated for the drug is anything other than intravenous, and if an intravenous formulation is also available, studies comparing the pharmacokinetics following intravenous and the alternative route of dosing should be done early to estimate bioavailability.

Following single-dose studies, multiple-dose studies are initiated, usually in the same type of subject enrolled in the single-dose trials. Such testing proceeds when data from the single-dose studies suggest that the tolerated doses are likely to produce the desired pharmacologic effects and that the severity of the adverse effects at these doses would not present an unacceptable risk. Based on the pharmacokinetic data and the range of doses that were tolerated, several multidose regimens are tested, usually sequentially. Fewer dose levels are tested than in the single-dose studies. As with the single-dose study, the early multiple-dose studies will include intensive pharmacokinetic sampling. Sampling is usually done during the first dosing interval and then over one or more other dosing intervals to confirm when steady state is reached and how much accumulation of drug occurs between the first dose and when at steady state. While the degree of drug accumulation can be predicted based on the half-life determined in Phase I and the dosing interval used, multiple-dose pharmacokinetics definitively determines this accumulation. Some studies in Phase II may also explore different dosing intervals. Also, Phase II provides the first opportunity to explore rigorously the nature of relationships of pharmacokinetics and outcome.

For drugs given more frequently than once per day, it is useful to compare pharmacokinetically morning and evening dosing intervals to test for clinically important diurnal variation. This can be done in a separate study rather than the first multidose study performed. If there are good biochemical markers that might predict the desired clinical outcome, such as blockade of a targeted

---

*Depending on assay requirements and distribution of drug into red blood cells, the concentration of drugs is measured in blood or plasma. For the remainder of this chapter, concentration will be used as a general term for either.

receptor or minimization of a particular toxicity, these, too, will be evaluated relative to the concentration of drug, which can be useful in planning dosing intervals in subsequent studies. These studies also include subjects dosed with placebo, or sometimes an active comparator, at each dose level in order to compare the frequency of adverse events.

Phase II: testing whether a drug has the desired effects predicted from preclinical studies

From the range of doses tested in Phase I, several doses are chosen to test in Phase II. Phase II is always done in the type of patient for whom the drug is intended. Ideally, a range of doses is chosen that would be predicted to cover a range of effects from a minimal effect to one where the beneficial effects reach a maximum without inducing unacceptable toxicity. There are several important practical problems with this approach, depending on how the drug is going to be used. If a drug is intended to be an addition to the current standard of care, such an approach is feasible. However, if a drug is meant to substitute for a component of an established regimen, the risk of underdosing and losing efficacy has to be minimized. An example of a typical Phase II trial is one published by Vincenti *et al.* with belatacept in renal transplantation [10]. This trial led to larger Phase III studies [11]. Another Phase II-type study tested whether mycophenolate mofetil would allow for the elimination of calcineurin inhibition in the immediate post-transplant period. In that study the rate of acute rejection was deemed too high and thus this approach was apparently abandoned for further development [12]. In addition, the cost to perform the trials and competitive pressures to enter the final phase of testing as quickly as possible provide commercial disincentives to such a thorough approach.

The initial target population for a new drug is chosen before starting clinical development based on medical considerations of who is most likely to derive the hypothesized benefit of the new drug and on commercial considerations, taking into account the size of the population. It is for this latter reason that most drugs for transplant patients are initially developed in renal transplant patients. However, sometimes Phase II can be used to explore the effect of a new drug in several populations to determine if one type of patient may derive more benefit than others. Usually, the size of Phase II is determined by scientific need and the commercial pressure to minimize the time to regulatory approval, and in this regard compromises are made in both directions.

The keystone of Phase II is a clinical trial, or several clinical trials, that test the safety and efficacy of a new drug at the doses most likely to produce the best balance of safety and efficacy as determined from the preliminary trials outlined above. In general, these key Phase II trials are randomized and, if possible, double blind. These trials may not be powered to the same degree as studies in Phase III. However, they should have enough statistical rigor to give one confidence that the results, if positive, will be corroborated in Phase III, and that finding a null result is not likely if indeed the drug is truly effective. The actual choice of the value of type I and type II error acceptable in a Phase II study is based on several factors. For example, if a drug has the potential to fill an entirely unmet medical need and has great commercial value, then one would want to minimize type II error and be willing to accept a somewhat larger type I error. However, when a drug may have less medical importance and have less of a perceived commercial value one would want a Phase II trial to minimize type I error and accept a larger type II error. Another goal of the larger Phase II studies is to identify logistical issues that might bear on the Phase III studies, so that the Phase III studies can be designed accommodating such issues if they arise.

Phase III: confirming the hypothesis

The main goal of Phase III is to conduct trials that can give a statistically rigorous appraisal of the efficacy of a drug and that provide a safety database extensive enough to make a judgment whether the demonstrated risks are outweighed by the clinical benefits observed. These trials form the primary basis for regulatory approval. In general, a minimum of two such trials, showing consistent results, are required for approval, but there are notable exceptions in solid organ transplantation. For example, after mycophenolate mofetil was approved for use in renal transplantation, only one Phase III trial each in cardiac and hepatic transplant patients was deemed adequate for approval in those populations because it was assumed that the basic mechanism leading to efficacy was the same regardless of the organ transplanted [13, 14]. Also, a sizeable safety database had accumulated. Essentially all Phase III studies in transplantation are randomized. Ideally, all would be double blind; but, as discussed later, this is not always practical. The randomization is often blocked by site, which insures that roughly an equal number of subjects from each site will be assigned to each treatment group. Blocking simply means that, within a certain number of patients to be entered, all treatments will be assigned equally. For example, if there are two treatment arms in a trial, blocking may be in groups of six so that, for each six patients entered, three will be assigned to one treatment and three to the other, although not in any particular order within the block. Blocking by site is not always possible, especially when most sites are not expected to enter many patients. In such a case, randomization is not by site but is centralized. When certain factors are known to affect outcome, or when one wants to test an effect in a special subset of the expected sample to enter the study, the randomization can be stratified so that the distribution of patients with a certain characteristic is balanced across study groups.

The population studied in a Phase III study should be as reflective as possible of the total population for whom treatment is intended. If certain patients are excluded then the results are not strictly applicable to them. All trials have entry criteria that patients must meet to get into a study that define the population from which the trial's sample will be derived. These usually exclude the sickest patients, because they are not likely to respond to therapy and/or not likely to survive long enough to make a meaningful assessment of a therapy's effect. Patients with very abnormal laboratory tests and those at the extremes of age and weight are usually excluded. Finally, patients in Phase III studies are usually followed more frequently with more monitoring of their condition than patients in the usual practice setting. For all these reasons the results of a clinical trial are likely to be better than what will eventually be observed in clinical practice if a drug reaches the market.

The most important part of designing Phase III trials is the choice of the primary endpoint. With rare exception [15], if the primary endpoint is not met then the results will not lead to approval. There is good statistical rationale for this, in that the validity of the type I error is dependent on prespecifying what the endpoint is and what the hypothesis being tested is. The calculated type I error is not valid if a new endpoint is chosen after unblinding or during an open-label study, because the choice could be influenced by knowledge of the result. Once one knows the results, it is a flagrant misuse of inferential statistics to choose an endpoint because it looks like the drug has a desired effect. Some liken this latter practice to betting on a winning horse after the race is run.

Most Phase III clinical trials are not powered to detect differences in subsets of the sample studied, such as the elderly, recipients of organs from donors meeting extended criteria, or patients with hepatitis C undergoing liver transplantation. Also, a finding in such subsets typically is not set as the primary endpoint. However, subset analyses are done to explore whether there is a signal for a different outcome in certain patients compared with the study sample as a whole. A result in a subset that is qualitatively similar to the overall result provides added confidence that the result is applicable to the entire sample studied. Performing a separate trial only in a special population could establish definitively efficacy and safety in that population, as long as the population was well defined by specific criteria.

Patients should be followed for the full duration of the observation period set by a trial, even if a patient withdraws from the assigned treatment. While time to event endpoints (such as time to the first acute rejection) is able to accommodate data from patients lost to follow-up, so-called "time to event analysis" is rarely the primary endpoint of a Phase III trial forming the basis of regulatory approval. When the primary endpoint is a proportion of patients experiencing some event, such as rejection or graft loss or death at some time point, such as at 1 year post-transplant, if one does not actually know the status of a patient at that time then one has to infer it. If one infers that the patient did not experience the event, then the result of the study will be shifted in a positive direction assuming that the event is an undesirable one. However, if one assumes that the patients with missing information experienced the event, then the result will be shifted in a negative direction. Regulatory agencies usually adopt the latter approach because it is more conservative. Therefore, it is more difficult to demonstrate a statistically significant result, in that it assumes that the null hypothesis is true for the missing patients. For continuous variables, such as glomerular filtration rate (GFR), if one does not have data at the time of interest, such as the change from baseline to 1 year post-transplant, then one has to assign some value at 1 year. A common way of doing this is to carry the last observation forward. However, this can result in an inefficient trial at best and a wrong conclusion at worst, especially if the variable was changing at the time of the last value. Some have suggested a modeling approach that incorporates the observed data to estimate the "outcome" [16]. However, such modeling makes certain assumptions that may or may not be acceptable to a reviewer. In any case, the validity of a trial is vitiated if too much data are missing.

When the concentration of a drug is found to be important to achieving efficacy or minimizing toxicity, Phase III studies may employ a strategy of adjusting doses to meet target concentrations of both the control and experimental agents. However, achieving target concentrations is not easy, and concentrations achieved are not always the targeted ones. The concentrations achieved must be taken into account in the prescribing information that is written into the label at the time of regulatory approval [17].

There are several operational decisions that need to be made in designing Phase III studies. They should include a broad selection of patients, so that the sample is as reflective of the population for whom the drug is intended. To some extent this determines where studies are conducted. Most regulatory agencies accept trials conducted in a wide range of countries, but also require that the sample includes patients typical of their jurisdiction. Thus, for a drug to be approved in the USA the study population has to include a representative sample of African Americans because of the well-known differences in outcome in this group compared with Caucasians. Similarly, some Asian countries require studies in an Asian population. Both men and women need to be included in adequate number to get a sense of whether gender has an effect on outcome. Sometimes a balance is not possible if the target population naturally has an imbalance in gender. For example, heart transplantation is carried out more frequently in men than in women because men are more susceptible to a major cause of end-stage heart disease, namely coronary artery disease. With the exception of pediatric patients, the sample should include a wide range of ages. Pediatric patients are usually studied separately, because a separate dosing strategy needs to be developed and the types of toxicity that may be observed could be different from adults. Sometimes, as in liver transplantation where very young children and infants are transplanted because of biliary atresia, a separate study to determine appropriate dosing may be performed in a highly delineated group.

One of two basic types of hypothesis is tested in Phase III studies. The first is that the test drug provides a different result from the control, such as a difference in the rate of acute rejection or a difference in survival. The hypothesis tested in this trial is often called a superiority hypothesis, since one treatment will be superior to others if the null hypothesis is rejected. In this type of trial a two-tailed level of significance is required because one needs to determine if the test drug is better or worse than the control. An α level of <0.05 is typical. Occasionally, a trial may have two primary endpoints and a test drug could be declared different from the control if either of the two endpoints is met. In such a case, a correction to the *p*-value must be made which essentially reduces the significance level of the type I error allowed for each endpoint. This is different from the more common situation, described below, in which two co-primary endpoints must be met to declare a test drug better than the control. The main analysis is conducted in the intent to treat population (ITT), which consists of all randomized patients. The analysis is repeated in a "per protocol" (PP) population, which is a subset of the ITT population, which includes only subjects who adhered to the protocol in predefined ways, such as receiving the assigned treatment for some defined period of time. The result in the PP population is expected to be similar to that in the ITT population, but if a difference is seen between treatment arms in the ITT population then the difference observed would be expected to be of greater magnitude in the PP population. Some trials define the ITT population as all randomized patients who receive at least one dose of study drug. However, when the assigned treatment could affect whether a patient does in fact receive the assigned drug, as is always the case in a nonblinded study, this definition should not be used. In a blinded study, where the treatment assignment could not influence whether a patient actually got dosed, this definition might be acceptable if it were prespecified as the primary analysis population. However, as a matter of practice, the definition of ITT being the same as all randomized patients is the one usually adhered to. Because of the importance of the ITT population, randomization of patients into a trial should occur as close to initiation of treatment as possible. If randomization is too remote from the start of therapy then there is a risk that patients may not actually receive the therapy. If enough patients do not receive the intended therapy, then evaluating the impact of study drug may be hampered and can even influence the outcome of a study [13].

The second type of hypothesis tested in some Phase III studies is that the experimental drug is not inferior to an active control. For example, in renal transplantation, where acute rejection rates now achieved are quite low, it is exceedingly difficult to show that a new drug reduces the rejection rate beyond what the control regimen does. However, there may be some advantage to having a choice of agents that affect the same clinical outcome. In this case a so-called noninferiority trial is carried out. The hypothesis is that the test drug does not produce a result that is worse than the control by a clinically significant margin. In the analysis, a confidence interval of the observed difference in outcome is calculated. Suppose the observed difference in rates of acute rejection for test treatment A and control B is $R_A - R_B = 2\%$. Perhaps it would be acceptable to use the test drug in place of the control because of some other advantage, such as tolerability. This would be acceptable if one were reasonably certain that the acute rejection rate of drug A in the general population of renal transplant patients was less than 4% higher than obtained by the control. This acceptable difference is referred to as the inferiority margin. Then drug A would be an acceptable choice if the upper limit of the 95% confidence interval of $R_A - R_B$ is less than 4%, whereas drug A would not be an acceptable choice if the upper limit of the confidence interval were ≥4%. Noninferiority trials are more subject to bias than superiority trials, and great care must be taken to minimize the occurrence of noncompliance, withdrawals, and lost to follow-up, all of which can make two study arms appear similar independent of a drug effect. In a noninferiority trial the choice of control must be made with care. Strong data must exist, usually from randomized controlled studies, that the control has a positive effect on the outcome of the endpoints tested in the trial.

In transplant trials, it is quite common that two co-primary endpoints are chosen, both of which have to be met in order to declare that a test drug is acceptable for use. For example, one might want to test whether a new drug improves some outcome such as renal function without adversely affecting patient survival. Two hypotheses would be tested: that the new drug is different to the control for the first endpoint and not worse than the control for patient survival, by some acceptable inferiority margin. In such cases, no adjustment of the acceptable type I error (*p*-values) has to be met to declare that the test drug provided a successful outcome.

Usually, a Phase III study will have a number of prespecified secondary endpoints of particular interest, such as time to event analyses, the proportion of patients requiring treatment of rejection, a comparison of the number and severity of rejection episodes, or the incidence of a particular adverse event, such as post-transplant diabetes mellitus. The main reason for prespecifying these is to ensure that the proper data are collected and to the degree that statistical testing is done, to avoid predicating the choice of comparisons with knowledge of the outcome. While *p*-values are often calculated for these endpoints, unless proper adjustments are made for multiple comparisons, which is rarely done, these *p*-values are really nominal and do not provide an accurate assessment of the type I error.

Phase III studies also collect data on safety. This is done in two ways. The first method is generic to all clinical trials, and is the collection of adverse events, which consist of any change or worsening of a patient's clinical condition. These are collected and analyzed in a standard fashion. While it is common to report *p*-values for observed differences in events collected that way, this is inappropriate, since no correction for multiple comparisons is made, and usually the events which appear to occur at different rates in the experimental and control groups are the ones subsequently chosen for testing. However, sometimes particular prespecified events of interest are analyzed and more details are collected. For example, the incidence of certain infections may be of interest and the protocol may include specific ways of collecting data about these and specific criteria for defining these. Similarly, the incidence of hypertension or post-transplant diabetes mellitus may be of interest and what constitutes these entities may be defined in a protocol. While statistical analyses of these have the same issue described above for secondary endpoints, the protocol-defined definitions result in a more accurate assessment of incidence than routine collection of adverse events does.

The analysis of safety from Phase III studies is limited because of the size of the Phase III population. Events that are rare will almost never be detected in clinical development programs. For example, if the true incidence of an event is 1/1000

in the population represented by the control group, at a type I error of 0.05 and a type II error of 0.1, about 30,100 patients would have to be studied to detect a relative risk of 2.0 and about 3900 patients would be required to detect a relative risk of 5 [18]. Studies in the transplant population are never this large. In addition, if an event occurs with a high background rate, then detecting a causal relationship between a drug and the event is also difficult. These types of events are usually detected after approval, when a much larger number of patients receive the drug.

Phase III trials are conducted in a double-blind manner whenever possible. Blinding eliminates bias that can occur if patients or investigators know what drug a patient is on, although this can be imperfect if one of the drugs has unique observable effects. Blinding also offers the advantage of allowing for changes in analysis plans as the trial proceeds, as long as the necessary data are being collected. While this practice is not ideal, Phase III trials take several years to complete and sometimes a new perspective on what is important vis-à-vis endpoints emerge over this time period. Such changes are not possible if some rigor is to be maintained in an open-label study, because it is not possible to exclude that a change in analysis is made based on some sense of the result of the trial. However, sometimes blinding is not possible or at least very difficult to maintain. This is especially true when dosing is dictated by concentrations of drug. The only way to maintain the blind is to keep the personnel making the dose adjustments based on these concentrations separate from those doing the evaluations. Dummy adjustments also have to be built into the placebo dosing as well. While this has been done in a Phase II study [19], it is not really feasible in a Phase III study. If a nonblinded study is conducted, several precautions can be made to increase the rigor and to decrease observer bias. Sometimes it is feasible to have evaluations done by a person who is blind to treatment, such as the reading of biopsies or the questioning of patients about adverse events. The randomization should be either centralized or blocked, such that study personnel would not be able to guess what treatment assignment a prospective patient is likely to receive. Also, under no circumstance should an unblinded study meant for regulatory approval undergo an interim analysis, since the results can easily influence the behavior of patients and investigators for the remainder of the trial. Suppose an interim analysis of an unblinded study suggested that the control treatment is somewhat better than the test drug. Although this finding could be spurious and have occurred by chance alone, it might influence patients assigned to the experimental group to drop out of the trial prematurely and switch to the control group. This would confound the ultimate ITT analysis of the trial, rendering the results useless in supporting regulatory approval. There is a possible example of this in pulmonary transplantation, where a 1 year result, presented at an international congress and published in abstract form, showed an improved survival in patients receiving the test drug [20]. The primary endpoint was the development of bronchiolitis obliterans syndrome at 3 years. By 3 years, more patients in the control arm had dropped out of the study and were either lost to follow-up or had switched to the experimental therapy. The experimental therapy had been approved for other indications and was thus available, and it was impossible to make an "unambiguous conclusion regarding the relative efficacies of the two therapies" [21].

A distinction must be made between testing the effect of a particular drug and testing the effect of a regimen. The difference between these two approaches is that in the former the only change in the experimental and control group is that one group receives the experimental agent and the other does not. When testing regimens, however, regimens differing by more than one agent may be tested, but the contribution of each component to the outcome cannot be evaluated.

During Phase II and often in Phase III a technique known as population pharmacokinetics is increasingly applied to gain a better understanding of the pharmacokinetics and how it relates to clinical effects [22]. While beyond the scope of this chapter, population pharmacokinetics allows one to characterize the pharmacokinetics of a drug by using sparse data from a large number of subjects, and to establish what covariates have significant influences on the pharmacokinetics of a drug [23,24]. When such evaluations are performed in Phase II they can be quite helpful in choosing the dose or doses to test in advanced Phase II studies or in Phase III. When derived from Phase III studies, such results can help modulate or fine tune recommendations for dosing.

In addition to the operational aspects of carrying out a study, it is common for studies to be monitored by an independent panel of clinical and statistical experts called independent data monitoring committees or drug safety monitoring boards [25]. The members of these boards are independent of the study's sponsor and of the investigators and institutions carrying out the study. These bodies may have several purposes, the main one being to ensure the safety of patients. Sometimes these committees are also charged with monitoring a study to determine if an efficacy result is so overwhelmingly positive that it would be unethical to keep the trial going or, conversely, if after a certain number of patients are studied it would be nearly impossible for the trial to reach a definitive result, a so-called futility analysis. Typically, these committees review unblinded data to make these determinations. A detailed discussion about the methods employed to statistically review such data but still maintain the integrity of the trial is beyond the scope of this chapter. However, the methods need to be set up with care so that a study would be stopped early for an efficacy finding only when the chances of being wrong are very low. Just as important, if the study is completed as planned, which usually is the case, the statistical analysis of interim results needs to be set up so that type I error is not unduly compromised in the final analysis. Several methods are available to accomplish this. The most commonly used one prospectively establishes a set of stopping rules and specifies very low type I errors for the early analyses so that only a small adjustment to the p-value at the end of the study is required [26, 27]. One problem with stopping a study early for efficacy is that it limits the amount of safety data available to make an assessment of the balance of risk and benefit. Futility considers type II error to determine, given a set of results at some interim time, whether the trial has a chance to still meet its primary endpoint. If not, then it might not be proper to continue subjecting patients to the trial. Stopping a trial early in this regard also has the potential of saving resources for the sponsor and the institutions carrying out the trial. Establishing a set of stopping rules for safety is harder because safety signals can come in a wide variety of manifestations. Sometimes certain safety signals can be anticipated based on earlier clinical trials, and rules may be established for these. In general, the rules for stopping a trial for safety reasons and the degree of certainty required are somewhat less than for efficacy. Stopping a trial for safety reasons might also require consideration of efficacy to decide if the safety signal warrants a change in the study conduct or stopping it altogether. Finally, it is essential that the details of the deliberations and analyses carried out by monitoring committees be kept confidential and not revealed to anyone involved in the study, unless a decision is taken to terminate a study early. Only the general conclusion regarding whether a trial can go on or whether some specific change in the conduct of the study is warranted is shared publicly.

Findings from Phase II-type studies are inconsistently borne out in Phase III either because efficacy is not confirmed or because of safety findings that were not detected in Phase II. For example, an early study of daclizumab in cardiac transplant patients demonstrated a reduction in acute rejection [28]. When daclizumab was studied in a large, multicenter trial, the results on rejection were similar but there were more deaths in the daclizumab group [29]. This may have been a result of the trial design, because some patients received daclizumab with cytolytic therapy which may have predisposed such patients to infections. Nevertheless, the findings would not have led to regulatory approval.

Other supportive studies

In a development program, other supportive studies, usually pharmacokinetic in nature, are carried out. These include drug interaction studies, the effect of inducers or inhibitors of particular enzymes systems, the effect of food on pharmacokinetics, and studies in patients with severe impairment in the organs of elimination, a study of mass balance or how much of an administered drug and its metabolites is excreted in urine and feces. These studies lead to instructions on how to dose in particular settings and whether a drug needs to be taken in the fasted state or not.

Further considerations of endpoints

One of the most important aspects of clinical development programs is the choice of endpoints in each clinical study. As already discussed, the main endpoints of Phase I studies are defined around pharmacokinetics and signals for toxicity. In Phase II studies, a variety of endpoints are analyzed and there is some flexibility in choosing these. A key set of endpoints in Phase II, especially if one is developing a drug to substitute for a component of the standard of care, is to establish the presence of the desired immunologic effect in patients. That way, one would have some comfort in initiating trials in which patients would not get the full standard regimen. In Phase III studies geared to obtaining regulatory approval, the primary endpoint of each study has to be generally acceptable as medically important and significant by regulatory bodies and clinicians alike, and amenable to the practicalities of carrying out studies to evaluate it. A primary endpoint has to be defined for each study, and it serves to answer the primary question being asked by the study or the primary hypothesis being tested. Most studies also have a variety of secondary endpoints which serve to provide supportive evidence that the findings related to the primary endpoint are likely to be correct. Other secondary endpoints may be designed to examine ancillary questions or to generate hypotheses that could be tested in future studies. When choosing a primary endpoint for Phase III studies, one has to be very conscious of how indications are written from a regulatory point of view. One has to have a well-defined population to which the results pertain and well-defined events that comprise the primary endpoint.

The use of surrogate endpoints can be useful to make the process of development more efficient when following the actual event of interest takes a long time. However, the degree of certainty to which a surrogate endpoint actually reflects what would happen if the actual event of interest were accounted for is important. The most stringent definition is that the surrogate must correlate with the actual endpoint and changes in the surrogate should predict changes in the actual endpoint. An intervention that has an effect on the surrogate must have the same effect on the endpoint. Both conditions are necessary, since an association of an event or biological marker is not proof of causality: "A correlate does not a surrogate make" [30]. Some would insist that all the changes that an intervention would induce be reflected by the surrogate endpoint. While a prospective clinical trial could validate a surrogate, this approach would defeat the purpose of using the surrogate in the first place (but could enable the surrogate for use in future trials). Other methods to validate surrogate endpoints should rely on a combination of sound biological reasoning and other empirical methods, such as meta-analysis. A hierarchy of validity of surrogate endpoints has been proposed to consider their use [30], and some have proposed adoption of a surrogate based on the preponderance of evidence and reaching a certain level of certainty as to the surrogate endpoint's validity [31]. The use of surrogates as the sole basis of regulatory approval is allowed in cases of urgent medical need, but in such cases more rigorous studies have to be carried out after approval to actually prove that the original conclusion regarding the benefit of a drug is borne out. This approach has been used in drugs approved for AIDS and in oncology, but not in transplantation.

While not usually suitable for definitive evidence of efficacy, endpoints such as biological markers are very useful in Phase II to show that the effects discovered in preclinical work carry over into patients. While modulating the biological effect may or may not lead to a clinical effect, evidence that a biological effect occurred can be important in moving a project forward. The biomarker can provide a level of comfort that a new agent might be efficacious and thus justify experiments in people.

In transplantation, the traditional primary endpoint in Phase III studies has been the incidence of biopsy-proven acute rejection. However, in recent years with standard therapy, the incidence of acute rejection achieved is acceptable to most clinicians and further improvements, with the exception of achieving tolerance, would add little clinical value. In addition, statistically demonstrating an improvement becomes increasingly difficult, since the difference between a new therapy and control would be small and thus require very large sample sizes to have enough power to demonstrate a statistically significant difference. Furthermore, there is the possibility that added immunosuppression leading to less acute rejection might in fact lead to an increased incidence of opportunistic infections and malignancy. While the former would be relatively easy to measure in a clinical trial lasting 1 year, malignancy would not. Demonstrating noninferiority for acute rejection is less of a problem, but the added medical value of such trials is limited. Thus, for both medical and logistical reasons, investigators are seeking to establish new endpoints that could warrant regulatory approval [32]. Some are functional. For example, in renal transplantation, GFR at various times after transplantation has received attention recently [33, 34]. In cardiac transplantation, the development of post-transplant coronary artery disease has achieved some prominence [35], but has not been used as a primary endpoint. Post-transplant coronary artery disease has not been proven to be a surrogate for graft survival that would meet regulatory muster, in that a decrease in post-transplant coronary artery disease has not resulted in improved survival [36]. Since calcineurin inhibitors are a cause of deteriorating renal function in organ transplantation in general, regimens being tested that might reduce this outcome have been explored in recent years. If rejection rates are acceptably low, renal function per se would seem a reasonable primary endpoint [37, 38]. Long-term graft survival and function is of obvious interest. However, long-term studies exceeding 1 year, or at most 2 years, are extremely difficult to carry out successfully, primarily due to attrition [39, 40], and from patients crossing over to the standard of care, which is often the control, after discontinuing an experimental treatment. Acute humoral rejection has been studied and is recognized as an important source of damage to allografts, and has also received some attention as an endpoint [32].

The ultimate outcome of development

The process of clinical drug development proceeds through a series of steps, each one shaped by data from earlier ones. It is an iterative process of hypothesis generation and testing. When completed, a body of data has accumulated that allows sponsors and regulatory agencies to determine which patients benefit from therapy and to write prescribing information that can guide physicians as to the use of the drug. Because clinical practice differs from clinical trials in major ways, the prescribing information provides guidelines for clinical use that physicians must adapt to specific clinical situations. A development program really establishes a starting point, based on studies of high quality, to institute a new therapy. A large amount of information, some very rigorously obtained and analyzed and some not so much, always becomes available from trials and observational data not included in a formal development program. It is the responsibility of the clinical community to continually evaluate the data so provided with critical judgment and to make judicious modifications of therapy accordingly.

References

1 Buöen C, Holm S, Mikael TS. Evaluation of the cohort size in phase 1 dose escalation trials based on laboratory data. *J Clin Pharmacol* 2003;43:470–476.

2 Posvar EL, Sedman AJ. New drugs: first time in man. *J Clin Pharmacol* 1989;29:961–966.

3 Chappell WR, Mordenti J. Extrapolation of toxicological and pharmacological data from animals to humans. In Testa B (ed.) *Advances in Drug Research*, vol. 20. San Diego: Academic Press; 1991, pp. 1–116.

4 Mahmood I, Green MD, Fisher JE. Selection of the first-time dose in humans: comparison of different approaches based on interspecies scaling of clearance. *J Clin Pharmacol* 2003;43:692–697.

5 Mordenti J, Osaka G, Garcia K *et al.* Pharmacokinetics and interspecies scaling of recombinant human factor VIII. *Toxicol Appl Pharmacol* 1996;136:75–78.

6 Mordenti J, Thomsen K, Licko V *et al.* Efficacy and concentration-response of murine anti-VEGF monoclonal antibody in tumor-bearing mice and extrapolation to humans. *Toxicol Pathol* 1999;27:14–21.

7 Mordenti J, Chen SA, Moore JA *et al.* Interspecies scaling of clearance and volume of distribution data from five therapeutic proteins. *Pharm Res* 1991;8:1351–1359.

8 Food and Drug Administration. Estimating the maximum safe starting dose in initial clinical trials for therapeutics in adult healthy volunteers; 2005. http://www.fda.gov/downloads/Drugs/GuidanceComplianceRegulatoryInformation/Guidances/UCM078932.pdf (accessed 8 August 2009).

9 EMEA. Guidline on strategies to identify and mitigate risks for first-in-human clinical trials with investigational medicinal products; 2007 (accessed 8 August 2009).

10 Vincenti F, Larsen C, Durrbach A *et al.* Costimulation blockade with belatacept in renal transplantation. *N Engl J Med* 2006;353:770–781.

11 Vincenti F, Charpentier B, Vanrenterghem Y *et al.* A phase III study of belatacept-based immunosuppression regimens versus cyclosporine in renal transplant recipients (BENEFIT study). *Am J Transplant* 2010;10(3):535–546.

12 Vincenti F, Ramos E, Brattstrom C *et al.* Multicenter trial exploring calcineurin inhibitors avoidance in renal transplantation. *Transplantation* 2001;71:1282–1287.

13 Kobashigawa J, Miller L, Renlund D *et al.* A randomized active-controlled trial of mycophenolate mofetil in heart transplant recipients. *Transplantation* 1998;66:507–515.

14 Wiesner R, Rabkin J, Klintmalm G *et al.* A randomized double-blind comparative study of mycophenolate mofetil and azathioprine in combination with cyclosporine and corticosteroids in primary liver transplant recipients. *Liver Transplant* 2001;7:442–450.

15 Food and Drug Administration. Transcript: Open Session, Subcommittee of the Antiviral Drugs Advisory Committee, 14 January 1998.

16 Jonsson EN, Sheiner L. More efficient clinical trials through use of scientific model-based statistical tests. *Clin Pharmacol Ther* 2002;72:603–614.

17 Ekberg H, Mamelok RD, Pearson TC *et al.* The challenge of achieving target drug concentrations in

clinical trials: experience from the symphony study. *Transplantation* 2009;87:1360–1366.

18 Mamelok RD. Drug discovery and development. In *Clinical Pharmacology* (Carruthers SG, Hoffman BB, Melmon KL, Nierenberg DW eds), 4th edn. New York: McGraw Hill, 2000, pp. 1289–1305.

19 Van Gelder T, Hilbrands LB, Vanrenterghem Y *et al.* A randomized double-blind, multicenter plasma concentration controlled study of the safety and efficacy of oral mycophenolate mofetil for the prevention of acute rejection after kidney transplantation. *Transplantation* 1999;68:261–266.

20 Corris P, Glanville A, McNeil K *et al.* One year analysis of an ongoing international randomized study of mycophenolate mofetil vs azathioprine in lung transplantation. *J Heart Lung Transplant* 2001;20:149–150.

21 McNeil K, Glanville AR, Wahlers T *et al.* Comparison of mycophenolate mofetil and azathioprine for prevention of bronchiolitis obliterans syndrome in de novo lung transplant recipients. *Transplantation* 2006;81:998–1003.

22 Ette EI, Williams PJ. Population pharmacokinetics 1: background, concepts and models. *Ann Pharmacol* 2004;38:1702–1706.

23 Van Hest RM, Mathot RAA, Pescovitz MD *et al.* Explaining variability in mycophenolic acid exposure to optimize mycophenolate mofetil dosing: a population pharmacokinetic meta-analysis of mycophenolic acid in renal transplant patients. *J Am Soc Nephrol* 2006;17:871–880.

24 Van Hest RM, van Gelder T, Bouw R *et al.* Time-dependent clearance of mycophenolic acid in renal transplant recipients. *Br J Clin Pharmacol* 2007;63:741–752.

25 Food and Drug Administration. Establishment and operations of clinical trial data monitoring committees; 2006. http://www.fda.gov/downloads/RegulatoryInformation/Guidances/UCM127073.pdf (accessed 21 August 2009).

26 Evans SR, Li L, Wei LJ. Data monitoring in clinical trials using prediction. *Drug Inf J* 2007;41:733–742.

27 Green SJ, Fleming TR, O'Fallon JR. Policies for study monitoring and interim reporting of results. *J Clin Oncol* 1987;5:1477–1484.

28 Beniaminovitz A, Itescu S, Lietz K *et al.* Prevention of rejection in cardiac transplantation by blockade of the interleukin-2 receptor with monoclonal antibody. *N Engl J Med* 2000;342:613–619.

29 Hershberger RE, Starling RC, Eisen HJ *et al.* Daclizumab to prevent rejection after cardiac transplantation. *N Engl J Med* 2005;352:2705–2713.

30 Fleming TR. Surrogate endpoints and FDA's accelerated approval process. *Health Aff* 2005;24:67–78.

31 Woodcock J. http://www.fda.gov/ohrms/dockets/ac/04/slides/2004-4079S2_03_Woodcock.ppt; 2004 (accessed 7 August 2009).

32 Vincenti F. http://cme.medscape.com/viewarticle/465463; 2003 (accessed 15 August 2009).

33 Abramowicz D, Manas D, Lao M *et al.* Cyclosporine withdrawal from a mycophenolate mofetil-containing immunosuppressive regimen in stable kidney transplant recipients: a randomized, controlled study. *Transplantation* 2002;74:1725–1734.

34 Weir MR, Ward MT, Blahut SA *et al.* Long-term impact of discontinued or reduced calcineurin inhibitor in patients with chronic allograft nephropathy. *Kidney Int* 2001;59:1567–1573.

35 Mehra MR, Benza R, Deng MC *et al.* Surrogate markers for late cardiac allograft survival. *Am J ransplant* 2004; 4:1184–1191.

36 Eisen HJ, Tuzcu EM, Dorent R *et al.* Everolimus for the prevention of allograft rejection and vasculopathy in cardiac-transplant recipients. *N Engl J Med* 2003; 349:847–858.

37 Ekberg H, Tedesco-Silva H, Demirbas A *et al.* Reduced exposure to calcineurin inhibitors in renal transplantation. *N Engl J Med* 2003;357:2562–2575.

38 Neuberger JM, Mamelok RD, Neuhaus P *et al.* Delayed introduction of reduced-dose tacrolimus and renal function in liver transplantation: the 'ReSpECT' study. *Am J Transplant* 2009;9:327–336.

39 Mele TS, Halloran PF. The use of mycophenolate mofetil in transplant recipients. *Immunopharmacology* 2000;47:215–245.

40 Eisen HJ, Kobashigawa J, Keogh A *et al.* Three-year results of a randomized, double-blind, controlled trial of mycophenolate mofetil versus azathioprine in cardiac transplant recipients. *J Heart Lung Transplant* 2005;24:517–525.

PART 3
Agents

PART 1
Agents

CHAPTER 12
Corticosteroids

Olivia R. Blume, Sarah E. Yost, and Bruce Kaplan
University of Arizona Medical Center, Tucson, AZ, USA

History

- Since the first days of organ transplantation in the 1950s, corticosteroids have been used for immunosuppression and as an adjunct to irradiation. Prior to the 1950s there had been several successful living-related renal transplant procedures from twin donors [1]. In 1959, Dameshek and Schwartz from the Peter Bent Brigham Hospital had found that 6-mercaptopurine, which is an imidazole derivative of azathioprine, had antibody blocking effects in rabbits. The first cadaveric renal transplant was performed in 1962 at the Peter Bent Brigham Hospital, where azathioprine was used as the first immunosuppressive drug. Initially, corticosteroids were used for maintenance immunosuppression in prevention and treatment of rejection in patients on irradiation or azathioprine monotherapy. It was then common practice to use both azathioprine and steroids in combination. Shortly afterward, introduction of antilymphocyte globulin with living-related donors had resulted in 45 % 1 year graft survival, which improved to 80 % 1 year graft survival after refinement in patient selection. The only issue with antithymocyte globulin was that it was not readily available; therefore, it was common practice to use both azathioprine and corticosteroids.

- *Induction* More than 40 agents have been used for induction medication alone or in combination. Corticosteroids are usually used in combination and have been found that when used with alemtuzumab, has lowest risk of graft failure [2]. This is followed by alemtuzumab alone, thymo with steroids, thymo alone, basilizimab, and steroids alone. Lymphocyte-depleting strategies, when given concurrently with steroids, are more efficient in preventing graft failure.

- *Maintainence* Steroid avoidance, minimization, and withdrawal had been common practice even from the beginning of transplantation owing to the long list of side effects and complications. Weight gain, hyperglycemia, peptic ulcer osteoporosis, and muscle wasting are an incomplete list which will be covered in this chapter [3].

Chemistry/structure

See Figure 12.1 [4].

Mechanism of action

- *Effects on lymphocytes* The mechanisms by which corticosteroids act are by altering lymphocyte function by negative regulation of cytokine gene expression [1]. Corticosteroids repress cytokine gene expression at glucocorticoid binding sites of two transcription factors, which are activator protein-1 (AP-1) and nuclear factor κB (NF-κB). AP-1 induces cytokine genes and growth factors

Immunotherapy in Transplantation: Principles and Practice, First Edition. Edited by Bruce Kaplan, Gilbert J. Burckart and Fadi G. Lakkis.
© 2012 Blackwell Publishing Ltd. Published 2012 by Blackwell Publishing Ltd.

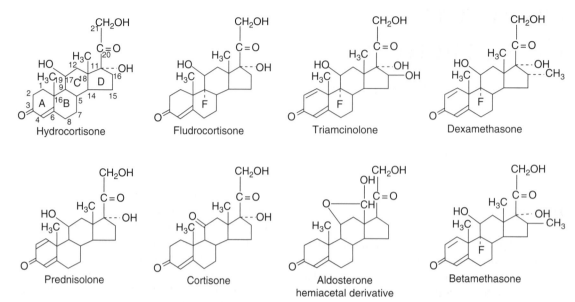

Figure 12.1 *Structure and nomenclature of corticosteroids.* Prednisone has high oral bioavailability which, when given, is rapidly hydrolyzed via the liver which reduces the 11-oxo group to form prednisolone. Prednisolone binds to transcortin (70%) and exhibits saturable nonlinear binding. From [4], Schimmer BP, Parker KL. Adrenocorticotropic hormone; adrenocortical steroids and their synthetic analogs; inhibitors of the synthesis and actions of adrenocortical hormones. In *Goodman & Gilman's The Pharmacological Basis of Therapeutics* (Brunton LL, Lazo JS, Parker KL eds), 11th edn. New York: McGraw-Hill; ©2006. Reproduced with permission by The McGraw-Hill Companies.

such as the IL-2 cytokine, whereas NF-κB is an important regulator of the genes used for many cytokine and cell adhesion molecules. Corticosteroids cause transcriptional interference with transcriptional regulatory proteins which bind to AP-1 sites as well as induce a protein that inhibits NF-κB activity. Corticosteroids indirectly affect B lymphocytes by increasing catabolism of immunoglobulins. This is caused by inhibition of cytokines IL-1 through IL-6, which prevents accessory or helper T cell activities. Also, this is explained by inhibition of CD40 ligand expression and transcription in activated T cells. Moderate and high doses of corticosteroids used for treatment of rejection treatment prevent cytokine action, which prevents cytotoxic T cell responses as well. See Figure 12.2.

- *Side effects*
  - *Weight gain*: Ghrelin is a 28 amino acid peptide which stimulates growth hormone and adrenocorticotropin secretion from the pituitary. It is mainly produced and secreted in the stomach,

using a gastro-hypophyseal feedback loop for regulation. Ghrelin signals the central nervous system to increase metabolism when necessary. There is evidence that decreased ghrelin may be involved in mechanisms leading to obesity and type 2 diabetes mellitus [5]. Two groups were studied that included patients with history of Cushing's disease and healthy patients who were given 30 mg prednisolone once daily for 5 days. It was found that plasma ghrelin had increased 3–24 months after surgical removal of adenomas found in Cushing disease patients. Healthy patients who were given exogenous prednisolone were shown to have decreased plasma ghrelin after 5 days of therapy. The findings have shown that there is a decrease in plasma ghrelin during hypercortisolism, indicating a feedback mechanism between ghrelin levels and the pituitary–adrenal axis. Therefore, ghrelin levels are low under the influence of corticosteroids and increased in their absence. This explains the weight gain seen as a

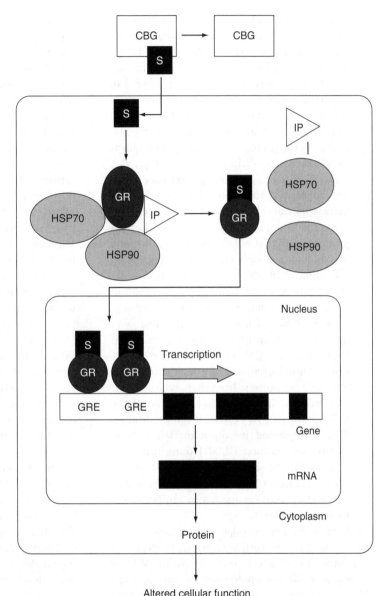

Figure 12.2 *Glucocorticoid receptor.* The glucocorticoid receptor (GR) resides in the cytoplasm in inactive form before it binds to steroid hormone (S), which is closely associated with heat-shock protein 70 (HSP70). GR then changes in conformation for activation/ translocation of nucleus allowing for transcription of target genes. Within the gene are introns and extrons allowing transcription and mRNA processing. From [4], Schimmer BP, Parker KL. Adrenocorticotropic hormone; adrenocortical steroids and their synthetic analogs; inhibitors of the synthesis and actions of adrenocortical hormones. In *Goodman & Gilman's The Pharmacological Basis of Therapeutics* (Brunton LL, Lazo JS, Parker KL eds), 11th edn. New York: McGraw-Hill; © 2006. Reproduced with permission by The McGraw-Hill Companies.

side effect in patients who use prednisone as part of immunosuppressive therapy.

o *Hyperglycemia*: Steroids and calcineurin inhibitors have been shown to cause development of post-transplantation diabetes mellitus [6]. It has been demonstrated that corticosteroids cause insulin resistance similar to type 2 diabetes mellitus. A study by Hjelmesaeth *et al.* demonstrated that the risk of developing post-transplant diabetes mellitus is dose dependent [7]. The risk is 5 % per 0.01 mg/(kg day) increase in prednisolone dosage and it was found that changing from high-dose to low-dose steroids was associated with a decreased incidence. Also, it is important to note that post-transplant diabetes mellitus has been found in higher incidence (21.1% versus 5.1 %) with patients who weigh >70 kg [8].

- It was found with adrenalectomized rats that excess corticosteroids can affect glucose metabolism by increasing hepatic glucose production and decreasing insulin sensitivity [9]. This can lead to hyperglycemia and eventually lead to steroid-diabetes. The exact mechanism responsible for alteration of glucose metabolism is still unclear, but there are several proposed mechanisms. Corticosteroids can up-regulate gluconeogenic enzymes such as phosphoenolpyruvate carboxykinase and glucose-6-phosphatase, causing hyperglycemia. Also, glycerol release is increased in fat cells during gluconeogenesis. In turn, a second major effect that corticosteroids produce is inhibition of glucose uptake and metabolism in peripheral tissues by decreasing the number of glucose transporters. Insulin action can be altered as well by alteration of insulin receptor and post-receptor functioning.

- As is known, chronic hyperglycemia over time can cause insulin resistance as well [9]. Impairment of glucose uptake is often the cause of insulin resistance by desensitization of glucose transporters from hyperglycemia. It was recently discovered that the role of the hexosamine pathway causes insulin resistance. This is explained by phosphorylation from non-insulin-sensitive GLUT-1 transporter into non-insulin-sensitive hexokinase. Following a series of reactions, alteration of insulin signaling in target cells occurs, which inhibits translocation of GLUT-4.

o *Peptic ulcer*: The pathogenesis of peptic ulcer as a side effect of corticosteroids is unclear and is found to be a common complaint patients disclose while on prednisone as part of their immunosuppressive therapy [10]. Data have been found that cases of peptic ulcer commonly occur in the early period after transplantation, occurring mostly during the first 90 days. It was found that 116 of 1734 patients studied from January 1964 through 1983 at the University of California, San Francisco, had peptic ulcer after transplantation. This is a 6.7% incidence. Prior to development of H2 receptor antagonists in the 1980s, the incidence of peptic ulcer in transplant patients was the second major complication found after transplantation [11]. This study conducted by Steger *et al.* compared a group of patients on azathioprine and prednisone with a group of patients on cyclosporin, low-dose azathioprine, and low-dose prednisone. In both groups, endoscopy was performed for surveillance 7–14 days after transplantation. It was found that there was no difference between these groups and the incidence of peptic ulcer (13.5–18%), which can indicate that this complication is multi-factorial. Factors could include increased gastric acid secretion in the post-operative period while on dialysis, elevated plasma histamine after surgery, and increased gastrin concentrations after surgery as well. Therefore, prophylactic therapy with H2 antagonists after surgery is of high importance to prevent this complication.

o *Osteoporosis*: Bone loss while on corticosteroid therapy can occur over a span of 12 months and is a well-known side effect [12]. Weinstein *et al.* [13] have shown that corticosteroids increase osteoclast function and cause increased rate of apoptosis of osteoblasts and inhibition of collagen synthesis, which are required for bone growth. The study suggests that these factors account for a decline in bone formation and trabecular width. Glucocorticoids also may have indirect negative effects on bone by inhibition of insulin-like growth factor-1. Bone loss also occurs due to calcium losses by other organ systems. Corticosteroids decrease serum calcium by inhibiting intestinal calcium absorption and allowing for renal calcium loss.

o *Muscle wasting*: Also a common side effect found with patients on corticosteroids is muscle wasting, which has been studied in mouse models of acute diabetes [14]. Adrenalectomized mice with acute diabetes showed progressive muscle wasting when given a physiologic dose of glucocorticoids. Factors affecting muscle wasting are described by glucocorticoid receptor activation (Figure 12.1), which competes with IRS-1 for PI3K, reducing IRS-1-associated PI3K activity. Diabetes, acidosis, sepsis, uremia, fasting, and excess angiotensin II are catabolic conditions which activate muscle proteolysis. The mechanism to explain this is described by glucocorticoid receptor activation, which competes with IRS-1 for PI3K, reducing IRS-1-associated PI3K activity. This in turn leads to reduction of p-Akt which in turn activates proteolytic mechanisms causing muscle atrophy. It is unclear, however, if pharmacologic doses of glucocorticoids solely cause this.

Pharmacokinetics/ pharmacodynamics

• *Bioavailability, binding, elimination* Methylprednisolone/ prednisolone are both poorly water soluble, but prednisolone has high oral bioavailability [15]. When methylprednisolone is given intravenously, water-soluble salts of esters form which are rapidly hydrolyzed in the liver to alcohol form. Peak concentration is reached in 31 min. Methylprednisolone is primarily bound to albumin when given, and is not affected by inflammatory states or renal impairment to reveal dose-linear pharmacokinetics. Methlyprednisolone metabolism occurs via reversible oxidation of the 11-hydroxyl group in the liver, and has an elimination half-life of 2–3 h excreted by the kidney. Prednisone has high oral bioavailability, which when given is rapidly hydrolyzed via the liver which reduces the 11-oxo group to form prednisolone. Prednisolone although highly bioavailable (92 %, peak concentration 1.3 h), has decreased clearance in the settings of inflammation or renal failure [16]. Prednisolone binds to transcortin (70 %) and exhibits saturable nonlinear binding. Owing to the saturable nature of prednisolone to transcortin, as concentrations of prednisolone fall, clearance decreases. Prednisone has an elimation half-life of 2.6–3 h and is not dialyzable. Over a 5 h dialysis period, only 7–17.5 % of the dose is removed.

• *Interactions* Multiple drugs, including prednisolone, use the CYP450 system for metabolism, so prednisolone can have many drug interactions. Prednisolone uses 3A4 substrate for metabolism [16]. For transplantation, however, both cyclosporin and tacrolimus, which is used commonly for immunosuppression, do not affect the pharmacokinetics of prednisolone or methylprednisolone. It is notable that corticosteroid withdrawal studies show that concurrent use of prednisone with mycophenolate mofetil (MMF) can increase activity of UDP-glucuronosyltransferase (UGT-GT) [17]. UGT-GT is an enzyme found mainly in the liver which can, in turn, inactivate the active form of MMF. This was found in a study performed by Schuetz *et al.*, where activity of UDP-GT was increased in rat hepatocyte cells both in culture and in in-vivo rodent animal models [18]. Also, these pharmacokinetic differences for lower active MMF exposure can be attributed to poor gastrointestinal absorption in the perioperative phase.

• *Special circumstances affecting pharmacokinetics* As mentioned earlier, renal failure mainly affects the clearance of oral prednisone by decreasing clearance [16]. Methylprednisolone is not affected. There is decreased clearance of both prednisolone and methylprednisolone in hepatic failure, since both utilize the CYP3A system. Pediatric patients were found to increase clearance of prednisolone only, although there is not much data about elderly patients and pharmacokinetics.

Solumedrol adsorption, distribution, metabolism, excretion

Solumedrol is well absorbed and the bioavailability of rectal is 14.2 % and topical is variable from 1 to 36 % [19]. The volume of distribution is 1.5 L/kg [20, 21]. Solumedrol undergoes extensive liver metabolism via reversible oxidation of the 11-hydroxyl group [22]. Solumedrol is excreted by the kidneys primarily as metabolites. The total body clearance is 16–21 L/h. The elimination half-life is 2–3 h [20, 21, 23]. The time to peak concentration in the intravenous form is 31 min and intra-articular form it is 16 days [20, 23, 24].

Prednisone adsorption, distribution, metabolism, excretion

The oral bioavailability of prednisone is 92 % [25, 26]. The time to peak concentration is 1.3 h and the mean maximum serum concentration of prednisolone, the active metabolite, is 233 ng/mL [25].

The protein binding is 70% and the active metabolite, prednisolone, is nonlinearly bound to transcortin and albumin [27, 28]. The volume of distribution of prednisone is 0.4–1 L/kg. Prednisone is metabolized by the liver to the 11-oxo group of prednisone to form the biologically active steroid prednisolone. Historically, prednisolone has been recognized as the primary metabolite of prednisone; however, some work has established that prednisone and prednisolone undergo complex reversible metabolism. After oral doses of prednisone or prednisolone, the plasma concentration–time profiles for both agents are superimposable [25, 28]. The elimination half-life is 2.6–3 h [25]. Prednisone is not dialyzable, however, when prednisone is administered before dialysis: as noted above, 7–17.5% of the dose was removed over a 5 h dialysis period [28].

Therapeutic drug monitoring

As of today, there is no clinical reason for therapeutic drug monitoring for the corticosteroids.

Pharmacogenomics

One of the factors affecting transplant outcomes includes the evolving complexities presented by our growing knowledge about pharmacogenomics. Ethnic and genetic factors have been shown to influence the dose requirements for tacrolimus, with African Americans requiring higher doses secondary to the CYP3A5*1 allele that is present in 70–80% of African American individuals. Patients require two to three times more tacrolimus to reach therapeutic concentrations. For these patients the number of pills and cost of tacrolimus are significantly higher than individuals who do not express CYP3A5. Patients who have a delay in achieving target tacrolimus concentrations within the first few weeks after transplant have a higher risk for rejection [29]. Studies are underway to evaluate this allele expression in regard to corticosteroids.

Drug–drug interactions

The following drug interactions are classified as contraindicated for current use. A major drug interaction may be life threatening and/or require medical intervention to minimize or prevent serious adverse effects. A moderate interaction may result in exacerbation of the patient's condition and/or require an alteration in therapy. Finally, a minor interaction would have limited clinical effects.

Current use of rotavirus vaccine and corticosteroids is contraindicated because of the increased risk of infection by the live vaccine [30]. Quetiapine and corticosteroids can lead to decreased serum concentrations of quetiapine and is defined as a major interaction [31]. Concurrent use of phenobarbital, butabarbital, and phenytoin can have a moderate effect of reducing the therapeutic effect of corticosteroids [16, 32, 33]. The concurrent use of floroquinolones and corticosteroids may result in an increased risk for tendon rupture [34]. Transplant medications can also interact with corticosteroids. The combination of cyclosporine and corticosteroids may result in cyclosporine toxicity and steroid excess. Monitor cyclosporine levels and adjust cyclosporine dosage as necessary. Monitor patients for increased cyclosporine toxicity (renal dysfunction, neurotoxicity). Also, monitor patients for corticosteroid excess and adjust methylprednisolone dosage as necessary [35]. The combination with tacrolimus may result in increased tacrolimus concentrations, and so monitor and look for signs of tacrolimus toxicity (nephrotoxicity, hyperglycemia, hyperkalemia). Tacrolimus doses may need to be reduced when methylprednisolone is used concomitantly [36]. The concurrent use of azole antifungals and prednisone may result in increased prednisone plasma concentrations and increased risk for prednisone side effects [37, 38].

References

1 Morrissey PE, Madras PN, Monaco AP. History of kidney and pancreas transplantation. In: Norman DJ, Turka LA (eds), *Primer on Transplantation*, 2nd edn. New Jersey: American Society of Transplantation; 2001, pp. 411–413.

2 Cai J, Terasaki PI. Induction immunosuppression improves long-term graft and patient outcome in organ transplantation: an analysis of United Network for Organ Sharing Registry Data. *Transplantation* 2010;90:1511–1515.

3 Srinivas TR, Meier-Kriesche H. Mimimizing immuno-suppression, an alternative approach to reducing side effects: objectives and interim result. *Clin J Am Soc Nephrol* 2008;3:S101–S116.

4 Schimmer BP, Parker KL. Adrenocorticotropic hormone; adrenocortical steroids and their synthetic analogs; inhibitors of the synthesis and actions of adrenocortical hormones. In *The Pharmacological Basis of Therapeutics* (Brunton LL, Lazo JS, Parker KL eds), 11th edn. New York: McGraw-Hill; 2006, pp. 1595, 1597.

5 Otto B, Tschöp M, Heldwein W *et al*. Endogenous and exogenous glucocorticoids decrease plasma ghrelin in humans. *Eur J Endocrinol* 2004;151:113–117.

6 Mathew JT, Rao M, Job V *et al*. Post-transplant hyperglycemia: a study of risk factors. *Nephrol Dial Transplant* 2003;18:164–171.

7 Hjelmesæth J, Hartmann A, Kofstad J *et al*. Glucose intolerance after renal transplantation depends upon prednisolone dose and recipient age 1. *Transplantation* 1997;64(7):979–983.

8 Boudreaux JP, McHugh L, Canafax DM *et al*. The impact of cyclosporine and combination immunosuppression on the incidence of posttransplant diabetes in renal allograft recipients. *Transplantation* 1987;44 (3):376–380.

9 Jin JY, Jusko WJ. Pharmacodynamics of glucose regulation by methylprednisolone. *I. Adrenalectomized rats. Biopharm Drug Dispos* 2009;30:21–34.

10 Feduska NJ, Amend WJ, Vincenti F *et al*. Peptic ulcer disease in kidney transplant recipients. *Am J Surg* 1984;148:51–57.

11 Steger AC, Timoney SA, Griffen S *et al*. The influence of immunosuppression on peptic ulceration following renal transplantation and the role of endoscopy. *Nephrol Dial Transplant* 1990;5:289–292.

12 Kumar R. Glucocorticoid-induced osteoporosis. *Curr Opin Nephrol Hypertens* 2001;10:589–595.

13 Weinstein RS, Jilka RL, Parfitt AM, Manolagas SC. Inhibition of osteoblastogenesis and promotion of apoptosis of osteoblasts and osteocytes by glucocorticoids: potential mechanisms of their deleterious effects on bone. *J Clin Invest* 1998;102:274–282.

14 Hu Z, Wang H, Lee IH *et al*. Endogenous glucocorticoids and impaired insulin signaling are both required to stimulate muscle wasting under pathophysiological conditions in mice. *J Clin Invest* 2009;119:3059–3069.

15 Srinivas TR, Meier-Kriesche HU, Kaplan B. Pharmacokinetic principles of immunosuppressive drugs. *Am J Transplant* 2005;5:207–217.

16 Micromedex: Corticosteroids; 2011. http://www.thomsonh.com (accessed 31 March 2011).

17 Cattaneo D, Perico N, Gaspari F *et al*. Glucocorticoids interfere with mycophenolate mofetil bioavailability in kidney transplantation. *Kidney Int* 2002;62:1060–1067.

18 Schuetz EG, Hazelton GA, Hall J *et al*. Induction of digitoxigenin monodigitoxoside UDP-glucuronosyltransferase activity by glucocorticoids and other inducers of cytochrome P-450p in primary monolayer cultures of adult rat hepatocytes and in human liver. *J Biol Chem* 1986;261:8270–8275.

19 Kelly R, Keipert JA. Selecting a topical corticosteroid. *Curr Ther* 1979;20:89–95.

20 Al-Habet SM, Rogers HJ. Methylprednisolone pharmacokinetics after intravenous and oral administration. *Br J Clin Pharmacol* 1989;27:285–290.

21 Stjernholm MR, Katz FH. Effects of diphenylhydantoin, phenobarbital, and diazepam on the metabolism of methylprednisolone and its sodium succinate. *J Clin Endocrinol Metab* 1975;41:887–893.

22 Gilman AG, Rall TW, Nies AS, Taylor P (eds.). *Goodman and Gilman's The Pharmacological Basis of Therapeutics, 8th edn*. New York, NY: Pergamon Press; 1990.

23 Derendorf H, Möllmann H, Krieg M *et al*. Pharmacodynamics of methylprednisolone phosphate after single intravenous administration to healthy volunteers. *Pharm Res* 1991;8:263–268.

24 Mattila J. Prolonged action and sustained serum levels of methylprednisolone after a local injection of methylprednisolone acetate. *Clin Trials J* 1983;20:18–23.

25 Ferry JJ, Horvath AM, Bekersky I *et al*. Relative and absolute bioavailability of prednisone and prednisolone after separate oral and intravenous doses. *J Clin Pharmacol*. 1988;28:81–87.

26 Anderson RJ, Gambertogolio JG, Schrier RW. *Clinical Use of Drugs in Renal Failure*. Springfield, IL: Charles C Thomas Publisher; 1976.

27 Chen PS, Mills IH, Bartter FC. Ultrafiltration studies of steroid protein binding. *J Endocrinol* 1961;23:129–137.

28 Frey B, Frey FJ. Clinical pharmacokinetics of prednisone and prednisolone. *Clin Pharmacokinet* 1990; 19:126–146.

29 MacPhee IA, Fredericks S, Tai T *et al*. The influence of pharmacogenetics on the time to achieve target tacrolimus concentrations after kidney transplantation. *Am J Transplant* 2004;4:914–919.

30 Grabenstein JD. Drug interactions involving immunologic agents. Part 1. Vaccine–vaccine, vaccine–

immunoglobulin, and vaccine–drug interactions. *DICP* 1990;24:67–81.

31 Product Information: Seroquel®, quetiapine fumurate. Wilmington, DE: AstraZeneca Pharmaceuticals; 01/2001.

32 Gambertoglio JG, Holford NH, Kapusnik JE *et al.* Disposition of total and unbound prednisolone in renal transplant patients receiving anticonvulsants. *Kidney Int* 1984;25:119–123.

33 Petereit LB, Meikle AW. Effectiveness of prednisolone during phenytoin therapy. *Clin Pharmacol Ther* 1977;22:912–916.

34 Levaquin® [package insert]. Raritan, NJ: Ortho-McNeil Pharmaceutical, Inc.; 2002.

35 Baciewicz AM, Baciewicz FA. Cyclosporine pharmacokinetic drug interactions. *Am J Surg* 1989;157: 264–271.

36 Prograf® [package insert]. Deerfield, IL: Astellas Pharm US, Inc.; 2006.

37 Glynn AM, Slaughter RL, Brass C *et al.* Effects of ketoconazole on methylprednisolone pharmacokinetics and cortisol secretion. *Clin Pharmacol Ther* 1986;39: 654–659.

38 Lebrun-Vignes B, Archer V, Diquet B *et al.* Effect of itraconazole on the pharmacokinetics of prednisolone and methylprednisolone and cortisol secretion in healthy subjects. *Br J Clin Pharmacol* 2001;51: 443–450.

CHAPTER 13

Azathioprine

Barry J. Browne

Abdominal Transplantation, Balboa Institute of Transplantation, San Diego, CA, USA

History

Alexis Carrel [1] and C.C. Guthrie [2] developed the surgical techniques required for organ transplantation at the turn of the twentieth century. Early attempts at clinical renal transplantation began thereafter with a series of unsuccessful cadaveric and living donor kidney transplants carried out in Europe [3–5], which were doomed due to poorly understood immunologic barriers. It was not until Medawar's pioneering work with skin grafts [6, 7] that the immunologic basis of graft rejection was first recognized. These obstacles were circumvented in the 1950s through the use of identical-twin donors and led to the first successful kidney transplant at the Peter Bent Brigham Hospital in Boston in 1954 [8]. The modern era of successful clinical transplantation began in earnest with the introduction of azathioprine (AZA) by Roy Calne [9] and Joseph Murray [10], coupled with the empirical addition of corticosteroids by Goodwin *et al.* [11] in the early 1960s.

The groundwork leading to the development of AZA started in 1942 with the Nobel Prize winning work of Elion and Hitchings [12, 13] published over the following three decades. Elion and Hutchings were charged with examining purine and pyrimidine analogs to be used in the treatment of leukemic disorders. Schwartz and Dameshek [14] went on to show that one of these compounds, 6-mercaptopurine (6-MP), demonstrated immunosuppressive prop-

erties without bone marrow suppression in a nontransplant model. They [15], along with Meeker *et al.* [16], then reported success in a rabbit skin transplant model. Calne *et al.* [9] and Zukoski *et al.* [17] independently reported immunosuppressive efficacy in a dog model of kidney transplantation using 6-MP. In Calne's series, two of his dogs survived the first month post-transplant but then succumbed to pneumonia. Remarkably, neither animal displayed any histologic evidence of acute rejection.

During the early years of experimentation with 6-MP, Burroughs Wellcome Pharmaceuticals developed a number of analogs to 6-MP in an attempt to increase oral bioavailability and decrease metabolic deactivation. It was also hoped that bone marrow suppression and gastrointestinal distress might also be attenuated. AZA [6(1-methyl-4-nitro-5-imidazolyl)thiopurine] was developed primarily to decrease the rate of inactivation by enzymatic *S*-methylation, nonenzymatic oxidation, or conversion to thiourate by xanthine oxidase. It was hoped that the imidazolyl side-chain would protect the sulfhydryl group of 6-MP, thereby lengthening the half-life (Figure 13.1). In vivo, however, AZA is cleaved almost immediately into 6-MP and 6-thioinosinic acid by red blood cell glutathione. Nonetheless, early results in dogs seemed to favor AZA over 6-MP [18,19], although long-term successes were rare [20]. Similarly poor results were obtained in early clinical trials using AZA monotherapy [21, 22]. While AZA appeared to be effective at preventing allograft rejection, it

Immunotherapy in Transplantation: Principles and Practice, First Edition. Edited by Bruce Kaplan, Gilbert J. Burckart and Fadi G. Lakkis.
© 2012 Blackwell Publishing Ltd. Published 2012 by Blackwell Publishing Ltd.

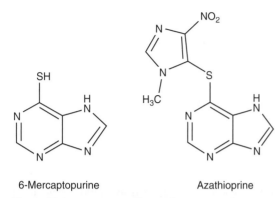

6-Mercaptopurine   Azathioprine

Figure 13.1 Comparative chemical structures of
6-mercaptopurine and azathioprine.

was ineffective at reversing rejection once it had
begun. Cognizant of Goodwin's experiences with
corticosteroids and evidence that rejection could be
reversed with high-dose steroids [23], Starzl and
coworkers began a series of clinical transplants in
which recipients received a cocktail of AZA
combined with steroids [24,25]. Between 1962 and
1964, 64 living related donor transplants were
carried out, with 23 % of these patients surviving at
least 25 years. Starzl's results from his series at the
University of Colorado led to a rapid expansion of
transplant centers across the USA and Europe and
encouraged the development of transplantation
utilizing cadaveric organs. The first cadaveric
transplant with similar long-term survival was
done in Paris by Hamburger's group in 1964 [26].

As success became more common in renal
transplantation, early attempts at liver
transplantation [27] and cardiac transplantation
[28] soon followed, but with only limited success.
Dual therapy for kidney transplantation with AZA
and steroids became the standard immunosuppressive regimen worldwide, and AZA became
commercially available as Imuran in 1968. The use
of antilymphocyte serum was pioneered by Starzl
et al. in 1967 [29]. This event opened the door to
complicated sequential polypharmaceutical regimens
in the management of transplant patients which
have become the norm in modern-day management. As such, it has become increasingly more
difficult to specifically attribute either efficacy or
toxicity to specific agents within each transplant

center's specific immunosuppressive protocol.
Despite a rapid escalation in clinical experience, the
results of renal transplantation using AZA/
prednisone (Pred) were not significantly better
than dialysis [30], whose technological and
pharmacologic improvements mirrored that of
transplantation in the 1960s. One-year patient
survival peaked at 80 %, with graft survival at
1 year of about 50 % [31, 32].

The report by Calne et al. [33] on the efficacy of
the new calcineurin inhibitor cyclosporin A (CsA)
in 1979 marked the beginning of the end of
the AZA/Pred era of immunosuppression. The
introduction of this new agent offered four
therapeutic approaches: (1) monotherapy with the
de novo introduction of CsA, (2) dual therapy with
substitution of CsA for AZA in combination with
Pred, (3) triple therapy involving the addition of
CsA to the existing AZA/Pred cocktail, and (4)
creation of a sequential protocol utilizing a number
of combinations. All four of these approaches were
attempted and resulted in better outcomes than
those seen with conventional AZA/Pred. Because
of significant side effects observed with early CsA
monotherapy, Morris et al. converted patients after
90 days from CsA to AZA/Pred [34] without noting
any significant drop in efficacy. Starzl's group at the
University of Pittsburgh substituted CsA for AZA in
combination with Pred [35] and reported a 1 year
graft survival rise from 50 % to 90 %. Najarian's
group at the University of Minnesota combined all
three agents in lower doses [36] and reported
similar results.

By the end of the 1980s, CsA-based immunosuppression had become standard and the role of
AZA was reduced to an adjuvant medication used
primarily in an attempt to reduce the dose required
to maintain graft function in patients intolerant to
full-dose CsA. This role was nearly eliminated in
the 1990s owing to the introduction of three new
immunosuppressants: (1) CsA microemulsion
(Neo), (2) tacrolimus (Tac), and most importantly
(3) mycophenolate mofetil (MMF). With the
conversion from CsA to Neo, dose regulation of CsA
levels became more reliable and dual therapy with
Pred reduced rejection rates to single digits [37].
Equally good results were achieved using the new

calcineurin inhibitor Tac, which has a unique structure, but similar pharmacokinetic profile to Neo [38]. The death knell for AZA in transplantation was heralded by the publication of the Tricontinental Mycophenolate Mofetil Renal Transplantation Study Group's paper comparing MMF with AZA in combination with CsA and Pred [39]. Although there was no difference in graft survival at 1 year, MMF was able to reduce the incidence of acute rejection by about one-half during the early post-transplant period. Interestingly, there is no substantive data to support the use of MMF over AZA following the first 3 months after transplantation. Nonetheless, MMF in combination with either Tac or Neo has become the most common immunosuppressant used following renal transplantation. The current use of AZA is limited primarily to situations in which financial expediency supersedes that of clinical efficacy. With MMF now available in a generic formulation, it is likely that the use of AZA in clinical transplantation will become even more marginalized. The only situation in which is AZA is indicated in preference to MMF is in fertile women, owing to the significant risk of birth defects with MMF [40], although AZA may also be teratogenic [41]. Following delivery, it is probably prudent to continue AZA in breastfeeding mothers owing to minimal drug concentrations of AZA transferred in breast milk [42, 43].

Chemistry and mode of action

AZA is an imidazolyl derivative of 6-MP and, thus, shares many, but not all, of the characteristics displayed by 6-MP. 6-MP is the sulfate derivative of hypoxanthine, and this explains the rationale for its clinical use as an immunosuppressant. As purine analogs, both AZA and 6-MP primarily inhibit DNA and RNA synthesis by interfering with the precursors of purine synthesis and suppressing de novo purine synthesis. Both compounds suppress lymphocyte proliferation in vitro and the production of interleukin-2, thereby inhibiting T cell proliferation [44]. Following intravenous or oral administration, about 90 % of AZA is rapidly cleaved by sulfhydryl-containing compounds, such

as cysteine and glutathione, into 6-MP and the nitroimidizole group. In order to become biologically active, 6-MP is acted upon by hypoxanthine-guanine phosphoribosyl transferase (HGPRT) within erythrocytes and leukocytes to produce 6-thioguanosine 5'-monophosphate (TGMP) [45]. The human HGPRT gene is constitutively expressed in all cells and located at position Xq26 of the X chromosome. Somatic mutations arise regularly in T cells and occur at increased frequency in conditions where T cell proliferation is increased, such as in response to an allograft [46–48]. Because these mutations alter the cellular phenotype and inhibit the phosphoribosylation of AZA into active metabolites, patients with these mutations tend to be resistant to AZA-induced cytotoxicity but may also be at increased risk of acute rejection episodes [49].

6-MP may also be metabolized prior to activation by intracellular xanthine oxidase (XO) into thiouric acid (6-TU) and thioxanthine [50] within the liver and gastrointestinal tract. Thioxanthine can then be further metabolized into 6-TU, explaining why 6-TU is the primary metabolite identified in plasma and urine following both AZA and 6-MP administration [51, 52]. Because of the pivotal role played by XO in detoxification of 6-MP, any drug that decreases XO activity results in increased potency of AZA. Co-administration of allopurinol is particularly potent, increasing plasma 6-MP levels fivefold and markedly increasing toxicity [53, 54].

A competing pathway involves a second enzyme, thiopurine methyl transferase (TPMT), which metabolizes 6-MP via S-methylation to 6-methyl-mercaptopurine (6-MMP). TPMT is present in most tissues, including hematopoietic tissues (spleen and bone marrow) and erythrocytes [55, 56]. Because XO is absent in hematopoietic tissue and there are no known deficiency states, TPMT activity plays a crucial role in both the efficacy and toxicity of AZA [57]. Although TPMT can deactivate AZA at the 6-MP stage of metabolism, its action on TGMP leads to production of S-methyl-thioinosine 5'-monophosphate (SM-IMP) which potently interferes with de novo purine synthesis. Because lymphocyte replication relies primarily on de novo synthesis, this pathway explains a primary immunosuppressive

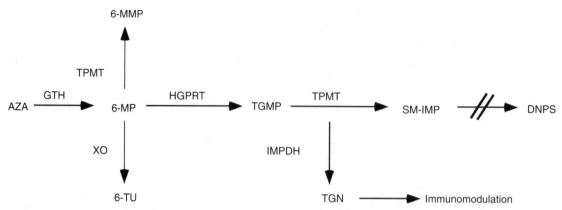

Figure 13.2 Mechanism of action of azathiprine. Following cleavage by glutathione (GTH), HGPRT phosphorylates 6-MP into TGMP. Depending on TPMT activity, the pathway diverges creating two distinct mechanisms of action. High TPMT activity favors methylation to SM-IMP, which inhibits de novo purine synthesis (DNPS). Low TPMT activity favors a pathways leading to an array TGN, which in turn leads to long-lasting immunomodulation.

action of AZA in preventing allograft rejection. But inhibition of purine synthesis only partly explains the clinical efficacy of AZA.

TGMP is also acted upon by inosine monophosphate dehydrogenase (IMPDH) and a series of kinases and reductases to form an array of thioguanine nucleotides (TGNs). One such nucleotide, deoxy-6 thioguanosine 5′-triphosphate (DGS) can trigger cell-cycle arrest during the S-phase of cell division, leading to apoptosis and cell death via the mismatch repair pathway [58]. This effect, which is strongly identified in murine leukemic cells, may explain the early promising results found with AZA in the treatment of acute lymphoblastic leukemia [59]. TGNs can be stable in vivo for days, allowing for delayed uptake into DNA [60]. Thus, it may take weeks to reach steady state at therapeutically tolerated doses [61]. This delay in action may partially explain the failure of AZA to effectively prevent acute rejection in the peri-operative time frame, yet it may be as effective or even more effective than MMF in the long-term. As the levels of TGN increase, they may also play a role in decreasing inflammation associated with T cell activation by blocking the expression of TNFRS7, TRAIL, and alpha integrin [62]. AZA may also decrease inflammation by attenuating the number of circulating monocytes exposed to the allograft. In a murine model of inflammation caused by newborn calf serum, the absolute number of circulating monocytes was reduced by 50% in animals receiving AZA. More specific examination showed that AZA administration resulted in the prolongation of the S-phase of the cell cycle for promonocytes, thereby impairing their conversion into mature monocytes [63]. A schematic of the major pathways leading to immunosuppression is shown in Figure 13.2.

T cell apoptosis can also be accelerated by the inhibition caused by AZA and its metabolites on Rac1 activation upon CD28 costimulation. 6-Thio-GTP competitively binds to Rac1 in place of GTP. This in turn suppresses the activation of Rac1 target genes, including MEK, NF-κB, and bcl-xL, and leads to a mitochondrial pathway of apoptosis [64]. So, CD28 costimulation leads to immune activation in the absence of AZA, but costimulation can result in apoptosis and down-regulation of the immune response in the presence of AZA.

Although many of the clinical effects seen with AZA can be attributed to its conversion to 6-MP, AZA's behavior is more complicated than what would be expected from a simple prodrug. Using equimolar concentrations of both drugs, Nathan *et al.* [65] and Elion [66] studied the inhibition of anti-sheep red blood cell (SRBC) antibody production and generated dose–response curves. In both series of experiments, AZA was found to be more potent and less toxic than 6-MP. Release of the nitroimidizole group during cleavage by glutathione may explain some of the increased potency of AZA, since nitridazole, an antiparasitic drug with a nitroimidazole group, is known to exhibit immunosuppressive activity [67]. It is more likely, however, that the myriad of fragments produced by alternative metabolic pathways interfere with immune mechanisms outside those explained by interference with purine metabolism. Indeed, when oral pretreatment with glutathione was added to accelerate the metabolism of AZA to 6-MP, the dose–response curves of both drugs became identical when measuring antiSRBC antibodies [68]. The native molecule may also confer greater immunosuppressive activity, since in-vitro tests of potency also favor AZA over 6-MP [69,70]. It remains unclear as to why AZA exhibits less toxicity than 6-MP.

Pharmacokinetics

Because of the complexity in the metabolism of AZA, pharmacokinetic evaluation and interpretation has been difficult. When given intravenously (IV), AZA is rapidly taken up by erythrocytes and hepatocytes, where 90% conversion to 6-MP occurs. Following conversion to 6-MP, its elimination is best described by a two-compartment body model. In a cohort of uremic patients given a 100 mg IV dose of AZA, the rapid phase mean half time of elimination ($t_{1/2}$) was 6.1 min, while the second phase $t_{1/2}$ was 50 min [71]. The clearance was 6.9 L/min, with both AZA and 6-MP being undetectable at 6 h. Time to peak 6-MP level (C_{max}) was 5 min with clearance calculated at 8 L/min. Neither renal nor hepatic insufficiency significantly affects early metabolism [72], simplifying dosing for both renal and hepatic transplant patients. In addition, hemodialysis does not appreciably affect the pharmacokinetics, efficacy, or toxicity of AZA [73], although hepatic insufficiency adversely

affects its potency, resulting in decreased intracellular levels of TGNs [74]. This difference may explain the disparity in clinical success seen between kidney and liver transplantation in the pre-CsA era.

AZA is an effective oral agent with a bioavailability of 47% [75], although there is wide intra- and inter-patient variability. There is extensive first-pass metabolism in the intestinal mucosa and liver, resulting in 6-MP concentrations being 10 times higher in these organs than in plasma [76]. Both C_{max} and $t_{1/2}$ are increased to 74 min and 1.9 h respectively. The primary breakdown product, 6-TU, is physiologically inert and peaks at 3.8 h in plasma [77]. Because 6-TU is excreted in the urine, its plasma levels correlate well with serum creatinine ($r = 0.98$) and limit its usefulness in therapeutic drug monitoring (TDM). Measurement of 6-MP levels has also been shown to be of little clinical value owing to a six- to eight-fold variability in area under the concentration curve (AUC) calculations that is seen not only between patients, but also within individual patients [78]. Not surprisingly, there is also no correlation between dose and AUC [79].

A number of attempts have been made to measure and correlate the most active moiety, TGN, with clinical outcome. Although some utility has been suggested [80], most investigators have found little clinical benefit [81]. Despite wide variations in intra-individual AZA AUC, total TGN levels within erythrocytes are relatively constant in stable renal transplant patients with coefficients of variation between 4.4% and 29.8%. Unfortunately, there was no clinical correlation observed between TGN levels and toxicity as measured by total white blood cell count [60]. The failure to correlate any measurable metabolite to either efficacy or toxicity has effectively precluded the use of TDM in patients receiving AZA.

Pharmacogenomics

The primary use-limiting side effect of AZA is myelosuppression. This is not unexpected, since the drug was initially developed for use in treating childhood leukemias [82]. Bone marrow toxicity occurs from abnormal accumulation of TGNs due to either too much drug being administered or, more commonly, defects in 6-MP metabolism from decreased TPMT activity [83–85]. Genetic polymorphism in human red blood cells was identified as the etiology of decreased TPMT activity in 1980 [86]. Large inter-individual differences were known to be inherited in an autosomal co-dominant fashion [87]. Clinically relevant genotypes can be divided into three categories based on physiologic activity: homozygous wild type (TPMTw), homozygous mutant (TMPTm), and heterozygous (TPMTh). Ninety percent of most populations examined exhibit TPMTw and behave as expected when given AZA with enzyme levels greater than 13.7 U/mL pRBC. Less than 1% are TMPTm and have low (<5.0 U/ml pRBC) or unmeasurable levels of TMPT activity. This patient group is at high risk of life-threatening side effects if given AZA and would likely benefit from pre-dose screening. The remaining 10% display TPMTh and require dose reductions of approximately two-thirds to stay within the therapeutic window and avoid significant leukopenia. This polymorphism has been identified in all ethnic groups examined, including Caucasians, African Americans, and Asians [88–90].

Weinshilboum and Woodson were able to partially purify and then characterize TPMT in 1983 [91, 92]. TPMT*1, the wild type, is most common. At least 17 mutant genotypes have been identified although three alleles – TPMT*2, TPMT*3A, and TPMT*3C – account for 90% of clinically relevant cases of impaired or absent enzyme activity [93–95]. TPMT is encoded by a 27 kb gene on chromosome 6p22.3 [96] and has 8 exons which encode the protein [97]. TMPT*2 was the first identified variant allele and contains a single nucleotide transversion resulting in the substitution of alanine for proline [98]. The increased flexibility in the tertiary structure leads to protein instability and decreased catalytic activity. Two single nucleotide polymorphisms in exon 7 and exon 10 are responsible for TPMT*3A, the most common variant seen in Caucasians. In this allele, alanine is substituted for threonine at codon 154 and cysteine is replaced by tyrosine at codon 240 [99]. TPMT*3C

is most common allele identified in Africans [100] and Southeast Asians [101], with decreased TPMT activity.

Although clinical testing by polymerase chain reaction is readily available to identify patients with abnormal TPMT activity, pre-transplant screening is not generally advocated for a number of reasons. The primary reason has been the near abandonment of AZA in the de novo prophylaxis of allograft recipients. The use of AZA is most commonly advocated when cost containment is paramount. In this circumstance, the additional cost of pre-transplant screening is probably not justified [102]. In instances where the therapeutic benefits of using AZA are thought to outweigh the benefits of alternative drugs such as MMF, screening may be of value due to the high costs associated with inpatient treatment of leukopenia in industrialized countries [103]. Routine genetic screening is probably best reserved for patients receiving AZA as primary therapy for medical disorders of the skin [104], gastrointestinal tract [105], and other organ systems [106, 107].

Clinical considerations

The introduction of AZA in the early 1960s revolutionized clinical transplantation and opened the door to effective chemoprophylaxis of allograft rejection. But in spite of nearly 50 years of clinical experience, the appropriate role that AZA should play both in current and future immunosuppressive regimens remains unclear. Owing to the rapid expansion and absence of standardized protocols following the introduction of CsA in the early 1980s and Tac in the 1990s, the scientific data regarding the impact of AZA in the age of polypharmacy is difficult, if not impossible, to interpret. The only certainty is that AZA will probably never return to the predominant position it once held as the cornerstone of immuno-suppressive therapy. With the introduction of MMF and its recent release in generic formulations, it is possible that the use of AZA will disappear completely from use in transplantation in the near future.

Although I have not written a prescription for AZA since 1995, it is not my intention to write AZA's obituary, and recent reports suggest that AZA can still play a role in clinical transplantation, particularly in the management of extra-renal transplants. In a review of the liver transplant literature by Germani *et al.* [108], the data suggest that both acute rejection and hepatitis C recurrence is lower in patients treated with AZA compared with MMF. Likewise in lung transplantation, Celik *et al.* [109] found no difference in acute rejection rates, but they did see a decrease in bronchiolitis obliterans in patients treated with AZA. In heart transplantation, however, MMF use decreases both early rejection and late rejection while increasing life expectancy [110].

Following the approval of MMF for use in kidney transplantation, the de novo use of AZA has effectively been eliminated in the USA. This occurred without the benefit of data comparing MMF with AZA when combined with either Neo or Tac [111] and heralded the beginning of successful aggressive pharmaceutical marketing within transplantation. Since then, randomized control trials [112] as well as paired kidney evaluation [113] failed to confirm the belief that MMF is superior to AZA when the drugs are used in combination with Neo and steroids. Both short- and long-term follow-up utilizing registry data [114], however, tend to favor MMF when compared with historical controls. Perhaps the most difficult impediment to comparing the advantages and disadvantages of two drugs is that adequate TDM for both AZA and MMF is suboptimal, making appropriate study design problematic. It is now unlikely that an adequately powered study will ever be completed to definitively identify which of the two drugs confers the best efficacy or the best side-effect profile. Because AZA continues to be used extensively for the treatment of nontransplant immunologic disorders, much of the work aimed at optimizing the therapeutic benefits of AZA is now being carried out under the direction of other medical subspecialties. Perhaps a better understanding of the mechanisms of action combined with novel approaches to TDM may pave the way for the return of AZA as a mainstay in transplantation medicine.

References

1 Carrel A. La technique operatoire des anastomoses vasculires, et la transplantation des visceres. *Lyon Med* 1902;98:859.

2 Guthrie CC. *Blood Vessel Surgery and its Application*. New York: Longmans Green; 1912.

3 Kuss R, Teinturier J, Milliez P. Quelques essais de greffe de rein chez l'homme. *Mem Acad Chir* 1951;77:755.

4 Servelle M, Soulie P, Rougeulle J *et al.* La greffe du rein. *Rev Chir* 1951;70:186–189.

5 Dubost C, Oeconomos N, Nenna A, Milliez P. Resultats d'une tentative de greffe renale. *Bull Soc Med Hop Paris* 1951;67:1372.

6 Medawar PB. The behavior and fate of skin autografts and skin homografts in rabbits. *J Anat* 1944;78:176–199.

7 Medawar PB. Second study of behavior and fate of skin homografts in rabbits. *J Anat* 1945;79:157.

8 Merrill JP, Murray JE, Harrison JH, Guild WR. Successful homotransplantation of the human kidney between identical twins. *JAMA* 1956;160:277–282.

9 Calne RY, Alexandre GP, Murray JE. A study of the effects of drugs in prolonged survival of homologous renal transplants in dogs. *Ann N Y Acad Sci* 1962;99: 743–761.

10 Murray JE, Merrill JP, Harrison JH *et al.* Prolonged survival of human-kidney homografts by immunosuppressive drug therapy. *N Eng J Med* 1963;268:1315–1323.

11 Goodwin WE, Mims MM, Kaufmann JJ. Human renal transplantation: III. Technical problems encountered in six cases of kidney homotransplantation. *Trans Am Assoc Genitourin Surg* 1962;54:116–125.

12 Elion GB, Singer S, Hitchings GH. Purine metabolism of a diaminopurine-resistant strain *Lactobacillus casei*. *J Biol Chem* 1953;200:7–16.

13 Elion GB, Bieber S, Hitchings GB. The fate of 6-mercaptopurine in mice. *Ann N Y Acad Sci* 1955;60: 297–303.

14 Schwartz R, Dameshek W. Drug induced immunological tolerance. *Nature* 1959;183:1682–1683.

15 Schwartz R, Dameshek W. The effects of 6-mercaptopurine on homograft reactions. *J Clin Invest* 1960; 39:952–958.

16 Meeker W, Condie R, Weiner D *et al.* Prolongation of skin homograft survival in rabbits by 6-mercaptopurine. *Proc Soc Exp Biol Med* 1959;102:459–461.

17 Zukoski CF, Lee HM, Hume DM. The prolongation of functional survival of canine renal homografts by 6-mercaptopurine. *Surg Forum* 1960;11:470–472.

18 Calne RY. Inhibition of the rejection of renal homografts in dogs with purine analogues. *Transplant Bull* 1961;28:445.

19 Calne RY, Murray JE. Inhibition of the rejection of renal homografts in dogs by Burroughs Wellcome 57-222. *Surg Forum* 1961;12:118.

20 Murray JE, Sheil AGR, Moseley R *et al.* Analysis of mechanism of immunosuppressive drugs in renal homotransplantations. *Ann Surg* 1964;160:449–473.

21 Murray JE, Merrill JP, Dammin GJ *et al.* Kidney transplantation in modified recipients. *Ann Surg* 1962;156:337–355.

22 Murray JE, Merril JP, Harrison JH *et al.* Prolonged survival of human-kidney homografts by immuno-suppressive drug therapy. *N Eng J Med* 1963;268:1315–1323.

23 Marchioro TL, Axtell HK, LaVia MF *et al.* The role of adrenocortical steroids in reversing established homograft rejection. *Surgery* 1964;55:412–417.

24 Starzl TE. *Experience in Renal Transplantation*. Philadelphia, PN: Saunders; 1964.

25 Starzl TE, Marchioro TL, Waddell WR. The reversal of rejection in human renal homografts with subsequent development of homograft tolerance. *Surg Gynecol Obstet* 1963;117:385–395.

26 Starzl TE, Schroter GP, Hartmann NJ *et al.* Long term (25-year) survival after renal homotransplantations: the world experience. *Transplant Proc* 1990;22:2361–2365.

27 Starzl TE, Marchioro TL, Von Kaulla KN *et al.* Homotransplantation of the liver in humans. *Surg Gynecol Obstet* 1963;117:659–676.

28 Lower RR, Dong E, Jr, Shumway NE. Long-term survival of cardiac homografts. *Surgery* 1965;58:110–119.

29 Starzl TE, Marchioro TL, Porter KA *et al.* The use of heterologous antilymphoid agents in canine renal and liver homotransplantation and in human renal homotransplantations. *Surg Gynecol Obstet* 1967;124:301–318.

30 Disney AP, Correll RL. Report of the Australian and New Zealand combined dialysis and transplant registry. *Med J Aust* 1981;7:117–122.

31 Kerman RH, Floyd M, Van Buren CT, Kahan BD. Improved allograft survival of strong immune responder–high risk recipients with adjuvant antithymocyte globulin therapy. *Transplantation* 1980;30:450–454.

32 Kuhlback B. Effect on patient and graft survival of reducing the methylprednisolone dose after renal transplantation. *Scand J Urol Nephrol Suppl* 1981;64:191–194.

33 Calne RY, Rolles K, White DJ *et al.* Cyclosporin A initially as the only immunosuppressant in 34 recipients of cadaveric organs: 32 kidneys, 2 pancreases, and 2 livers. *Lancet* 1979;2:1033–1036.

34 Morris PJ, French ME, Dunnill MS *et al.* A controlled trial of cyclosporine in renal transplantation with conversion to azathioprine and prednisolone after three months. *Transplantation* 1983;36:273–277.

35 Rosenthal JT, Hakala TR, Iwatsuki S *et al.* Cadaveric renal transplantation under cyclosporine-steroid therapy. *Surg Gynecol Obstet* 1983;157:309–315.

36 Simmons RL, Canafax DM, Strand M *et al.* Management and prevention of cyclosporine nephrotoxicity after renal transplantation: use of low doses of cyclosporine, azathioprine, and prednisone. *Transplant Proc* 1985;17(4 Suppl 1):266–275.

37 Browne BJ, Op't Holt C, Emovon OE. Diurnal cyclosporine dosing optimizes exposure and reduces the risk of acute rejection after kidney transplantation. *Clin Transplant* 2001;15(6 Suppl):55–58.

38 Takahara S. Efficacy of FK506 in renal transplantation. *Ann N Y Acad Sci* 1993;696:235–44.

39 The Tricontinental Mycophenolate Mofetil Renal Transplantation Study Group. A blinded, randomized clinical trial of mycophenolate mofetil for the prevention of acute rejection in cadaveric renal transplantation. *Transplantation* 1996;61:1029–1037.

40 Pisoni CN, D'Cruz DP. The safety of mycophenolate mofetil in pregnancy. *Expert Opin Drug Saf* 2008;7:219–222.

41 Cleary BJ, Källén B. Early pregnancy azathioprine use and pregnancy outcomes. *Birth Defects Res A Clin Mol Teratol* 2009;85:647–54.

42 Sau A, Clarke S, Bass J *et al.* Azathioprine and breastfeeding: is it safe? *BJOG* 2007;114:498–501.

43 Christensen LA, Dahlerup JF, Nielsen MJ *et al.* Azathiprine treatment during lactation. *Ailment Pharmacol Ther* 2008;1:90–91.

44 Bach JF. *The Mode of Action of Immunosuppressive Agents*. Oxford: North Holland Publishing Company; 1975.

45 Lennard L. The clinical pharmacology of 6-mercaptopurine. *Eur J Clin Parmacol* 1992;43:329–339.

46 Falta MT, Atkinson MA, Allegretta M *et al.* Azathioprine associated T-cell mutations in insulin-dependent diabetes mellitus. *Scand J Immunol* 2000;51:626–633.

47 Albertini RJ, Castle KL, Borcherding WR. T-cell cloning to detect the mutant 6-thioguanine-resistant lymphocytes present in human peripheral blood. *Proc Natl Acad Sci U S A* 1982;79:6617–6621.

48 Tates AD, van Dam FJ, van Mossel H *et al.* Use of the clonal assay for the measurement of frequencies of HPRT mutants in T-lymphocytes from five control populations. *Mutation Res* 1991;253:199–213.

49 Ansari AA, Mayne A, Sundstrom JB *et al*. Frequency of hypoxanthine guanine phosphoriboslytransferase (*HPRT⁻*) T cells in the peripheral blood of cardiac transplant recipients: a noninvasive technique for the diagnosis of allograft rejection. *Circulation* 1995;92: 862–874.

50 Elion GB. The purine path to chemotherapy. *Science* 1989;244:41–47.

51 Elion GB, Callahan S, Rundles RW, Hitchings GH. Relationship between metabolic fates and antitumor activities of thiopurines. *Cancer Res* 1963;23: 1207–1217.

52 Hamilton L, Elion GB. The fate of 6-mercaptopurine in man. *Ann N Y Acad Sci* 1954;60:304–314.

53 Berns A, Rubenfeld S, Rymzo WT, Jr, Calabro JJ. Hazard of combining allopurinol and thiopurine. *N Eng J Med* 1972;286:730–731.

54 Zimm S, Collins JM, O'Neill D *et al*. Inhibition of first-pass metabolism in cancer chemotherapy: interaction of 6-mercaptopurine and allopurinol. *Clin Pharmacol Ther* 1983;34:810–817.

55 Van Loon JA, Weinshilboum RM. Thiopurine methyltransferase biochemical genetics: human lymphocyte activity. *Biochem Genet* 1982;20:637–658.

56 Woodson LC, Dunnette JH, Weinshilboum RM. Pharmacogenetics of human thiopurine methyltransferase: kidney–erythrocyte correlation and immunotitration. *J Pharmacol Exp Ther* 1982;222:174–181.

57 Krynetski EY, Evans WE. Pharmacogenetics as a molecular basis for individualized drug therapy: the thiopurine *S*-methyltransferase paradigm. *Pharm Res* 1999;16: 342–349.

58 Swann PF, Waters TR, Moulton DC *et al*. Role of postreplicative DNA mismatch repair in the cytotoxic action of thioguanine. *Science* 1996;273:1109–1111.

59 Inamochi H, Higashigawa M, Shimono Y *et al*. Delayed cytotoxicity of 6-mercaptopurine is compatible with mitotic death caused by DNA damage due to incorporation of 6-thioguanine into DNA as 6-thioguanine nucleotide. *J Exp Clin Cancer Res* 1999;18:417–424.

60 Chan GL, Erdmann GR, Gruber SA *et al*. Azathioprine metabolism: pharmacokinetics of 6-mercaptopurine, 6-thiouric acid and 6-thioguanine nucleotides in renal transplant patients. *J Clin Pharmacol* 1990;30:358–363.

61 Sandborn WJ, Tremaine WJ, Wolf DC *et al*. Lack of effect of intravenous administration on time to respond to azathioprine for steroid-treated Crohn's disease. North American Azathioprine Study Group. *Gastroenterology* 1999;117:527–535.

62 Thomas CW, Myhre GM, Tschumper R *et al*. Selective inhibition of inflammatory gene expression in activated T lymphocytes: a mechanism of immune suppression by thiopurines. *J Pharmacol Exp Ther* 2005;312: 537–545.

63 Van Furth R, Gassmann AE, Diesselhoff-Den Dulk MM. The effect of azathioprine (Imuran) on the cell cycle of promonocytes and the production of monocytes in the bone marrow. *J Exp Med* 1975;141:531–46.

64 Tiede I, Fritz G, Strand S *et al*. CD28-dependent Rac1 activation is the molecular target of azathioprine in primary human CD4⁺ T lymphocytes. *J Clin Invest* 2003;111:1133–1145.

65 Nathan HC, Bieber S, Elion GB, Hitchings GH. Detection of agents which interfere with the immune response. *Proc Soc Exp Biol* 1961;107:796.

66 Elion GB. Biochemistry and pharmacology of purine analogues. *Fed Proc* 1967;26:898.

67 Solbach W, Wagner H, Rollinghoff M. Effect of nitridazole on cellular immunity in vivo and in vitro. *Clin Exp Immunol* 1978;32:411–418.

68 Elion GB. Significance of azathioprine metabolites. *Proc R Soc Med* 1972;65:257.

69 Bach JF, Dardenne M, Fournier C. In vitro evaluation of immunosuppressive drugs. *Nature (Lond)* 1969; 222:998.

70 Forbes IJ, Smith JL. Effects of anti-inflammatory drugs on lymphocytes. *Lancet* 1967;2:334.

71 Odlind B, Hartvig P, Lindström B *et al*. Serum azathioprine and 6-mercaptopurine levels and immunosuppressive activity after azathioprine in uremic patients. *Int J Pharmacol* 1986;8:1–11.

72 Chan GL, Canafax DM, Johnson CA. The therapeutic use of azathioprine in renal transplantation. *Pharmacotherapy* 1987;7:165–177.

73 Schusziarra V, Ziekursch V, Schlamp R, Siemensen HC. Parmacokinetics of azathioprine under haemodialysis. *Int J Pharmacol Biopharm* 1976;14:298–302.

74 Armstron VW, Oellerich M. New developments in the immunosuppressive drug monitoring of cyclosporine, tacrolimus, and azathioprine. *Clin Biochem* 2001;34: 9–16.

75 Van Os EC, Zins BJ, Sandborn WJ *et al*. Azathioprine pharmacokinetics after intravenous, oral, delayed release oral and rectal foam administration. *Gut* 1996;39:63–68.

76 Kurowski V, Iven H. Plasma concentrations and organ distribution of thiopurines after oral application of azathioprine in mice. *Cancer Chemother Pharmacol* 1991;28:7–14.

77 Chan GL, Erdmann GR, Gruber SA *et al*. Pharmacokinetics of 6-thiouric acid and 6-mercaptopurine in renal allograft recipients after oral

administration of azathioprine. *Eur J Clin Pharmacol* 1989;36:265–271.

78 Bergan S, Rugstad HE, Bentdal O *et al*. Kinetics of mercaptopurine and thioguanine nucleotides in renal transplant recipients during azathioprine treatment. *Ther Drug Monit* 1994;16:13–20.

79 Ohlman S, Albertioni F, Peterson C. Day-to-day variability in azathioprine pharmacokinetics in renal transplant recipients. *Clin Transplant* 1994;8:217–223.

80 Bergan S, Rugstad HE, Bentdal O *et al*. Monitored high-dose azathioprine treatment reduces acute rejection episodes after renal transplantation. *Transplantation* 1998;66:334–339.

81 Escousse A, Guedon F, Mounie J *et al*. 6-Mercaptopurine pharmacokinetics after use of azathioprine in renal transplant recipients with intermediate or high thiopurine methyltransferase activity phenotype. *J Pharm Pharmacol* 1998;50:1261–1266.

82 Elion GB. The George Hitchings and Gertrude Elion Lecture. The pharmacology of azathioprine. *Ann N Y Acad Sci* 1993;685:400–4007.

83 Evans WE, Horner M, Chu YQ *et al*. Altered mercaptopurine metabolism, toxic effects, and dosage requirement in a thiopurine-deficient child with acute lymphocytic leukemia. *J Pediatr* 1991;119:985–989.

84 Lennard L, Lilleyman JS, Van Loon J, Weinshilboum RM. Genetic variation in response to 6-mercaptopurine for childhood acute lymphoblastic leukaemia. *Lancet* 1990;336:225–229.

85 McLeod HL, Miller DR, Evans WE. Azathioprine-induced myelosuppression in a thiopurine methyltransferase deficient heart transplant recipient. *Lancet* 1993;341:1151.

86 Weinshilboum, Sladek SL. Mercaptopurine pharmacogenetics: monogenic inheritance of erythrocyte thiopurine methyltransferase activity. *Am J Hum Genet* 1980;32:651–662.

87 Chrzanowska M, Kurzawski M, Droździk M *et al*. Thiopurine *S*-methyltransferase phenotype–genotype correlation in hemodialyzed patients. *Pharmacol Rep* 2006;58:973–978.

88 Lowenthal A, Meyerstein N, Ben-Zvi Z. Thiopurine methyltransferase activity in the Jewish population of Israel. *Eur J Clin Pharmacol* 2001;57:43–46.

89 Hon YY, Fessing MY, Pui CH *et al*. Polymorphism of the thiopurine *S*-methyltransferase gene in African-Americans. *Hum Mol Genet* 1999;8:371–376.

90 Ameyaw MM, Collie-Duguid ES, Powrie RH *et al*. Thiopurine methyltransferase alleles in British and Ghanaian populations. *Hum Mol Genet* 1999;8:367–370.

91 Woodson LC, Ames MM, Selassie CD *et al*. Thiopurine methyltransferase. Aromatic thiol substrates and inhibition by benzoic acid derivatives. *Mol Pharmacol* 1983;24:471–478.

92 Woodson LC, Weinshilboum RM. Human kidney thiopurine methyltransferase. *Purification and biochemical properties. Biochem Pharmacol* 1983;32:819–826.

93 Otterness D, Szumlanski C, Lennard L *et al*. Human thiopurine methyltransferase pharmacogenetics: gene sequence polymorphisms. *Clin Pharmacol Ther* 1997;62:60–73.

94 Spire-Vayron de la Moureyre C, Debuysère H, Sabbagh N *et al*. Detection of known and new mutations in the thiopurine *S*-methyltransferase gene by single-strand conformation polymorphism analysis. *Hum Mutat* 1998;12:177–185.

95 Tai HL, Krynetski EY, Yates CR *et al*. Thiopurine *S*-methyltransferase deficiency: two nucleotide transitions define the most prevalent mutant allele associated with loss of catalytic activity in Caucasians. *Am J Hum Genet* 1997;58:694–702.

96 Krynetski EY, Tai HL, Yates CR *et al*. Genetic polymorphism of thiopurine *S*-methyltransferase: clinical importance and molecular mechanisms. *Pharmacogenetics* 1996;6:279–290.

97 McLeod HL, Krynetski EY, Relling MV, Evans WE. Genetic polymorphism of thiopurine methyltransferase and its clinical relevance for childhood acute lymphoblastic leukemia. *Leukemia* 2000;14:567–572.

98 Krynetski EY, Schuetz JD, Galpin AJ *et al*. A single point mutation leading to loss of catalytic activity in human thiopurine *S*-methyltransferase. *Proc Natl Acad Sci U S A* 1995;92:949–953.

99 Tai HL, Krynetski EY, Schuetz EG *et al*. Enhanced proteolysis of thiopurine *S*-methyltransferase (TPMT) encoded by mutant alleles in humans (*TPMT*3A*, *TPMT*2*): mechanisms for the genetic polymorphism of TPMT activity. *Proc Natl Acad Sci U S A* 1997;94:6444–6449.

100 McLeod HL, Pritchard SC, Githang'a J *et al*. Ethnic differences in thiopurine methyltransferase pharmacogenetics: evidence for allele specificity in Caucasian and Kenyan individuals. *Pharmacogenetics* 1999;9:773–776.

101 Collie-Duguid ES, Pritchard SC, Powrie RH *et al*. The frequency and distribution of thiopurine methyltransferase alleles in Caucasian and Asian populations. *Pharmacogenetics* 1999;9:37–42.

102 Compagni A, Bartoli S, Buehrlen B *et al*. Avoiding adverse drug reactions by pharmacogenetic testing: a systematic review of the economic evidence in the

case of TMPT and AZA-induced side effects. *Int J Technol Assess Health Care* 2008;24:294–302.

103 Marra CA, Esdaile JM, Anis AH. Practical pharmacogenetics: the cost effectiveness of screening for thiopurine *S*-methyltransferase polymorphisms in patients with rheumatological conditions treated with azathioprine. *J Rheumatol* 2002;29:2507–2512.

104 Vestergaard T, Bygum A. An audit of thiopurine methyltransferase genotyping and phenotyping before intended azathioprine treatment for dermatological conditions. *Clin Exp Dermatol* 2010;35(2):140–144.

105 Gardiner SJ, Gearry RB, Begg EJ *et al*. Thiopurine dose in intermediate and normal metabolizers of thiopurine methyltransferase may differ three-fold. *Clin Gastroenterol Hepatol* 2008;6:654–660.

106 Askanase AD, Wallace DJ, Weisman MH *et al*. Use of pharmacogenetics, enzymatic phenotyping, and metabolite monitoring to guide treatment with azathioprine in patients with systemic lupus erythematosus. *J Rheumatol* 2009;36:89–95.

107 Heneghan MA, Allan ML, Bornstein JD *et al*. Utility of thiopurine methyltransferase genotyping and phenotyping, and measurement of azathioprine metabolites in the management of patients with autoimmune hepatitis. *J Hepatol* 2006;45:584–591.

108 Germani G, Pleguezuelo M, Villamil F *et al*. Azathioprine in liver transplantation: a reevaluation of its use and a comparison with mycophenolate mofetil. *Am J Transplant* 2009;9:1725–1731.

109 Celik MR, Lederer DJ, Wilt J *et al*. Tacrolimus and azathioprine versus cyclosporine and mycophenolate mofetil after lung transplantation: a retrospective cohort study. *J Heart Lung Transplant* 2009;28:697–703.

110 Aguero J, Almenar L, Martínez-Dolz L *et al*. Influence of immunosuppressive regimens on short-term morbidity and mortality in heart transplantation. *Clin Transplant* 2008;22:98–106.

111 Knight SR, Russell NK, Barcena L, Morris PJ. Mycophenolate mofetil decreases acute rejection and may improve graft survival in renal transplant recipients when compared with azathioprine: a systematic review. *Transplantation* 2009;87:785–794.

112 Remuzzi G, Lesti M, Gotti E *et al*. Mycophenolate mofetil versus azathioprine for prevention of acute rejection (MYSS) a randomized trial. *Lancet* 2004;364:503–512.

113 Shah S, Collett D, Johnson R *et al*. Long-term graft outcome with mycophenolate mofetil and azathioprine: a paired kidney analysis. *Transplantation* 2006;82:1634–1639.

114 Meier-Kriesche HU, Steffen BJ, Hochberg AM *et al*. Mycophenolate mofetil versus azathioprine therapy is associated with a significant protection against long-term renal allograft function deterioration. *Transplantation* 2003;75:1341–1346.

CHAPTER 14

Pharmacokinetic and Pharmacodynamic Properties of Mycophenolate

David Hager[1], Arjang Djamali[2], and Bruce Kaplan[3]

[1]University of Wisconsin Hospital and Clinics, Madison, WI, USA

[2]University of Wisconsin-Madison, Madison, WI, USA

[3]University of Arizona Medical Center, Tucson, AZ, USA

Introduction

Mycophenolate mofetil (MMF) has had an unprecedented course in its development and rapid acceptance by the transplant community. It was approved by the US Food and Drug Administration (FDA) based on its effects on the rate of acute rejection as opposed to graft survival, as was the standard in the past. This approval followed the results from three large registration trials that spanned 55 transplant centers and 1500 patients [1–3]. By the late 1990s, 80% of renal transplant patients were taking MMF at discharge [4].

Currently, mycophenolic acid (MPA), the active moiety of mycophenolate, is available in two main compounds, which are a prodrug MMF (Cellcept, Roche Pharmaceuticals) and an enteric-coated salt, mycophenolate sodium (EC-MPS, Myfortic, Novartis Pharmaceuticals). The EC-MPS product was designed to delay the absorption of MPA till the drug reaches the small intestine. Both, however, are rapidly converted to MPA, such that no parent compound is detectible in the blood after dosing. Although new generic forms are arriving on the market, this chapter will focus on MMF and EC-MPS, since these drugs have been studied more thoroughly.

History

MPA was originally isolated from a penicillium fungus in 1893 and described in an Italian paper [5]. It was later evaluated for its antineoplastic, antiviral, and antifungal activity [6–13]. It took until 1969 for its immunosuppressive properties to be described by a Japanese group looking to develop an antibiotic [13]. In the 1970s, ongoing research was examining the effect of purine synthesis deficiency on the immune response [14]. Patients lacking adenosine deaminase (ADA) had combined disruption of both T and B lymphocytes. Since ADA's primary role is to convert adenosine pools to guanosine nucleotides, it was determined that creating a relative deficiency of guanosine nucleotides can inhibit deoxyribonucleic acid synthesis and cell division. In order to mimic this state, the search for a compound able to inhibit inosine-5′-monophosphate dehydrogenase (IMPDH) began, since this enzyme was known to regulate guanosine pools. These studies rediscovered MPA and its known inhibition of IMPDH. Development of MMF as a drug for the prevention of acute rejection in renal transplantation started in 1988 and culminated in FDA approval for that indication in June of 1995 [15].

Immunotherapy in Transplantation: Principles and Practice, First Edition. Edited by Bruce Kaplan, Gilbert J. Burckart and Fadi G. Lakkis.
© 2012 Blackwell Publishing Ltd. Published 2012 by Blackwell Publishing Ltd.

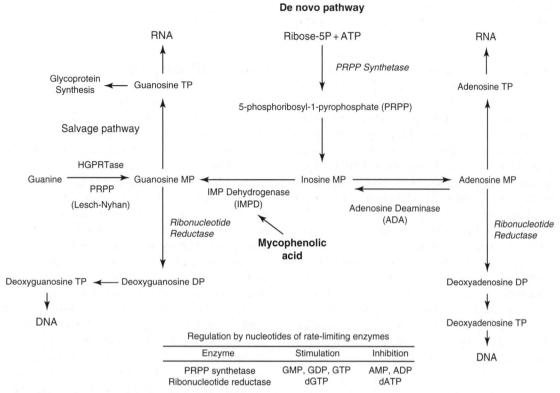

De novo pathway

Figure 14.1 Purine biosynthesis pathway and location of MPA mechanism of action. ATP, adenosine triphosphate; DNA, deoxyribonucleic acid; DP, diphosphate; GDP, guanosine diphosphate; HGPRTase, hypoxanthine-guanine phosphoribosyl transferase; MP, monophosphate; RNA, ribonucleic acid; TP, triphosphate. From [14], Allison A, Eugui E. Mechanisms of action of mycophenolate mofetil in preventing acute and chronic allograft rejection. *Transplantation* 2005;80(2 Suppl):S181–S190. Reproduced with permission by LWW.

Chemistry/structure

MMF is a prodrug and the morpholinoethyl ester of MPA [16]. Esterification was perused as a means to improve the bioavailability of MPA that has a substituted benzofuranone core with a hexenoic acid side chain [17, 18]. This structure, with its bicyclic ring, fits underneath the hypoxanthine ring of xanthosine monophosphate (XMP), trapping IMPDH in this intermediate state [19]. Other variants of MPA have been explored, mostly to prevent MPA glucuronidation, but alterations to MPA have been difficult given the complex hydrogen binding and spatial constraints within the active site [18].

Mechanism of action

MPA is a potent, selective, noncompetitive, and reversible inhibitor of the highly conserved protein IMPDH [20]. IMPDH, in the absence of MPA, catalyzes the conversion of insosine monophosphate (IMP) to XMP through the cofactor nicotinamide adenine dinucleotide (NAD) [19]. This represents the rate-limiting enzyme in the de novo synthesis of guanine nucleotides [21]. MPA noncompetitively blocks IMPDH by occupying the NAD and catalytic water site. This creates a relative depletion of guanosine nucleotides and a relative excess of adenosine nucleotides, resulting in feedback inhibition of phophoribosylpyrophosphate synthetase (Figure 14.1) [22].

The reduction of deoxyguanosine triphosphate inhibits DNA synthesis and T and B cell survival [23].

MPA displays selectivity to T and B cells through two mechanisms. First, T and B cells are dependent on the de novo pathway for the synthesis of guanine nucleotides, while all other cells in the body can access these nucleotides through the salvage pathway [24]. Second, IMPDH exists in two isoforms: type I and type II [25]. Type I IMPDH is a housekeeping enzyme found in almost all human cells. Type II IMPDH, however, is found only in activated T and B cells. MPA has fivefold specificity for this second isoform, lending more selectivity to the desired cell target [26].

MPA may have other mechanisms to create immunosuppression. One mechanism involves reduced synthesis of selectins and integrins by inhibiting guanosine nucleotides [27]. Additionally, depletion of guanosine triphosphate depletes tetrahydrobioptrin, a rate-limiting cofactor in the production of inducible nitric oxide synthase (iNOS) [14]. High levels of iNOS have been associated with rejection episodes in renal allografts.

Preclinical efficacy and safety

Animal studies of MMF, originally named RS-61443, demonstrated the vast potential for MPA to improve graft survival in transplant recipients. Islet allografts in mice, heart allografts in rats, and kidney allografts in dogs were all prolonged either with MMF alone or in combination with cyclosporine and prednisone [7, 28–30]. Dogs given 40 mg/kg had prolonged graft survival, but significantly more gastrointestinal adverse effects. Additionally, MMF was demonstrated to reverse acute rejection in a rat heart allograft and kidney allograft dog model better than steroid boluses. Based on these results, a phase I trial in 48 renal transplant recipients was conducted [31]. Patients received doses between 100 mg/day and 3.5 g/day in eight dosing groups. A correlation between doses greater than 2 g/day and lower rates of rejection was found along with safety, with only one adverse event (hemorrhagic gastritis) related to MMF. Gastrointestinal adverse effects, therefore, were present, but the drug was highly effective in preventing rejection and had no hepatotoxicity, nephrotoxicity, or neurotoxicity.

Clinical efficacy and safety

Three multi-center prospective, randomized double-blind trials formed the basis for FDA and European approval for MMF. These trials had a similar design, combining MMF 2 g/day or 3 g/day with cyclosporine and corticosteroids with an endpoint of biopsy-proven acute rejection (BPAR) or treatment failure, defined as graft loss, death, or withdrawal all at 6 months. One significant difference between the three studies was the US and Tricontinental study groups compared MMF with azathioprine (AZA), while the European study group compared MMF with placebo. Induction was used in the US Renal Transplantation study, but not in either the European study or Tricontinental study. The US Renal Transplant MMF Study Group trial contained 499 patients and found an incidence of the primary endpoint of 31.1% in the 2 g/day group ($p=0.0015$) and 31.3% in the 3 g/day group ($p=0.0021$), compared with 47.6% in the AZA group [1]. The European MMF Cooperative Study Group trial randomized 491 patients. Owing to the lack of induction and a comparison with placebo, MMF further reduced the incidence of BPAR or treatment failure within the two study groups from 56.0% in the placebo group to 30.3% and 38.8% in the MMF 2 g/day and MMF 3 g/day groups respectively ($p<0.001$ for both groups compared with placebo) [2]. In the Tricontinental MMF Renal Transplantation Study Group trial of 503 patients, the incidence of the primary endpoint was 50.0% in the control group compared with 38.2% in the MMF 2 g/day ($p=0.0287$) and 34.8% in the MMF 3 g/day ($p=0.0045$) groups [3]. A pooled analysis conducted by Halloran et al. confirmed MMF was significantly better than placebo or AZA in reducing graft loss due to BPAR by greater than 50% ($p<0.002$) [32]. However, statistically significant improvement in patient or graft survival at 1 year could not be demonstrated in these three trials or in the pooled analysis. Adverse drug events did increase withdrawals from 5.2% in the AZA/placebo group compared with 8.7% and 14.7% in the MMF 2 g/day and MMF 3 g/day groups respectively.

MPA for the prevention of rejection in transplant recipients now has more than a decade of clinical experience. The Tricontinental study group reported an analysis of the impact of MMF at the end of 3 years and showed a reduction in graft loss due to acute rejection from 9.9% in the AZA group to 5.8% and 3% in the MMF 2 g/day and 3 g/day groups respectively [33]. Early rejection, within the first 6 months, seems to be of critical importance, because, of patients who experienced BPAR within that timeframe 31.5% went on to lose their grafts compared with only 6.6% of patients who did not have early rejection. A retrospective analysis of data from 1988 to 1997 of 66 774 renal transplant patients in the US registry confirmed these results. Acute rejection was the strongest risk factor for late graft loss with a risk ratio (RR) of 2.41 ($p < 0.001$) and MMF reduces this risk compared with AZA [34]. MMF was found to reduce the relative risk for chronic allograft nephropathy by 27% independent of this reduction in acute rejection (RR 0.73, $p < 0.001$).

From a safety perspective, MMF was generally well tolerated in most studies. Commonly reported adverse events include nausea, vomiting, diarrhea, and abdominal pain. In renal transplant patients, 20–40% of patients required dose reduction or withdrawal due to these adverse drug events. Slightly higher rates of cytomegalovirus may be related to MMF use, especially at 3 g/day. While overall rates of post-transplant lymphoproliferative

disorder increased with MMF compared with AZA or placebo in the three registration trials, it remained less than 2% and the antiviral properties of MMF may be protective in selected populations [1–3, 33]. No other relationship has been demonstrated with increased malignancies, including skin cancer [35]. Leukopenia was higher in MMF 3 g/day treated patients compared with AZA patients, but lower in patients MMF 2 g/day patients.

Pharmacokinetics

The absorption of MMF is near complete and rapid in both healthy individuals and renal transplant recipients at least 3 months post-transplantation. It begins by being hydrolyzed by esterases on epithelial cells in the stomach, small intestine, blood, or liver to the active moiety MPA (see Table 14.1 for absorption, distribution, metabolism, and excretion) [16]. This occurs rapidly, as no MMF is detectable following oral administration or within 10 min of cessation of an intravenous infusion, which indicates a $t_{1/2}$ of less than 2 min [36]. In comparative kinetic studies with intravenous MMF in healthy volunteers, the area under the curve AUC_∞ of oral MMF was 93.5% (range 60.8–167%), demonstrating equivalent bioavailability. In a pooled analysis of 129 healthy individuals given 1 g of MMF, the absorption had an early peak (t_{max}) around 1 h (0.8±0.4 h) [37]. In these single-dose studies, a secondary peak was noted between 6 and

Table 14.1 Absorption, distribution, metabolism, and excretion parameters for MPA at a glance.

	Description	Pharmacokinetic parameter
Absorption	Rapid	$t_{max} < 1$ h
	Extensive	$f = 94\%$
Distribution	Almost entirely in plasma 99.9% versus 0.01% found in cellular components	$V_d = 3.6–4$ L
	Highly bound to plasma protein 99%	
Metabolism	MPA metabolized to:	Elimination $t_{1/2} = 17.6$ h
	MPAG (98%)	
	7-O-glucoside	
	AcMPAG	
	6-O-desmethyl-MPA	
Excretion	As MPAG >90% in urine, 6% fecal	

12 h after the dose, a result of the enterohepatic cycling. The $t_{1/2}$ in healthy individuals supports the twice daily dosing of MMF at 16 h (16±6 h). The C_{max} and AUC_∞ were reported as 24.5±9.5 mg/L and 63.9±16 mg/(Lh) respectively. In renal transplant patients at least 3 months out from transplantation, MMF pharmacokinetics are similar. More than 90 % of a given dose of mycophenolate is eliminated through the urine, with fecal elimination making up the remaining 5–10 % [38].

Patients immediately following renal transplantation display different pharmacokinetics, resulting from alterations in renal function, gastrointestinal absorption, hemodynamics, and drug interactions [37,39]. C_{max} and AUC_{12} of MMF in early post-transplant recipients are substantially lower than in healthy patients (6.6±6.6 mg/L versus 32.8±8.2 mg/L and 21.4±17.5 versus 51.5±15.1 mg/(Lh) respectively) [37]. The t_{max} is also significantly delayed from less than 1 h in healthy patients to 4.5±5.4 h in first-day transplant patients. Poor absorption is not the sole reason for decreased drug availability in this context, since intravenous MMF has similar AUC_{12} values to that of oral mycophenolate given on day 1 [37]. Further studies have analyzed these kinetic parameters at day 20. In one of these studies, C_{max} and AUC_{12} remained nearly 50 % of normal healthy volunteers (13.0±8.4 mg/L versus 23.2 ±11.9 mg/L and 36.6±5.15 mg/(Lh) versus 61.3±28.7 mg/(Lh)) [31]. The rise in the AUC_{12} is very gradual over the first 3 months post-transplantation and MPA AUC can increase 30–50 % during this time [37]. The effect of MPA binding to plasma protein will be described later; however, serum albumin concentrations increase over this time period post-transplant and likely increased binding sites allow for higher maximum concentrations and slower clearance contributing to higher AUC_{12} values.

MPA is metabolized to MPA 7-O-glucuronide (MPAG) through hepatic glucuronidation [40]. This occurs by uridine diphosphate glucuronosyltransferases (UGTs) found in the digestive tract, liver, and kidney. MPAG is an inactive metabolite that is then excreted into the bile by transport mechanisms, including multidrug resistance-associated protein 2, which allows for enterohepatic cycling, as gut bacteria containing glucuronidases convert MPAG back to MPA to be reabsorbed. This accounts for up to 10–60 % of the total dose-interval MPA AUC [37]. The conversion of MPA to MPAG is extensive, as only small amounts of MPA (mean of 0.6 % of the administered dose) were recovered in urine studies of radioactively labeled MMF given to healthy patients [37]. At least two other minor metabolites are formed, a 7-O-glucoside and an acyl-glucuronide. The acyl-glucuronide metabolite, which constitutes 0.3 % of the administered dose found in the urine, is important in that it is an active metabolite with comparative IMPDH inhibition to MPA [41]. The acyl-glucuronide metabolite has also been linked to cytokine release, hypersensitivity, drug toxicity, and immune response [42].

The pharmacokinetics of MPAG also vary depending on time since the transplant and between transplant recipients and healthy individuals, although to a lesser degree than MPA kinetics. The t_{max} of MPAG in healthy patients occurs approximately 1 h after the peak of MPA, which demonstrates a precursor–successor kinetic relationship [37]. MPAG AUC_∞ in healthy patients was five times higher than MPA AUC_∞; however, C_{max} and $t_{1/2}$ were similar. Immediately post-transplant the patients have a substantially delayed MPAG t_{max} compared with healthy volunteers (8.65±6 h versus 1.7±0.5 h), but have similar C_{max} and AUC values. In comparison, late post-transplant patients have t_{max} values more consistent with healthy volunteers (2.8±0.8 h versus 1.7±0.5 h), but now have almost a twofold higher total MPAG exposure (420±140 mg/(Lh) versus 234±87 mg/(Lh)), which is likely related to lower renal clearance.

The distribution of MPA in whole blood is nearly entirely (99.99 %) in the plasma. Only 0.01 % is found within the cellular component [43,44]. While in-vitro data demonstrated that only free MPA can inhibit IMPDH, between 97 and 99 % of MPA is protein bound [43]. A number of factors then can alter protein binding and potentially contribute some drug–drug interactions. Factors known to alter MPA protein binding include disease states that alter the availability of albumin binding sites, as in severe renal or liver dysfunction or severe hypoalbuminemia [45, 46]. Liver cirrhosis, when compensated, does not seem to alter the pharmacokinetic profile of MPA or MPAG, potentially due to enhanced renal glucuronidation, although decreased oral absorption of MMF has been described in liver transplant recipients post-operatively [44–46]. The free fraction of MPA can be altered more than twofold, with alterations in serum albumin from 4 g/dL to 2.4 g/dL [43]. In liver transplant patients, this explains the increase in MPA AUC over the first month post-transplant [45, 46]. Additionally, competition from excessive, but clinically possible, concentrations of urea or MPAG could displace MPA [39, 44, 46, 47]. Factors confirmed unable to alter protein binding include MPA concentration and therapeutic concentrations of warfarin, digoxin, phenytoin, cyclosporine, tacrolimus, and prednisone.

The effects of renal impairment on the pharmacokinetics of mycophenolate are worth discussion given the frequency with which this drug is administered to patients with this condition and because of its significant effects on both protein binding and overall clearance. Uremia displaces MPA from serum albumin, creating an increase in both the free fraction of MPA and increased free MPA AUC values [43]. In contrast, in single-dose studies analyzing the effect of glomerular filtration rate (GFR) with MPA clearance, no correlation was found, which confirms the previous statement of primary liver clearance of MPA [37]. MPAG, however, is eliminated by the kidney and demonstrates a statistically significant decline in elimination as GFR decreases, with a linear correlation coefficient of 0.86. High concentrations of MPAG are not correlated to adverse effects, and since only free MPA is pharmacologically active, there is no rationale for reduced doses in patients with renal dysfunction. Since high concentrations of MPAG displace MPA in vitro, severe renal dysfunction could increase patient exposure to free MPA [43]. Owing to the previously mentioned extensive protein binding of MPA to plasma proteins, little MPA is cleared during hemodialysis and does not require dose adjustment [48].

EC-MPS was demonstrated to be equivalent to MMF based on MPA exposure in renal and heart transplant patients. Significant differences exist, as the absorption of MPA is more delayed (t_{max} 2 h versus 0.3 h), the rate of absorption is lower (3.0 versus 4.1 h^{-1}) and more variable in EC-MPS-treated patients than in MMF-treated patients (inter-individual variability 123% versus 76%, intra-individual variability 64% versus 42%; Plate 14.1) [50, 51]. Delayed absorption results in a higher C_{trough} in EC-MPS-treated patients (2.6 mg/L versus 1.6 mg/L) [50]. Safety and efficacy have been confirmed to be equivalent, but EC-MPS pharmacokinetics may preclude reliable implementation of trough level (C_0) or even abbreviated therapeutic drug monitoring protocols [52–54].

Pharmacodynamics

Efficacy

The data have not consistently demonstrated a significant correlation between MPA AUC and reduced episodes of rejection. This was due to a number of complicating factors, including low rates of rejection in the population studied, insufficient sampling, and failure to investigate levels of co-administered immunosuppressive agents [47]. The first study to convincingly demonstrate the relationship examined 150 renal transplant patients in a randomized concentration-controlled trial (RCCT) with MMF and cyclosporine [55]. In that study, both pre-dose MPA C_0 and MPA AUC_{12} significantly correlated with prevention of rejection ($p=0.01$ and $p<0.001$ respectively). Patients were randomly assigned to one of three AUC_{12} groups: 16.1, 32.2, or 60.6 (mg h)/L; 27.5% of patients in the low MPA group experienced rejection, compared with 14.9% in the intermediate group and 11.5% in the high group. Further studies have attempted to define cut-off values for which pharmacokinetic parameters above a given target minimize the risk for rejection. In a study of 33 adult renal transplant patients where MPA pharmacokinetics were analyzed, of the seven rejections during the study period five of them occurred in the group where MPA AUC_{12} values were less than 30 (mg h)/L [39]. In a study of pediatric renal transplant patients, an AUC_{12} of 33.8 (mg h)/L in the initial post-transplant period had a sensitivity of 75 % and a specificity of 64 % for discrimination of patients with acute rejection, while an MPA C_0 value of 1.2 mg/L had a sensitivity of 83 % and a specificity of 64 % [56]. The authors concluded that the goal range for MPA AUC_{0-12} is 30–60 (mgh)/L or a C_0 MPA concentration of 1–3.5 mg/L for cyclosporine and steroid-containing regimens in the early post-transplant period. This would limit rates of acute rejection to less than 10 % [57].

One application of this guideline was the APOMYGRE study completed in 2007, which compared fixed-dose MMF at 2 g/day with a concentration-controlled group with a target concentration of 40 (mgh)/L using a three-concentration Bayesian approach. The concentration-controlled group had significantly reduced BPAR (7.7 % versus 24.6 %, $p<0.01$), but there was no difference in patient or graft survival [58]. In the fixed dose-concentration controlled (FDDC) study, 901 patients were randomized to 2 g/day of MMF or a concentration-controlled regimen with a goal concentration of 30–60 (mgh)/L. There was no difference in the composite endpoint of BPAR, graft loss, death, or discontinuation of mycophenolate therapy between the concentration-controlled group and the fixed-dose group (25.6 % versus 25.7 %) [52]. A relationship was found, however, between MPA AUC on day 3 with BPAR in the first month and in the first year ($p=0.009$ and $p=0.006$ respectively) [52]. In the final of the three largest randomized trials published to date, the Opticept study randomized 720 patients to one of three groups, two with concentration-controlled dosing of MMF with either standard or reduced calcineurin dosing and a group on fixed-dose mycophenolate and standard calcineurin dosing [53]. Target MPA levels were on the basis of a C_0 of 1.3 mg/L in the cyclosporine-treated patients and 1.9 mg/L in tacrolimus-treated patients. Based on an intention to treat analysis, there was no difference in rates of treatment failure between the concentration-controlled and fixed-dose groups. Many difficulties exist in completing these studies, as routinely in both the Opticept and FDCC studies the clinicians were reluctant to increase doses, particularly in the immediate post-operative period. In addition, much more heterogeneity was allowed in these trials than in the APOMYGRE study, which may mask the benefit of therapeutic drug monitoring [59, 60].

Safety

The safety and adverse drug event relationship with mycophenolate pharmacokinetics is even less clear. The most common clinical complication from mycophenolate use, gastrointestinal toxicity, has not been consistently related to MPA exposure [37, 39, 54]. In van Gelder *et al.*'s prospective study, withdrawals due to adverse effects increased as target concentration increased in each group: 16.1 (mgh)/L (7.8 %), 32.2 (mgh)/L (23.4 %), and 60.6 (mgh)/L (44.2 %); but since dose adjustments were not allowed, withdrawals were falsely elevated [61]. Another prospective study of 100 renal transplant patients more than 3 months post-transplant found patients with anemia and leukopenia had significantly higher MPA AUC_{12} than those not experiencing these effects [62].

In a study of 31 renal transplant patients, C_{30} but not C_0 or MPA AUC values were significantly related to adverse effects [55]. Others reported no correlation between hematological adverse effects and C_0 or MPA AUC in 39 renal transplant patients at 1 year follow-up [63]. In a subsequent report from Mourad *et al.*, MPA AUC_{12} and C_0 correlated with toxicity. The threshold of toxicity was identified at 3 mg/L (sensitivity 38.7 %; specificity 91.5 %) for MPA C_0 and at 37.6 (mgh)/L for MPA AUC_{12} (sensitivity 83.3 %; specificity 59.6 %) [64]. Free MPA AUC or C_0 may correlate better with hematological complications. A study in 45 pediatric renal transplant patients found free MPA AUC_{12} greater than 0.4 (mgh)/L correlated with increased risk for infection or leukopenia in the 1–3 week time period [59]. This resulted in a diagnostic sensitivity of 92.3 % and specificity of 61.0 % for infections and leukopenia. Finally, acyl-MPAG levels have also been related to adverse effects, including anemia, although not consistently [60, 65, 66].

In summary, there is no consensus on what pharmacokinetic parameter or value is specifically related to adverse drug events. In the three most recent randomized, prospective trials (APOMYGRE, FDCC, and Opticept), no correlation between MPA

C_0 or AUC was observed [52, 53, 58]. However, when MPA AUC_{12} values exceed 60 (mgh)/L there is no further benefit in preventing rejection and potentially higher adverse effects [61]. Owing to the wide variability in inter-patient pharmacokinetics in transplant patients as a result of differing renal function, immunosuppressive regimen, time from transplant, and MPA metabolism, further research in this area is warranted [44].

Drug–drug interactions

Mycophenolate, owing to its metabolism by glucuronidation and, therefore, outside the CYP450 system, was not expected to have many clinically significant drug interactions [37]. In recent years more interactions are beginning to be described in the literature. Given the complex interactions involved in enterohepatic cycling and MPA binding, this is no longer surprising. Given the widespread use of concomitant immunosuppressive agents, the first discussion of drug interactions must focus on the effect of cyclosporine compared with tacrolimus on MPA kinetics. It has been demonstrated that patients receiving tacrolimus have higher dose-adjusted MPA AUC values than those receiving cyclosporine [67–69]. The proposed mechanism is that biliary secretion of MPAG is inhibited by cyclosporine's effect on the multidrug resistance-associated protein 2 transporter present in the canalicular membrane of hepatocytes [44, 70–73]. This reduced secretion inhibits enterohepatic circulation of MPAG back to MPA and, therefore, reduces overall exposure to MPA approximately 30–40% when compared with patients receiving tacrolimus or sirolimus [74–78]. If cyclosporine is tapered or discontinued, MPA concentrations can increase 50–100% [44]. Tacrolimus may also increase mycophenolate exposure through inhibition of UGT [68].

Another potential interaction as a result of enterohepatic cycling by MPA is in its interactions with antibiotics and antacids. Norfloxacin and metronidazole specifically reduce MPA AUC values [79]. Reductions in MPAG AUC and MPAG urinary excretion values were also found. This reduced exposure may be the result of reduced gut bacteria and, therefore, a reduction in glucuronidase enzyme available to covert MPAG back to MPA to be reabsorbed. As a result of the gastrointestinal side effects related to mycophenolate and the chronic nature of its administration, the effect of antacids and food on mycophenolate kinetics has been examined. In a study of 10 patients with rheumatoid arthritis, high-fat meals and an aluminum hydroxide/magnesium hydroxide antacid were co-administered with MMF and a full pharmacokinetic analysis was completed [80]. Feeding decreased MPA C_{max} and increased t_{max}, but had little impact on AUC_{24}. MPAG kinetics were altered, potentially a result of food-enhanced hepatic glucuronidation. Since MPA is the active moiety and total drug exposure is unchanged, co-administration is unlikely to be clinically significant. Antacid co-administration reduced both C_{max} and AUC_{24} for both MPA and MPAG. This consistent reduction in total exposure is the result of reduced absorption; and given the structure of MPA, chelation is the likely mechanism. Similar examples of potential chelation interactions include: sevelamer (reduced MPA AUC by 25%), calcium polycarbophil (reduced MPA AUC by 50%), cholestyramine (impact unknown), and iron (reduced MPA AUC in healthy volunteers 90%, no interaction in renal transplant patients) [37, 44, 81–85]. It is possible, therefore, that MPA exposure is reduced in these cases, thereby reducing the efficacy of mycophenolate.

Proton pump inhibitors (PPIs) are often prescribed to organ transplant recipients owing to the risk of peptic ulcer disease. In a prospective study of 22 heart transplant patients, pantoprazole (40 mg) reduced plasma MPA concentration and total MPA AUC by 34% based on its withdrawal [86]. The concentrations were lower at 0.5 and 1 h after MMF dosing, but not at 2 h after dosing. The authors concluded that reduced gastric acid secretion inhibits hydrolysis of MMF, thereby decreasing the plasma concentrations of MPA. Consistent with these results, Miura *et al.* demonstrated that lansoprazole significantly reduced plasma concentrations of MPA at 1 year after renal transplantation [87]. In a recent study including enteric-coated mycophenolate sodium, pantoprazole (40 mg twice daily) reduced MMF MPA AUC and C_{max} significantly, but did not alter the pharmacokinetics in the EC-MPS group (Plate 14.2) [88]. This difference is likely related to MMF's poor solubility and absorption at elevated intragastric pH. Larger prospective trials are needed to confirm the clinical impact of this interaction and the potential need for dose elevation in PPI-treated patients.

Another potential source of drug interactions with mycophenolate is induction of UGT conversion of MPA, the active moiety, to MPAG, the inactive metabolite. One common instance in which this could occur is mycophenolate use with corticosteroids. In a study of 26 renal transplant patients, their steroid doses were tapered off over a 21 month period [89]. At the end of the study period the patients who remained on steroids acted as a control group and were compared with the withdrawal group. Exposure to MPA increased in the steroid-withdrawal group over the length of the study, with the control group having similar exposure at 21 months as the withdrawal group had at 6 months. Other studies have found that lower doses of corticosteroids may not interact [90]. In a study of 30 renal transplant patients, mycophenolate was co-administered with tacrolimus, steroids, and either telmisartan, valsartan, or candesartan cilexeil [91]. Telmisartan has been previously described as a peroxisome proliferator-activated receptor γ (PPAR-γ) activator, while valsartan and candesartan cilexeil lack this ability. While PPAR-γ activity may have benefits in transplant patients owing to its capacity to help regulate insulin sensitivity and lower blood pressure, significant lowering of MPA kinetics also occurred through PPAR-γ induction of UGT. The dose-adjusted AUC_{12} MPA was 29% lower than that of MPA without angiotensin receptor blockade ($p = 0.0353$). Further research on this interaction and its implications for increased therapeutic drug monitoring is warranted.

Therapeutic drug monitoring

Standardized dosing for MMF and EC-MPS has been used for more than a decade with excellent results in not only decreasing acute rejection, but also in late rejection and graft failure [34, 92]. Desire to tailor immunosuppressive therapy to minimize the potential risks of adverse drug events and infection have driven research to find therapeutic drug level targets for MPA. This is in part due to the large inter-patient and intra-patient variability in MPA pharmacokinetics, which has been outlined above. In addition to drug–drug interactions, altered protein binding, renal disease, hepatic disease, and time from transplantation, a patient's race, body weight, gender, genetic polymorphisms, or even the presence of diarrhea can alter MPA pharmacokinetics [47, 93]. Dose-interval MPA AUC values can vary between patients by 10-fold given the same doses of MMF [57]. This variability was associated with a risk of rejection, which results in an average length of stay of 8.3 days and an estimated cost between $15 000 and $18 000 [94].

In 2006, based on the data in the RCCT trial, a target AUC between 30 and 60 (mgh)/L was agreed upon by a panel of invited experts on therapeutic drug monitoring [61, 95]. Little change in these goals has occurred since (Table 14.2) [93]. The APOMYGRE study demonstrated lower rates of rejection in the group with MPA AUC > 45 (mgh)/L. In the FDCC trial, rates of rejection were higher when MPA AUC was < 30 (mgh)/L at day 3. An MPA C_0 concentration range of 1.5–3 mg/L has been suggested, but waits confirmation. This panel also recommended therapeutic drug monitoring for patients at high immunologic risk, in immunosuppression minimization/avoidance protocols, with delayed graft function, with altered pharmacokinetics, and suspected noncompliance [93]. The remaining challenges to therapeutic drug monitoring are the degree of overlap between therapeutic and potentially toxic MPA AUC values, relatively high intra-patient variability, relatively low rates of acute rejection currently with tacrolimus-based immunosuppressive regimens, and the difficulty in obtaining full 12 h MPA AUC [53, 93, 94]. The best guidance to practical solutions to these problems may lie in the APOMYGRE study, as these investigators successfully used a three time-point Bayesian estimator that was widely adhered to by clinicians who then were able to significantly alter MPA AUC values and prevent rejection [58, 93]. Further

Table 14.2 Summary of pivotal dose-monitoring trials in kidney transplant recipients.

Study	N	CNI[a]	Sampling strategy	MPA AUC pharmacokinetic parameter	Endpoints		p-value
					Primary	Secondary	
RCCT [61]	150	CsA	Eight-concentration AUC inpatient,	C_0	BPAR C_0		$p=0.001$
			five-concentration abbreviated AUC outpatient	AUC_{12}	BPAR AUC_{12}		$p<0.001$
APOMYGRE [58]	137	CsA	Three-concentration, Bayesian model	AUC_{12}	Composite[b]		$p=0.03$
						Presumed rejection	$p=0.01$
						BPAR	$p<0.001$
FDDC [52]	901	Tac or CsA	Three-concentration, abbreviated AUC	AUC_{12}	Composite[c]		NS
						BPAR or presumed rejection	NS
						Graft loss	NS
						Death	NS
Opticept [53]	720	Tac or CsA	C_0	C_0	Composite[d]		NS
					Change in GFR		NS
						Composite at 24 months	NS
						BPAR	NS
						Presumed rejection	NS

[a]CNI: calcineurin inhibitor; CsA: cyclosporine; Tac: tacrolimus.
[b]BPAR, graft loss, discontinuation of MMF.
[c]BPAR, graft loss, death, discontinuation of MMF at 12 months.
[d]BPAR, graft loss, death or withdrawal at 12 months.

research may find that pharmacodynamic monitoring through IMPDH activity is of more value, as the intra-individual variability is low [96]. Additionally, high and low IMPDH activity have already been tied to rejection and toxicity respectively [97, 98].

Pharmacogenomic considerations

Potential genetic polymorphisms of interest would concern the transport mechanisms essential to its absorption and distribution, notably multidrug resistance-associated protein 2 and UGTs or the therapeutic target IMPDH. The regulation of UGT1 and UGT2 genes has been reported and may vary between patients. UGT1A9 can glucuronidate MPA and is widely present in the kidney, as well as in liver and intestine where MPA is glucuronidated to MPAG [99]. Indeed, UGT1A9 is responsible for 40–50 % of intestinal MPAG production. Single nucleotide polymorphisms (SNPs) with a clinical impact on UGT1A9 activity were studied in 95 renal transplant patients [100]. The T-275A and C-2152T SNPs of the UGT1A9 gene promoter resulted in significantly lower MPA AUC. This is thought to be the result of decreased enterohepatic recirculation of MPA. IMPDH genetic variants were studied in 191 renal transplant patients and two SNPs were found to be significantly associated with increased incidence of BPAR in the first year after transplantation [101]. A similar study in liver transplant patients related increased IMPDH2 expression and increased hematological and gastrointestinal adverse effects [102]. Further research is ongoing to define the role of these polymorphisms in the clinical care of transplant recipients [103].

Conclusion

In conclusion, MMF gained FDA approval in 1995 based on three large international trials in renal transplant patients for the prevention of acute rejection. Mycophenolate is now available commercially in two products, the prodrug MMF (Cellcept, Roche) and EC-MPS (Myfortic, Novartis). Generic forms of MMF are also commercially available. MPAG is the primary metabolite of MPA and is excreted almost exclusively in the urine (>90%). MPA is distributed almost entirely in the plasma 99.99%, with only 0.01% found in cellular components. Pharmacokinetics of MPA and MPAG vary based on a variety of factors, including time from transplantation, changes in serum albumin concentration, and the presence of severe renal dysfunction. Drug interactions contribute to pharmacokinetic variability in transplant patients on mycophenolate-containing regimens. While mycophenolate is not metabolized through the hepatic cytochrome P450 system, the potential for drug interactions exists through alterations in enterohepatic cycling, chelation, pH-dependent absorption, and increased conversion to MPAG, the inactive metabolite. Studies have been ongoing to relate pharmacokinetic parameters, specifically MPA exposure (AUC) and trough levels (C_0) to outcomes in renal transplant patients. While MPA AUC_{0-12} values between 30 and 60 (mg h)/L seem to be efficacious in the prevention of acute rejection, strategies for monitoring and dose adjustments have not been universally successful or accepted. Part of this difficulty lies in the overlapping toxicities, mainly hematological and gastrointestinal, at therapeutic doses. Pharmacogenetic studies of mycophenolate are still in the early stages; however, genetic polymorphisms in multidrug resistance-associated protein 2, UGT, and IMPDH may contribute to its pharmacokinetic and pharmacodynamic variability. Mycophenolate has gained wide acceptance in the transplant community based on its relatively low and tolerable side-effect profile, along with its established efficacy in reducing acute rejection, while improving long-term outcomes. Further research will focus on individualization of this therapy to minimize these adverse effects and maximize patient outcomes.

References

1 Sollinger H. Mycophenolate mofetil for the prevention of acute rejection in primary cadaveric renal allograft recipients. U.S. Renal Transplant Mycophenolate Mofetil Study Group. *Transplantation* 1995;60(3):225–232.

2 European Mycophenolate Mofetil Cooperative Study Group. Placebo-controlled study of mycophenolate mofetil combined with cyclosporin and corticosteroids for prevention of acute rejection. *Lancet* 1995; 345(8961):1321–1325.

3 The Tricontinental Mycophenolate Mofetil Renal Transplantation Study Group. A blinded, randomized clinical trial of mycophenolate mofetil for the prevention of acute rejection in cadaveric renal transplantation. *Transplantation* 1996;61(7):1029–1037.

4 Kaufman D, Shapiro R, Lucey M et al. Immunosuppression: practice and trends. *Am J Transplant* 2004;4(Suppl 9):38–53.

5 Gosio B. Sperimentate su culture pure di bacilli del carbonchio demonstraratonotevole potere antisettica. *CR Acad Med Torino* 1893;61:484.

6 Suzuki S, Kimura T, Ando K et al. Antitumor activity of mycophenolic acid. *J Antibiot (Tokyo)* 1969; 22(7):297–302.

7 Eugui E, Mirkovich A, Allison A. Lymphocyte-selective antiproliferative and immunosuppressive activity of mycophenolic acid and its morpholinoethyl ester (RS-61443) in rodents. *Transplant Proc* 1991;23(2 Suppl 2):15–18.

8 Franklin T, Cook J. The inhibition of nucleic acid synthesis by mycophenolic acid. *Biochem J* 1969; 113(3):515–524.

9 Carter SB, Franklin TJ, Jones DF et al. Mycophenolic acid: an anti-cancer compound with unusual properties. *Nature.* 1969;223(5208):848–850.

10 Brewin T, Cole M, Jones C et al. Mycophenolic acid (NSC-129185): preliminary clinical trials. *Cancer Chemother Rep* 1972;56(1):83–87.

11 Williams R, Lively D, DeLong D et al. Mycophenolic acid: antiviral and antitumor properties. *J Antibiot (Tokyo)* 1968;21(7):463–464.

12 Florey HW, Gilliver K, Jennings MA. Mycophenolic acid: an antibiotic from *Penicillium breicompactum*. *Lancet* 1946;1:46–49.

13 Mitsui A, Suzuki S. Immunosuppressive effect of mycophenolic acid. *J Antibiot (Tokyo)* 1969;22(8): 358–363.

14 Allison A, Eugui E. Mechanisms of action of mycophenolate mofetil in preventing acute and chronic allograft rejection. *Transplantation* 2005;80 (2 Suppl):S181–S190.

15 Sollinger H. A few memories from the beginning… *Transplantation* 2005;80(2 Suppl):S178–S180.

16 Lee W, Gu L, Miksztal A *et al*. Bioavailability improvement of mycophenolic acid through amino ester derivatization. *Pharm Res* 1990;7(2):161–166.

17 Allison A, Almquist S, Muller C, Eugui E. In vitro immunosuppressive effects of mycophenolic acid and an ester pro-drug, RS-61443. *Transplant Proc* 1991;23(2 Suppl 2):10–14.

18 Sintchak M, Nimmesgern E. The structure of inosine 5′-monophosphate dehydrogenase and the design of novel inhibitors. *Immunopharmacology* 2000;47(2–3): 163–184.

19 Sintchak MD, Fleming MA, Futer O *et al*. Structure and mechanism of inosine monophosphate dehydrogenase in complex with the immunosuppressant mycophenolic acid. *Cell* 1996;85(6):921–930.

20 Allison A. Mechanisms of action of mycophenolate mofetil. *Lupus* 2005;14(Suppl 1):s2–s8.

21 Mele T, Halloran P. The use of mycophenolate mofetil in transplant recipients. *Immunopharmacology* 2000; 47(2–3):215–245.

22 Garcia R, Leoni P, Allison A. Control of phosphoribosylpyrophosphate synthesis in human lymphocytes. *Biochem Biophys Res Commun* 1977;77(3):1067–1073.

23 Thelander L, Reichard P. Reduction of ribonucleotides. *Annu Rev Biochem* 1979;48:133–158.

24 Allison A, Hovi T, Watts R, Webster A. Immunological observations on patients with Lesch–Nyhan syndrome, and on the role of de-novo purine synthesis in lymphocyte transformation. *Lancet* 1975;2(7946):1179–1183.

25 Natsumeda Y, Carr S. Human type I and II IMP dehydrogenases as drug targets. *Ann N Y Acad Sci* 1993; 696:88–93.

26 Eugui E, Almquist S, Muller C, Allison A. Lymphocyte-selective cytostatic and immunosuppressive effects of mycophenolic acid in vitro: role of deoxyguanosine nucleotide depletion. *Scand J Immunol* 1991;33(2): 161–173.

27 Allison A, Kowalski W, Muller C *et al*. Mycophenolic acid and brequinar, inhibitors of purine and pyrimidine synthesis, block the glycosylation of adhesion molecules. *Transplant Proc* 1993;25(3 Suppl 2): 67–70.

28 Platz K, Bechstein W, Eckhoff D *et al*. RS-61443 reverses acute allograft rejection in dogs. *Surgery* 1991;110(4):736–740; discussion 740–741.

29 Morris R, Hoyt E, Murphy M *et al*. Mycophenolic acid morpholinoethylester (RS-61443) is a new immunosuppressant that prevents and halts heart allograft rejection by selective inhibition of T- and B-cell purine synthesis. *Transplant Proc* 1990;22(4):1659–1662.

30 Hao L, Lafferty K, Allison A, Eugui E. RS-61443 allows islet allografting and specific tolerance induction in adult mice. *Transplant Proc* 1990;22(2):876–879.

31 Sollinger H, Deierhoi M, Belzer F *et al*. RS-61443 – a phase I clinical trial and pilot rescue study. *Transplantation* 1992;53(2):428–432.

32 Halloran P, Mathew T, Tomlanovich S *et al*. Mycophenolate mofetil in renal allograft recipients: a pooled efficacy analysis of three randomized, double-blind, clinical studies in prevention of rejection. The International Mycophenolate Mofetil Renal Transplant Study Groups. *Transplantation* 1997;63(1):39–47.

33 Neyts J, Andrei G, De Clercq E. The novel immunosuppressive agent mycophenolate mofetil markedly potentiates the antiherpesvirus activities of acyclovir, ganciclovir, and penciclovir in vitro and in vivo. *Antimicrob Agents Chemother* 1998;42(2):216–222.

34 Ojo AO, Meier-Kriesche HU, Hanson JA *et al*. Mycophenolate mofetil reduces late renal allograft loss independent of acute rejection. *Transplantation* 2000;69(11):2405–2409.

35 Wang K, Zhang H, Li Y *et al*. Safety of mycophenolate mofetil versus azathioprine in renal transplantation: a systematic review. *Transplant Proc* 2004;36(7):2068–2070.

36 Bullingham R, Monroe S, Nicholls A, Hale M. Pharmacokinetics and bioavailability of mycophenolate mofetil in healthy subjects after single-dose oral and intravenous administration. *J Clin Pharmacol* 1996;36(4):315–324.

37 Bullingham R, Nicholls A, Kamm B. Clinical pharmacokinetics of mycophenolate mofetil. *Clin Pharmacokinet* 1998;34(6):429–455.

38 Lintrup J, Hyltoft-Petersen P, Knudtzon S, Nissen N. Metabolic studies in man with mycophenolic acid (NSC-129185), a new antitumor agent. *Cancer Chemother Rep* 1972;56(2):229–235.

39 Shaw L, Kaplan B, DeNofrio D *et al*. Pharmacokinetics and concentration-control investigations of mycophenolic acid in adults after transplantation. *Ther Drug Monit* 2000;22(1):14–19.

40 Sweeney M, Hoffman D, Esterman M. Metabolism and biochemistry of mycophenolic acid. *Cancer Res* 1972;32(9):1803–1809.

41 Shipkova M, Armstrong VW, Wieland E *et al.* Identification of glucoside and carboxyl-linked glucuronide conjugates of mycophenolic acid in plasma of transplant recipients treated with mycophenolate mofetil. *Br J Pharmacol* 1999;126(5):1075–1082.

42 Maes BD, Dalle I, Geboes K *et al.* Erosive enterocolitis in mycophenolate mofetil-treated renal-transplant recipients with persistent afebrile diarrhea. *Transplantation* 2003;75(5):665–672.

43 Nowak I, Shaw L. Mycophenolic acid binding to human serum albumin: characterization and relation to pharmacodynamics. *Clin Chem.* 1995;41(7):1011–1017.

44 Staatz C, Tett S. Clinical pharmacokinetics and pharmacodynamics of mycophenolate in solid organ transplant recipients. *Clin Pharmacokinet* 2007;46(1):13–58.

45 Jain A, Venkataramanan R, Kwong T *et al.* Pharmacokinetics of mycophenolic acid in liver transplant patients after intravenous and oral administration of mycophenolate mofetil. *Liver Transpl* 2007;13(6):791–796.

46 Jain A, Sharma R, Ryan C *et al.* Potential immunological advantage of intravenous mycophenolate mofetil with tacrolimus and steroids in primary deceased donor liver transplantation and live donor liver transplantation without antibody induction. *Liver Transpl* 2008;14(2):202–209.

47 Van Gelder T, Shaw L. The rationale for and limitations of therapeutic drug monitoring for mycophenolate mofetil in transplantation. *Transplantation* 2005; 80(2 Suppl):S244–S253.

48 Shaw L, Mick R, Nowak I *et al.* Pharmacokinetics of mycophenolic acid in renal transplant patients with delayed graft function. *J Clin Pharmacol* 1998; 38(3):268–275.

49 Budde K, Glander P, Krämer BK *et al.* Conversion from mycophenolate mofetil to enteric-coated mycophenolate sodium in maintenance renal transplant recipients receiving tacrolimus: clinical, pharmacokinetic, and pharmacodynamic outcomes. *Transplantation* 2007; 83(4):417–424.

50 De Winter BC, van Gelder T, Glander P *et al.* Population pharmacokinetics of mycophenolic acid: a comparison between enteric-coated mycophenolate sodium and mycophenolate mofetil in renal transplant recipients. *Clin Pharmacokinet* 2008;47(12):827–838.

51 Cattaneo D, Cortinovis M, Baldelli S *et al.* Pharmacokinetics of mycophenolate sodium and comparison with the mofetil formulation in stable kidney transplant recipients. *Clin J Am Soc Nephrol* 2007; 2(6):1147–1155.

52 Van Gelder T, Silva HT, de Fijter JW *et al.* Comparing mycophenolate mofetil regimens for de novo renal transplant recipients: the fixed-dose concentration-controlled trial. *Transplantation* 2008;86(8):1043–1051.

53 Gaston RS, Kaplan B, Shah T *et al.* Fixed- or controlled-dose mycophenolate mofetil with standard- or reduced-dose calcineurin inhibitors: the Opticept trial. *Am J Transplant* 2009;9(7):1607–1619.

54 Oellerich M, Shipkova M, Schütz E *et al.* Pharmacokinetic and metabolic investigations of mycophenolic acid in pediatric patients after renal transplantation: implications for therapeutic drug monitoring. German Study Group on Mycophenolate Mofetil Therapy in Pediatric Renal Transplant Recipients. *Ther Drug Monit* 2000;22(1):20–26.

55 Mourad M, Malaise J, Chaib Eddour D *et al.* Correlation of mycophenolic acid pharmacokinetic parameters with side effects in kidney transplant patients treated with mycophenolate mofetil. *Clin Chem.* 2001;47(1):88–94.

56 Weber L, Lamersdorf T, Shipkova M *et al.* Area under the plasma concentration–time curve for total, but not for free, mycophenolic acid increases in the stable phase after renal transplantation: a longitudinal study in pediatric patients. German Study Group on Mycophenolate Mofetil Therapy in Pediatric Renal Transplant Recipients. *Ther Drug Monit* 1999;21(5):498–506.

57 Shaw L, Korecka M, DeNofrio D, Brayman K. Pharmacokinetic, pharmacodynamic, and outcome investigations as the basis for mycophenolic acid therapeutic drug monitoring in renal and heart transplant patients. *Clin Biochem* 2001;34(1):17–22.

58 Le Meur Y, Büchler M, Thierry A *et al.* Individualized mycophenolate mofetil dosing based on drug exposure significantly improves patient outcomes after renal transplantation. *Am J Transplant* 2007;7(11):2496–2503.

59 Weber LT, Shipkova M, Armstrong VW *et al.* The pharmacokinetic–pharmacodynamic relationship for total and free mycophenolic acid in pediatric renal transplant recipients: a report of the German study group on mycophenolate mofetil therapy. *J Am Soc Nephrol* 2002;13(3):759–768.

60 Shipkova M, Armstrong V, Oellerich M, Wieland E. Acyl glucuronide drug metabolites: toxicological and analytical implications. *Ther Drug Monit* 2003;25(1):1–16.

61 Van Gelder T, Hilbrands LB, Vanrenterghem Y *et al.* A randomized double-blind, multicenter plasma

concentration controlled study of the safety and efficacy of oral mycophenolate mofetil for the prevention of acute rejection after kidney transplantation. *Transplantation* 1999;68(2):261–266.

62 Kuypers D, Claes K, Evenepoel P *et al.* Clinical efficacy and toxicity profile of tacrolimus and mycophenolic acid in relation to combined long-term pharmacokinetics in de novo renal allograft recipients. *Clin Pharmacol Ther* 2004;75(5):434–447.

63 Kuriata-Kordek M, Boratyńska M, Klinger M *et al.* The efficacy of mycophenolate mofetil treatment in the prevention of acute renal rejection is related to plasma level of mycophenolic acid. *Transplant Proc* 2002;34(7):2985–2987.

64 Mourad M, Malaise J, Chaib Eddour D *et al.* Pharmacokinetic basis for the efficient and safe use of low-dose mycophenolate mofetil in combination with tacrolimus in kidney transplantation. *Clin Chem.* 2001;47(7):1241–1248.

65 Kuypers DR, Vanrenterghem Y, Squifflet JP *et al.* Twelve-month evaluation of the clinical pharmacokinetics of total and free mycophenolic acid and its glucuronide metabolites in renal allograft recipients on low dose tacrolimus in combination with mycophenolate mofetil. *Ther Drug Monit* 2003;25(5):609–622.

66 Heller T, van Gelder T, Budde K *et al.* Plasma concentrations of mycophenolic acid acyl glucuronide are not associated with diarrhea in renal transplant recipients. *Am J Transplant* 2007;7(7):1822–1831.

67 Smak Gregoor P, van Gelder T, Hesse C *et al.* Mycophenolic acid plasma concentrations in kidney allograft recipients with or without cyclosporin: a cross-sectional study. *Nephrol Dial Transplant* 1999; 14(3):706–708.

68 Zucker K, Tsaroucha A, Olson L *et al.* Evidence that tacrolimus augments the bioavailability of mycophenolate mofetil through the inhibition of mycophenolic acid glucuronidation. *Ther Drug Monit* 1999;21(1):35–43.

69 Zucker K, Rosen A, Tsaroucha A *et al.* Unexpected augmentation of mycophenolic acid pharmacokinetics in renal transplant patients receiving tacrolimus and mycophenolate mofetil in combination therapy, and analogous in vitro findings. *Transpl Immunol* 1997; 5(3):225–232.

70 Kobayashi M, Saitoh H, Tadano K *et al.* Cyclosporin A, but not tacrolimus, inhibits the biliary excretion of mycophenolic acid glucuronide possibly mediated by multidrug resistance-associated protein 2 in rats. *J Pharmacol Exp Ther* 2004;309(3):1029–1035.

71 Van Gelder T, Klupp J, Barten M *et al.* Comparison of the effects of tacrolimus and cyclosporine on the

pharmacokinetics of mycophenolic acid. *Ther Drug Monit* 2001;23(2):119–128.

72 Deters M, Kirchner G, Koal T *et al.* Influence of cyclosporine on the serum concentration and biliary excretion of mycophenolic acid and 7-*O*-mycophenolic acid glucuronide. *Ther Drug Monit* 2005;27(2):132–138.

73 Hesselink DA, van Hest RM, Mathot RA *et al.* Cyclosporine interacts with mycophenolic acid by inhibiting the multidrug resistance-associated protein 2. *Am J Transplant* 2005;5(5):987–994.

74 Filler G, Zimmering M, Mai I. Pharmacokinetics of mycophenolate mofetil are influenced by concomitant immunosuppression. *Pediatr Nephrol* 2000;14(2): 100–104.

75 Picard N, Prémaud A, Rousseau A *et al.* A comparison of the effect of ciclosporin and sirolimus on the pharmokinetics of mycophenolate in renal transplant patients. *Br J Clin Pharmacol* 2006;62(4):477–484.

76 Kaplan B, Meier-Kriesche HU, Minnick P *et al.* Randomized calcineurin inhibitor cross over study to measure the pharmacokinetics of co-administered enteric-coated mycophenolate sodium. *Clin Transplant* 2005;19(4):551–558.

77 El Haggan W, Ficheux M, Debruyne D *et al.* Pharmacokinetics of mycophenolic acid in kidney transplant patients receiving sirolimus versus cyclosporine. *Transplant Proc* 2005;37(2):864–866.

78 Hohage H, Zeh M, Heck M *et al.* Differential effects of cyclosporine and tacrolimus on mycophenolate pharmacokinetics in patients with impaired kidney function. *Transplant Proc* 2005;37(4):1748–1750.

79 Naderer O, Dupuis R, Heinzen E *et al.* The influence of norfloxacin and metronidazole on the disposition of mycophenolate mofetil. *J Clin Pharmacol* 2005; 45(2):219–226.

80 Bullingham R, Shah J, Goldblum R, Schiff M. Effects of food and antacid on the pharmacokinetics of single doses of mycophenolate mofetil in rheumatoid arthritis patients. *Br J Clin Pharmacol* 1996;41(6):513–516.

81 Pieper AK, Buhle F, Bauer S *et al.* The effect of sevelamer on the pharmacokinetics of cyclosporine A and mycophenolate mofetil after renal transplantation. *Nephrol Dial Transplant* 2004;19(10):2630–2633.

82 Kato R, Ooi K, Ikura-Mori M *et al.* Impairment of mycophenolate mofetil absorption by calcium polycarbophil. *J Clin Pharmacol* 2002;42(11):1275–1280.

83 Morii M, Ueno K, Ogawa A *et al.* Impairment of mycophenolate mofetil absorption by iron ion. *Clin Pharmacol Ther* 2000;68(6):613–616.

84 Mudge DW, Atcheson B, Taylor PJ *et al.* The effect of oral iron administration on mycophenolate mofetil

absorption in renal transplant recipients: a randomized, controlled trial. *Transplantation* 2004;77(2):206–209.

85 Lorenz M, Wolzt M, Weigel G *et al.* Ferrous sulfate does not affect mycophenolic acid pharmacokinetics in kidney transplant patients. *Am J Kidney Dis* 2004;43(6):1098–1103.

86 Kofler S, Shvets N, Bigdeli AK *et al.* Proton pump inhibitors reduce mycophenolate exposure in heart transplant recipients – a prospective case-controlled study. *Am J Transplant* 2009;9(7):1650–1656.

87 Miura M, Satoh S, Inoue K *et al.* Influence of lansoprazole and rabeprazole on mycophenolic acid pharmacokinetics one year after renal transplantation. *Ther Drug Monit* 2008;30(1):46–51.

88 Rupprecht K, Schmidt C, Raspé A *et al.* Bioavailability of mycophenolate mofetil and enteric-coated mycophenolate sodium is differentially affected by pantoprazole in healthy volunteers. *J Clin Pharmacol* 2009;49(10):1196–1201.

89 Cattaneo D, Perico N, Gaspari F *et al.* Glucocorticoids interfere with mycophenolate mofetil bioavailability in kidney transplantation. *Kidney Int* 2002;62(3): 1060–1067.

90 Gregoor PJ, de Sévaux RG, Hené RJ *et al.* Effect of cyclosporine on mycophenolic acid trough levels in kidney transplant recipients. *Transplantation* 1999; 68(10):1603–1606.

91 Miura M, Satoh S, Kagaya H *et al.* Effect of telmisartan, valsartan and candesartan on mycophenolate mofetil pharmacokinetics in Japanese renal transplant recipients. *J Clin Pharm Ther* 2009;34:683–692.

92 Meier-Kriesche H-U, Steffen BJ, Hochberg AM *et al.* Long-term use of mycophenolate mofetil is associated with a reduction in the incidence and risk of late rejection. *Am J Transplant* 2003;3(1):68–73.

93 Kuypers DR, Le Meur Y, Cantarovich M *et al.* Consensus report on therapeutic drug monitoring of mycophenolic acid in solid organ transplantation. *Clin J Am Soc Nephrol* 2010;5(2):341–358.

94 Cox V, Ensom M. Mycophenolate mofetil for solid organ transplantation: does the evidence support the need for clinical pharmacokinetic monitoring? *Ther Drug Monit* 2003;25(2):137–157.

95 Van Gelder T, Le Meur Y, Shaw L *et al.* Therapeutic drug monitoring of mycophenolate mofetil in transplantation. *Ther Drug Monit* 2006;28(2):145–154.

96 Knight S, Morris P. Does the evidence support the use of mycophenolate mofetil therapeutic drug monitoring in clinical practice? A systematic review. *Transplantation* 2008;85(12):1675–1685.

97 Glander P, Hambach P, Braun KP *et al.* Pre-transplant inosine monophosphate dehydrogenase activity is associated with clinical outcome after renal transplantation. *Am J Transplant* 2004;4(12):2045–2051.

98 Barraclough K, Staatz C, Isbel N, Johnson D. Therapeutic monitoring of mycophenolate in transplantation: is it justified? *Curr Drug Metab* 2009; 10(2):179–187.

99 Picard N, Ratanasavanh D, Prémaud A *et al.* Identification of the UDP-glucuronosyltransferase isoforms involved in mycophenolic acid phase II metabolism. *Drug Metab Dispos* 2005;33(1): 139–146.

100 Kuypers D, Naesens M, Vermeire S, Vanrenterghem Y. The impact of uridine diphosphate-glucuronosyltransferase 1A9 (*UGT1A9*) gene promoter region single-nucleotide polymorphisms *T–275A* and *C–2152T* on early mycophenolic acid dose-interval exposure in de novo renal allograft recipients. *Clin Pharmacol Ther Oct* 2005;78(4):351–361.

101 Wang J, Yang JW, Zeevi A *et al.* *IMPDH1* gene polymorphisms and association with acute rejection in renal transplant patients. *Clin Pharmacol Ther* 2008; 83(5):711–717.

102 Vannozzi F, Filipponi F, Di Paolo A *et al.* An exploratory study on pharmacogenetics of inosine-monophosphate dehydrogenase II in peripheral mononuclear cells from liver-transplant recipients. *Transplant Proc* 2004;36(9):2787–2790.

103 Wavamunno M, Chapman J. Individualization of immunosuppression: concepts and rationale. *Curr Opin Organ Transplant* 2008;13(6):604–608.TABLES

CHAPTER 15

Cyclosporine: Molecular Action to Clinical Therapeutics

Bradford Strijack[1] and Paul A. Keown[2]

[1] Division of Nephrology, Department of Medicine, University of British Columbia, Vancouver, BC, Canada
[2] Departments of Medicine and Pathology and Laboratory Medicine, University of British Columbia, Vancouver, BC, Canada

Introduction

The success of organ transplantation has increased dramatically during the past decades, driven by innovations in biology, pharmacology, medicine, and surgery. Almost 40% of patients with chronic kidney disease in Canada and Australia and 30% of those in the USA are now maintained with a functioning transplant, while other developed countries have somewhat lower transplantation rates due to societal, logistical, or economic factors [1–4]. Patient and graft survival now exceed 95% and 90% respectively during the first year, and over 80% of patients remain free from acute rejection [1–4]. Complications have diminished in frequency and severity; life-threatening bacterial, fungal, and viral infections are now uncommon, and there has been a corresponding improvement in both quality of life and overall cost effectiveness [5–8].

Arguably the singular and most important innovation in this transition was the discovery of cyclosporine A (CsA) by Dr. Jean Borel [9]. This novel therapeutic agent contributed to the understanding of biological processes of lymphocyte activation and graft injury and enabled the selective inhibition of key molecular steps in alloantigen response, both of which have been critical in this evolution [10–12]. The use of this agent transformed the safety and success of transplantation, particularly mitigating the incidence and severity of acute rejection during the critical first 3 months post-transplant when the graft is at greatest risk of acute immunological injury [13]. At the same time, the important organo-toxicity, narrow therapeutic index, and profound pharmacological heterogeneity of CsA challenged prior rather simplistic concepts of immunosuppression, requiring exceptional therapeutic caution and expertise to maximize clinical benefit and long-term success, and introducing pharmacokinetics, pharmacodynamics, and pharmacogenomics to clinical practice [14, 15].

Over the three decades since its discovery, the use of this exceptional agent has gradually declined as new agents within its drug class and with other mechanisms of action have been adopted into practice, and its clinical role has changed from the single major agent to a selected component of combination therapy [16,17]. Biological induction immunosuppression is now often used to minimize the risks of delayed graft function and rejection, while potent purine inhibitors or mTOR (mammalian target of rapamycin) antagonists are used to complement its effect in pharmacological maintenance immunosuppression [18, 19]. The role of CsA is now more closely confined to specific therapeutic indications in developed countries, to minimize viral infection or metabolic disorders in

Immunotherapy in Transplantation: Principles and Practice, First Edition. Edited by Bruce Kaplan, Gilbert J. Burckart and Fadi G. Lakkis.
© 2012 Blackwell Publishing Ltd. Published 2012 by Blackwell Publishing Ltd.

subjects at particular risk of these complications. This chapter will summarize the molecular actions and pharmacology of the drug; it will document the current treatment and guidelines; and it will review the principal toxicities of this therapy.

Origin and action

Structure and binding

The lipophilic cyclic undecapeptide CsA and its naturally occurring derivatives were obtained from the fermentation products of the fungal species *Tolypocladium inflatum* Gams, and the unique molecular structure and physicochemical properties of these analogs are integral to their biological actions and pharmacological behavior [20]. Several analogs exhibit diverse in vitro biological activities, but only CsA and the natural analogs (Thr²)-cyclosporine (CsC), (Val²)-cyclosporine (CsD), (Nval²)-cyclosporine (CsG), and (Nva²)-cyclosporine (CsM), produced by substitution of the α-aminobutyric acid at the 2 position, selectively inhibit the immune response in vivo [11]. These molecules consist of 10 known aliphatic amino acids and one novel C9 amino acid 4-butenyl-4-methyl-threonine (MeBmt) arranged in a cyclic structure, with a molecular weight of approximately 1200 kDa. Solid-state X-ray diffraction and nuclear magnetic resonance studies in nonaqueous solution show that the molecule is characterized by two structural motifs. Residues 1, 2, 9, 10, and 11 represent the receptor-binding domain, while residues 4–8 function as the effector domain (Plate 15.1). Residues MeBmt¹ to MeLeu⁶ comprise an antiparallel β-sheet which is stabilized by three transannular hydrogen bonds, while the residues Ala⁷ to MeVal¹¹ form a loop in which the 9–10 peptide bond is in the *cis* position. An additional extra-annular hydrogen bond links the NH of DAla⁸ to the carbonyl oxygen of MeLeu⁶. Molecular substitution within either of these regions substantially alters the biologic effects of the compound.

CsA binds to several proteins in the eukaryotic cell, of which the most important are the cyclophilins [11]. These proteins, one of three families of peptidyl-prolyl *cis–trans* isomerases, are widely distributed in prokaryotic and eukaryotic cells, and their evolutionary structural conservation implies an important role in cell biology and function [22]. Twenty different cyclophilins have been described in humans, which have a variety of intracellular functions, including tertiary protein folding, intracellular signaling, protein trafficking, and the regulation of activity of other proteins. The principal cytoplasmic isoform, cyclophilin A (CypA), is the most abundantly expressed in mammalian tissue, is located primarily in the cytoplasm, and is directly under the transcriptional control of the transcription factors p53 and hypoxia inducible factor-1a [22, 23]. Expression is upregulated in inflammatory conditions such as rheumatoid arthritis, autoimmune disease, and cancer, and there is a strong correlation between overexpression of the CypA gene and malignant transformation in some cancers [22–25]. Seven other mammalian cyclophilin isoforms contain rotamase domains and exhibit substantial homology with CypA, but differ in subcellular localization and CsA binding affinity [22]. CypB resides in the endoplasmic reticulum and may mediate translocation into this structure. CypC is expressed predominantly within the same organelle, but shows restricted tissue distribution and is found principally in the kidney. CypD possesses a signal sequence thought to target it to mitochondria, where it serves as a component of the permeability transition pore formed by the adenine nucleotide translocase and the voltage-dependent anion channel at contact sites between the inner and outer membrane, and a further protein termed Cyp-40 has been identified which is a component of the inactive steroid receptor and is found in Hsp90-containing protein complexes.

Signal inhibition

CsA binds CypA with high affinity, blocking tertiary protein folding through its peptidyl-prolyl *cis–trans* isomerase function at high concentrations. This appears to be incidental to the immunosuppressive action of the drug, however, and the formation of the molecular complex between CsA, CypA, calcineurin A and B, and calmodulin is the most important and extensively studied function leading to selective inhibition of lymphocyte signal transduction [11, 26] (Plate 15.2). T cell receptor engagement is followed by a coordinated sequence of signaling events characterized by protein tyrosine kinase activation and propagation through two discrete pathways involving respectively calcium/calcineurin signaling and MAP kinase activation through Ras, Rac, and small GTPases. The bimolecular CsA–CypA complex interacts via the CsA effector domain with the calcium- and calmodulin-dependent serine/threonine phosphatase calcineurin, a rate-limiting step in lymphocyte activation, resulting in the silencing or activation of key oncogenes and genes regulating differentiation and proliferation [26]. Blockade of the enzymatic functions of calcineurin prevents dephosphorylation of the antigen-inducible transcription factors NFAT1, elk-1, and the cAMP-response element binding protein (CREB). Translocation of nuclear factor of activated T cells (NFAT) to the nucleus is prevented, abrogating transcription of the cytokine gene complex and of the proto-oncogenes c-myc, c-fos, and n-ras. Interleukin 2 gene expression is under the coordinate control of NFAT and AP1, and is markedly inhibited under these circumstances, along with expression of the genes for IL-3, IL-4, IL-5, IL-8, IL-13, GM-CSF, and interferon-γ (IFNγ), and the transcription factor EGR3 in T cells [28]. CsA blocks the expression of CD5 and Igk in B cells and of IL-4, IL-5, and TNF-α in mast cells and TNF-α and GM-CSF in NK cells. As a consequence of these events, expression of G_0/G_1 switch genes is silenced, entry into the cell cycle is arrested at the G_0 or G_1 phase, DNA, RNA, and protein synthesis is inhibited, and growth factor production is abrogated. Activation structures such as CD40L, FasL, and IL-2Rα (CD25) are not expressed on the lymphocyte surface, and the generation of specific antibody and cytotoxic T lymphocytes directed against donor antigens is attenuated.

CsA impedes the downstream organization of inflammatory events within the graft [29] by blocking the dynamic upregulation of adhesion molecules and MHC determinants on the high endothelial venule which occur under the influence of IFNγ, tumor necrosis factor (TNF), and other inflammatory cytokines. Chemokine-mediated lymphocyte trafficking, transendothelial migration, and accumulation within the graft are attenuated, preventing the

T cell clustering necessary for interaction between graft antigen and the T cell receptor [30]. IL-17 secretion from Th17 naive and memory cells is inhibited [31], and the resulting cascade of inflammatory events, including macrophage infiltration, eosinophil degranulation, and neutrophil chemotaxis, superoxide anion production, and lysozyme release, are also suppressed, minimizing direct tissue injury. CsA influences NK cell phenotype and function, which may have important implications for graft-versus-leukemia effects. CD56$^+$CD16$^+$KIR$^+$ cells are reduced owing to decreased proliferation of the CD56(dim) NK-cell subpopulation; NFAT dephosphorylation and nuclear translocation are reduced, while NKp30 is increased and NKp44 and NKG2D reduced [32].

Other actions

Other biological actions of CsA provide an intriguing insight into the complex roles of cyclophilins in intracellular signaling networks relating to viral disease and inflammation, and offer a focus for new drug discovery in these settings [33, 34].

CsA and certain non-immunosuppressive cyclosporine analogs compete with the Gag polyproteins of the human immunodeficiency virus (HIV) for binding to CypA, thereby preventing incorporations of this isomerase into the virions. This results in a variable reduction of reverse transcription after cell infection which may be dependent on viral genotype, cell type, and state of replication [35]. CsA blocks HIV-1 infectivity via two independent mechanisms, the first involving HIV-1 CA in target cells and the second involving HIV-1 Env in producer cells. CsA decreases gp120 and gp41 incorporation into HIV-1 virions and the fusion of these virions with susceptible target cells is impaired [36]. Certain non-immunosuppressive analogs of CsA, including Debio-025 or SCY-635, have also been shown to alter replication steps of hepatitis C virus (HCV). Based on this, virtual screening using structure- and pharmacophore-based design has been used to identify nonpeptidic cyclophilin ligands that may suppress viral replication through their ability to inhibit the cis–trans isomerase activity of CypA, providing a novel strategy for rational design and development of peptidic drugs [37, 38]. Recent studies indicate that CypA has an essential role in supporting HCV-specific RNA replication and protein expression. CypA interacts with several virally expressed proteins, including the nonstructural (NS) proteins NS2, NS5A, and NS5B, and may regulate diverse activities ranging from polypeptide processing to viral assembly. As a consequence, Cyp inhibition is an active area for exlporing novel therapeutics for the treatment of chronic HCV infection [39, 40].

Cyclophilins are also implicated in a broad array of disorders ranging from cancers to atherogenesis. Biological mechanisms of atherogenesis appear to differ from those pathways critical for immuno-suppression, and include inhibition of intracellular cyclophilin peptidylprolyl isomerase and chaperone activities, inhibition of pro-inflammatory extra-cellular CypA, and NFAT-independent trans-criptional effects. CsA demonstrates complex and often bidirectional effects on these steps, and influences lipoprotein metabolism, bile acid production, endothelial cells, smooth muscle cells, and macrophages, all of which are critical to the atherosclerotic process [41–43].

Clinical pharmacology

Formulations
Sandimmune, the first-generation oral preparation, was developed as a crude oil-in-water emulsion. Absorption, which required emulsification by bile salts in the intestine, permitting digestion by pancreatic enzymes, was slow and unpredictable, reflecting complex interactions in the gastro-intestinal tract, producing wide bioavailability ranging from 2 to 90 % (median 30 %) [44]. Neoral, the second-generation preparation, was developed as a stable microemulsion formulation combining a lipophilic solvent, a hydrophilic solvent, and a surfactant. Available in both liquid and gel caplet forms, this exhibited superior bioavailability and consistency, improved linear dose–exposure relationships over a wide therapeutic range, and greater therapeutic efficacy, and quickly became the preferred formulation [45]. Several generic products are also now available, and are used increasingly in

developed and emerging economies, though concerns of comparative bioavailability and unanticipated costs have limited widespread use [46, 47]. Efforts have been made to develop third-generation preparations using modified polysac-charide vehicles or nanoparticles, attempting to improve the apical-to-basolateral permeability of CsA in the intestine, enhance absorption, and improve pharmacological performance [48]. While these preparations show promise in animal models, they have not yet been adopted clinically. CsA is also available as an intravenous formulation stabilized with cremophore at a concentration of 100 mg/mL, which is administered either by intermittent or continuous infusion over 4–24 h. Cremophore may cause severe anaphylactoid reactions, hyperlipidemia, erythrocyte aggregation, and peripheral neuropathy, and other preparations are in development using Intralipid, liposomes, or miscelles as nanoparticles.

Pharmacology
The pharmacology of cyclosporine is well described by Dunn *et al.* [49]. CsA is absorbed preferentially from the jejunum and ileum via a zero-order process in which the rate of absorption is constant and independent of drug concentration at the absorption site (Figure 15.1). Pre-systemic metabolism occurs in the intestinal epithelium under the influence of the cytochrome P450 enzyme family, reducing the amount of parent drug available for uptake. A variable proportion is also recycled into the gut lumen by the multiple drug resistance (MDR) gene product P-glycoprotein in the epithelial cell membrane [13]. The residual unchanged parent compound is absorbed into the portal system; only a small amount is transported via the lymphatics.

Absorption from the microemulsion Neoral is rapid and approximately dose-linear owing to the homogeneous dispersion of uniform particles (<0.15 μm) at the absorptive surface [49]. The absorption lag is short, the peak concentration (C_{max}) occurs at approximately 1.5 h, and delayed or secondary absorption peaks are uncommon. C_{max} is increased by more than 60 % and overall bioavaila-bility by 30–50 % compared with first-generation formulations. Between- and within-patient

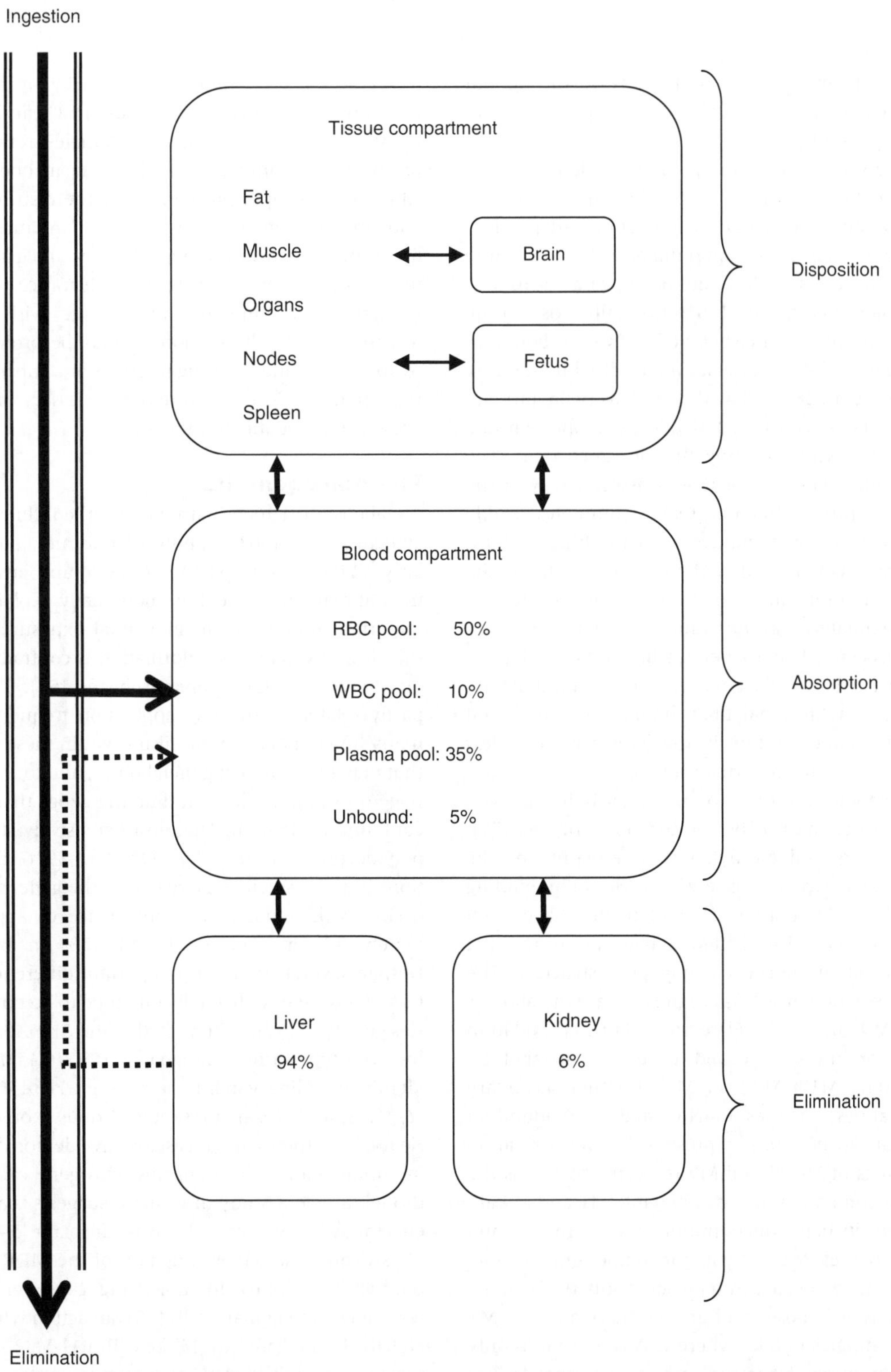

Ingestion

Tissue compartment

Fat

Muscle ← → Brain

Organs

Nodes ← → Fetus

Spleen

Disposition

Blood compartment

RBC pool: 50%

WBC pool: 10%

Plasma pool: 35%

Unbound: 5%

Absorption

Liver

94%

Kidney

6%

Elimination

Elimination

Figure 15.1 Principal routes and compartments reflecting absorption, disposition and elimination of cyclosporine.

variability in t_{max}, C_{max}, and exposure throughout the dosing interval (AUC_{0-12}) are reduced by up to 75 % [14–16].

Disposition of CsA is independent of the formulation employed. Partitioning within the blood compartment obeys a temperature-dependent equilibrium in which approximately 50 % is bound to erythrocytes, 10 % to leukocytes, and 30–40 % to plasma proteins; only 1–6 % normally exists in the free state [49]. In plasma, 98 % of CsA is bound to proteins: 33–46 % is associated with high-density lipoproteins, 28–35 % with low-density lipoprotein, and 6–19 % with very low density lipoprotein in a ratio inversely reflecting the clearance rates. The remaining 11–23 % of CsA is associated with the non-lipoprotein fraction. CsA accumulates readily in body fat, liver, pancreas, heart, lung, kidney, spleen, lymph nodes, and blood, where the concentration in mononuclear leukocytes is approximately 1000 times higher than in erythrocytes. It does not readily cross the blood–brain barrier or placenta: drug concentrations are low in cerebrospinal fluid, brain, and spinal cord and the concentration in the fetus represents less than 5 % of the maternal drug load.

Metabolism of CsA occurs primarily in the liver, with lesser rates in bowel and other organs [50], and occurs by demethylation of derivatives on the molecular face opposite the cyclophilin binding site [51]. More than 25 metabolites have been documented in human blood, bile, and urine, all of which retain the cyclic oligopeptide structure. The first oxidation products are the primary metabolites M1, M9, and M4N (Plate 15.3). Further oxidation then produces a second group of metabolites, including M19, M49, or M4N9. Other secondary derivatives, such as M4N69 and M69 found in human urine, may represent further oxidation products of M4N9 and M9 respectively. CsA is the major component in plasma, while M1 and M9 are present in high concentration in erythrocytes and other tissues. M1 is the major component in urine, where unchanged CsA represents only 0.1 % of the administered dose, and an acid derivative of M1 predominates in bile, where CsA is present in only trace amounts. All natural and synthetic metabolites are less immunosuppressive than the parent molecule. CsA is eliminated primarily by biliary excretion, with median $t_{1/2}$ of 6–8 h. Clearance is higher in children and slower in females, reflecting partly the accumulation of the drug in body fat. Alterations in lipid profile modify the distribution and metabolism of CsA, while CsA increases lipoprotein concentration, thereby reciprocally modulating its own distribution. Clearance of CsA is significantly impaired in patients with liver disease and the elimination $t_{1/2}$ may be prolonged by fourfold. Longer dosing intervals or a substantial reduction in dose is therefore necessary in the presence of hepatic dysfunction.

Pharmacogenetics

Metabolism occurs primarily under the influence of cytochrome P-4503A family of enzymes, particularly CYP3A4 and CYP3A5. Genetic and environmental may, therefore, both potentially explain the important differences in individual exposure with this drug. Despite this, information is contradictory on the role of CYP polymorphisms [52]. This is partly related to the low population frequency of many functional polymorphisms within these genes that may influence drug metabolism, and to the carriage of multiple alleles in differing genes that may confound evaluation. The most extensively studied polymorphism is the CYP3A4*1B (A-392G transition) in the 5′-regulatory region of the gene, which occurs with a population prevalence of approximately 5 % in Caucasians and 67 % in Blacks. Despite several studies, no important differences in CsA exposure have been documented to accompany this genotype [52]. With regard to the CYP3A5 gene, the wild-type form is designated as CYP3A5*1, and identified coding variants, including CYP3A5*2, *4, *6, *8, *9, and *10, are present in various exons [53]. Again, few studies in Caucasians have demonstrated important kinetic relationships with gene carriage, though a recent study in Chinese suggests that this effect may be evident early post-transplant [54].

CsA causes selective inhibition of the MDR gene product P-glycoprotein, a leading cause of drug resistance in malignant cells [55], an action which is effectively mediated by [3′-keto-Bmt1]-Val2 cyclosporine, a non-immunosuppressive cyclosporine D derivative. Results regarding the functional influence of polymorphisms in the MDR1 gene are conflicting, however. Small cohort studies are susceptible to confounding by factors such as ethnic origin or multible gene effect, and offer limited insight. Larger studies of four MDR1 SNPs with extensive pharmacokinetic parameters in stable Caucasian transplant patients on cyclosporine therapy found an association between the dose-adjusted C_{max} and the dose-adjusted AUC[0–4] and the *MDR1 1236 C.T SNP*. However, this association was weak, and haplotype analysis showed only a trend toward higher exposure to cyclosporine and better intestinal absorption in the mutated haplotype [52]. Overall, therefore, pharmacogenomic typing has not achieved the promise anticipated some years ago, and has an uncertain role in predicting therapeutic response [52, 56].

Interactions

Pharmacological interactions are common with CsA, and may have important clinical implications [57] (Table 15.1). Many drugs can modulate cytochrome P450 enzyme activity, altering the metabolism and clearance of CsA [58]. Phenytoin, rifampin, and nafcillin are prototypic of drugs which induce mixed-function oxidases: they cause a fall in CsA levels within 72h of administration and may lead to graft rejection unless the interaction is recognized and corrected. Less commonly, drugs such as cholestyramine or the somatostatin analog octreotide influence CsA absorption through direct or indirect means. In contrast, erythromycin, ketoconazole, diltiazem, colchicine, and certain fluoroquinolones and antiretroviral agents inhibit the cytochrome P450 enzyme system. These agents increase CsA

Table 15.1 Principal pharmacokinetic interactions that alter levels of cyclosporine or co-administered agents. Indicator schema adapted from University of North Carolina drug interaction reports. http://www.med.unc.edu/medicine/edursrc/drug_int.htm.

Increase in cyclosporine levels	
Calcium channel blockers	diltiazem[1B], nicardipine[1B], verapamil[1B], voriconazole[1B]
Antifungal agents	ketoconazole[1B], fluconazole[1B], itraconazole[1B]
Macrolide antibiotics	clarithomycin[1B], erythromycin[1B],
Proton pump inhibitors	lanzoprazole[6G], rabeprazole[6G]
Other drugs	cimetidine[1B], allopurinol[1F], cochicine[1F], methylprednisolone[5F], metoclopramide[1D], amiodarone[1B], grapefruit juice[1D]
Antidepressants	fluoxetine, fluvozamine[1B], sertraline[1B], venlafaxine[1B], mirtazapine[1B], paroxetine[1B]
Decrease in cyclosporine levels	
Anticonvulsants	carbemazepine[3B], phenobarbital[3B], pentobarbital[3B], phenytoin[3B], primidone[3B], phosphenytoin[3B]
Antibiotics	rifampin[3B], nafcillin[3B]
Other drugs	orlistat[3D], rifabutin[3B], octreotide[5D], ticlopidine[3BD]
Increase in other agents or biological effects	
Statins	atorvastatin[2B], lovastatin[2B], simvastatin[2B]
Anticoagulants	warfarin[5F], dabigatran[2D], etexilate[2D]
Other drugs	methotrexate[2F], colchicines[2F], digoxin[2C]

Effect on drug concentrations: (1) increased level of CsA; (2) increased level of other drug; (3) decreased level of CsA; (4) decreased level of other drug; (5) variable effect on drug level; (6) effect on drug in same class (tacrolimus) but data not substantiated for CsA.

Mechanism of drug interaction: (A) displacement from plasma proteins; (B) altered liver metabolism; (C) altered renal metabolism; (D) altered absorption or metabolism in the gastrointestinal tract; (E) toxicity or enhanced pharmacologic activity; (F) unknown; (G) altered metabolism in carriers of selected genotypes.

exposure within days and may cause acute nephrotoxicity, requiring a reduction in CsA dose by 50 % or more. Less potent interactions have been reported with the macrolide derivatives josamycin, ponsinomycin, roxithromycin, with fluconazole and with verapamil. Nifedipine and nitrendipine have no demonstrable influence on CsA pharmacokinetics. Oral contraceptives are weak inhibitors of cytochrome P450 enzymes, and may increase CsA concentration in recipients of renal and liver transplants. CsA and prednisolone are metabolized by the same hepatic microsomal enzymes, and human liver microsomal studies show a bidirectional inhibition of CsA and corticosteroid metabolism. High-dose intravenous methylprednisolone may transiently increase CsA trough levels, but this interaction is of uncertain clinical importance [59].

CsA may also alter the concentration and potency of other therapeutic agents with important consequences. This effect is typified by the interaction with mycophenolate mofetil (MMF), where CsA inhibits the biliary secretion and/or hepatic extraction of MPAG, leading to a reduced rate of enterohepatic recirculation of MPA. Several concurrent mechanisms, such as cyclosporine-induced changes in renal tubular MPAG excretion and enhanced elimination of free MPA through competitive albumin binding with MPAG, can also contribute to the altered MPAG pharmacokinetics observed in the presence and absence of cyclosporine [60]. Despite their metabolism through the CYP3A4 pathway, statins do not increase systemic exposure of CsA. However, CsA may enhance the concentration of HMG-CoA reductase inhibitors leading to rhabdomyolysis, and patients receiving this drug show substantially higher systemic exposure of all statins, whether metabolised by CYP3A4 or by CYP2C9. The mechanism for this interaction does not seem to be simply inhibition of CYP3A4 activity, but may also result from inhibition of statin transport in the liver [61].

Pharmacodynamic drug interactions may influence the immunosuppression or toxicity of CsA, and of complementary immunosuppression [62, 63]. Median effect analysis in experimental animals shows that immune suppression is additive with azathioprine and mycophenolate, and synergistic

with sirolimus. In contrast, ciprofloxacin antagonizes CsA in vitro by increasing IL-2 gene transcription, and may increase the risk of acute rejection in vivo [64]. Nonsteroidal anti-inflammatory drugs reduce intra-renal blood flow by inhibiting the production of vasodilatory prostaglandins, and may lead to acute renal dysfunction in patients receiving CsA. These are generally avoided, although short courses may be required for treatment of acute gout or other rheumatologic conditions. Septra, cimetidine, and ranitidine may also elevate serum creatinine, although this occurs by inhibition of tubular secretion rather than by impairment of glomerular filtration. It may reduce the clearance of prednisone and digoxin, and potentiate hyperkalemia. Finally, pharmacokinetic or pharmacodynamic interactions may occur with natural products and herbal remedies, now increasingly used as alternative therapies, though detailed analysis is complicated by the highly variable strengths and contents of these preparations [65].

Therapeutic monitoring

Analytical methods

CsA can be monitored on venous or capillary blood, mononuclear cells, tissues, and other matrices [66, 67] using a variety of techniques that offer different performance characteristics of accuracy, precision, sensitivity, and specificity [15, 68]. High-performance liquid chromatography (HLPC) was first used to quantitate the parent molecule and the principal metabolites. It is sensitive and specific, but time consuming and operator dependent, and is now used in only a minority of centers for routine purposes [69]. Newer chromatographic methods, including tandem mass spectrometry, offer rapid throughput, high precision, and multidrug analytical capability.

Immunoassays are widely used in normal clinical practice because of their simplicity, sensitivity, precision, and operator independence. Current assays utilize an antibody specific for the parent CsA molecule, and are available from a variety of manufacturers [70]. Fluorescence polarization immunoassay (FPIA) methods are common, followed by enzyme-multiplication immunoassay technique (EMIT) or radioimmunoassay (RIA), while many laboratories are now using the cloned enzyme donor immunoassay (CEDIA), antibody-conjugated magnetic immunoassay (ACMIA) or ADVIA systems [69–71]. Current immunoassays exhibit a variable positive bias (deviation) compared with HPLC, due to the detection of CsA metabolites. Bias is reported to be greatest (range: 17–38 %) for fluorescence polarization methods, and lower for RIA, EMIT, CDEIA, and ACMIA (range: −5 to +13 %) methods [70].

The metabolic ratio (metabolite to parent drug concentration) of CsA is lower at maximum (C_{max}) than at minimum (C_{min}, trough, C_0) concentration [72–74]. The reporting bias of immunoassay is therefore substantially reduced when CsA concentrations are measured within the first hours of the dosing interval, improving the diagnostic performance of these methods and approximating more closely the values obtained by chromatography. The use of specific point specimens requires rigorous attention to sample timing, however [75].

A window of up to 1 h or more may be accepted for trough samples, but because of the rapid changes in blood CsA concentration during the first hours of the dosing interval, specific samples must be taken within 15 min of the designated time otherwise kinetic inaccuracy rises and the prognostic value is decreased [68].

Measuring exposure and elimination

Maximum concentration (C_{max}) of CsA normally occurs in the blood compartment within the first 2 h of the dosing interval, and exposure can be described by a gamma distribution (of which the classical first-order absorption model is a special case), providing an opportunity for Bayesian monitoring of cyclosporine therapy [76, 77]. CsA concentration profiles become more uniform throughout the first 2 weeks, with a reduction in T_{max} from approximately 2.5 h to 1.5 h and a decrease in within- and between-patient coefficient of variation for most important pharmacokinetic parameters (Figure 15.2). A small number of renal transplant patients exhibit delayed

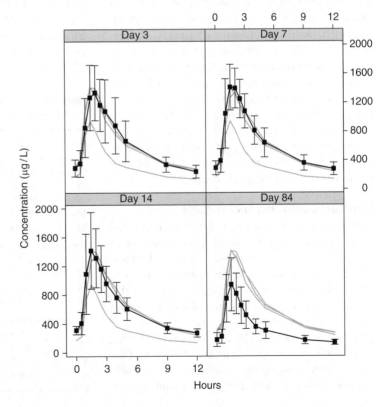

Figure 15.2 Mean cyclosporine concentration profiles during the first 3 months post-transplant [78].

or secondary peaks, and relative drug absorption may vary by up to fivefold, perhaps due to differential activity of the intestinal cytochrome P450 system or the multidrug resistance (MDR) gene product P-glycoprotein, which influence first-pass metabolism.

Drug exposure varies between studies depending on therapeutic practice [78, 79]. In a prospective Canadian study, the area under the full concentration time curve, AUC[0–12], was 9249 μg h/L and the abbreviated curve, AUC[0–4], was approximately half this value within the first week post-transplant. In an international study, exposure was approximately 15–20 % lower, with an AUC[0–12] of 7462 μg h/L and AUC[0–4] 3803 μg h/L by day 3, reflecting perhaps the lower dosing schedules in Europe [78]. AUC[0–4], capturing the drug absorption phase, was 52 % of the AUC[0–12] values across both studies and all study days. Relative exposure (measured as exposure per unit dose) increased by 80 % and 100 % respectively during the first 3 months post-transplant, permitting an important reduction in dose. Whether improved bioavailability reflects increased intestinal absorption, inhibition/saturation of enzyme systems, or both remains to be determined. Patients could be distinguished as low, intermediate, or high absorbers within 72 h of commencing therapy, after which the absorption characteristics generally remain consistent over time [78, 79] (Figure 15.2). This may be valuable in early identification of patients at risk during the first post-transplant week, a period of critical antigen recognition, and aid in adjusting treatment to minimize rejection risk.

Limited sampling techniques

Therapeutic monitoring is frequently performed using trough concentrations of whole blood taken prior to the morning oral dose. However, because of the extensive inter- and intra-patient variability in CsA absorption, disposition, and elimination, the use of a single pre-dose specimen does not provide an adequate assessment of drug exposure in patients receiving CsA [78–80]. The measurement of individual timed specimens and the integration of this data using linear, nonlinear, or Bayesian models, known as limited or sparse sampling, was

therefore proposed by Johnston and others as a simpler way to determine drug exposure throughout the dosing interval [15, 68, 77, 81, 82].

Studies using limited sampling methods in both de novo and stable transplant patients have shown that models combining blood samples taken during the first 6 h of the dosing interval closely predict the area under the complete concentration–time curve [77, 80, 83, 84]. Bias and prediction error are lowest with five-point and four-point models, but certain three-point, two-point, and even single-point models can accurately predict individual CsA exposure in adult and pediatric transplant recipients with an R^2 value of 0.80 or greater [80, 85–87] (Table 15.2). The greatest variability in CsA exposure between and within patients occurs in the first 4 h of the dosing interval, and absorption profiling during this interval is more simple, relevant, and effective for estimating drug exposure and predicting biological effects than measurement of exposure at other points during the dosing interval. Four-point sampling at 0, 1, 2, and 4 h provides a 97 % correlation with the full 12 h AUC, while just two points at 0 and 2 h show a correlation of 95 % and a <10 % mean predictive error.

Table 15.2 Examples of selected algorithm coefficients for prediction of AUC[0–4] according to day post-transplant.

Day	Algorithm and coefficients	R^2
One-point predictors		
3	$466.9 + 2.49 \times C_2$	0.85
7	$1214.1 + 2.01 \times C_2$	0.67
14	$785.1 + 2.34 \times C_2$	0.85
84	$452.3 + 2.27 \times C_2$	0.85
Two-point predictors		
3	$644.6 + 1.16 \times C_1 + 2.00 \times C_3$	0.91
7	$464.1 + 1.04 \times C_1 + 2.29 \times C_3$	0.93
14	$118.2 + 0.93 \times C_1 + 2.84 \times C_3$	0.94
84	$243.4 + 0.97 \times C_1 + 2.59 \times C_3$	0.92
Three-point predictors		
3	$318.7 + 0.71 \times C_1 + 1.11 \times C_2 + 1.29 \times C_3$	0.96
7	$265.4 + 0.87 \times C_1 + 0.79 \times C_2 + 1.62 \times C_3$	0.97
14	$274.3 + 0.76 \times C_1 + 1.09 \times C_2 + 1.38 \times C_3$	0.98
84	$129.5 + 0.77 \times C_1 + 1.13 \times C_2 + 1.31 \times C_3$	0.98

Pharmacodynamic monitoring

The biological effect of CsA is conditioned by pharmacodynamic and pharmacokinetic factors, and both must be considered in a comprehensive therapeutic monitoring program. In vitro sensitivity to CsA shows inter-individual and clonal variation, and is greater in transplant recipients than in normal controls, though the molecular explanation for this latter observation is not clear. For these reasons, direct measurement of biological effect would be highly desirable. In vitro studies have shown that the concentration of CsA within the dosing interval is inversely related to lymphocyte calcineurin activity or IL-2 production, key measures of T cell activation. Maximum inhibition of these parameters occurs approximately 2 h after dosing, consistent with the peak concentration of CsA in peripheral blood. Whole blood calcineurin activity may prove a valuable assay, and a single trough measure may be a useful surrogate for the inhibition of this enzyme by CsA during the whole dosing interval. Genetic polymorphisms in the genes encoding NFAT may also be interesting candidates for studying interpatient differences in calcineurin inhibitor (CNI) efficacy and toxicity, while differences in isoforms and tissue distribution of the calcineurin protein may help to explain variable drug responses [88]. Although no simple measures yet fulfill the stringent criteria of performance and practicality required for routine and effective pharmacodynamic monitoring of CsA, the search for these is now a major new area of research.

Clinical therapeutics

Formulation and administration

Treatment strategies for the use of CsA vary by therapeutic indication, center, and region based on clinical preference, costs, and risks. Neoral is available in various strengths of 10–100 mg soft-gelatin capsules, and an oral solution of 100 mg/mL [44]. The solution may be diluted with fruit juice or other vehicles, though grapefruit juice has a well-known interaction in raising the CsA concentration and should be avoided. Oral therapy in organ transplantation is normally commenced at a dose of 4–5 mg/kg twice daily, while a higher dose or a shorter dosing interval may be required in children, and in subjects with external bile drainage, gastrointestinal disease, or a decreased elimination half-life. Doses are also often slightly lower in liver, heart, and bone marrow recipients, and in treatment of autoimmune disorders. Cyclosporine may be administered intravenously when gastrointestinal function is impaired, and is used at a dose approximately one-quarter the oral dose. Pre-transplant pharmacokinetic monitoring or genotyping may be used to identify patients and to predict the dose and dosing interval required in subjects at risk of inadequate drug exposure who have a high probability of rejection and graft loss, although the precise clinical utility of this approach remains to be determined [52]. CsA microemulsion may be used alone for autoimmune indications, but this is rarely the case in organ transplantation, where current treatment strategies employ dual or triple therapy with a purine inhibitor such as MMF or azathioprine, an mTOR antagonist such as sirolimus or everolimus, and/or prednisone. CsA microemulsion is normally administered twice daily, at constant times, but preliminary evidence suggests that a double dose once daily may be equally effective for maintenance therapy. Dosing is adjusted based on a combination of measured drug concentrations and clinical parameters, including renal and hepatic function, blood pressure, lipids and glycemia, evidence of graft rejection, infection, and malignancy.

Initial use and impact

The introduction of CsA immunosuppression revolutionized solid organ transplantation. Despite the difficulties with dosing and toxicity, the reduction in mortality and graft loss was compelling, leading to the rapid adoption of CsA as foundation therapy [89–91]. Subsequent prospective, concentration-controlled studies in renal transplantation showed that Neoral further decreased the both the risk (44 % versus 60 %) and recurrence of acute rejection, and enabled more predictable and cost-effective therapy [45, 92]. Nested pharmacokinetic evaluation showed superior bioavailability of CsA from Neoral, the dose-normalized AUC in the first 3 months was increased by one-third to one-half, and dose-normalized peak CsA blood concentrations stabilized within this time. The UK multicenter study confirmed these results [92]; target CsA levels were achieved quickly (2 days), acute rejection was again significantly reduced (34 % versus 47 %), and treatment failures declined (45 % versus 58 %).

Neoral proved particularly valuable in liver transplantation, where absorption was enhanced up to sixfold and blood levels were comparable to those achieved with intravenous administration within the first 48 h so that intravenous therapy could be avoided in 90 % of patients [93]. Graft survival rose above 90 % owing to the reduced frequency and severity of acute rejection, without incremental toxicity. Preliminary studies in pancreas, heart, and heart–lung transplantation confirmed these observations, and exposure was increased by approximately twofold and C_{max} by threefold in patients with cystic fibrosis.

Concentration-controlled therapy

CsA exposure was shown to be significantly lower in patients who experienced acute graft rejection and higher in those with CsA nephrotoxicity, and intermediate exposure was associated with a low risk of both outcomes [87, 94]. Patients with AUC[0–4] levels of 4400–5500 µg h/L by day 3 posttransplant had no CsA nephrotoxicity and only a 3 % risk of acute rejection, compared with 45 % rejection in those below this range, and optimum CsA exposure did not delay recovery of graft function. The Canadian multicenter trial extended these observations [79], showing that CsA exposure in the first week was significantly lower in patients with acute rejection than in those who were rejection free, whether measured by AUC[0–12] or AUC[0–4] (Figure 15.3). More importantly, the study demonstrated that a single-point measure of

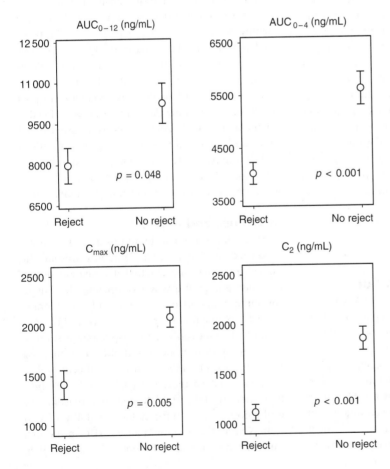

Figure 15.3 Mean cyclosporine exposure measured by AUC_{0-12}, AUC_{0-4}, C_{max} or C_2 at 1 week post-transplant in patients with or without acute graft rejection [79].

C_2 or C_{max} was highly predictive of acute rejection, providing both a simple measure and therapeutic threshold for clinical therapy.

Single-point monitoring was adopted into clinical practice as a surrogate of AUC[0–4] for simplicity, efficacy, and cost. Studies in kidney, liver, and thoracic transplantation validated the use of C_2 monitoring, showing correlation with acute rejection and to a lesser extent with nephrotoxicity, while many others confirmed the lack of prognostic value of C_0 [87, 93, 95–101]. The importance of C_2 monitoring was examined in large multicenter trials in patients receiving induction with the anti-CD25 monoclonal basiliximab. The international study, conducted in eight countries, showed that relative absorption of CsA could be determined as early as 72 h post-transplant using a simple index derived from C_2 divided by the weight-adjusted CsA morning dose as a surrogate for CsA bioavailability, dividing patients into low, intermediate, or high absorber categories, a characteristic that remains consistent throughout the period of follow-up [78] (Figure 15.3). The US multicenter study reinforced these findings, confirming a highly significant influence of C_2 and the lack of prognostic value of trough levels in patients receiving basiliximab [102]. The international prospective "Mozart" study (Monitoring of 2-hour absorption in renal transplantation) reinforced the relationship between C_2 exposure and freedom from acute rejection in a large, heterogeneous international study population receiving complementary MMF and prednisone [103]. The overall rate of biopsy-proven acute rejection in this study (11%) was the lowest reported to that point for any international trial in patients receiving simple triple therapy with Neoral; it was achieved without any increase in toxicity or adverse events, and was comparable or superior to the results reported with potent biological induction.

Defining optimal blood CsA concentrations was more difficult for maintenance therapy. However, empirical observation in kidney transplantation suggested that low CsA exposure was associated with increased risks of subclinical and chronic rejection, while high exposure contributed to adverse effects and functional graft deterioration. C_2 levels were again noted to be significantly lower in patients with biopsy-proven subclinical acute rejection, and a target range of 1100–1200 µg/L by 6 months post-transplant was proposed to ensure optimum immune suppression. Studies examining CsA exposure and chronic rejection in stable long-term kidney transplant recipients receiving Neoral and steroids showed that 50% of subjects with a C_2 below 960 µg/L had acute rejection compared with only 10% of those with a C_2 between 960 and 1322 µg/L [104]. Reduction in CsA dose to achieve C_2 target levels of 1000 µg/L decreased hypertension, improved graft function, and ameliorated the general symptoms of well-being, tremor, and gum hyperplasia without adverse clinical or biological effects [105,106]. In children, David-Neto *et al.* showed that tremor and hypertrichosis were closely correlated with C_2, C_4, C_{max}, and AUC[0–4] and that a $C_{max} > 878$ µg/L or AUC[0–4] > 4158 µg h/L respectively were the best predictors of the these complications [107]. In contrast, gingival hyperplasia appeared to be unrelated to CsA levels but was closely related to the use of nifedipine.

Studies performed in maintenance liver and heart recipients demonstrated a similar correlation between C_2 and AUC[0–4] which substantially exceeded the predictive capacity of C_0. Liver recipients randomized to a maintenence C_2 of 300–600 µg/L experienced a significant reduction in Neoral dose and serum creatinine and an improved clinical benefit compared with those maintained within a C_0 range of 100–200 µg/L. De novo and stable cardiac graft recipients randomized to an identical C_2 range (300–600 µg/L) saw a parallel and significant reduction in CsA daily dose and serum creatinine (138 versus 168 µmol/L) without evidence of acute rejection or ventricular dysfunction [101, 108]. Cross-over studies showed that resumption of C_0 monitoring with a target of 100–200 µg/L resulted in an increase in Neoral dose and in C_0 and C_2 levels, as well as a reduction in clinical benefit with no gain in rejection risk or survival.

Informed by these studies, target C_2 levels for the first week post-renal transplantation were set at 1700 µg/L to minimize the risk of graft rejection, renal toxicity, and other adverse events. Corresponding C_2 target levels in liver transplantation was lower at 1000 µg/L, reflecting the direct delivery of

CsA to the liver via the portal system, while targets for other organs were established between these values, often reflecting the increased risk of renal toxicity in cardiothoracic transplantation. Targets were then gradually reduced for each organ to reach maintenance values at 3 months. Current data suggest that the target levels may be lower for patients receiving other potent complementary immunosuppressants, but detailed trials are required to explore other therapeutic combinations. Whether these relationships extend to generic formulations of CsA is unclear without comparable pharmacokinetic or clinical data, but should not be assumed uncritically owing to the differing behavior of these formulations under diverse physiological conditions.

Current therapeutic strategies

Immunosuppressive management has changed markedly in the decade since these studies were reported [16, 17, 109]. The use of induction agents has increased by over twofold, so that almost 75 % of kidney transplants and half of intestine, heart, and lung transplants in the USA now receive biological therapy [110]. The most common biological agent in the USA is rabbit antithymocyte globulin, while the anti-CD25 monoclonal antibodies basiliximab and daclizumab predominate in other parts of the world [18]. MMF has replaced azathioprine as the baseline purine antagonist, and now less than 1 % of subjects in the USA and Europe commence on this latter therapy. And, finally, there has been a strong and continuing trend to the avoidance or elimination of steroids [16, 17, 110].

While CNIs remain a foundational therapy, there has been a progressive decline in the use of CsA from approximately 79 % of kidney patients in 1996 to only 15 % in 2005, with adoption of tacrolimus rising from 13 % to 76 % in this same time interval. This trend reflects not only the greater simplicity of tacrolimus use, but also its superior performance in preventing graft rejection in both observational and comparative studies, associated with improved graft survival and function and with reduced hirsutism, gum hyperplasia, hypertension, and hyperlipidemia [111–115]. While these differences in effectiveness were most evident in

combination with azathioprine, improved freedom from rejection and superior graft function was also observed with MMF [115]. Studies from the Symphony trial comparing tacrolimus and azathioprine, CsA and MMF, and tacrolimus and MMF showed a lower risk of acute rejection and of need for antithymocyte globulin rescue therapy with tacrolimus, and in particular subjects with delayed graft function experienced superior outcomes after 3 years [116–118].

The dose of MMF required was lower, but the risks of post-transplant diabetes mellitus were almost fourfold higher in the group receiving tacrolimus and MMF (11 % versus 3 %) [118], consistent with the known risk of this complication in subjects treated with tacrolimus [119]. Other studies also suggest that while steroid-free treatment is possible with CsA and may offer benefit, this is accompanied by a measureable risk of rejection and is perhaps more easy to achieve with tacrolimus [120–122]. The Freedom trial, conducted in subjects receiving Neoral and enteric-coated mycophenolic acid, showed that the risk of acute graft rejection, graft loss, or death was lower at 1 year in treatment groups with early steroid withdrawal or without steroid therapy (19 % versus 30 % versus 36 %) [123]. However, graft function measured by glomerular filtration was comparable and the use of antidiabetic and lipid-lowering medications was lower in the group without steroids [123]. In general, CsA is therefore currently employed principally in selected subjects at high risk of post-transplant diabetes mellitus following renal transplantation to minimize the risk of this complication.

Similar trends in transplantation of the liver and other organs were spurred by evidence of superior efficacy of tacrolimus measured by patient and graft survival, rejection risk, and severity [124]. Early randomized comparative studies showed that 62 % of subjects randomized to tacrolimus after liver transplantation were alive by 3 years of follow-up compared with 42 % in the CsA limb [125, 126]. Interestingly, these differences were not observed in subjects with hepatitis C [127, 128], and interest in the use of CsA has been rekindled by this finding in combination with in vitro studies demonstrating the antiviral effect of CsA on suppressing the HCV replicon RNA level, protein expression, and the multiplication of the HCV genome in vitro and the in vivo increase in the rate of sustained viral response [129, 130]. Neither the potential benefit of CsA in reducing HCV reactivation nor in reducing the risk of post-transplant diabetes are fully confirmed, however, so the preferred agent in liver transplantation remains unclear [131].

Clinical toxicology

Adverse effects of CsA involve many organ systems and, in general, reflect the dose and duration of treatment (Table 15.3).

Table 15.3 Principal complications of cyclosporine therapy in solid organ transplantation.

Skin and appearance
Hypertrichosis, hirsutism, gingival hyperplasia, cranio-facial abnormalities

Neurological
Peripheral tremor, hyperesthesia, seizures, confusion, visual loss, extraparymidal syndromes, posterior reversible leukoencephalopathy

Cardiovascular
Accelerated atherosclerosis, hypertension, thromboembolism, hemolytic uremic syndrome

Renal
Delayed graft function, reduced renal plasma flow, acute tubular injury, acute renal dysfunction, thrombotic microangiopathy, chronic nephrotoxicity

Metabolic
Hyperkalemia, type 4 renal tubular acidosis, hyperuricemia, new-onset diabetes, hypercholesterolemia

Infection
Cytomegalovirus, Epstein–Barr virus, *Clostridium difficile*, bacterial infection, fungal infection, pneumocystis carinii, mucormycoses

Malignancy
Skin cancer, vulvo-vaginal cancer, Kaposi's sarcoma, non-Hodgkin lymphoma, renal cell cancer, melanoma, leukemia, hepatobiliary cancer, testicular and bladder cancer, colon cancer, esophageal cancer

Skin and appearance

Hypertrichosis, the most frequent and serious cutaneous complication, occurs in 10–50% of patients receiving CsA. Folliculodystrophy, hyperpigmentation, or other cutaneous eruptions occur more rarely, and their relationship to CsA is less certain [132]. Hair growth occurs on the scalp, eyebrows, preauricular area, upper lip, limbs, and trunk and is most noticeable in females and dark-skinned individuals. The etiology is unclear and treatment is empiric. Blood concentrations of sex hormones and sex-hormone-binding globulin are generally normal, but experimental studies show that CsA stimulates growth of murine hair epithelial cell and epidermal keratinocytes over a wide dose range, an effect partially attributable to the downregulation of certain protein kinase C isozymes in hair epithelial cells or inhibition of translocation to the membrane or cytoskeleton of hair epithelial cells [133].

Gingival hyperplasia occurs in a similar proportion of subjects receiving CsA and may be related to inhibition of type 1 plasminogen activator or enhanced endothelin expression [134, 135]. Papillary enlargement is most marked in the interdental papillary region on the labial side of the anterior teeth of the maxilla, but it may affect the entire maxilla and mandible with an increase in gingival fibroblasts and collagen and variable lymphocytic infiltrate. Phenytoin, nifedipine, and calcium channel blockers may accentuate the effect of CsA, sometimes to a remarkable degree [136]. Hyperplasia is related to the development of plaque and calculus in patients with poor dental hygiene and is most common in children [137]. Scrupulous dental care is essential, and gum hypertrophy gradually resolves approximately 3 months after withdrawal of the drug.

Craniofacial abnormalities, though rare, range from a subtle coarsening and accentuation of the facial features to a severe facial dysmorphism and are the most disturbing long-term structural complications in the child [138]. Abnormal osseous development in the lower third of the face produces shortening of posterior facial height and the mandibular body, a deep mandibular plane angle, and mandibular retrognathia.

Skeletal

The impact of transplantation upon renal osteodystrophy is variable, depending on the immunosuppression employed, the physiologic status of the patient, and the the timing of intervention [139, 140]. Linear growth is retarded by high-dose prednisone, which may inhibit somatomedin release and accelerate epiphyseal closure, with measurable reduction in 40 % of children [141]. The steroid-sparing effect of CsA reduced these problems, enabling improvement in body habitus, fat distribution, and muscle mass. Bone maturation occurs at a more normal rate following renal transplantation, with growth acceleration at 2–3 years in up to 80 % of children receiving CsA and a decline in the devastating complication of avascular necrosisoccurs to less than 5 % of renal transplant recipients.

Although CsA faciliates linear growth, it has an important effect on skeletal remodelling. Bone metabolism reflects a complex interaction of signals influencing osteoclast and osteoblast growth and differentiation, and experimental studies in the rodent show that CsA causes profound osteoporosis with a loss of trabecular volume which is not associated with changes in serum calcium, magnesium, parathormone, or vitamin D levels but is dependent on the dose and duration of drug administration. CsA and other CNIs inhibit osteoclast differentiation in bone marrow cell cultures and osteoclastic bone resorption in bone organ cultures induced by parathyroid hormone, calcitriol, prostaglandins, and cytokines, which may occur through inhibition of NFAT activation and translocation following receptor activator of nuclear factor κ-B ligand (RANKL) stimulation [142]. These findings suggest that calcineurin is an essential downstream mediator of the RANKL-induced signal transduction pathway for osteoclast differentiation, and that activation of the NFATc1 transcription factor is sufficient to induce osteoclast differentiation and to express bone resorptional function [142]. This may contribute to the bone loss following renal and, more particularly, nonrenal transplantation, where mean bone density frequently remains at or below the fracture threshold and vertebral compression fractures occur in an important proportion of heart or liver graft recipients [143].

Neurological

Neurological complications are common after transplantation, so it is difficult to distinguish causal relationships to specific therapeutic agents [144–146]. Peripheral tremor and hyperesthesia of the hands and face are common with CsA treatment and are usually dose related. Acute myopathy, acute ascending motor paralysis, and a prolonged post-anesthetic neuromuscular blockade have been reported, but a causal relationship to CsA is not firmly established. Cephalalgia is common in patients receiving CsA, and may be severe, persistent, or recurrent [147]. Subtle organic mental disorders may present as anxiety, lethargy, memory loss, insomnia, and sleep–wake reversal. Seizures, drowsiness, confusion, hallucinations, visual disturbances, and mental changes have been reported, and complex status epilepticus and selective neurological defects such as dysphasia, dysarthria, akinetic mutism, extrapyramidal syndromes, hemiplegia, and cortical blindness may also be seen and accompanied by focal lacunar changes in the white matter and cortices of the cerebral hemispheres [145]. Posterior reversible leukoencephalopathy syndrome has been reported in up to 5 % of pediatric patients receiving CsA, and may present with a sudden episode of neurological symptoms accompanied by radiological changes in the gray matter, frontal and temporal lobes, and even the cerebellum [148] (Figure 15.4). Most neurological sequelae resolve following a reduction in the dose or discontinuation of CsA.

Cardiovascular

CsA has important effects on the vascular tree, leading to endothelial injury, accelerated atherosclerosis, and hypertension. It induces morphological and phenotypic endothelial changes suggestive of a partial endothelial-to-mesenchymal transition and contributing to endothelial cell death; it alters circulating endothelial cells and endothelial microparticles; and it results in vascular dysfunction characterized by impairment of endothelin-dependent vasorelaxation and enhanced sensitivity

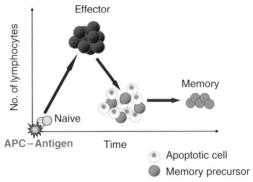

Plate 1.1 *Schematic representation of the immune response to a foreign antigen.* Naive T cells (yellow) are activated and proliferate exponentially upon encountering foreign antigen presented by antigen-presenting cells (APC). Proliferated T cells differentiate into effector lymphocytes (red), the majority of which die by apoptosis upon eliminating the foreign antigen. Those that survive become memory lymphocytes (green). Memory T cells behave similarly to naive T cells upon re-encountering antigen, except that their response is faster and larger in magnitude. One can envision that effective regulation or suppression of the immune response can be achieved by different means: by inhibiting T cell proliferation or T cell differentiation, or by enhancing T cell death.

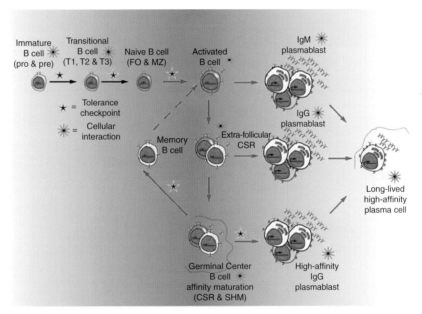

Plate 4.1 *Fate map of B cell development.* B cells develop in the bone marrow and then migrate to the secondary lymphoid organs. Localization within the bone marrow, circulatory system/lymphatics, and secondary lymphoid organs (spleen and lymph nodes) is depicted by a gray scale, where the most intense gray represents the secondary lymphoid organs. Immature and transitional B cells engage with IL-7-producing and Baff/BLys-expressing stromal cells in the bone marrow. Activated B cells interact with activated T cells or dendritic cells in the secondary lymphoid organs, whereas Germinal Center B cells interact with follicular dendritic cells and T-follicular helper cells. Plasmablast cells interact with stromal components that express Baff/BLys in extrafollicular spaces of the secondary lymphoid organs, whereas the long-lived plasma cells interact with IL-6-producing stromal cells in the bone marrow. The tolerance checkpoints indicate developmental intermediates that can be affected by the presence of auto-antigen. BCR = B cell receptor (membrane or secreted); CSR = class switch recombination; FO = follicular B cell; MZ = marginal zone B cell; SHM = somatic hypermutation; Transitional B cell = migrating immature B cell.

Immunotherapy in Transplantation: Principles and Practice, First Edition. Edited by Bruce Kaplan, Gilbert J. Burckart and Fadi G. Lakkis.
© 2012 Blackwell Publishing Ltd. Published 2012 by Blackwell Publishing Ltd.

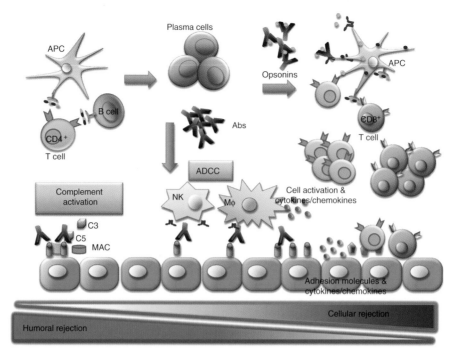

Plate 4.2 *B cells and antibodies in transplantation rejection.* Antibodies and B cells can induce transplantation rejection by a number of potential mechanisms arising from: (1) B cells functioning as antigen-presenting cells and engaging in T cell–B cell interactions, thereby facilitating T cell activation and B cell differentiation into antibody-secreting cells; (2) the ability of antibodies to bind to vascular endothelial cells in the graft and eliciting humoral or antibody-mediated rejection; (3) antibodies generating immune complexes and opsonins that result in enhanced antigen uptake and presentation, thereby facilitating alloreactive T cell activation and cellular rejection. None of these activities is mutually exclusive. Thus, antibodies can play differential roles in promoting the continuum of humoral and cellular rejection.

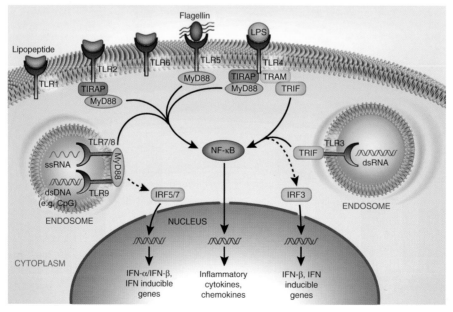

Plate 5.1 TLRs and their major signaling adaptors. With permission from the American Society of Nephrology, from Shirali AC, Goldstein DR. *J Am Soc Nephrol* 2008;19:1444–1450.

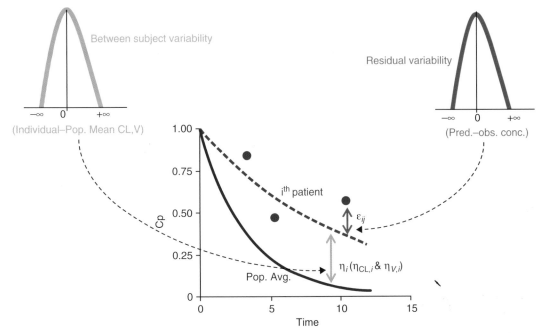

Assume between-occasion variability = 0

Plate 9.1 Conceptual framework for nonlinear mixed-effects modeling.

Plate 14.1 Comparison of EC-MPS and MMF pharmacokinetics at day 0, day 14, and 3 months. From [49], Budde K, Glander P, Krämer BK, Fischer W, Hoffmann U, Bauer S *et al*. Conversion from mycophenolate mofetil to enteric-coated mycophenolate sodium in maintenance renal transplant recipients receiving tacrolimus: clinical, pharmacokinetic, and pharmacodynamic outcomes. *Transplantation* 2007;83(4):417–424. Reproduced with permission by LWW.

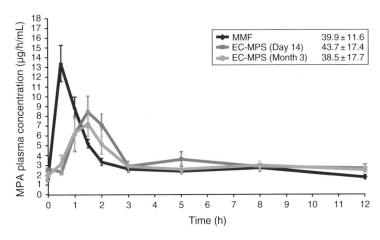

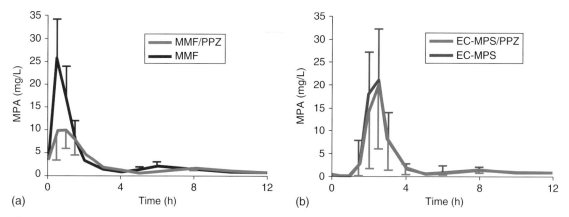

Plate 14.2 Comparison of the effect of PPIs on MPA AUC in (a) MMF- and (b) EC-MPS-treated patients. From [87], Rupprecht K, Schmidt C, Raspé A, Schweda F, Shipkova M, Fischer W *et al*. Bioavailability of mycophenolate mofetil and enteric-coated mycophenolate sodium is differentially affected by pantoprazole in healthy volunteers. *J Clin Pharmacol* 2009;49(10):1196–1201. Reproduced with permission by Sage.

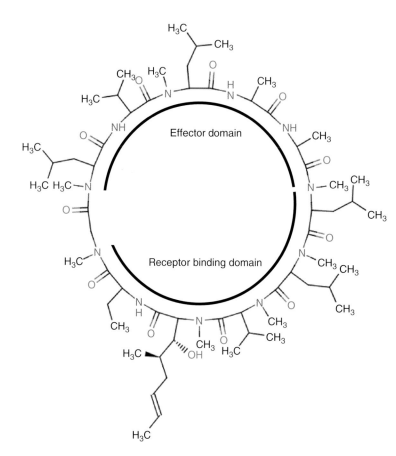

Plate 15.1 Molecular structure of cyclosporine A. From Lim E, Pon A, Djoumbou Y, Knox C, Shrivastava S, Guo AC, Neveu V, Wishart DS. T3DB: a comprehensively annotated database of common toxins and their targets. *Nucleic Acids Res* 2010;38(suppl 1):D781–D786. http://www.t3db.org/toxins/T3D3498.

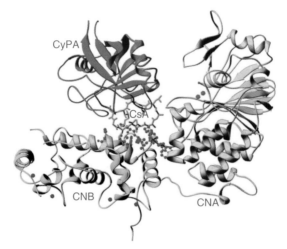

Plate 15.2 Ribbon representation of the structural association between cyclosporine A (CsA) and the trimolecular complex comprising cyclophilin A (CyPA), calcineurin A (CAN) and calcineurin B (CNB). CsA is oriented through its interaction with CyPA to interface with both the catalytic (CNA) and regulatory (CNB) subunits of calcineurin through a binding site unique to calcineurin, inhibiting the phosphatase activity of these molecules and subsequent downstream biological events. Huai Q, Kim H-Y, Liu Y, Zhao Y, Mondragon A, Liu JO, Ke H. *Proc Natl Acad Sci U S A* 2002;99:12037–12042.

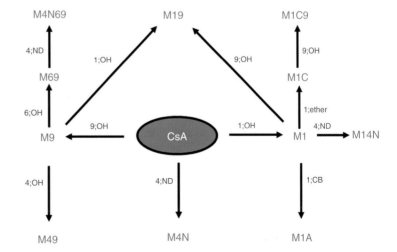

Plate 15.3 Biotransformation of cyclosporine and principal metabolites.

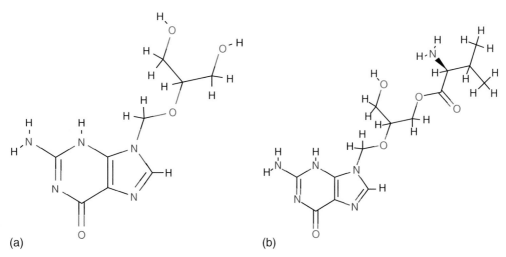

Plate 21.1 Chemical structures of ganciclovir (a) and valganciclovir (b) [9, 10]. Ganciclovir is a cyclic analog of guanosine. Ganciclovir is also known as DHPG or 9-[(1,3-dihydroxy-2-propoxy)methyl]guanine. Valganciclovir is the hydrochloride salt of the L-valyl ester of ganciclovir. Valganciclovir is a mixture of two diastereomers that are converted to ganciclovir. The chemical name for valganciclovir is L-valine, 2-[(2-amino-1,6-dihydro-6-oxo-9H-purin-9-yl)methoxy]-3-hydroxypropyl ester, monohydrochloride.

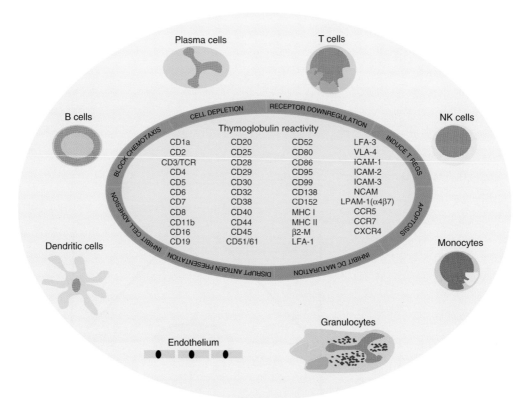

Plate 22.1 Thymoglobulin specificity and mechanism of action. Summarized are the immune-response antigens, adhesion molecules, cell trafficking molecules, and a variety of other cell surface receptors that are known to interact with thymoglobulin [1, 13–15]. Also represented are the different cell types of the immune system that could be bound by thymoglobulin via interactions with these receptors. A variety of biological effects are listed, which contribute to the overall mechanism of action and can be attributed to the interaction between thymoglobulin and cells involved with an immune response.

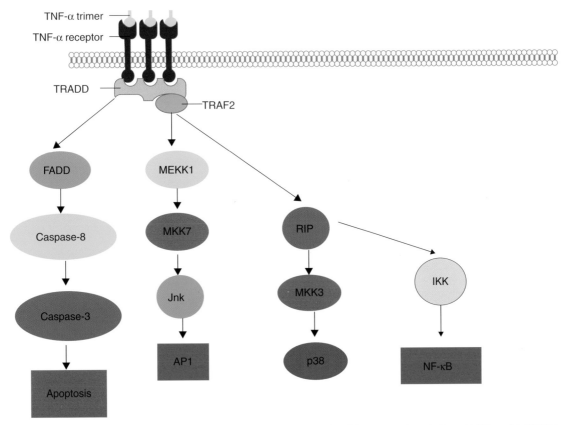

Plate 26.1 Simplified diagram demonstrating signaling pathways initiated by TNF-α. Association of TNF-α with TNFR1 leads to the recruitment of the TNFR-associated death domain (TRADD) and to the subsequent recruitment of the Fas-associated death domain (FADD) with sequential activation of caspase-8 and caspase-3, which induces apoptosis. Another pathway activated through TRADD is the JUN N-terminal kinase (JNK), through sequential activation of several MAP kinases (including MEKK1 and MKK7), leading to activation of several transcription factors, such as activator protein 1 (AP1). TNF-α binding has also been linked to activation of p38, via recruitment of RIP and MKK3. One of the major consequences of TNF-α binding is activation of NF-κB. Modified from Tracey D, Klareskog L, Sasso EH, Salfeld JG, Tak PP. *Pharmacol Therapeut* 2008;117:244–279.

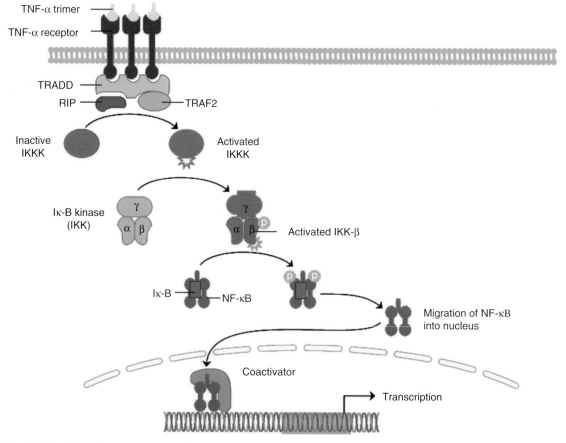

Plate 26.2 Schematic representation of NF-κB activation by TNF-α. Modified from Aggarwal BB. Signalling pathways of the TNF superfamily: a double-edged sword. *Nat Rev* 2003;3:745–756.

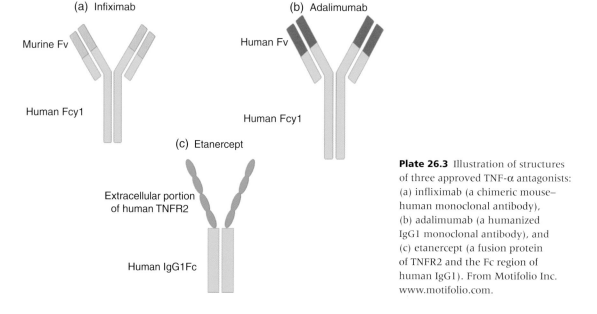

Plate 26.3 Illustration of structures of three approved TNF-α antagonists: (a) infliximab (a chimeric mouse–human monoclonal antibody), (b) adalimumab (a humanized IgG1 monoclonal antibody), and (c) etanercept (a fusion protein of TNFR2 and the Fc region of human IgG1). From Motifolio Inc. www.motifolio.com.

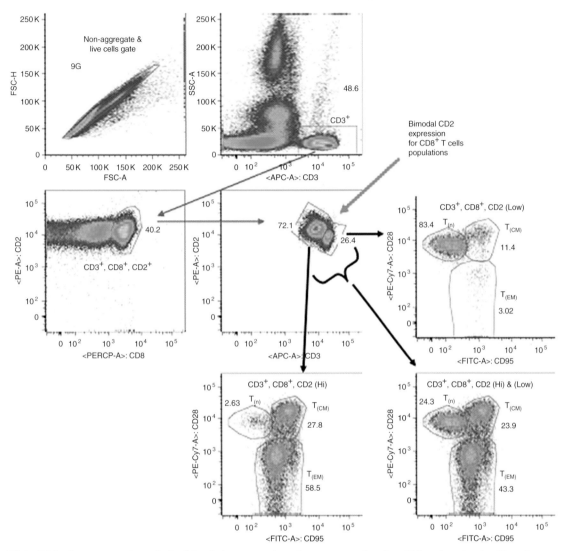

Plate 28.1 Flow cytometric analysis of T cells by maturation phenotype as related to CD2 surface density. Note that T cells segregate into a bimodal distribution based on CD2 and CD3 with mature/memory cells being relatively CD2 high and CD3 low and naive T cells being relatively CD2 low and CD3 high. Modified from [61].

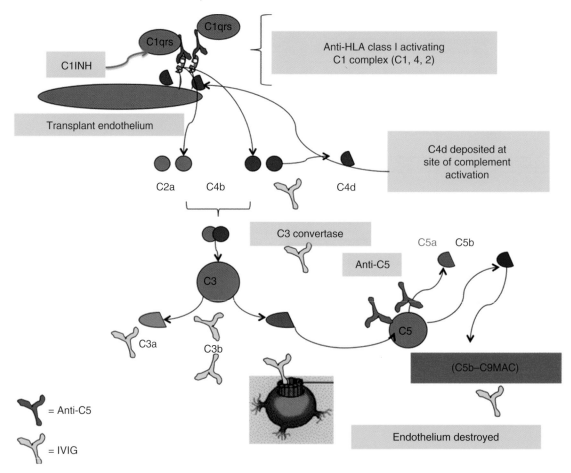

Plate 29.1 Anti-HLA antibodies binding to targets on vascular endothelial cells of the allograft result in activation of the classic complement cascade. C1,4,2 forms the C3 convertase that activates C3. C3 activation results in activation of C5 to C5a and C5b. C5b interacts with C6–9 to form the membrane attack complex (MAC) that destroys the endothelium. C5a and the MAC are the most inflammatory of all complement proteins. Complement activation augments other procoagulant and inflammatory pathways that ultimately results in allograft dysfunction and loss. IVIG and the protease inhibitor C1 inhibitor (C1INH) are natural regulators of complement-mediated inflammation. C1INH blocks the assembly of the C1qrs complex, thus resulting in early termination of complement activation by antigen–antibody complexes. For IVIG, the sites of action are mediated by both Fab and Fc fragments and are shown in the figure. Importantly, IVIG inhibits C3b, C3a and C3 convertase, which blocks generation of C5a and the MAC, thus blunting inflammation induced by complement-*activating antibodies. IVIG also has a potent "scavenger" effect by absorbing activated complement components. A potentially important inhibitor of complement activation and injury is the monoclonal antibody to C5 that could work in conjunction with IVIG.

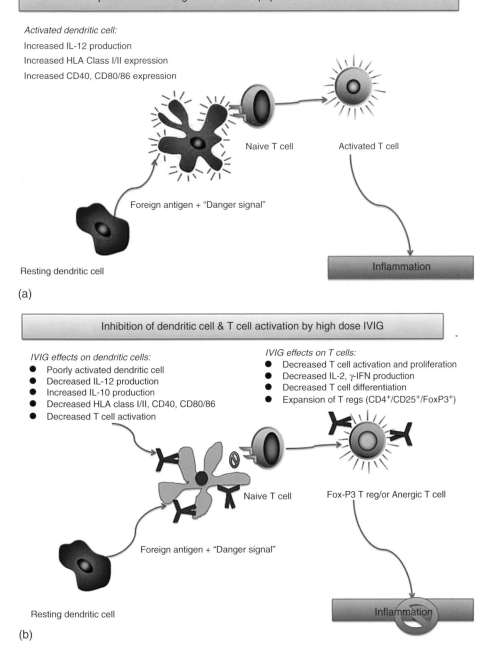

Plate 29.2 (a) The activation of resting dendritic cells (DCs) by antigen and danger signals such as TNF-α. This results in upregulation of proinflammatory cytokine production (IL-12) and expression of HLA Class I/II with the concomitant upregulation of the co-stimulatory molecules (CD80/86 and CD40). This results in a potent activating signal to resting T cells with subsequent effector functions. (b) The potent inhibitory effects of high-dose IVIG on DC function. These include reduction of HLA ClassI/II expression, reduction in CD80/86 expression, reduction in IL-12 secretion, and increase in IL-10 secretion. The end result is a poor activating signal to T cells that can result in T cell anergy or deviation to a T regulatory cell profile. In addition, IVIG can have direct effects on T cells, decreasing IL-2 and γ-IFN production, decreasing T cell differentiation and expanding T regulatory cells directly through the actions of T regitopes present in the Fc portion of IgG molecules (see text for explanation). The net result is a decrease in T cell activation, proliferation, and inflammation.

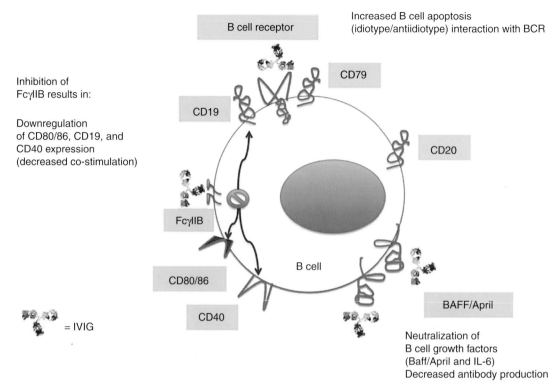

Plate 29.3 The described effects of IVIG on B cell function. First, interaction of antiidiotypic antibodies with cognate idiotypes on the B cell receptor can result in apoptosis of these cells, thus reducing specific antibody-producing cells. Interaction of IVIG with FcgIIB on B cells results in negative signaling that reduces CD80/86, CD40, and CD19 expression on B cells. This substantially reduces the APC activity of B cells. IVIG also contains antibodies that neutralize important growth factors, such as anti-BAFF and anti-April activity, that can impede conversion of B cells to plasma cells.

Figure 15.4 Cortical changes associated with cyclosporine-induced cerebral blindness. (a) CT scan on day 81 revealed hypoattenuation of occipital lobes. (b, c) T2-weighted magnetic resonance image on day 82 revealed high signal intensity in the white matter, the gray matter of the right frontal lobe, and both occipital lobes. (d, e) Fluid-attenuated inversion recovery magnetic resonce image revealed abnormal findings more clearly. From [149] (Uoshima N, Karasuno T, Yagi T *et al.* Late onset cyclosporine-induced cerebral blindness with abnormal SPECT imagings in a patient undergoing unrelated bone marrow transplantation. *Bone Marrow Transplant* 2000;26:105).

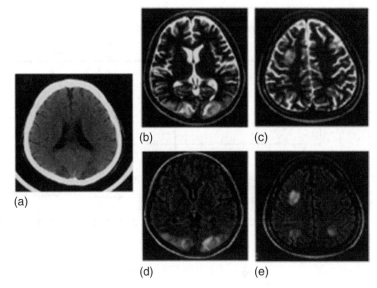

to vasospasm, and through these and related mechanisms may potentiate endothelial proliferation and vascular injury [150–152]. Clinical sequelae include microvascular injury and, rarely, diffuse fulminant hemolytic uremic syndrome with thrombocytopenia, microangiopathic hemolytic anemia, acute renal failure, and variable hepatic dysfunction. CsA also enhances procoagulant activity and accentuates the hypercoagulable state following renal transplantation [153], so that pulmonary thromboembolism, systemic venous thrombosis, and other thromboembolic complications in larger vessels are more common in the early postoperative period in patients receiving CsA.

These endothelial effects, combined with enhanced sympathetic activity, renal vasoconstriction, and salt retention, and altered baroreceptor reflexes contribute to the increase in arterial pressure observed in 70–90 % of adults or children receiving CsA [154–156]. Hypertension is aggrevated by elevated blood CsA levels, or impaired renal allograft function secondary to CsA nephrotoxicity. Proximal tubular reabsorption is increased, plasma renin and aldosterone activity are suppressed, and tubular insensitivity to aldosterone inhibits potassium excretion. Plasma atrial natriuretic peptide levels are generally elevated, perhaps as a compensatory response. Although sodium transport

systems are normal, erythrocyte and leukocyte magnesium levels are markedly decreased in hypertensive patients receiving CsA by comparison with either normal subjects or renal transplant recipients treated with azathioprine. Cardiac output is usually normal, but systemic vascular resistance is elevated as a result of these changes.

Hypertension in patients on CsA is frequently severe and resistant to therapy. Calcium channel blockers are often the first-line therapy, and may be associated with improvements in glomerular filtration rate. Inhibitors of the renin–angiotensin system (RAS), including angiotensin-converting enzyme inhibitors and angiotensin receptor blockers, are widely used both for their antihypertensive and antiproteinuric effects, but may cause significant adverse effects, including decreased glomerular filtration, hyperkalemia, and anemia [154]. Beta blockade and other agents with direct vasodilatory activity may then be employed in a formal stepped-care approach if required.

Nephrotoxicity

Nephrotoxicity is perhaps the most important adverse consequence of CsA use, and its pathogenesis and presentation have been recently reviewed by Naesens *et al.* [157]. CsA produces an acute decrease in renal cortical and medullary

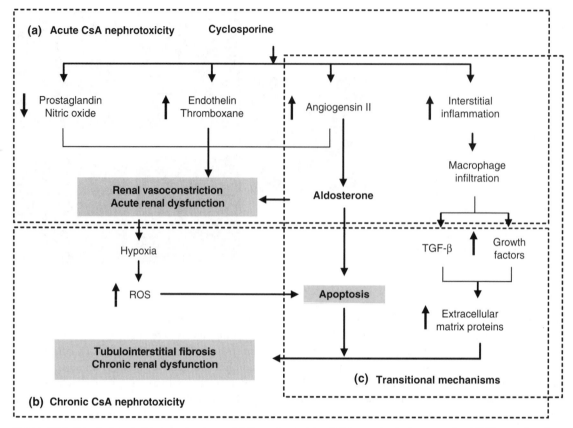

Figure 15.5 Principal postulated mechanisms of CsA nephrotoxicity. ROS: reactive oxygen species; TGFβ: transforming growth factor-β. Adapted from [160].

blood flow, a fall in glomerular capillary perfusion, and mesangial cell contraction which reverse rapidly on withdrawal of the drug. These events are accompanied by a dose-dependent decrease in glomerular filtration, with an elevation in the blood urea nitrogen/creatinine ratio, oliguria, and the virtual disappearance of sodium from the urine, reflecting a simultaneous increase in proximal tubular reabsorption [158]. Vasoconstriction is mediated by neurohumoral mechanisms which inhibit myogenic autoregulation, producing renal cortical vasoconstriction and an increase in vascular resistance [159, 160] (Figure 15.5). Dysfunction results from an increase in vasoconstrictor factors that include endothelin and thromboxane and activation of the RAS, as well as a reduction of

vasodilator factors like prostacyclin, prostaglandin E2, and nitric oxide (NO). Selective inhibition of thromboxane synthesis prevents the increase in TxA2 and, depending upon the strain employed, causes a parallel rise in renal blood flow and glomerular filtration [161]. In addition, free-radical formation plays a role in acute CNI nephrotoxicity, as well as sympathetic nerve activation in native kidneys. It is currently not known whether these effects are related to calcineurin/NFAT-dependent mechanisms, but the similarities between CNIs with different molecular structure and intracellular binding sites suggest this may be the case [157].

CsA causes both acute and chronic structural changes within the kidney [157]. The earliest of these is the isometric vacuolization evident in the proximal tubular epithelium, perhaps releflecting the direct toxicity of high concentations of CsA to proximal straight and convoluted tubular epithelium, while the thick ascending limb of Henle's loop and the cortical collecting tubules are relatively resistant. Injury may reflect ischemia, the reduction of both active and uncoupled mitochondrial respiration, or may involve the cytoplasmic calcium-dependent cystein protease calpain, which is present in high concentrations in the proximal tubular epithelium. While striking, this histologic injury is not of principal importance in the pathogenesis of the CsA effect, as proximal tubular cell function is enhanced and reabsorption of sodium and other substances transported in this segment is increased under the action of CsA. Continued high-dose CsA administration, however, is followed by more serious structural changes, including the loss of proximal tubular epithelial cell integrity leading to tubular atrophy, a variable interstitial mononuclear cell infiltrate, interstitial injury with secondary interstitial fibrosis, and vascular sclerosis with luminal narrowing [157]. Several factors have been implicated in this progression, including the effect of calcineurin–NFAT on smooth muscle cells, the release of vasoactive substances, and modulation of endothelin release and endothelin-receptor function. CsA-triggered thromboxane and leukotriene production may lead to enhanced platelet aggregation on the vessel wall with the release of platelet-derived growth factor and other trophic factors, contributing to medial hypertrophy and sustained parenchymal ischemia. Production of TGFβ and other fibrogenic factors may then increase production of extracellular matrix components [157]. Finally, the release of free radicals in the vessel or ischemic interstitium may potentiate the vascular injury and fibrotic reaction [162, 163].

CsA produces three distinct forms of clinical renal injury [157]. The most common, acute nephrotoxicity, parallels that in the experimental animal. CsA reduces renal blood flow and glomerular filtration, increases proximal tubular reabsorption, and produces a mild, incomplete distal tubular acidosis in the native or transplanted kidney. Tubular injury is signaled by increased excretion of urinary

enzymes *N*-acetyl β-D-glucosaminidase, γ-GT and β-2 microglobulin. Acute CsA nephrotoxicity occurs in a high proportion of subjects within the first 6 months after renal transplantation, and may be difficult to distinguish from mild acute rejection. Discrimination generally relies on a combination of clinical and histologic features supplemented by therapeutic CsA monitoring.

Thrombotic microangiopathy is a less common, though more fulminant, form of renal injury. This occurs spontaneously in less than 5 % of patients within the first month following renal transplantation and may follow an episode of acute rejection or viral infection, or drug interaction. The clinical course is characterized by thrombocytopenia, red cell fragmentation, hyperbilirubinemia, and acute graft failure [157]. Endothelial injury is evidenced by increased factor VIII or thrombomodulin production, and microscopy shows endothelial injury with platelet deposition, or myocyte necrosis with additional degenerative and vacuolar changes of myocytes and prominent accumulation of hyaline within medial portions of the vessel wall, confined to arterioles and the terminal portions of the interlobular arteries. Acute microangiopathic vasculopathy often resolves following temporary withdrawal of CsA.

Chronic toxicity produces progressive functional deterioration with more extensive histologic change. Renovascular resistance is elevated, due largely to an increase in preglomerular resistance, and there is a gradual erosion of renal functional reserve. Morphologic changes include an occlusive afferent arteriolopathy with downstream collapse or sclerosis of glomeruli and ischemic nephrons with patchy fibrosis of the surrounding interstitium. The incidence and severity of chronic CsA nephrotoxicity following renal transplantation have declined markedly as the induction and maintenance doses of CsA have been reduced. Renal graft function remains stable during the first 5–10 years post-transplant in patients receiving CsA, and chronic CsA toxicity is a less frequent cause of late renal allograft loss. Chronic CsA nephrotoxicity may occur also in the native kidney. Progression to dialysis is reported in an increasing number of heart and lung transplant recipients by 5 years post-transplant, and a similar decline is seen in both pediatric and adult liver transplant recipients. Longitudinal follow-up in these patients shows an increasing number of sclerotic glomeruli. Remnant glomeruli demonstrate hypertrophy, and an elevated single nephron filtration rate assumedly compensates for the declining number of functional glomeruli. Strategies to prevent this progression include careful monitoring of CsA dose and blood levels, avoidance of combinatorial nephrotoxins, and the potential replacement of CsA treatment by an mTOR antagonist in the stable recipient [157].

Metabolic

CsA impairs urate clearance by increasing tubular reabsorption and reducing the filtered load of urate. Fractional urate clearance falls within the first 3 months post-transplant and may not be reversible even after discontinuation of the drug, suggesting irreversible tubular damage. Hyperuricemia occurs in up to 90 % of CsA recipients, related to both the degree of renal functional impairment and the use of diuretics, although there appears to be no clear correlation with trough blood CsA concentration. New gouty arthritis occurs in up to 10 % of cases treated with CsA and is more common in older males [164]. A similar incidence of hyperuricemia is reported following extrarenal transplantation, leading to the rapid development of polyarticular disease and tophaceous deposits in approximately 10 % of patients. Uric acid stone formation is rare post-transplant, and whether hyperuricemia contributes to hypertension and a progressive deterioration in renal function via interstitial injury in this setting is not yet established.

New-onset diabetes mellitus (NODM) occurs post-transplant in up to 24 % of patients receiving CsA and prednisone [165]. It is characterized by a variety of clinical manifestations, ranging from predominant insulin resistance requiring only lifestyle intervention, to beta-cell failure requiring insulin treatment [166]. The etiology is multifactorial, and diabetogenic immunosuppressive drugs are of major importance, though CsA is significantly less problematic than tactrolimus in this effect [119]. NODM is an important risk factor, and graft survival is reduced by up to 20 % at

5 years following renal transplantation. Both CsA and prednisone contribute to carbohydrate intolerance [166]. CsA is directly toxic to the endocrine pancreas in the experimental animal and to islet cells in humans. Insulin release is inhibited by CsA in the rodent, the larger animal, and non-human primate, and returns to normal only following withdrawal of the drug. Although literature is sparse, CsA appears to impair peripheral insulin sensitivity, amino acid uptake, and fatty acid oxidation. Corticosteroids, in turn, influence insulin receptor number and affinity, peripheral glucose uptake, and activation of the glucose/fatty acid cycle. Careful measures of glycemic control have now been incorporated by many transplant uints, and guidelines for selection of therapy and management of complications have been developed [165].

Hypercholesterolemia occurs in at least 60 % of patients receiving CsA within the first 3 months following transplantation, and declines with time to less than 15 % at 2 and 3 years post-transplant. Severe hypertriglyceridemia is reported in approximately 15 % of patients, but only 7 % remain hypertriglyceridemic at 3 years. High-density lipoprotein (HDL) cholesterol levels are usually normal or high, although HDL3 is reported to be low. Hyperlipidemia contributes to accelerated cardiovascular disease and chronic graft injury, and is a major risk factor in this setting [167]. Both corticosteroids and CsA contribute to this effect via increased hepatic lipoprotein synthesis and cholesterol production, and the metabolism of triglyceride-rich very-low-density lipoprotein to low-density lipoprotein (LDL). CsA produces hypercholesterolemia in experimental animal models, but trough levels correlate poorly with absolute cholesterol values in man. Management is often challenging by virtue of the immunosuppressive requirements and drug interactions. Reduction in the prednisone dosage, conversion to alternate-day therapy, or complete withdrawal of prednisone are frequently successful in decreasing cholesterol levels, and while HMG-CoA reductase inhibitors lower total cholesterol and LDL by 20–30 % they may cause acute rhabdomyolysis in patients on CsA [167].

Conclusion

The use of CsA has revolutionized clinical transplantation during the last decade, both by increasing the success rate and reducing morbidity and mortality. The typical steroid-related complications of infection, growth retardation, and osteoporosis are disappearing, but have been replaced by new concerns of hypertension, nephrotoxicity, and lymphoproliferative disease that reflect the potency and toxicity of CsA. The rapid development and introduction of new pharmacologic and biologic agents has gradually improved clinical outcomes and the risk/benefit ratio of immunosuppressive treatment. Although CsA is no longer the principal treatment for many grafts, synergistic combinations incorporating CsA and other drugs operating at differing sites in the immune cascade are selectively employed to provide long-term immunosuppression with minimal toxicity in specific situations.

References

1 Canadian Organ Replacement Register C. Annual Report: Treatment of end-stage organ failure in Canada 2000 to 2009. Ottawa, Ontario: Canadian Institute for Health Information; 2010.

2 Australia and New Zealand Dialysis and Transplant Registry A. ANZDATA Registry Report 2010, Australia and New Zealand Dialysis and Transplant Registry, Adelaide, South Australia; 2010.

3 United States Renal Data System. Annual Data Report 2010. Bethesda, MD; 2010.

4 European Renal Association, European Dialysis and Transplant Association. ERA–EDTA Annual Report 2008. ERA–EDTA; 2011.

5 Parasuraman R, Yee J, Karthikeyan V, del Busto R. Infectious complications in renal transplant recipients. *Adv Chronic Kidney Dis* 2006;13(3):280.

6 Keown P. Improving quality of life – the new target for transplantation. *Transplantation* 2001;72(12 Suppl):S67.

7 Yao G, Albon E, Adi Y *et al.* A systematic review and economic model of the clinical and cost-effectiveness of immunosuppressive therapy for renal transplantation in children. *Health Technol Assess* 2006;10(49):iii.

8 Winkelmayer WC, Weinstein MC, Mittleman MA *et al.* Health economic evaluations: the special case of end-stage renal disease treatment. *Med Decis Making* 2002;22(5):417.

9 Borel JF. History of the discovery of cyclosporin and of its early pharmacological development. *Wien Klin Wochenschr* 2002;114(12):433.

10 Keown PA, Essery-Rice G, Hellstrom A *et al.* Inhibition of human in vivo cytotoxic T lymphocyte generation by cyclosporine following organ transplantation. *Transplantation* 1985;40(1):45.

11 Galat A, Bua J. Molecular aspects of cyclophilins mediating therapeutic actions of their ligands. *Cell Mol Life Sci* 2010;67(20):3467.

12 Cai W, Hu L, Foulkes JG. Transcription-modulating drugs: mechanism and selectivity. *Curr Opin Biotechnol* 1996;7(6):608.

13 Stiller C. An overview of the first decade of cyclosporine. *Transplant Proc* 1996;28 (4):2005.

14 Keown P, Stiller C, Ulan R *et al.* Immunological and pharmacological monitoring in the clinical use of cyclosporin A. *Lancet* 1981;1(8222):686.

15 Keown P. New concepts in cyclosporine monitoring. *Curr Opin Nephrol Hypertens* 2002;11(6):619.

16 Knoll G. Trends in kidney transplantation over the past decade. *Drugs* 2008;68(Suppl 1):3.

17 Gaston R. Current and evolving immunosuppressive regimens in kidney transplantation. *Am J Kidney Dis* 2006;47(4 Suppl 2):S3.

18 Kirk AD. Induction immunosuppression. *Transplantation* 2006;82(5):593.

19 Halloran P. Immunosuppressive drugs for kidney transplantation. *N Engl J Med* 2004;351(26):2715.

20 Wenger RM. Cyclosporine and analogues – isolation and synthesis – mechanism of action and structural requirements for pharmacological activity. *Fortschr Chem Org Naturst* 1986;50:123.

21 Lim E, Pon A, Djoumbou Y *et al.* T3DB: a comprehensively annotated database of common toxins and their targets. *Nucleic Acids Res* 2010;38(suppl 1):D781. http://www.t3db.org/toxins/T3D3498.

22 Lee J, Kim SS. An overview of cyclophilins in human cancers. *J Int Med Res* 2010;38(5):1561.

23 Le Hir M, Su Q, Weber L *et al.* In situ detection of cyclosporin A: evidence for nuclear localization of cyclosporine and cyclophilins. *Lab Invest* 1995;73(5):727.

24 Kim H, Kim WJ, Jeon ST *et al.* Cyclophilin A may contribute to the inflammatory processes in rheumatoid arthritis through induction of matrix degrading enzymes and inflammatory cytokines from macrophages. *Clin Immunol* 2005;116(3):217.

25 Wang L, Wang CH, Jia JF *et al.* Contribution of cyclophilin A to the regulation of inflammatory

processes in rheumatoid arthritis. *J Clin Immunol* 2010;30(1):24.

26 Mascarell L, Truffa-Bachi P. New aspects of cyclosporin a mode of action: from gene silencing to gene up-regulation. *Mini Rev Med Chem* 2003;3(3):205.

27 Huai Q, Kim H-Y, Liu Y *et al*. Crystal structure of calcineurin–cyclophilin–cyclosporine shows common but distinct recognition of immunophilin–drug complexes. *Proc Natl Acad Sci U S A* 2002;99:12037.

28 Kiani A, Rao A, Aramburu J. Manipulating immune responses with immunosuppressive agents that target NFAT. *Immunity* 2000;12(4):359.

29 Cornell L, Smith R, Colvin R. Kidney transplantation: mechanisms of rejection and acceptance. *Annu Rev Pathol* 2008;3:189.

30 Datta A, David R, Glennie S *et al*. Differential effects of immunosuppressive drugs on T-cell motility. *Am J Transplant* 2006;6(12):2871.

31 Zhang C, Zhang J, Yang B, Wu C. Cyclosporin A inhibits the production of IL-17 by memory Th17 cells from healthy individuals and patients with rheumatoid arthritis. *Cytokine* 2008;42(3):345.

32 Wang H, Grzywacz B, Sukovich D *et al*. The unexpected effect of cyclosporin A on CD56-CD16⁻ and CD56⁺CD16⁺ natural killer cell subpopulations. *Blood* 2007; 110(5):1530.

33 Chen S, Zhao X, Tan J *et al*. Structure-based identification of small molecule compounds targeting cell cyclophilin A with anti-HIV-1 activity. *Eur J Pharmacol* 2007;565(1–3):54.

34 Satoh K, Shimokawa H, Berk BC. Cyclophilin A: promising new target in cardiovascular therapy. *Circ J* 2010;74(11):2249.

35 Saini M, Potash MJ. Novel activities of cyclophilin A and cyclosporin A during HIV-1 infection of primary lymphocytes and macrophages. *J Immunol* 2006; 177(1):443.

36 Sokolskaja E, Olivari S, Zufferey M *et al*. Cyclosporine blocks incorporation of HIV-1 envelope glycoprotein into virions. *J Virol* 2010;84(9):4851.

37 Guichou JF, Viaud J, Mettling C *et al*. Structure-based design, synthesis, and biological evaluation of novel inhibitors of human cyclophilin A. *J Med Chem* 2006;49(3):900.

38 Pang X, Zhang M, Zhou L *et al*. Discovery of a potent peptidic cyclophilin A inhibitor Trp-Gly-Pro. *Eur J Med Chem* 2011;46(5):1701.

39 Ciesek S, Steinmann E, Wedemeyer H *et al*. Cyclosporine A inhibits hepatitis C virus nonstructural protein 2 through cyclophilin A. *Hepatology* 2009; 50(5):1638.

40 Fischer G, Gallay P, Hopkins S. Cyclophilin inhibitors for the treatment of HCV infection. *Curr Opin Investig Drugs* 2010;11(8):911.

41 Kockx M, Jessup W, Kritharides L. Cyclosporin A and atherosclerosis – cellular pathways in atherogenesis. *Pharmacol Ther* 2010;128(1):106.

42 Kim SH, Lessner SM, Sakurai Y, Galis ZS. Cyclophilin A as a novel biphasic mediator of endothelial activation and dysfunction. *Am J Pathol* 2004;164(5):1567.

43 Jin ZG, Melaragno MG, Liao DF *et al*. Cyclophilin A is a secreted growth factor induced by oxidative stress. *Circ Res* 2000;87(9):789.

44 Beauchesne PR, Chung NS, Wasan KM. Cyclosporine A: a review of current oral and intravenous delivery systems. *Drug Dev Ind Pharm* 2007;33(3):211.

45 Keown P, Niese D. Cyclosporine microemulsion increases drug exposure and reduces acute rejection without incremental toxicity in de novo renal transplantation. International Sandimmun Neoral Study Group. *Kidney Int* 1998;54(3):938.

46 Helderman JH, Kang N, Legorreta AP, Chen JY. Healthcare costs in renal transplant recipients using branded versus generic ciclosporin. *Appl Health Econ Health Policy* 2010;8(1):61.

47 Johnston A, Belitsky P, Frei U *et al*. Potential clinical implications of substitution of generic cyclosporine formulations for cyclosporine microemulsion (Neoral) in transplant recipients. *Eur J Clin Pharmacol* 2004; 60(6):389.

48 Czogalla A. Oral cyclosporine A – the current picture of its liposomal and other delivery systems. *Cell Mol Biol Lett* 2009;14(1):139.

49 Dunn CJ, Wagstaff AJ, Perry CM *et al*. Cyclosporin: an updated review of the pharmacokinetic properties, clinical efficacy and tolerability of a microemulsion-based formulation (Neoral®) in organ transplantation. *Drugs* 2001;61(13):1957.

50 Kelly P, Kahan BD. Review: metabolism of immunosuppressant drugs. *Curr Drug Metab* 2002;3(3):275.

51 Masuda S, Inui K. An up-date review on individualized dosage adjustment of calcineurin inhibitors in organ transplant patients. *Pharmacol Ther* 2006;112 (1):184.

52 Thervet E, Anglicheau D, Legendre C, Beaune P. Role of pharmacogenetics of immunosuppressive drugs in organ transplantation. *Ther Drug Monit* 2008;30(2):143.

53 Thervet E, Legendre C, Beaune P, Anglicheau D. Cytochrome P450 3A polymorphisms and immunosuppressive drugs. *Pharmacogenomics* 2005;6(1):37.

54 Hu YF, Qiu W, Liu ZQ *et al*. Effects of genetic polymorphisms of CYP3A4, CYP3A5 and MDR1 on

cyclosporine pharmacokinetics after renal transplantation. *Clin Exp Pharmacol Physiol* 2006;33(11):1093.

55 Demeule M, Laplante A, Sepehr-Araé A *et al*. Inhibition of P-glycoprotein by cyclosporin A analogues and metabolites. *Biochem Cell Biol* 1999;77(1):47.

56 Mourad M, Wallemacq P, De Meyer M *et al*. Biotransformation enzymes and drug transporters pharmacogenetics in relation to immunosuppressive drugs: impact on pharmacokinetics and clinical outcome. *Transplantation* 2008;85(7 Suppl):S19.

57 Kuypers DR. Influence of interactions between immunosuppressive drugs on therapeutic drug monitoring. *Ann Transplant* 2008;13(3):11.

58 Pal D, Mitra AK. MDR- and CYP3A4-mediated drug-drug interactions. *J Neuroimmune Pharmacol* 2006;1(3):323.

59 Lam S, Partovi N, Ting L, Ensom M. Corticosteroid interactions with cyclosporine, tacrolimus, mycophenolate, and sirolimus: fact or fiction? *Ann Pharmacother* 2008;42(7):1037.

60 Kuypers DR, Ekberg H, Grinyó J *et al*. Mycophenolic acid exposure after administration of mycophenolate mofetil in the presence and absence of cyclosporin in renal transplant recipients. *Clin Pharmacokinet* 2009;48(5):329.

61 Asberg A, Hartmann A, Fjeldså E *et al*. Bilateral pharmacokinetic interaction between cyclosporine A and atorvastatin in renal transplant recipients. *Am J Transplant* 2001;1(4):382.

62 Bai S, Stepkowski S, Kahan B, Brunner L. Metabolic interaction between cyclosporine and sirolimus. *Transplantation* 2004;77(10):1507.

63 Podder H, Stepkowski SM, Napoli KL *et al*. Pharmacokinetic interactions augment toxicities of sirolimus/cyclosporine combinations. *J Am Soc Nephrol* 2001;12(5):1059.

64 Wrishko RE, Levine M, Primmett DR *et al*. Investigation of a possible interaction between ciprofloxacin and cyclosporine in renal transplant patients. *Transplantation* 1997;64(7):996.

65 Williamson EM. Drug interactions between herbal and prescription medicines. *Drug Saf* 2003;26(15):1075.

66 Taylor PJ, Tai CH, Franklin ME, Pillans PI. The current role of liquid chromatography–tandem mass spectrometry in therapeutic drug monitoring of immunosuppressant and antiretroviral drugs. *Clin Biochem* 2011;44(1):14.

67 Mendonza A, Gohh R, Akhlaghi F. Determination of cyclosporine in saliva using liquid chromatography–tandem mass spectrometry. *Ther Drug Monit* 2004;26(5):569.

68 Kahan B, Keown P, Levy G, Johnston A. Therapeutic drug monitoring of immunosuppressant drugs in clinical practice. *Clin Ther* 2002;24(3):330.

69 Morris RG, Holt DW, Armstrong VW *et al*. Analytic aspects of cyclosporine monitoring, on behalf of the IFCC/IATDMCT Joint Working Group. *Ther Drug Monit* 2004;26(2):227.

70 Wallemacq PE. Therapeutic monitoring of immunosuppressant drugs. Where are we? *Clin Chem Lab Med* 2004;42(11):1204.

71 Soldin SJ, Hardy RW, Wians FH *et al*. Performance evaluation of the new ADVIA Centaur system cyclosporine assay (single-step extraction). *Clin Chim Acta* 2010;411(11–12):806.

72 Steimer W. Performance and specificity of monoclonal immunoassays for cyclosporine monitoring: how specific is specific? *Clin Chem* 1999;45(3):371.

73 Fernández-Marmiesse A, Hermida J, Tutor JC. Comparison of predose vs 2-h postdose blood metabolites/cyclosporine ratios in kidney and liver transplant patients. *Clin Biochem* 2000;33(5):383.

74 Garrido MJ, Hermida J, Tutor JC. Relationship between cyclosporine concentrations obtained using the Roche Cobas Integra and Abbott TDx monoclonal immunoassays in pre-dose and two hour post-dose blood samples from kidney transplant recipients. *Ther Drug Monit* 2002;24(6):785.

75 Morris RG. Cyclosporin therapeutic drug monitoring – an established service revisited. *Clin Biochem Rev* 2003;24(2):33.

76 Debord J, Risco E, Harel M *et al* Application of a gamma model of absorption to oral cyclosporin. *Clin Pharmacokinet* 2001;40(5):375.

77 Leger F, Debord J, Le Meur Y *et al* Maximum a posteriori Bayesian estimation of oral cyclosporin pharmacokinetics in patients with stable renal transplants. *Clin Pharmacokinet* 2002;41(1):71.

78 International Neoral Renal Transplant Study Group. Cyclosporine microemulsion (Neoral) absorption profiling and sparse-sample predictors during the first 3 months after renal transplantation. *Am J Transplant* 2002;2(2):148.

79 Canadian Neoral Renal Transplant Study Group. Absorption profiling of cyclosporine microemulsion (neoral) during the first 2 weeks after renal transplantation. *Transplantation* 2001;72(6):1024.

80 Primmett DR, Levine M, Kovarik JM *et al*. Cyclosporine monitoring in patients with renal transplants: two- or three-point methods that estimate area under the curve are superior to trough levels in predicting drug exposure. *Ther Drug Monit* 1998;20(3):276.

81 David O, Johnston A. Limited sampling strategies. *Clin Pharmacokinet* 2000;39(4):311.

82 David OJ, Johnston A. Limited sampling strategies for estimating cyclosporin area under the concentration–time curve: review of current algorithms. *Ther Drug Monit* 2001;23(2):100.

83 Monchaud C, Rousseau A, Leger F *et al*. Limited sampling strategies using Bayesian estimation or multilinear regression for cyclosporin AUC(0–12) monitoring in cardiac transplant recipients over the first year post-transplantation. *Eur J Clin Pharmacol* 2003; 58(12):813.

84 Rousseau A, Monchaud C, Debord J *et al*. Bayesian forecasting of oral cyclosporin pharmacokinetics in stable lung transplant recipients with and without cystic fibrosis. *Ther Drug Monit* 2003;25(1):28.

85 Meier-Kriesche HU, Kaplan B, Brannan P *et al*. A limited sampling strategy for the estimation of eight-hour neoral areas under the curve in renal transplantation. *Ther Drug Monit* 1998;20(4):401.

86 Meier-Kriesche HU, Alloway R, Gaber AO *et al*. A limited sampling strategy for the estimation of 12-hour SangCya and neoral AUCs in renal transplant recipients. *J Clin Pharmacol* 1999;39(2):166.

87 Clase C, Mahalati K, Kiberd B *et al*. Adequate early cyclosporin exposure is critical to prevent renal allograft rejection: patients monitored by absorption profiling. *Am J Transplant* 2002;2(8):789.

88 Press RR, de Fijter JW, Guchelaar HJ. Individualizing calcineurin inhibitor therapy in renal transplantation – current limitations and perspectives. *Curr Pharm Des* 2010;16(2):176.

89 The Canadian Multicentre Transplant Study Group. A randomized clinical trial of cyclosporine in cadaveric renal transplantation. Analysis at three years. *N Engl J Med* 1986;314(19):1219.

90 Merion RM, White DJ, Thiru S *et al*. Cyclosporine: five years' experience in cadaveric renal transplantation. *N Engl J Med* 1984;310(3):148.

91 A randomized clinical trial of cyclosporine in cadaveric renal transplantation. *N Engl J Med* 1983;309(14):809.

92 Pollard SG, Lear PA, Ready AR *et al*. Comparison of microemulsion and conventional formulations of cyclosporine A in preventing acute rejection in de novo kidney transplant patients. The U.K. Neoral Renal Study Group. *Transplantation* 1999;68(9):1325.

93 Levy GA. Neoral use in the liver transplant recipient. *Transplant Proc* 2000;32(3A Suppl):2S.

94 Mahalati K, Belitsky P, Sketris I *et al*. Neoral monitoring by simplified sparse sampling area under the concentration–time curve: its relationship to acute rejection and cyclosporine nephrotoxicity early after kidney transplantation. *Transplantation* 1999;68(1):55.

95 Internation Neoral Renal Transplantation Study Group. Randomized, international study of cyclosporine microemulsion absorption profiling in renal transplantation with basiliximab immunoprophylaxis. *Am J Transplant* 2002;2(2):157.

96 Cantarovich M, Besner JG, Barkun JS *et al*. Two-hour cyclosporine level determination is the appropriate tool to monitor Neoral therapy. *Clin Transplant* 1998;12(3):243.

97 Oellerich M, Armstrong VW. Two-hour cyclosporine concentration determination: an appropriate tool to monitor neoral therapy? *Ther Drug Monit* 2002; 24(1):40.

98 Glanville AR, Morton JM, Aboyoun CL *et al*. Cyclosporine C_2 monitoring improves renal dysfunction after lung transplantation. *J Heart Lung Transplant* 2004;23(10):1170.

99 Morton JM, Aboyoun CL, Malouf MA *et al*. Enhanced clinical utility of de novo cyclosporine C_2 monitoring after lung transplantation. *J Heart Lung Transplant* 2004;23(9):1035.

100 Delgado DH, Rao V, Hamel J *et al*. Monitoring of cyclosporine 2-hour post-dose levels in heart transplantation: improvement in clinical outcomes. *J Heart Lung Transplant* 2005;24(9):1343.

101 Mathias HC, Ozalp F, Will MB *et al*. A randomized, controlled trial of C_0- vs C_2-guided therapeutic drug monitoring of cyclosporine in stable heart transplant patients. *J Heart Lung Transplant* 2005;24(12):2137.

102 Pescovitz MD, Barbeito R, Simulect US01 Study Group. Two-hour post-dose cyclosporine level is a better predictor than trough level of acute rejection of renal allografts. *Clin Transplant* 2002;16(5):378.

103 Thervet E, Pfeffer P, Scolari MP *et al*. Clinical outcomes during the first three months posttransplant in renal allograft recipients managed by C_2 monitoring of cyclosporine microemulsion. *Transplantation* 2003; 76(6):903.

104 Citterio F, Scatà MC, Romagnoli J *et al*. Results of a three-year prospective study of C_2 monitoring in long-term renal transplant recipients receiving cyclosporine microemulsion. *Transplantation* 2005; 79(7):802.

105 Cole E, Maham N, Cardella C *et al*. Clinical benefits of neoral C_2 monitoring in the long-term management of renal transplant recipients. *Transplantation* 2003; 75(12):2086.

106 Stefoni S, Midtved K, Cole E *et al*. Efficacy and safety outcomes among de novo renal transplant recipients

managed by C_2 monitoring of cyclosporine a microemulsion: results of a 12-month, randomized, multicenter study. *Transplantation* 2005;79(5):577.

107 David-Neto E, Lemos FB, Furusawa EA *et al.* Impact of cyclosporin A pharmacokinetics on the presence of side effects in pediatric renal transplantation. *J Am Soc Nephrol* 2000;11(2):343.

108 Hermann M, Enseleit F, Fisler AE *et al.* Cyclosporine C_0- versus C_2-monitoring over three years in maintenance heart transplantation. *Swiss Med Wkly* 2011;141:w13149.

109 U.S. Renal Data System U. *Annual Data Report: Atlas of End-Stage Renal Disease in the United States.* Bethesda, MD: National Institutes of Health, National Institute of Diabetes and Digestive and Kidney Diseases; 2006.

110 Meier-Kriesche HU, Li S, Gruessner RW *et al.* Immunosuppression: evolution in practice and trends, 1994–2004. *Am J Transplant* 2006;6(5 Pt 2):1111.

111 Pirsch JD, Miller J, Deierhoi MH *et al.* A comparison of tacrolimus (FK506) and cyclosporine for immuno-suppression after cadaveric renal transplantation. *Transplantation* 1997;63(7):977 [see comment].

112 Mayer AD, Dmitrewski J, Squifflet JP *et al.* Multicenter randomized trial comparing tacrolimus (FK506) and cyclosporine in the prevention of renal allograft rejection: a report of the European Tacrolimus Multicenter Renal Study Group. *Transplantation* 1997;64(3):436.

113 Margreiter R, European Tacrolimus vs Ciclosporin Microemulsion Renal Transplantation Study Group. Efficacy and safety of tacrolimus compared with ciclosporin microemulsion in renal transplantation: a randomised multicentre study. *Lancet* 2002;359 (9308):741.

114 Krämer BK, Del Castillo D, Margreiter R *et al.* Efficacy and safety of tacrolimus compared with ciclosporin A in renal transplantation: three-year observational results. *Nephrol Dial Transplant* 2008;23(7):2386.

115 Tanabe K. Calcineurin inhibitors in renal transplanta-tion: what is the best option? *Drugs* 2003;63(15):1535.

116 Johnson C, Ahsan N, Gonwa T *et al.* Randomized trial of tacrolimus (Prograf) in combination with azathio-prine or mycophenolate mofetil versus cyclosporine (Neoral) with mycophenolate mofetil after cadaveric kidney transplantation. *Transplantation* 2000;69(5):834.

117 Ahsan N, Johnson C, Gonwa T *et al.* Randomized trial of tacrolimus plus mycophenolate mofetil or azathio-prine versus cyclosporine oral solution (modified) plus mycophenolate mofetil after cadaveric kidney transplantation: results at 2 years. *Transplantation* 2001;72(2):245.

118 Gonwa T, Johnson C, Ahsan N *et al.* Randomized trial of tacrolimus+mycophenolate mofetil or azathio-prine versus cyclosporine+mycophenolate mofetil after cadaveric kidney transplantation: results at three years. *Transplantation* 2003;75(12):2048.

119 Heisel O, Heisel R, Balshaw R, Keown P. New onset diabetes mellitus in patients receiving calcineurin inhibitors: a systematic review and meta-analysis. *Am J Transplant* 2004;4(4):583.

120 Montagnino G, Tarantino A, Segoloni GP *et al.* Long-term results of a randomized study comparing three immunosuppressive schedules with cyclosporine in cadaveric kidney transplantation. *J Am Soc Nephrol* 2001;12(10):2163.

121 Pascual J, Galeano C, Royuela A, Zamora J. A syste-matic review on steroid withdrawal between 3 and 6 months after kidney transplantation. *Transplantation* 2010;90(4):343.

122 Barraclough K, Landsberg D, Shapiro R *et al.* A mat-ched cohort pharmacoepidemiological analysis of steroid free immunosuppression in renal transplan-tation. *Transplantation* 2009;87(5):672.

123 Vincenti F, Schena FP, Paraskevas S *et al.* A rando-mized, multicenter study of steroid avoidance, early steroid withdrawal or standard steroid therapy in kidney transplant recipients. *Am J Transplant* 2008; 8(2):307.

124 Mukherjee S, Mukherjee U. A comprehensive review of immunosuppression used for liver transplanta-tion. *J Transplant* 2009;2009:701464.

125 O'Grady JG, Burroughs A, Hardy P *et al.* Tacrolimus versus microemulsified ciclosporin in liver transplan-tation: the TMC randomised controlled trial. *Lancet* 2002;360(9340):1119.

126 O'Grady JG, Hardy P, Burroughs AK *et al.* Randomized controlled trial of tacrolimus versus microemulsified cyclosporin (TMC) in liver transplantation: poststudy surveillance to 3 years. *Am J Transplant* 2007;7(1):137.

127 McAlister VC, Haddad E, Renouf E *et al.* Cyclosporin versus tacrolimus as primary immunosuppressant after liver transplantation: a meta-analysis. *Am J Transplant* 2006;6(7):1578.

128 Haddad EM, McAlister VC, Renouf E *et al.* Cyclosporin versus tacrolimus for liver transplanted patients. *Cochrane Database Syst Rev* 2006;(4):CD005161.

129 Henry SD, Metselaar HJ, Lonsdale RC *et al.* Mycophenolic acid inhibits hepatitis C virus replica-tion and acts in synergy with cyclosporin A and interferon-alpha. *Gastroenterology* 2006;131(5):1452.

130 Firpi RJ, Zhu H, Morelli G *et al.* Cyclosporine sup-presses hepatitis C virus in vitro and increases the

chance of a sustained virological response after liver transplantation. *Liver Transpl* 2006;12(1):51.

131 Berenguer M, Royuela A, Zamora J. Immuno-suppression with calcineurin inhibitors with respect to the outcome of HCV recurrence after liver transplantation: results of a meta-analysis. *Liver Transpl* 2007;13(1):21.

132 Heaphy MR, Shamma HN, Hickmann M, White MJ. Cyclosporine-induced folliculodystrophy. *J Am Acad Dermatol* 2004;50(2):310.

133 Takahashi T, Kamimura A. Cyclosporin a promotes hair epithelial cell proliferation and modulates protein kinase C expression and translocation in hair epithelial cells. *J Invest Dermatol* 2001;117(3):605.

134 Ho YC, Lin HJ, Tsai CH, Chang YC. Regulation of type I plasminogen activator inhibitor in human gingival fibroblasts with cyclosporine A. *Oral Dis* 2010;16(4):396.

135 Tamilselvan S, Raju SN, Loganathan D *et al.* Endothelin-1 and its receptors ET_A and ET_B in drug-induced gingival overgrowth. *J Periodontol* 2007; 78(2):290.

136 Grassi FR, Pappalardo S, Baglìo OA *et al.* Gingival overgrowth in renal transplant recipients induced by pharmacological treatment. Review of the literature. *Minerva Stomatol* 2006;55(1–2):59.

137 Lucas VS, Roberts GJ. Oro-dental health in children with chronic renal failure and after renal transplantation: a clinical review. *Pediatr Nephrol* 2005; 20(10):1388.

138 Niles DG, Rynearson RD, Baum M *et al.* A study of craniofacial growth in infant heart transplant recipients receiving cyclosporine. *J Heart Lung Transplant* 2000;19(3):231.

139 Sprague SM. Mechanism of transplantation-associated bone loss. *Pediatr Nephrol* 2000;14(7):650.

140 Cunningham J. Posttransplantation bone disease. *Transplantation* 2005;79(6):629.

141 Cohen A, Addonizio LJ, Softness B *et al.* Growth and skeletal maturation after pediatric cardiac transplantation. *Pediatr Transplant* 2004;8(2):126.

142 Woo JT, Yonezawa T, Cha BY *et al.* Pharmacological topics of bone metabolism: antiresorptive microbial compounds that inhibit osteoclast differentiation, function, and survival. *J Pharmacol Sci* 2008;106(4):547.

143 Tamler R, Epstein S. Nonsteroid immune modulators and bone disease. *Ann N Y Acad Sci* 2006;1068:284.

144 Ponticelli C, Campise MR. Neurological complications in kidney transplant recipients. *J Nephrol* 2005;18(5):521.

145 Saner FH, Gensicke J, Olde Damink SW *et al.* Neurologic complications in adult living donor liver transplant patients: an underestimated factor? *J Neurol* 2010;257(2):253.

146 Yardimci N, Colak T, Sevmis S *et al.* Neurologic complications after renal transplant. *Exp Clin Transplant* 2008;6(3):224.

147 Maggioni F, Mantovan MC, Rigotti P *et al.* Headache in kidney transplantation. *J Headache Pain* 2009;10(6):455.

148 Ishikura K, Ikeda M, Hamasaki Y *et al.* Posterior reversible encephalopathy syndrome in children: its high prevalence and more extensive imaging findings. *Am J Kidney Dis* 2006;48(2):231.

149 Uoshima N, Karasuno T, Yagi T *et al.* Late onset cyclosporine-induced cerebral blindness with abnormal SPECT imagings in a patient undergoing unrelated bone marrow transplantation. *Bone Marrow Transplant* 2000;26:105.

150 Bouvier N, Flinois JP, Gilleron J *et al.* Cyclosporine triggers endoplasmic reticulum stress in endothelial cells: a role for endothelial phenotypic changes and death. *Am J Physiol Renal Physiol* 2009;296(1):F160.

151 Al-Massarani G, Vacher-Coponat H, Paul P *et al.* Impact of immunosuppressive treatment on endothelial biomarkers after kidney transplantation. *Am J Transplant* 2008;8(11):2360.

152 Nickel T, Schlichting CL, Weis M. Drugs modulating endothelial function after transplantation. *Transplantation* 2006;82(1 Suppl): S41.

153 Tomasiak M, Rusak T, Gacko M, Stelmach H. Cyclosporine enhances platelet procoagulant activity. *Nephrol Dial Transplant* 2007;22(6):1750.

154 Mangray M, Vella JP. Hypertension after kidney transplant. *Am J Kidney Dis* 2011;57(2):331.

155 Koomans HA, Ligtenberg G. Mechanisms and consequences of arterial hypertension after renal transplantation. *Transplantation* 2001;72(6 Suppl):S9.

156 Bouhaddi M, Delbosc B, Fortrat JO *et al.* Six-month cardiovascular changes in cyclosporine-treated recipients of corneal grafts: serial baroreflex responses. *Transpl Int* 2004;17(6):325.

157 Naesens M, Kuypers DR, Sarwal M. Calcineurin inhibitor nephrotoxicity. *Clin J Am Soc Nephrol* 2009;4(2):481.

158 Petric R, Freeman D, Wallace C *et al.* Effect of cyclosporine on urinary prostanoid excretion, renal blood flow, and glomerulotubular function. *Transplantation* 1988;45(5):883.

159 Burdmann EA, Andoh TF, Yu L, Bennett WM. Cyclosporine nephrotoxicity. *Semin Nephrol* 2003; 23(5):465.

160 Bobadilla NA, Gamba G. New insights into the pathophysiology of cyclosporine nephrotoxicity: a role of aldosterone. *Am J Physiol Renal Physiol* 2007;293(1):F2.

161 Petric R, Freeman D, Wallace C *et al*. Modulation of experimental cyclosporine nephrotoxicity by inhibition of thromboxane synthesis. *Transplantation* 1990; 50(4):558.

162 Zhong Z, Arteel GE, Connor HD *et al*. Cyclosporin A increases hypoxia and free radical production in rat kidneys: prevention by dietary glycine. *Am J Physiol* 1998;275(4 Pt 2):F595.

163 Longoni B, Boschi E, Demontis GC *et al*. Apoptosis and adaptive responses to oxidative stress in human endothelial cells exposed to cyclosporin A correlate with BCL-2 expression levels. *FASEB J* 2001;15(3):731.

164 Abbott KC, Kimmel PL, Dharnidharka V *et al*. New-onset gout after kidney transplantation: incidence,

risk factors and implications. *Transplantation* 2005;80(10):1383.

165 Wilkinson A, Davidson J, Dotta F *et al*. Guidelines for the treatment and management of new-onset diabetes after transplantation. *Clin Transplant* 2005; 19(3):291.

166 Hjelmesaeth J, Asberg A, Müller F *et al*. New-onset posttransplantation diabetes mellitus: insulin resistance or insulinopenia? Impact of immunosuppressive drugs, cytomegalovirus and hepatitis C virus infection. *Curr Diabetes Rev* 2005;1(1):1.

167 Mathis AS, Davé N, Knipp GT, Friedman GS. Drug-related dyslipidemia after renal transplantation. *Am J Health Syst Pharm* 2004;61(6):565.

CHAPTER 16
Tacrolimus

William E. Fitzsimmons
Astellas Pharma Global Development, Deerfield, IL, USA

History

Beginning in the early 1980s, Fujisawa Pharmaceutical Company initiated a systematic search for novel immunosuppressants in cultured broths of microorganisms isolated from soil samples. This screening system was based on suppression of the mixed lymphocyte reaction (MLR), since it was regarded as a correlate to allograft rejection based on the effects of known transplant immunosuppressants. In order to avoid nonspecific cytotoxicity, the mouse lymphoma EL-4 cell line was also employed in the screening process. In 1984, after testing a wide range of broths, an actinomycete, *Streptomyces* strain number 9993, was found to produce potent immunosuppression in the mouse MLR. This strain of *Streptomyces* was obtained from a soil sample collected at Mount Tsukuba in Japan. Since this microorganism differed from previously described *Streptomyces* bacteria, the strain was designated *Streptomyces tsukubaensis*, referring to the location of the soil sample. From this fermentation broth the pure crystalline form of FR900506 (FK506), tacrolimus, was isolated. This FR numbering system referred to Fujisawa Research, and the subsequent naming of FK refers to Fujisawa Kaihatsu (development) [1, 2].

In 1987, the first descriptions of the immunosuppressive effects of FK506 (tacrolimus) were published. Subsequently, differing opinions among academic investigators developed surrounding the relevance of arteritis seen in large animal transplant models [3–6].

In 1987, toxicologic studies of tacrolimus were initiated by Fujisawa Pharmaceutical Company in rats and baboons. Based on these studies, the pancreas and kidney were considered the target organs of toxicity [2].

Whereas traditionally drug development is initiated with normal volunteer Phase 1 trials, there was initial concern over the risk to healthy subjects with this potent immunosuppressant. Therefore, after extensive nonclinical evaluations, the first patient was treated with tacrolimus at the University of Pittsburgh under the direction of Dr. Thomas E. Starzl on 28 February 1989. Since patients losing their graft after liver transplant have few options (i.e., death or retransplant), the initial clinical use of this new immunosuppressant was targeted to patients rejecting their liver allograft despite conventional immunosuppression [6]. The pioneering efforts of the transplant team at the University of Pittsburgh facilitated the initiation of multicenter registration-driven Phase 3 trials for liver transplantation in 1990. Subsequently, tacrolimus (Prograf®) was approved by the FDA on 8 April 1994 for the prevention of rejection after liver transplantation. Important revelations during the clinical trials included:

1. the initial starting dosage of tacrolimus used in the Phase 3 clinical trials was higher than necessary;

Immunotherapy in Transplantation: Principles and Practice, First Edition. Edited by Bruce Kaplan, Gilbert J. Burckart and Fadi G. Lakkis.
© 2012 Blackwell Publishing Ltd. Published 2012 by Blackwell Publishing Ltd.

2. many patients could be managed with oral tacrolimus, avoiding the use of the intravenous (IV) formulation completely;

3. therapeutic drug monitoring (TDM) was essential to the optimization of therapy;

4. whole blood rather than plasma was the preferred biologic matrix for monitoring;

5. on-site assays for tacrolimus whole-blood levels allowed titration of therapy in the early post-transplant period;

6. the nonhuman primate model did not accurately predict the human dose.

Chemistry

Tacrolimus is a neutral macrolide lactone that contains a hemiketal-masked α,β-diketoamide incorporated in a 23-member ring (Figure 16.1)

with a molecular weight of 822 and a molecular formula of $C_{44}H_{69}NO_{12} \cdot H_2O$. Tacrolimus is practically insoluble in water and soluble in methanol, ethanol, ethyl acetate, acetone, chloroform, and diethyl ether. Although tacrolimus is structurally related to the immunosuppressant sirolimus, their mechanisms of action are quite distinct. The pharmacologic immunosuppressive activity of tacrolimus metabolites has demonstrated that demethylation at C31 does not substantially change the activity of parent tacrolimus, since this is not in the effector element. However, demethylation at C13 and/or C15 substantially reduces the immunosuppressive activity of the molecule (Figure 16.1) [2, 4, 7].

Based on the chemical characteristics of tacrolimus, and to solubilize the molecule for IV administration, the commercial formulation of IV Prograf® contains polyoxyl 60 hydrogenated castor oil (HCO-60) 200 mg and 80 % v/v dehydrated alcohol.

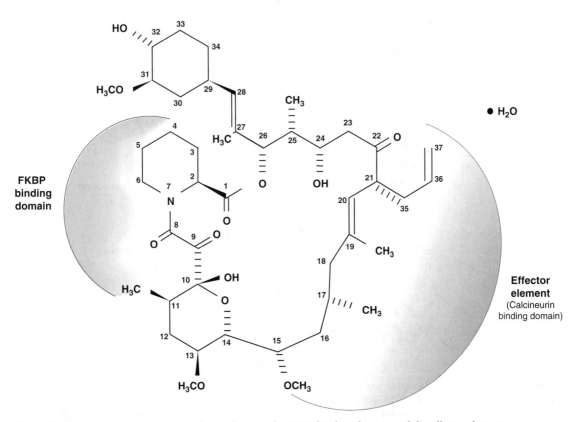

Figure 16.1 Chemical structure of tacrolimus showing the FKBP binding domain and the effector elements.

Tacrolimus appears as white crystals or crystalline powder. The partition coefficient in an octanol–water system is >1000. Tacrolimus does not display polymorphism and exists as one conformer, *cis*-form.

Mechanism of action

The mechanism of action of tacrolimus is within the T lymphocyte. Tacrolimus binds to an immunophilin, FK506-binding protein (FKBP) (Figure 16.2). FKBP catalyzes the conversion of the cis–trans isomers of the peptidyl-prolyl amide bond of peptide substrates. The binding of tacrolimus to FKBP inhibits this rotamase activity and is necessary but not sufficient to produce the immunosuppressant effect. The complex of FKBP and tacrolimus binds to calcineurin and is positioned to inhibit the phosphatase activity of calcineurin A. Key binding of the FKBP–tacrolimus complex to calcineurin and subsequent inhibition of the phosphatase activity of calcineurin A inhibits the dephosphorylation of

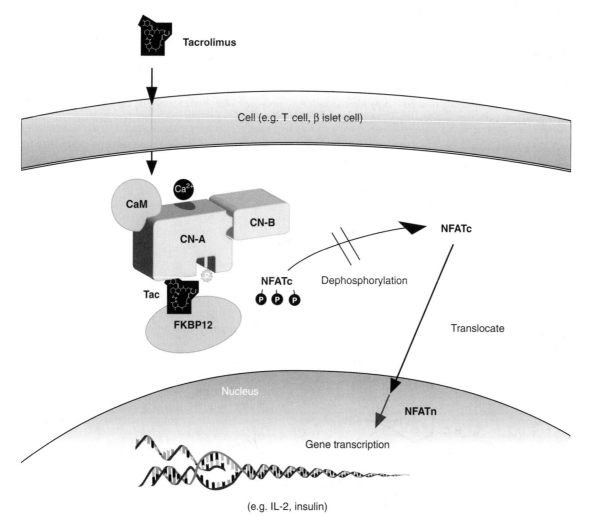

Figure 16.2 Intracellular mechanism of action of tacrolimus. Tacrolimus enters the cell, binds FKBP, and inhibits the phosphatase activity of calcineurin. This inhibits the dephosphorylation of NFAT, preventing its translocation from the cytoplasm to the nucleus, inhibiting gene transcription in the nucleus. CaM: calmodulin; Ca^{2+}: calcium ion; CN-A: calcineurin A; CN-B: calcineurin B; NFATc: cyctoplasmic nuclear factor of activated T cells; NFAT-n: nuclear form of nuclear factor of activated T cells; P: phosphate groups; FKBP: FK binding protein.

nuclear factor of activated T cells (NFAT). This inhibition prevents the translocation of NFAT from the cytoplasm to the nucleus of the T cell and subsequently inhibits the gene transcription for interleukin 2 (IL-2) and other transcription factors that are essential to early T cell activation (Figure 16.2). In-vitro tacrolimus inhibits the MLR, cytotoxic T cell generation, and production of T-cell-derived solubilized mediators such as IL-2, interleukin 3, and gamma interferon, and the expression of the IL-2 receptor. These effects are seen at concentrations that are approximately 100-fold lower than cyclosporine in these in-vitro systems. Tacrolimus suppresses T cell activation as well as T-helper-cell-dependent B cell proliferation. Tacrolimus-sensitive T cell activation events are those that cause a notable rise in intracellular calcium [2, 5, 8–10].

Pharmacokinetics/pharmacodynamics

Key pharmacokinetic characteristics are listed in Table 16.1.

Absorption

Commercial oral formulations of tacrolimus include an immediate-release hard gelatin capsule (Prograf®) for twice-daily administration and an extended/prolonged-release capsule (Advagraf®) for once-daily dosing. Capsule strengths include 0.5, 1.0, and 5.0 mg. The absorption of tacrolimus from the gastrointestinal tract after oral administration is incomplete and averages approximately 20 % absolute bioavailability. Absorption is found to occur throughout the gastrointestinal tract, including the duodenum, jejunum, and colon. Within the wall of the gastrointestinal tract, tacrolimus is metabolized by cytochrome P450 3A enzymes, as well as being affected by P-glycoprotein-mediated efflux.

One of the major factors affecting the oral absorption of tacrolimus is coadministration with food. Food has a significant effect in reducing both the rate and extent of absorption after oral administration [11]. This food effect is similar with both the immediate-release and extended-release

Table 16.1 Key pharmacokinetic characteristics.

Absorption	Oral bioavailability ~20 %
	Metabolized in the gut wall by CYP3A enzymes
Distribution	Strongly partitioned into red blood cells
	Highly (> 98 %) protein bound to albumin and α-1-acid glycoprotein
	Extensively distributed through the body
	Vd = 0.9–1.9 L/kg
Metabolism	Metabolized in the liver by CYP3A4 isozymes
	Demethylation and hydroxylation
	Eight metabolites identified
Elimination	Biliary secretion and fecal elimination accounts for > 90 %
	< 0.5 % of unchanged drug eliminated in feces and urine
	$t_{1/2}$ ~24–44 h
	Clearance ~0.03–0.08 L/(h/kg)

oral formulations, resulting in a reduction in the overall area under the curve (AUC) of approximately 25–37 % with a high-fat meal. The time to peak is prolonged and the peak concentration is also reduced. The administration of tacrolimus immediate-release capsules with a low-fat meal also results in a significant reduction in the rate and extent of absorption; however, the impact is slightly less than with a high-fat meal (26 % reduction in AUC with low fat compared with 33 % reduction with high fat). The timing of food intake relative to dosing has an impact on oral absorption of the immediate-release formulation. Ingestion of tacrolimus capsules 1 h before breakfast has a small effect: approximately a 12 % decrease in the AUC compared with the fasted state. However, administration either immediately following consumption of food or 1.5 h after beginning consumption of food has a similar significant effect in reducing the AUC [12].

Both grapefruit juice and pomelo have been reported to increase the blood levels of tacrolimus due to the inhibition of intestinal CYP3A4 [13–17].

Patient race also is a significant factor affecting the oral absorption of tacrolimus. The absolute bioavailability in African American subjects averaged approximately 12% compared with 19% in Caucasians. This effect translates into differences in dosing requirements to achieve similar target trough concentrations. The difference in oral absorption may be related to differences in the CYP3A5 genetic polymorphisms between the African population and Caucasian [18–22].

Formulation-dependent differences in oral absorption of tacrolimus are also seen depending upon the time post-transplant. When comparing extended-release to immediate-release tacrolimus, bioequivalence based on AUC was established in single and multiple dose normal volunteer studies as well as stable organ transplant patients. When liver and kidney transplant patients are studied at day 1 post-transplant there is a significant reduction in the AUC with the extended-release formulation compared with immediate release (approximately 50% reduction in liver transplant patients and 33% reduction in kidney transplant patients) [23].

The oral absorption of tacrolimus is dependent upon circadian rhythms. When the immediate-release formulation is administered in a twice-daily dosing frequency the AUC and peak concentration were significantly higher after the morning dose compared with evening dosing. The ratio of peak and AUC for evening/morning is 40% and 66% respectively. This diurnal variation in pharmacokinetics is also observed with the extended-release formulation with corresponding ratio of peak and AUC evening/morning of 79% and 65% respectively. The circadian effect may be due to diurnal differences in gastric emptying time or gastrointestinal perfusion [23–25].

Several anecdotal reports and small pilot studies describe the sublingual administration of tacrolimus, particularly during the early post-operative period for patients with gastrointestinal difficulties and inability to swallow oral capsules. Although absorption has been documented by measurement of blood levels, it is unclear whether this relates to absorption in the oral cavity, sublingual space, or subsequent ingestion and absorption from the gastrointestinal tract. Additionally, there are reports of very low tacrolimus blood levels after sublingual administration. Also, in the early post-operative period, tacrolimus capsules have been opened and

the contents flushed down the nasogastric (NG) tube in patients unable to swallow capsules. Blood levels have been documented with NG administration in anecdotal reports and small pilot studies, but the bioequivalence to intact capsules has not been demonstrated [26–30].

The extent of oral absorption of tacrolimus is not substantially affected by the rate of gastric emptying [31]. Increased tacrolimus absorption has been reported in the presence of significant diarrhea [32]. Additionally, the absorption of tacrolimus orally has been documented in the presence of bowel dissections and intestinal transplants [33, 34].

Tacrolimus appears to have pro-kinetic activity in the gastrointestinal tract. Faster gastric emptying of solids has been described in renal transplant patients in comparison with cyclosporine. This may provide a benefit to patients with gastroparesis [35].

Distribution

Within the blood, tacrolimus preferentially distributes into the red blood cells in a temperature-dependent partitioning with an average ratio of whole blood to plasma concentration of approximately 20–35. This binding to red blood cells creates a large reservoir for tacrolimus and is the primary reason that whole blood is the preferred biologic matrix for TDM. Patients with substantially reduced hematocrit may have an increase apparent clearance of tacrolimus. Within the plasma compartment, tacrolimus is highly bound to plasma proteins (approximately 98–99%), primarily albumin and α-1-acid glycoprotein. Patients with substantially reduced plasma proteins may have a larger free fraction of tacrolimus in the plasma with resultant higher clearance from the plasma [36] (Figure 16.3). Therefore, the pharmacologic effect for a given whole blood concentration may be greater than expected with hypoalbuminemia. Owing to the high red blood cell and plasma protein binding, there is a very small amount of free tacrolimus that is unbound and distributes to the tissues (Figure 16.3).

Tacrolimus is highly lipophilic; therefore, the drug that is not bound to red blood cells or plasma proteins distributes widely in the body. Tacrolimus is distributed into the placenta, maternal, cord, and

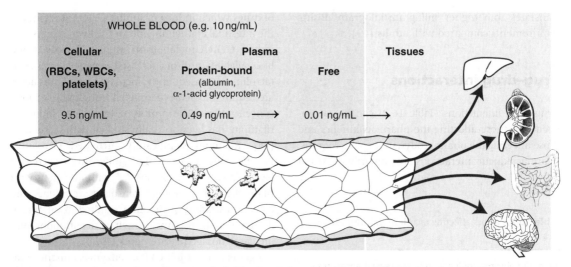

Figure 16.3 Distribution of tacrolimus in whole blood and plasma and free (unbound) drug that distributes to tissues.

neonatal blood. In addition, tacrolimus is distributed into human breast milk at concentrations reported between 23 and 57% of the maternal blood [37–39].

Metabolism

Tacrolimus is metabolized by the cytochrome P450 3A system in the liver. The molecule is demethylated and hydroxylated, with eight metabolites identified and characterized. The major metabolite in humans appears to be M1, 13-O-demethylated tacrolimus, which has negligible immunosuppressive activity [40]. Additionally, M3 (15-O-demethyl tacrolimus), a metabolite with no immunosuppressive activity, has been detected in liver transplant patients and subjects with mild hepatic dysfunction [41]. M2 (31-demethyl tacrolimus) has the same in vitro immunosuppressive activity as the parent compound [7]. In normal healthy volunteers, M1 (13-O-demethylated tacrolimus) was detected after a single dose in concentrations that allow pharmacokinetic characterization. The AUC of M1 was approximately 2–5% of the parent tacrolimus. The mean residence time of M1 (3.1–4.5 h) was less than the parent tacrolimus (24.0–29.3 h). M2 and M3 were also detected, but

the low concentrations did not allow characterization of the pharmacokinetic profile. The relative amounts of metabolite were M1 > M3 > M2 [18].

Elimination

Urinary excretion accounts for less than 3% of the total administered dose of tacrolimus. Less than 0.5% of the unchanged drug is detected in urine [42]. Renal clearance is less than 1% of the total body clearance; therefore, dosage adjustment is not necessary in patients with impaired renal function to achieve targeted whole blood concentrations. Biliary secretion and subsequent fecal elimination comprise the major route of elimination from the body. The elimination half-life of tacrolimus averages approximately 30–44 h in normal volunteers. The clearance of tacrolimus is prolonged in patients with severe hepatic impairment, with a half-life averaging between 119 and 198 h. Patients with significant hepatic impairment and patients receiving a reduced-size liver allograft from a living donor may require lower doses of tacrolimus to achieve targeted whole blood concentrations. In pediatric patients, the clearance of tacrolimus is increased, with a resultant terminal elimination half-life of approximately 11.5 h. This enhanced clearance translates into higher milligram/kilogram dosing requirements compared with adults [43].

Drug–drug interactions

Drug–drug interactions (Table 16.2) can be categorized into those affecting the pharmacokinetics and those affecting the pharmacodynamics of tacrolimus. Pharmacokinetic interactions are primarily the result

Table 16.2 Factors affecting tacrolimus absorption or clearance.

Increased absorption/decreased clearance – decreased dose requirements	Decreased absorption/ increased clearance – increased dose requirements
Physiologic/genetic	
Severe hepatic dysfunction	Pediatrics
Living donor liver transplant	
African descent	CYP3A 5*1 allele
Food/drink	
Grapefruit	Food (high fat > low fat
Pomelo	effect)
Pharmacologic	
Antacids (Mg–Al hydroxide)	St. John's wort
Ketoconazole	Corticosteroids
Fluronazole	Rifabutin
Clotrimazole	
Itraconazole	Rifampin
Voriconazole	Carbamazepine
Erythromycin	Phenytoin
Protease inhibitors (e.g.,	Phenobarbital
nelfinavir, ritonavir,	Caspofungin
telaprevir, and boceprevir)	
Troleandomycin	Sirolimus
Clarithromycin	
Diltiazem	
Nicardipine	
Nifedipine	
Verapamil	
Omeprazole	
Lansoprazole	
Ethinylestradiol	
Nefazodone	
Danazol	

of drugs which induce or inhibit CYP3A isozymes in the intestinal epithelium and/or the liver. Agents that induce CYP3A metabolism result in decreased oral bioavailability and/or increased hepatic clearance of tacrolimus. Consequently, increased tacrolimus doses are required to achieve targeted trough whole blood concentrations. The prototype for CYP3A inducers, rifampin, has been formally studied with tacrolimus [44]. Rifampin significantly increased tacrolimus hepatic clearance and significantly decreased bioavailability (14% versus 7% without versus with rifampin). In a renal transplant recipient, the co-administration of rifampin resulted in an abrupt decrease in tacrolimus trough concentrations and increased dosage requirements [45].

Agents that inhibit CYP3A enzymes enhance oral bioavailability and/or decrease hepatic clearance. Drug–drug interaction studies have been performed with the prototype potent CYP3A inhibitor ketoconazole [46]. Co-administration of ketoconazole significantly increased tacrolimus bioavailability (14% versus 30% without versus with ketoconzaole) but did not consistently affect the hepatic clearance. The magnitude of the drug–drug interaction with ketoconazole is greater in patients lacking the *1 CYP3A5 allele [47]. The clinical impact of this interaction on kidney transplant patients has been assessed. With long-term therapy, the dose of tacrolimus needed to obtain target trough whole blood concentrations was significantly reduced in ketoconazole-treated patients [48].

Pharmacodynamic interactions with tacrolimus include agents that enhance toxicity and those that increase efficacy through additive or synergistic immunosuppression. The primary focus for drug interactions enhancing the toxicity of tacrolimus has been agents affecting renal function. The combination of tacrolimus with nonsteroidal anti-inflammatory agents in the salt-depleted rat model of nephrotoxicty has shown that nonsteroidal anti-inflammatory drugs (both nonselective, diclofenac, and Cox-2 selective, rofecoxib) impaired renal function as measured by glomerular filtration rate (GFR) when combined with tacrolimus [49]. Additionally, there are case reports of acute renal failure associated with ibuprofen use in transplant recipients [50]. Other nephrotoxic agents also may potentiate the renal toxicity of tacrolimus, including aminoglycoside antibiotics, cyclosporine, and amphotericin B. The initial clinical trials in patients at the University of Pittsburgh combined tacrolimus with cyclosporine therapy [51]. Enhanced renal toxicity was seen, prompting the cessation of co-administration after the first 11 patients were treated [2].

Other pharmacodynamic interactions with tacrolimus include the potential increase in the neurotoxicity of ganciclovir, enhanced glucose intolerance in combination with corticosteroids, and enhanced gastrointestinal toxicity (i.e., diarrhea) with mycophenolate mofetil.

The combination of tacrolimus with other immunosuppressants has been studied in animal models of organ transplantation and clinical transplant studies. Combination therapy with mycophenolate mofetil results in additive immunosuppressive potency and a reduced incidence of acute allograft rejection in comparison with placebo or azathioprine. This combination regimen (tacrolimus plus mycophenolate mofetil) has become the most commonly used immunosuppression after renal transplantation. Additionally, tacrolimus has been studied with sirolimus, corticosteroids, azathioprine, and monoclonal or polyclonal antibody preparations. These pharmacodynamic interactions are the basis of combination immunosuppressant regimens that allow reduced dosing of each agent in order to optimize efficacy and minimize toxicity. The potency of the combination immunosuppressive regimen may also be an important risk factor for opportunistic infections (e.g., cytomegalovirus (CMV), herpes, JC, and BK viruses), as well as malignancies such as Epstein–Barr virus (EBV)-derived post-transplant lymphoproliferative disease and Kaposi's sarcoma with HHV8.

When switching immunosuppressive regimens, clinicians should be aware of the following:

• Discontinuation of corticosteroids may result in increased tacrolimus blood levels [52].

• Conversion from cyclosporine to tacrolimus in patients receiving mycophenolate mofetil may result in increased mycophenolic acid (MPA) levels

due to a lack of interaction with tacrolimus. Cyclosporine increases MPA levels owing to its effect on enterohepatic recirculation.

• When converting between tacrolimus and cyclosporine, one agent should be discontinued before starting the other owing to enhanced toxicity with the combination.

TDM

Owing to the narrow therapeutic index of tacrolimus, coupled with the inter- and intra-subject variability in pharmacokinetics, TDM was adopted as an important component of the safe and effective use of this immunosuppressant. The milligram/kilogram dosing of tacrolimus is not predictive of the blood levels (Figure 16.4). There is a high correlation of the tacrolimus trough to drug exposure as measured by AUC; therefore, trough concentration monitoring has become the standard practice for TDM. Early in the development of tacrolimus a prospective concentration-controlled trial in kidney transplant patients was performed [54]. This trial formed the basis for better definition of the therapeutic range, as increasing adverse events were seen with increasing trough concentrations and decreasing rates of acute rejection with increasing trough levels [55]. The first consensus

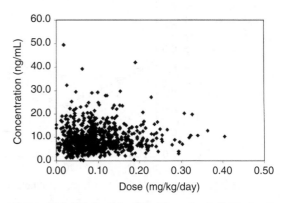

Figure 16.4 Relationship of tacrolimus immediate release dose (mg/kg/day) and steady-state trough whole blood concentration in liver transplant recipients [53]. Published with permission by Sage Publications Inc. Journals.

conference on tacrolimus TDM was held in 1995 and concluded that target tacrolimus trough concentrations should be in the range of 5–20 ng/mL. These general guidelines were further refined to provide more specific recommendations for target trough concentrations based on the following factors: organ transplanted, concomitant immuno-suppression, and time post-transplant (Table 16.3).

Table 16.3 Trough tacrolimus concentrations [43, 56, 57].

Organ	Time post-transplant (months)	Target trough (ng/mL)
Kidney*	0–12	4–11
	>12	3–9
Liver	0–1	10–20
	1–3	5–15
	>3	5–10
Heart	0–2	15–20
	2–6	10–15
	>6	5–10

*IL-2 receptor antibody induction, mycophenolate mofetil, steroids.

In general, higher concentrations are recommended early post-transplant, when patients are at the highest risk of acute cellular rejection, with decreasing concentrations later post-transplant. Additionally, depending on the use of concomitant monoclonal or polyclonal antibody induction, mycophenolate mofetil, and corticosteroids, the target trough concentration may be adjusted to take into account the total immunosuppressive load [53,56–58].

The relationship of trough concentration with toxicity, particularly renal dysfunction, is stronger (as reflected by odds ratios and P-values, as well as area under the receiver operating characteristic curves) than the relationship of tacrolimus trough concentrations with acute rejection after liver or kidney transplantation (Figure 16.5). Therefore, trough concentration monitoring is most useful for preventing nephrotoxicity of tacrolimus [53, 55]. In addition, meta-analyses of kidney transplant studies have shown that the incidence of new-onset diabetes after transplant is increased with increasing trough tacrolimus concentrations [59, 60]. Peak

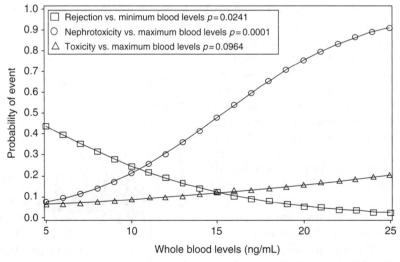

Figure 16.5 Logistic regression analysis of the probability of rejection, nephrotoxicity, and toxicity (defined as any adverse event that required a reduction in tacrolimus dose) as a function of trough whole blood tacrolimus concentration in the 0 to 7 day window prior to the event. This analysis is performed for liver transplant recipients in the first 12 weeks post-transplant [53]. Published with permission by Sage Publications Inc. Journals.

concentrations have not shown a significant relationship when evaluated after kidney transplantation for either rejection or toxicity.

The measurement of tacrolimus levels in whole blood is performed by either immunoassays or high-performance liquid chromatography–mass spectrometry with varying degrees of specificity and sensitivity. Clinicians should be aware of changes in the analytical methodology within their laboratories, since:

1. It has been shown that metabolites may cross-react with immunoassays, particularly in patients with hepatic dysfunction. The amount of metabolites in blood may be greater in patients than in normal volunteers and may increase over time post-transplant.

2. Low hematocrit (<30 %) may cause false elevations in concentrations measured by microparticle enzyme immunoassay (MEIA).

3. Low albumin concentrations (i.e., <3.0 g/dL) may also result in false elevated concentrations by MEIA.

4. Differences in calibrators/controls between methods may lead to bias differences.

5. Owing to differences in sensitivity, some assays may report "no detectable tacrolimus" while another method will quantify the concentration [57].

Pharmacodynamic monitoring

Several approaches have been explored for pharmacodynamic monitoring of the pharmacologic effect of tacrolimus and other immunosuppressants. These methodologies have included approaches that are not specific to calcineurin inhibition, such as the ImmuKnow® by Cylex, which detects cell-mediated immunity in the immunosuppressed patient populations, gamma interferon ELISPOT, T cell surface antigen expression, and intracellular cytokine synthesis in stimulated whole blood. Currently, none of these approaches has been implemented as a standard monitoring measure for the overall immunosuppressive effect of tacrolimus [57]. Several groups have also evaluated calcineurin phosphatase activity in peripheral blood mononuclear cells in patients treated with tacroli-

mus. The relationship with trough tacrolimus concentration is not highly correlated and there are limited data on the relationship with clinical outcome. One group has shown patients with nephrotoxicity having lower levels of calcineurin activity and patients with acute rejection have higher levels of calcineurin activity [61,62]. This approach to pharmacodynamic monitoring may hold potential for future applications.

Pharmacogenetics

Polymorphisms in genes coding for CYP-3A4 and -3A5 enzymes, as well as drug transporters such as ABCB1, have been evaluated for their impact on tacrolimus pharmacokinetics. The trough whole blood tacrolimus concentrations and associated dose requirements to achieve targeted trough concentrations have been demonstrated to be associated with the CYP3A5 polymorphism. Kidney, liver, heart, and lung transplant recipients have been shown to have higher dose-adjusted trough levels in patients who were homozygous CYP3A5*3/*3 compared with patients who were heterozygous or homozygous for the wild-type form, which is typically designated CYP3A5*1. Patients with the wild-type allele CYP3A5*1 have also been shown to require a higher daily tacrolimus dose than those with the CYP3A5*3/3* genotype. This may be due to intestinal metabolism of the CYP3A5 rather than hepatic. This effect of CYP3A5 polymorphism on the intestinal metabolism and bioavailability of tacrolimus may partly explain the difference in bioavailability seen in African Americans, compared with Caucasians, since the CYP3A5*3 allele is present in approximately 32 % of African Americans compared with 90 % or more of Caucasians. Therefore, the CYP3A5*1 wild type is more common in patients of African descent [57, 63].

Preclinical toxicology

Toxicities of tacrolimus have been observed in the nonhuman primate (cynomolgus monkey and baboon) models and rat models. Nephrotoxicity in the cynomolgus monkey has been evidenced by increases in serum urea, as well as histopathologic changes in the kidney, demonstrating mesangial cell proliferation and acute tubular necrosis [64]. In salt-depleted rats, tacrolimus decreases GFR, urinary osmolarity, and plasma magnesium, while increasing the plasma creatinine, fractional excretion of magnesium, urine volume, plasma renin activity, and alanine aminopeptidase. Histopathologically, the main lesion seen in the rat kidney is vacuolization in proximal tubules. This histopathologic injury is not observed in sodium-replete rats [65, 66].

After longer term treatment (i.e., 42 days) in salt-depleted rats, tubulo-interstitial scarring associated with increased plasma renin activity was seen. The fibrosis of chronic tacrolimus nephropathy has been suggested to involve the dual action of TGFβ1 on matrix deposition and degradation, and the renin–angiotensin system may play an important role [67].

In the pancreas, depletion of beta cells is seen in cynomolgus monkeys treated with tacrolimus for 90 days. In the rat, histopathological changes in the pancreas include vacuolation of the islets of Langerhans. The mechanism of the pancreatic toxicity of tacrolimus has been mechanistically explored in the rat model. Oral tacrolimus for 2 weeks at supra-therapeutic doses suppressed insulin production time dependently at the transcriptional step in pancreatic beta cells, while glucagon content in the pancreatic alpha cells was not affected. The decrease in insulin mRNA transcription insulin production was reversible after discontinuation of therapy. The differential effects of tacrolimus on alpha cells compared with beta cells affecting insulin but not affecting glucagon may be explained by the relatively high content of FKBP-12 in the beta cells, compared with the alpha cells, in conjunction with the relatively high content of calcineurin in the alpha cells compared with the beta cells [68].

The toxicities of tacrolimus that appear to be mediated through calcineurin phosphatase inhibition include central nervous system adverse effects (e.g., tremor), renal toxicity, and diabetogenicity [69] (Table 16.4). These effects not only appear to

Table 16.4 Tacrolimus adverse effects.

Calcineurin mediated
Nephrotoxicity (↑ serum creatinine)
Diabetogenicity (↑ fasting plasma glucose, Hgb A1c)
Neurotoxicity (e.g., tremor, headache, paresthesia)

Non-calcineurin mediated
Alopecia
Gastrointestinal (e.g., diarrhea)

Immunosuppression mediated
Opportunistic infections (e.g., CMV, BK, JC viruses)
Malignancy (e.g., skin cancer, EBV-driven lympho-proliferative disorders)

Metabolic/laboratory
Hyperkalemia
Hypomagnesemia

be related to the presence of calcineurin in the target organs, but may also be related to the relative ratios of FKBP-12 to calcineurin. High amounts of FKBP-12 and low amounts of calcineurin allow the more complete inhibition of calcineurin phosphatase activity, whereas lower amounts of FKBP-12 and higher amounts of calcineurin may be protective [68]. Other adverse effects of tacrolimus seen in clinical studies are listed in Table 16.4. In addition to those mediated by calcineurin phosphatase inhibition, some adverse events (e.g., viral opportunistic infections and EBV-driven lymphoproliferation) reflect immunodeficiency or the total immunosuppressive load.

Liver transplantation

The initial clinical studies of tacrolimus focused on the "rescue" use in patients with refractory liver rejection under standard therapy, including cyclosporine, steroids, and antibody therapy [6]. The positive clinical experience in case series in this setting led to the extension of tacrolimus use into the de novo prophylactic setting. After initial results from single-center experience at the University of Pittsburgh, Phase 3 trials were initiated comparing tacrolimus in combination with corticosteroids with cyclosporine-based immunosuppression [70–72]. These trials formed the basis for the first regulatory approval of tacrolimus in the USA and Europe. A meta-analysis of 16 randomized clinical trials comparing cyclosporine with tacrolimus was published by The Cochrane Collaboration and McAlister and coworkers [73, 74]. The results of this analysis indicated that tacrolimus was superior to cyclosporine in improving patient and graft survival and preventing acute rejection and steroid-resistant rejection. Lymphoproliferative disease and end-stage renal failure (dialysis dependence) was not different. De novo diabetes occurred with an increased frequency with tacrolimus. More patients were withdrawn from cyclosporine than from tacrolimus.

Kidney transplantation

The use of tacrolimus in kidney transplantation started at the University of Pittsburgh soon after its first clinical use in liver transplant recipients. For kidney transplant recipients, combination therapy with an anti-proliferative agent is common. Initially these regimens included azathioprine, but mycophenolate mofetil/MPA is most commonly used more recently. The Cochrane Collaboration and Webster et al. published meta-analyses of 123 reports from 30 randomized controlled trials where tacrolimus was compared with cyclosporine [59, 60]. The 6 month graft loss was significantly reduced with tacrolimus. This benefit in graft survival decreased with increasing target trough tacrolimus concentration. Tacrolimus was associated with a decreased risk of acute rejection and steroid-resistant rejection at 1 year post-transplant, but was also associated with more new onset of diabetes requiring insulin, tremor, headache, diarrhea, dyspepsia, and vomiting. There was a greater risk of constipation, hirsutism, and gingival hyperplasia with cyclosporine. There was no difference in infection or malignancy between the two immunosuppressants. The mean serum creatinine at 6 months post-transplant was significantly lower in the tacrolimus group. New onset of diabetes after transplantation increased with increasing trough tacrolimus concentration.

The largest prospective clinical study of immunosuppression after renal transplantation was reported by Ekberg et al. [75]. Tacrolimus with IL-2 receptor antibody induction, mycophenolate mofetil, and corticosteroids was compared with two different cyclosporine regimens and one regimen of sirolimus-based immunosuppression. At 1 year post-transplant, tacrolimus was associated with the highest mean calculated GFR, lowest biopsy-proven acute rejection rate, and highest graft survival in comparison with the other three groups.

Heart transplantation

Two multicenter prospective randomized controlled trials in adult recipients of heart transplantation have been performed comparing tacrolimus-based immunosuppression with cyclosporine-based immunosuppression for the prevention of acute rejection [76, 77]. Combination therapies have included azathioprine, mycophenolate mofetil, or sirolimus. In a meta-analysis of tacrolimus versus cyclosporine microemulsion, tacrolimus-treated patients had less acute rejection, discontinuations, and hypertension and more new-onset diabetes after transplantation [78].

Other solid organ transplants

The efficacy and safety of tacrolimus-based immunosuppression compared with cyclosporine-based immunosuppression has been assessed in prospective comparative trials of lung transplantation and simultaneous pancreas–kidney transplants. The benefits of the tacrolimus, particularly in combination with mycophenolate mofetil, have been demonstrated in these organs with historically high risks of rejection under cyclosporine-based therapy [79–82].

Graft-versus-host disease

Tacrolimus (IV and per os) has been studied for the prevention of graft-versus-host disease after allogeneic bone marrow transplantation (matched sibling and unrelated donor transplants). Three Phase 3 trials have been performed, in comparison with cyclosporine, demonstrating significant reductions in the rates of acute graft-versus-host disease [83–85].

Autoimmune diseases

Tacrolimus use has been extended to the treatment of T-cell-mediated autoimmune diseases. Oral tacrolimus has been studied in prospective multi-center controlled trials in rheumatoid arthritis. Significant improvement in ACR 20 as a measure of efficacy has been shown consistently at a dose of 3 mg/day in comparison with placebo or mizoribine [86–89]. Additionally, oral tacrolimus has demonstrated efficacy in the treatment of the following autoimmune diseases in prospective randomized controlled trials: plaque-type psoriasis, myasthenia gravis, nephrotic syndrome, Crohn's disease, and ulcerative colitis [90–95].

Topical tacrolimus (Protopic® ointment) has been shown to be safe and effective for the treatment of atopic dermatitis (eczema) and is commercially available [96].

Conclusion

The discovery of tacrolimus in 1984 has led to characterization of the ubiquitous immunophilin binding protein FKBP and the important role of calcineurin phosphatase activity in early T cell activation and other cellular functions in the kidney, brain, and pancreas. Although tacrolimus has a relatively narrow therapeutic index and substantial pharmacokinetic variability, it is established as one of the base immunosuppressants for the prevention of rejection after solid organ transplantation with uses extended to autoimmune diseases and hematopoietic stem cell transplantation. TDM has played a key role in the safe and effective use of tacrolimus in transplant immunosuppression.

References

1 Goto T, Kino T, Hatanaka H *et al*. FK-506: historical perspectives. *Transplant Proc* 1991;23:2713–2717.

2 Nishiyama M, Izumi S, Okuhara M. Discovery and development of FK506 (tacrolimus), a potent immunosuppressant of microbial origin. In *The Search for Anti-Inflammatory Drugs* (eds VJ Merluzzi, J Adams). Birkhauser: Boston; 1995, pp. 65–104.

3 Goto T, Kino T, Hatanaka H *et al*. Discovery of FK-506, a novel immunosuppressant isolated from *Streptomyces tsukubaenis*. *Transplant Proc* 1987;19(Suppl 6):4–8.

4 Kino T, Hatanaka H, Hashimoto M *et al*. FK-506, a novel immunosuppressant isolated from a *Streptomyces* I. Fermentation, isolation, and physico-chemical and biological characteristics. *The Journal of Antibiotics* 1987;40:1249–1255.

5 Kino T, Hatanaka H, Miyata S *et al*. FK-506, a novel immunosuppressant isolated from a *Streptomyces* II. Immunosuppressive effect of FK-506 in vitro. *J Antibiot* 1987;40:1256–1265.

6 Starzl TE, Fung J, Venkataramman R *et al*. FK506 for liver, kidney, and pancreas transplantation. *Lancet* 1989;2(8670):1000–1004.

7 Tamura K, Fujimura T, Iwasaki K *et al*. Interaction of tacrolimus (FK506) and its metabolites with FKBP and calcineurin. *Biochem Biophys Res Commun* 1994;202:437–443.

8 Harding MW, Galat A, Uehling DE. A receptor for the immunosuppressant FK506 is a *cis–trans* peptidyl-prolyl isomerase. *Nature* 1989;341:758–760.

9 Bierer BE, Mattila PS, Standaert RF *et al*. Two distinct signal transmission pathways in T lymphocytes are inhibited by complexes formed between an immunophilin and either FK506 or rapamycin. *Proc Natl Acad Sci U S A* 1990;87:9231–9235.

10 Griffith JP, Kim JL, Kim EE *et al*. X-ray structure of calcineurin inhibited by the immunophilin-immunosuppressant FKBP12–FK506 complex. *Cell* 1995;82:507–522.

11 Bekersky I, Dressler D, Mekki QA. Effect of low- and high-fat meals on tacrolimus absorption following 5 mg single oral doses to healthy human subjects. *J Clin Pharmacol* 2001;41:176–182.

12 Bekersky I, Dressler D, Mekki Q. Effect of time of meal consumption on bioavailability of a single oral 5 mg tacrolimus dose. *J Clin Pharmacol* 2001;41:289–297.

13 Fukatsu S, Fukudo M, Masuda S *et al*. Delayed effect of grapefruit juice on pharmacokinetics and pharmacodynamics of tacrolimus in a living-donor liver transplant recipient. *Drug Metab Pharmacokinet* 2006;21:122–125.

14 Peynaud D, Charpiat B, Vial T. Tacrolimus severe overdosage after intake of masked grapefruit in orange marmalade. *Eur J Clin Pharmacol* 2007;63:721–722.

15 Liu C, Shang YF, Zhang XF *et al.* Co-administration of grapefruit juice increases bioavailability of tacrolimus in liver transplant patients: a prospective study. *Eur J Clin Pharmacol* 2009;65:881–885.

16 Egashira K, Fukuda E, Onga T *et al.* Pomelo-induced increase in the blood level of tacrolimus in a renal transplant patient. *Transplantation* 2003;75:1057.

17 Egashira K, Ohtani H, Itoh S *et al.* Inhibitory effects of pomelo on the metabolism of tacrolimus and the activities of CYP3A4 and p-glycoprotein. *Drug Metab Dispos* 2004;32:828–833.

18 Mancinelli LM, Frassetto L, Floren LC *et al.* The pharmacokinetics and metabolic disposition of tacrolimus: a comparison across ethnic groups. *Clin Pharmacol Ther* 2001;69:24–31.

19 Renders L, Frisman M, Ufer M *et al.* CYP3A5 genotype markedly influences the pharmacokinetics of tacrolimus and sirolimus in kidney transplant recipients. *Clin Pharmacol Ther* 2007;81:228–234.

20 Roy JN, Lajoie J, Zijenah LS *et al.* CYP3A5 genetic polymorphisms in different ethnic populations. *Drug Metab Dispos* 2005;33:884–887.

21 Min DI, Ellingrod VL, Marsh S, McLeod H. CYP3A5 polymorphism and the ethnic differences in cyclosporine pharmacokinetics in healthy subjects. *Ther Drug Monit* 2004;26:524–528.

22 Fitzsimmons WE, Bekersky I, Dressler D *et al.* Demographic considerations in tacrolimus pharmacokinetics. *Transplant Proc* 1998;30:1359–1364.

23 EMEA Scientific Discussion. Advagraf® Product Monograph; 2007.

24 Min DI, Chen HY, Fabrega A *et al.* Circadian variation of tacrolimus disposition in liver allograft recipients. *Transplantation* 1996;62:1190–1192.

25 Park SI, Felipe CR, Pinheiro-Machado PG. Circadian and time-dependent variability in tacrolimus pharmacokinetics. *Fundam Clin Pharmacol* 2007;21: 191–197.

26 Garrity ER, Jr, Hertz MI, Trulock EP *et al.* Suggested guidelines for the use of tacrolimus in lung-transplant recipients. *J Heart Lung Transplant* 1999;18:175–176.

27 Reams BD, Palmer SM. Sublingual tacrolimus for immunosuppression in lung transplantation: a potentially important therapeutic option in cystic fibrosis. *Am J Respir Med* 2002;1:91–98.

28 Romero I, Jimenez C, Gil F *et al.* Sublingual administration of tacrolimus in a renal transplant patient. *J Clin Pharm Ther* 2008;33:87–89.

29 Van de Plas A, Dackus J, Christiaans MHL *et al.* A pilot study on sublingual administration of tacrolimus. *Transpl Int* 2009;22:358–359.

30 Goorhuis JF, Scheenstra R, Peeters PMJG, Albers MJ. Buccal vs. nasogastric tube administration of tacrolimus after pediatric liver transplantation. *Pediatr Transplant* 2006;10:74–77.

31 Kuypers DR, Claes K, Evenepoel P *et al.* The rate of gastric emptying determines the timing but not the extent of oral tacrolimus absorption: simultaneous measurement of drug exposure and gastric emptying by carbon-14-octanoic acid breath test in stable renal allograft recipients. *Drug Metab Dispos* 2004;32:1421–1425.

32 Eades SK, Boineau FG, Christensen ML. Increased tacrolimus levels in a pediatric renal transplant patient attributed to chronic diarrhea. *Pediatr Transplant* 2000; 4:63–66.

33 Olio DD, Gupte G, Sharif K *et al.* Immunosuppression in infants with short bowel syndrome undergoing isolated liver transplantation. *Pediatr Transplant* 2006; 10:677–681.

34 Patel N, Smith S, Handa A, Darby C. The use of oral tacrolimus in a case of short bowel syndrome. *Transpl Int* 2004;17:44–45.

35 Maes BD, Vanwalleghem J, Kuypers D *et al.* Differences in gastric motor activity in renal transplant recipients treated with FK-506 versus cyclosporine. *Transplantation* 1999;68:1482–1485.

36 Zahir H, McLachlan AJ, Nelson A *et al.* Population pharmacokinetic estimation of tacrolimus apparent clearance in adult liver transplant recipients. *Ther Drug Monit* 2005;27:422–430.

37 French AE, Soldin SJ, Soldin OP, Koren G. Milk transfer and neonatal safety of tacrolimus. *Ann Pharmacother* 2003;37:815–818.

38 Gardiner SJ, Begg EJ. Breastfeeding during tacrolimus therapy. *Obstet Gynecol* 2006;107(2 Pt 2):453–455.

39 Jain A, Venkataramanan R, Fung JJ *et al.* Pregnancy after liver transplantation under tacrolimus. *Transplantation* 1997;64:559–565.

40 Gonschior AK, Christians U, Braun F *et al.* Measurement of blood concentrations of FK506 (tacrolimus) and its metabolites in seven liver graft patients after the first dose by h.p.l.c.–MS and microparticle enzyme immunoassay (MEIA). *Br J Clin Pharmacol* 1994;38:567–571.

41 Tokunaga Y, Alak AM. FK506 (tacrolimus) and its immunoreactive metabolites in whole blood of liver transplant patients and subjects with mild hepatic dysfunction. *Pharm Res* 1996;13:137–140.

42 Möller A, Iwasaki K, Kawamura A *et al.* The disposition of ^{14}C-labeled tacrolimus after intravenous and oral administration in healthy human subjects. *Drug Metab Dispos* 1999;27:633–636.

43 Prograf® Package Insert. US labeling.

44 Hebert MF, Fisher RM, Marsh CL *et al.* Effects of rifampin on tacrolimus pharmacokinetics in healthy volunteers. *J Clin Pharmacol* 1999;39:91–96.

45 Chenhsu RY, Loong CC, Chou MH *et al.* Renal allograft dysfunction associated with rifampin-tacrolimus interaction. *Ann Pharmacother* 2000;34:27–31.

46 Floren LC, Bekersky I, Benet LZ *et al.* Tacrolimus oral bioavailability doubles with coadministration of ketoconazole. *Clin Pharmacol Ther* 1997;62:41–49.

47 Chandel N, Aggarwal PK, Minz M *et al.* CYP3A5*1/3* genotype influences the blood concentration of tacrolimus in response to metabolic inhibition by ketoconazole. *Pharmacogenet Genomics* 2009;19:458–463.

48 El-Dahshan KF, Bakr MA, Donia AF *et al.* Ketoconazole–tacrolimus coadministration in kidney transplant recipients: two-year results of a prospective randomized study. *Am J Nephrol* 2006;26:293–298.

49 Soubhia RMC, Mendes GEF, Mendonca FZ *et al.* Tacrolimus and nonsteroidal anti-inflammatory drugs: an association to be avoided. *Am J Nephrol* 2005;25: 327–334.

50 Sheiner PA, Mor E, Chodoff L *et al.* Acute renal failure associated with the use of ibuprofen in two liver transplant recipients on FK506. *Transplantation* 1994; 57:1132–1133.

51 Fung JJ, Todo S, Jain A *et al.* Conversion from cyclosporine to FK506 in liver allograft recipients with cyclosporine-related complications. *Transplant Proc* 1990;22(S1):6–12.

52 Van Duijnhoven EM, Boots JMM, Christians MHL *et al.* Increase in tacrolimus trough levels after steroid withdrawal. *Transpl Int* 2003;16:721–725.

53 Venkataramanan R, Shaw LM, Sarkozi L *et al.* Clinical utility of monitoring tacrolimus blood concentrations in liver transplant patients. *J Clin Pharmacol* 2001;41: 542–551.

54 Vincenti F, Laskow DA, Neylan J *et al.* One year follow-up of an open-label trial of FK506 for primary kidney transplantation. A report of the U.S. Multicenter FK506 Kidney Transplant Study Group. *Transplantation* 1996;61:1576–1581.

55 Kershner RP, Fitzsimmons, WE. Relationship of FK506 whole blood concentrations and efficacy and toxicity after liver and kidney transplantation. *Transplantation* 1996;62:920–926.

56 Bolin P, Shihab FS, Mulloy L *et al.* Optimizing tacrolimus therapy in the maintenance of renal allografts: 12 month results. *Transplantation* 2008;86: 88–95.

57 Wallemacq P, Armstrong VW, Brunet M *et al.* Opportunities to optimize tacrolimus therapy in solid organ transplantation: report of the European Consensus Conference. *Ther Drug Monit* 2009;31:139–152.

58 Jusko WJ, Thomson AW, Fung J *et al.* Consensus document: therapeutic monitoring of tacrolimus (FK506). *Ther Drug Monit* 1995;17:606–614.

59 Webster AC, Woodroffe RC, Taylor RS *et al.* Tacrolimus versus ciclosporin as primary immunosuppression for kidney transplant recipients: meta-analysis and meta-regression of randomised trial data. *BMJ* 2005; 331(7520):810.

60 Webster A, Woodroffe RC, Taylor RS *et al.* Tacrolimus versus cyclosporine as primary immunosuppression for kidney transplant recipients. *Cochrane Database Syst Rev* 2005;(4):CD003961.

61 Yano I. Pharmacodynamic monitoring of calcineurin phosphatase activity in transplant patients treated with calcineurin inhibitors. *Drug Metab Pharmacokinet* 2008;23:150–157.

62 Fukudo M, Yano I, Masuda S *et al.* Pharmacodynamic analysis of tacrolimus and cyclosporine in living-donor liver transplant patients. *Clin Pharmacol Ther* 2005; 78:168–181.

63 Anglicheau D, Legendre C, Beaune P. Cytochrome P450 3A polymorphisms and immunosuppressive drugs: an update. *Pharmacogenomics* 2007;8: 835–849.

64 Wijnen RMH, Ericzon BG, Tiebosch ATMG. Toxicology of FK506 in the cynomolgus monkey: a clinical, biochemical, and histopathological study. *Transpl Int* 1992;5(Suppl 1):S454–S458.

65 Andoh TF, Burdmann EA, Lindsley J *et al.* Functional and structural characteristics of experimental FK506 nephrotoxicity. *Clin Exp Pharmacol Physiol* 1995;22: 646–654.

66 Andoh TF, Burdmann EA, Lindsley J *et al.* Enhancement of FK506 nephrotoxicity by sodium depletion in an experimental rat model. *Transplantation* 1994;57:483–489.

67 Shihab FS, Bennett WM, Tanner AM, Andoh TF. Mechanism of fibrosis in experimental tacrolimus nephrotoxicity. *Transplantation* 1997;64:1829–1837.

68 Tamura T, Fujimura T, Tsutsumi T *et al.* Transcriptional inhibition of insulin by FK506 and possible involvement of FK506 binding protein-12 in pancreatic β-cell. *Transplantation* 1995;59:1606–1613.

69 Heit JJ. Calcineurin/NFAT signaling in the β-cell: from diabetes to new therapeutics. *BioEssays* 2007;29: 1011–1021.

70 Fung J, Abu-Elmagd K, Jain A *et al*. A randomized trial of primary liver transplantation under immunosuppression with FK506 vs cyclosporine. *Transplant Proc* 1991;23:2977–2983.

71 European FK506 Multicentre Liver Study Group. Randomised trial comparing tacrolimus (FK506) and cyclosporine in prevention of liver allograft rejection. *Lancet* 1994;344:423–428.

72 The US Multicenter FK506 Study Group. A comparison of tacrolimus (FK506) and cyclosporine for immunosuppression in liver transplantation. *N Engl J Med* 1994;331:1110–1115.

73 McAlister VC, Haddad E, Renouf E *et al*. Cyclosporin versus tacrolimus as primary immunosuppressant after liver transplantation: a meta-analysis. *Am J Transplant* 2006;6:1578–1585.

74 Haddad EM, McAlister VC, Renouf E *et al*. Cyclosporin versus tacrolimus for liver transplanted patients. *Cochrane Database Syst Rev.* 2006;(4):CD005161.

75 Ekberg H, Tedesco-Silva H, Demirbas A *et al*. Reduced exposure to calcineurin inhibitors in renal transplantation. *N Engl J Med* 2007;357:2562–2575.

76 Grimm M, Rinaldi M, Yonan NA *et al*. Superior prevention of acute rejection by tacrolimus vs. cyclosporine in heart transplant recipients – a large European trial. *Am J. Transplant* 2006;6:1387–1397.

77 Kobashigawa JA, Miller LW, Russell SD *et al*. Tacrolimus with mycophenolate mofetil (MMF) or sirolimus vs. cyclosporine with MMF in cardiac transplant patients: 1-year report. *Am J Transplant* 2006;6: 1377–1386.

78 Ye F, Ying-Bin X, Yu-Guo W, Hetzer R. Tacrolimus versus cyclosporine microemulsion for heart transplant recipients: a meta-analysis. *J Heart Lung Transplant* 2009;28:58–66.

79 Zuckerman A, Reichenspurner H, Birsan T *et al*. Cyclosporine A versus tacrolimus in combination with mycophenolate mofetil and steroids as primary immunosuppression after lung transplantation: one-year results of a two-center prospective randomized trial. *J Thorac Cardiovasc Surg* 2003;125:891–900.

80 Hachen RR, Yusen RD, Chakinala MM *et al*. A randomized, controlled trial of tacrolimus versus cyclosporine after lung transplantation. *J Heart Lung Transplant* 2007;26:1012–1018.

81 Keenan RJ, Konishi H, Kawai A *et al*. Clinical trial of tacrolimus versus cyclosporine in lung transplantation. *Ann Thorac Surg* 1995;60:580–585.

82 Malaise J, Sudek F, Boucek P *et al*. Tacrolimus compared with cyclosporine microemulsion in primary,

simultaneous pancreas–kidney transplantation: the EURO-SPK 3-year results. *Transplant Proc* 2005;37: 2843–2845.

83 Hiraoka A, Ohashi Y, Okamoto S *et al*. Phase III study comparing tacrolimus (FK506) with cyclosporine for graft-versus-host disease prophylaxis after allogeneic bone marrow transplantation. *Bone Marrow Transplant* 2001;28:181–185.

84 Nash RA, Antin JH, Karanes C *et al*. Phase 3 study comparing methotrexate and tacrolimus with methotrexate and cyclosporine for prophylaxis of acute graft-versus-host disease after marrow transplantation from unrelated donors. *Blood* 2000;96:2062–2068.

85 Ratanatharathorn V, Nash RA, Przepiorka D *et al*. Phase III study comparing methotrexate and tacrolimus (Prograf, FK506) with methotrexate and cyclosporine for graft-versus-host disease prophylaxis after HLA-identical sibling bone marrow transplantation. *Blood* 1998;92:2303–2314.

86 Ondo H, Abe T, Hashimoto H *et al*. Efficacy and safety of tacrolimus (FK506) in treatment of rheumatoid arthritis: a randomized, double-blind, placebo controlled dose-finding study. *J Rheumatol* 2004;31:243–251.

87 Kawai S, Hashimoto H, Kondo H *et al*. Comparison of tacrolimus and mizoribine in a randomized, double-blind controlled study in patients with rheumatoid arthritis. *J Rheumatol* 2006;33:2153–2161.

88 Yocum BE, Furst DE, Kaine JL *et al*. Efficacy and safety of tacrolimus in patients with rheumatoid *arthritis*: a double-blind trial. *Arthritis Rheum* 2003;48: 3328–3337.

89 Furst DE, Saag K, Fleishmann MR *et al*. Efficacy of tacrolimus in rheumatoid arthritis patients who have been treated unsuccessfully with methotrexate: a six-month, double-blind randomized dose ranging study. *Arthritis Rheum* 2002;46:2020–2028.

90 The European FK506 Multi-Centre Psoriasis Study Group. Systemic tacrolimus (FK506) is effective for the treatment of psoriasis in a double-blind, placebo-controlled study. *Arch Dermatol* 1996;132:419–423.

91 Nagane Y, Ytsugi Sawa K, Obara D *et al*. Efficacy of low-dose FK506 in the treatment of myasthenia gravis-a randomized pilot study. *Eur Neurol* 2005;53: 146–150.

92 Ogata H, Matsui T, Nakamura M *et al*. A randomized dose finding study of oral tacrolimus (FK506) therapy in refractory ulcerative colitis. *Gut* 2006;55: 1255–1262.

93 Sandborn WJ, Present DH, Isaacs KL *et al*. Tacrolimus for the treatment of fistulas in patients with Crohn's

disease, a randomized, placebo-controlled trial. *Gastroenterology* 2003;125:380–388.

94 Praga M, Barrio V, Juarez GF *et al.* Tacrolimus monotherapy in membranous nephropathy: a randomized controlled trial. *Kidney Int* 2007;71:924–930.

95 Choudhry S, Bagga A, Harri P *et al.* Efficacy and safety of tacrolimus versus cyclosporine in children with steroid-resistant nephrotic syndrome: a randomized controlled trial. *Am J Kidney Dis* 2009; 53:760–769.

96 El-Batawy MM, Bosseila MA, Mashaly HM, Hafez VS. Topical calcineurin inhibitors in atopic dermatitis: a systematic review and meta-analysis. *J Dermatol Sci* 2009;54:76–87.

CHAPTER 17

Inhibitors of Mammalian Target of Rapamycin

Barry D. Kahan

The University of Texas Medical School at Houston, Houston, TX, USA

Background

More than 25 years ago, sirolimus (SRL) was extracted from the soil actinomycete *Streptomyces hygroscopicus* discovered in the Vai Atari region of Rapa Nui (Easter Island, Chile). This zone, which is at the southeastern end of the island near the dormant volcano Rano Kao, was regarded as a holy site to the indigenous people. While sea captains had touched Rapa Nui, there was little attention to the island before the National Aeronautics and Space Administration announced that they would construct an emergency landing strip there for the space shuttle. Before that construction was completed, a Canadian medical mission joined by a team from the Centers for Disease Control documented the flora, fauna, and culture of this isolated land. They divided the island into sectors whose soil samples were extensively analyzed for antimicrobial activities by Ayerst Canada. Rapamycin, which was later renamed as SRL, was initially evaluated as an antifungal antibiotic before being documented to be an antineoplastic and immunosuppressive agent.

Chemistry of originator SRL and its derivatives

Structures

SRL (Rapamune®, Wyeth, Philadelphia, PA) is a large 31-member (MW 913.7 Da; Figure 17.1a) lipophilic, carboxylic lactone–lactam macrolide ($C_{51}H_{79}NO_{13}$) antibiotic that is practically insoluble in water (2.6 μg/mL), but is soluble in a variety of organic solvents. It is moderately sensitive to light and adheres to glass. The λ_{max} are 267, 277, and 288 nm. The melting point is 183–185 °C.

SRL contains a tricarbonyl array (carbons [C] 14–16) consisting of an amide, a ketone, and a hemi-ketal. In organic solvents, the compound exists as a mixture of *cis–trans* (~4:1) amide conformers. The detailed structural analysis is reviewed by Sehgal *et al.* [1], who pioneered the development of this drug. SRL is structurally related to tacrolimus (TRL; Figure 17.1b), although their mechanisms of action are entirely distinct.

Temsirolimus–CCl-779 (Wyeth, Philadelphia, PA; Figure 17.1c), an SRL ester formulation for intravenous (iv) administration, has greater but still limited water solubility (~120 μg/mL), requiring co-formulation with ethanol. This prodrug is rapidly hydrolyzed by plasma esterases to SRL [2]. It displays a fivefold increase in maximal concentration C_{max}, with decreased time to C_{max} (t_{max}), reduced half-life $t_{1/2}$ by fivefold, and substantially attenuated area under the concentration curve (AUC) with high inter-patient variability.

Everolimus (EVL; Certican; Novartis, Basle, SZ), which bears a 40-*O*-(2 hydroxyethyl) substitution on the SRL structure (Figure 17.1d), was designed to be rapidly absorbed, to reach peak concentrations at 1.3–1.8 h, and to more rapidly achieve a

Immunotherapy in Transplantation: Principles and Practice, First Edition. Edited by Bruce Kaplan, Gilbert J. Burckart and Fadi G. Lakkis.
© 2012 Blackwell Publishing Ltd. Published 2012 by Blackwell Publishing Ltd.

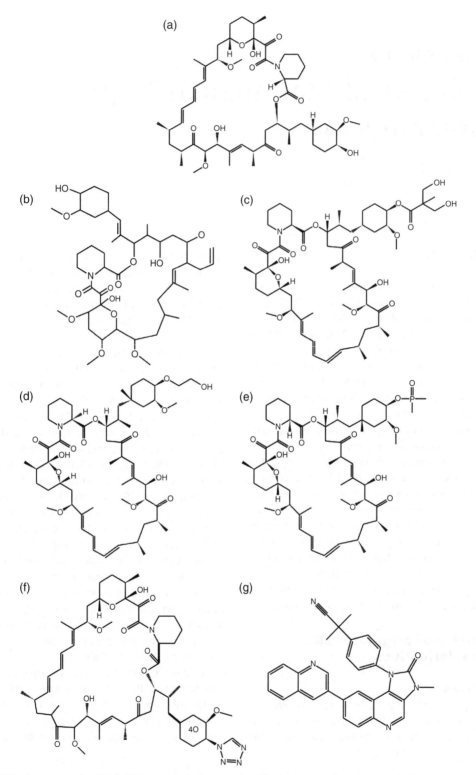

Figure 17.1 Structures of mTOR inhibitors: (a) sirolimus (SRL); (b) the structural congener tacrolimus; (c) temsirolimus; (d) everolimus (EVL); (e) deforolimus; (f) zotarolimus; (g) NVP-BEZ 235.

steady state within 7 days. EVL has eightfold greater solubility in water. It is not a prodrug of SRL.

C40 has been selected for structural modifications because it is away from the binding sites for FK binding protein (FKBP)12 and mammalian target of rapamycin (mTOR; vide infra [3]). Deforolimus (Ariad Pharmaceuticals; Figure 17.1e) bears a phosphonate substituted for a hydroxyl at C40, but it is not a prodrug. Rizzieri *et al.* [4] observed that deforolimus treatment showed good tolerance by patients with heavily treated hematologic malignancies and some evidence of antitumor activity. Using an accelerated titration design, the maximum tolerated dose of deforolimus was 18.75 mg/day and the agent showed encouraging antineoplastic activity at 12.5 mg/day. Zotarolimus (Abbott; Figure 17.1f), which has a tetrazole substitution at C40, displays a reduced half-life compared with SRL or EVL – namely, 9.4 versus 14 h after iv administration and an oral value of 7.9 versus 33.4 h with a fourfold reduced potency; this agent is being developed for impregation of stents [5].

Another orally available dual phosphoinositol-3-kinase (PI3K)/mTOR inhibitor which has been developed for cancer therapy is an imidazo-(4,5-*c*) quinoline derivative. It binds to the ATP cleft, displaying in vitro activity and in vivo tumor protection in gamma-irradiated mice (Figure 17.1g; NVP-BEZ 235) [6]. Deore *et al.* [7] described a novel cyanopyridyl-based molecule that appears to be a potent inhibitor of mTOR in vitro and exhibits activity in vivo.

In contrast to these compounds, most ester, carbamate, or carbonate modifications at C40 convert to SRL under physiologic conditions. Wagner *et al.* [8] reported that 40-epi-tetrazolylrapamycin and a 40-carbamate compound both inhibited in vitro mixed lymphocyte reactions (MLRs), and demonstrated equal efficacy to (albeit with less potency than) SRL for the treatment of adjuvant arthritis in rats. Both analogs showed shorter half-lives than SRL. The carbamate, but not the other compound, is a prodrug of SRL.

Formulations

The clinical oral nonaqueous solution of 1 mg/mL SRL contains Phosal 50 PG, phosphatidylcholine, propylene glycol, monodiglycerides, ethanol, soy, fatty acids, and ascorbyl palmitate, as well as Polysorbate 80 NF. The inactive ingredients in the tablet formulation of SRL include sucrose, lactose, polyethylene glycol 8000, calcium sulfate, microcrystalline cellulose, pharmaceutical glaze, talc, titanium dioxide, magnesium stearate, povidone, poloxamer 188, polyethylene glycol 20000, glycerol monooleate, carnauba wax, *dl*-α-tocopherol, and other ingredients. The tablet formulation shows a significant, albeit small and clinically unimportant, higher trough (C_{min}) value with similar 40 % intraindividual variability. The solution form showed higher C_{max} values and shorter t_{max}, but no difference in AUC or apparent bioavailability (CL/F) [9]. Finally, a randomized controlled trial demonstrated that the two preparations displayed similar efficacy for prophylaxis of acute renal graft rejection episodes and toxicity spectra – therapeutic equivalence [10].

SRL has been impregnated as a 13.7 μm thick polymer in a metallic scaffold cardiac stent of 140 μm thickness, which has been approved by the Food and Drug Administration (FDA) for insertion into angioplastied coronary arteries bearing lesions of <28 mm (Cypher, Cordis, Miami, FL). SRL has also been formulated as a microemulsion for treatment of inflammatory disorders of the ocular surface, but not those that require drug permeation [11]. Incorporation of the drug (10 % w/w) into polyethylene-glycol-block-poly (ε-caprolactone) microparticle micelles reportedly increases its distribution into plasma as well as enhances its permeability into and retention by tumors in experimental animals [12].

The compositions of the tablet and iv formulations of EVL were not presented in detail at the time of this writing, presumably because the drug was subsequently approved by the FDA. In initial studies, a gelatin capsule at a dosing strength of 0.25 mg was employed; the more recent tablet formulations of 0.25, 1.5, and 10 mg were shown to deliver dose-proportionate exposure in stable renal transplant patients [13]. Kovarik *et al.* [14] described a third formulation, a dispersible tablet in dose strengths of 0.1 and 0.25 mg, which was specifically formulated for the pediatric population. When tested in healthy subjects, the C_{max}, which occurred at 1 h, was 24 % lower than that achieved by the tablet formulation with a similar, approximately 37 % inter-individual variability. For half of the subjects, the AUC was similar for both formulations. There was a prominent food effect of fatty meals on this formulation, producing a 2.5 h delay in t_{max}, a 50 % decrease in C_{max}, and a 16 % reduced AUC. Steady state was reached on or before day 5. EVL has been impregnated into metallic CoCr stents of 81 µm thickness as a fluorinated copolymer of 7.8 µm (Xience, Abbott, N. Chicago, IL).

Quantitation

The most favorable medium for drug quantitation is whole blood collected into tubes with ethylenediaminetetraacetic acid (EDTA) as the anticoagulant.

Owing to complex interactions with other substances, SRL and its analogs are difficult to quantify in patient whole blood, requiring tedious procedures for sample clean-up, such as liquid or solid methods (Table 17.1).

Exploiting the modest ultraviolet (UV) absorption of SRL, Napoli and Kahan [16] introduced a high-pressure liquid chromatography (HPLC) method based on detection at 278 nm. The technique employed an isocratic mobile phase on two C8 analytical columns after ether liquid–liquid extraction and a hexane wash; des-methylsirolimus was the internal standard. This method showed interday coefficient of variation (CV) values for imprecision no greater than 8.9 % and intra-day values of 3.2 % with a sensitivity of 2 ng/mL. It was refined using the combination of

Table 17.1 Historical development and specifications of LC–UV, LC–MS, LC–MS/MS, and LC/LC–MS assays.

Technique	Linear range (ng/mL)	LOD[a] (ng/mL)	LOQ[b] (ng/mL)	Intra-assay %CV[c]	Inter-assay %CV
LC–UV	0–250	0.5	NR[d]	8.1 % (at 10 ng/mL) 1.9 % (at 50 ng/mL)	14.4 % (at 10 ng/mL) 9.8 % (at 50 ng/mL)
LC–UV	2–100	NR	2	6.4 % (at 3 ng/mL) 4.2 % (at 75 ng/mL)	7.8 % (at 3 ng/mL) 5.6 % (at 75 ng/mL)
LC–UV	1–50	NR	1	NR	11.0 % (at 4 ng/mL) 13.0 % (at 32 ng/mL)
LC–MS (ESI)[e]	0.25–500	25 pg	250 pg	15.4 % (at 1 ng/mL) 11.6 % (at 250 ng/mL)	19.5 % (at 1 ng/mL) 13.0 % (at 250 ng/mL)
LC–UV	1–50	0.4	NR	NR	9.8 % (at 5 ng/mL) 5.6 % (at 40 ng/mL)
LC–UV	NR	NR	6.5	<6.0 % (15–227 ng/mL)	<8.0 % (15–227 ng/mL)
LC–MS (ESI)	0.25–50	NR	0.25	NR	6.6–8.2 %
LC–MS/MS (ESI)	0.2–100	0.2	NR	10.3 % (at 0.2 ng/mL) 9.2 % (at 50 ng/mL)	2.7 % (at 0.2 ng/mL) 2.7 % (at 100 ng/mL)
LC–MS (ESI)	0.4–100	NR	0.4	4.6 % (at 5 ng/mL) 3.2 (at 100 ng/mL)	9.5 % (at 5 ng/mL) 7.8 % (at 100 ng/mL)
LC/-LC–MS	0.25–100	NR	0.25	NR	<10.0 % (>1 ng/mL)

Modified from Mahalati and Kahan [15], which contains each reference citation.
[a] Limit of detection.
[b] Limit of quantitation.
[c] Percentage coefficient of variation.
[d] Not reported.
[e] ESI: electrospray ionization.

C18 microbore columns, detection at 277 nm and a β-estradiol-3-methyl ether standard [17], which became the standard technique for this type of assay.

A more sensitive, high throughput, electrospray ionization (ESI) HPLC–tandem mass spectrophotometry (HPLC–MS/MS) technique was used initially to quantify SRL (TexMS; Houston, TX [18]). Butyl chloride extraction was followed by C18 chromatography and ionization with MS/MS detection.

A column-switching technique for extraction and sample clean-up followed by backflush onto the analytical HPLC column in tandem with MS/MS was developed for SRL by Christians *et al.* [19], for EVL by Vidal *et al.* [20], and for zotarolimus by Zhang *et al.* [21].

However, HPLC–MS/MS methods have intrinsic complexities of the instrumentation, demand extreme technical expertise, and require a chemical standard displaying similar ionization efficiency during the transfer of the analyte from the liquid to the gas phase as the parent compound. A major advance has been the simultaneous determination of SRL and cyclosporine (CsA) or TRL concentrations in pre-dose whole blood samples using HPLC–MS/MS methodologies [22, 23].

Immunoassays have gained widespread acceptance in the transplant community owing to their automated platforms and minimal requirements for technical expertise. The microparticle enzyme immunoassay (MEIA) on an iMx analyzer (Abbott; N. Chicago, IL) utilizes a whole blood sample, which is manually pretreated with a precipitation reagent followed by transfer of the supernate to the analysis well together with anti-sirolimus antibody-coated microparticles and an SRL/alkaline phosphatase conjugate. The result of the competition between drug in the patient sample and the drug conjugate is evaluated using a 4-methylumbelliferyl phosphate substrate that quantitates the fluorescent product. The lower limit of quantitation is 3.0 ng/mL, the imprecision is 11 %, and the analysis recovery is 94.2 %. Owing to cross-reactivity of the antibody reagent with metabolites, the overestimation has been reported to be as high as 42.5 ± 16.9 % (range: -12.7 ± 122.4 %) [24].

Subsequently, Holt *et al.* [25] characterized the microparticle assay versus HPLC–MS methodology. The former technique showed overall within-assay precision as estimated by percentage CV (%CV) of 8.6 %, with values of 11.0 %, 5.7 %, and 6.3 % at mean SRL concentrations in patient samples of about 5 ng/mL, 10 ng/mL, and 20 ng/mL. The sensitivity was 2 ng/mL. In their experience, there was a 20 % mean positive bias due to cross-reactivity with metabolites. Factors observed to influence the degree of overestimation of SRL by MEIA versus HPLC–MS included drug concentration, hemoglobin, and time post-transplantation.

It is important for the clinician to know the immunoassay platform being employed by the reference laboratory, for one method even showed a negative bias relative to HPLC–MS/MS. The newer Architect platform performs as expected with a positive bias. The clinician must recognize that inter-patient variations mitigate against the use of uniform conversion factors to evaluate results from various assays. While these variabilities seem daunting, automated methods have been useful for clinical practice provided that physicians establish therapeutic targets based on their in-center results and assure uniformity of measurement techniques.

Mechanism of action

Mammalian target of rapamycin (mTOR): chemistry and biology

mTOR, a 289 kDa evolutionarily conserved, atypical serine–threonine kinase, acts as a central node integrating information critical for cell growth proliferation, survival, and metabolism: ribosomal biogenesis, protein synthesis, gene transcription, mRNA turnover, vesicular trafficking, cytoskeletal organization, and autophagy. The mTOR cascade regulates 160 proteins, many of which are nuclear factors changing gene expression [26].

The structure of mTOR includes a C-terminal sequence (FATC), a regulatory domain (RD) upon which protein kinase B (Akt) acts, the catalytic domain, the FKBP12 binding domain (FKB), the FAT toxic domain scaffold, and the HEAT

(a)

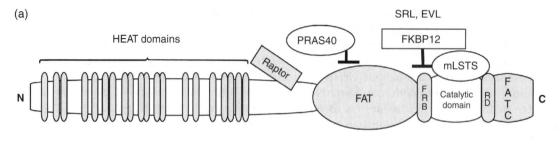

(b)

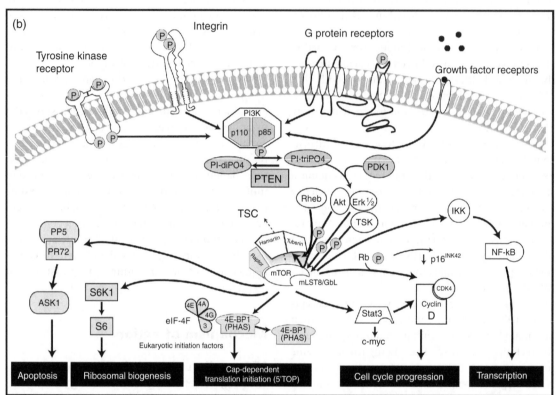

Figure 17.2 Mammalian target of rapamycin (mTOR). (a) Schematic structure of the kinase. HEAT: Huntington elongation factor 1A protein phosphatase 2A-TOR; FKB: FKBP12 binding domain; RD: regulatory domain; FATC: FAT C-terminal sequence; RAPTOR: regulator-associated protein; mLSTS: G protein β subunit protein. (b) Central role of mTOR in cellular responses. mTOR: mammalian target of rapamycin; IRS: insulin receptor substrate; PI3K: phosphinositol 3'-kinase; PTEN: phosphatase and tensin homolog; Akt: protein kinase B; IκK: inhibitory factor κ kinase; NFKB: nuclear factor KB; Raptor: regulatory associated protein of mTOR; GβL: G protein β-subunit-like protein; Cdk: cyclin-dependent kinase; PRB: phosphorylated retinoblastoma protein; eIF: eukaryotic initiation factor 4; PHAS: 4E-BP1, factor 4E-binding protein 1; S6k1: p70 ribosomal S6 kinase; Rheb: Ras-GTP binding protein homolog enriched in brain; 5'TOP: 5'terminal oligopyrimidine tract.

region (Huntington elongation factor 1A protein phosphatase 2A-TOR), which bears antiparallel α-helices that facilitate protein–protein interactions (Figure 17.2a). mTOR exists intracellularly as a large multiprotein complex (1.5–2.0 MDa): the rapamycin-sensitive regulatory complex TorC-1. It consists of mTOR, G protein beta subunit protein (mL ST8), a regulator-associated protein

(Raptor) as well as tuberous sclerosis complex (TSC), two inhibitory proteins which are dissociated upon activation of the small, G protein, Ras homolog enriched in brain (Rheb) that serves as a rheostat of mTOR. At the plasma membrane (its presumed location), Rheb also acts (as do other GTPases) to induce endocytosis and glucose import. In contrast, TSC, which is formed by the tuberous sclerosis proteins hamartin and tuberin, acts as a major inhibitor of mTOR (Figure 17.2b). Other pathways regulating mTOR are presently under extensive study.

ToRc1 has multiple downstream actions: it phosphorylates S6 kinase 1, for ribosomal biogenesis [27]; dissociates 4 elongation factor (4EF-4F)/4E binding protein 1 (4EBP1), which initiates protein translation of mRNAs bearing 5′ terminal oligopyrimidine tracts (5′TOP) [28]; and activates cyclin-dependent kinases hyper-phosphorylating retinoblastoma protein, which promotes gene transcription in addition to augmenting c-myc and cyclin D synthesis (Figure 17.2b [29]).

The upstream pathways that lead to mTOR include insulin growth factor (IGF)-1, phosphatidyl-inositol-3′ kinase (PI3K), protein kinase B (Akt), extracellular regulated kinase (ERK)1/2, and mitogen-activated kinase (MAPK) cascades. Receptor, integrin, and growth factor signals increase phosphatidyl-inositol phosphate (PIP)-3,4,5 levels via the activity of PI3K, recruiting pleckstrin homology phosphoinositide-dependent protein kinase (PDK1) to phosphorylate Akt. Akt together with p90 ribosomal S6 kinase 1 (rsk1) and the MAPK signaling molecules Erk1/2 block the normal inhibitory actions of TSC by phosphorylating distinct sites on mTOR.

An antagonistic pathway, which reverses the generation of phosphatidyl-inositol tri-phosphate (PIP$_3$) is regulated by the dual protein–lipid phosphatase and tensin homolog (PTEN). This enzyme has been shown to be inactivated or deleted in several advanced human cancers due to effects of the Ras oncogene, or to spontaneously activated receptor tyrosine kinase pathways, or to aberrant PI3K signaling, which thereby elevates Akt kinase activity, producing uncontrolled phosphorylation of downstream cascades.

Another negative feedback control loop on mTOR activity is provided by S6k1, which reduces the expression of insulin receptor substrate (IRS-1) and suppresses PI3K and Akt activation. This negative loop is augmented by forkhead box subfamily O (FoxO) transcription factors, which bind directly to TSC and thereby block the activities of Akt and Rheb [26].

Among the actions relevant to transplantation, mTOR serves as the downstream effector of epithelial–mesenchymal transitions which are generally recognized to be initiated and maintained by transforming growth factor-beta (TGFβ). Furthermore, mTOR has recently been shown to have multifunctional roles in innate immunity; namely, a critical role via PI3K and Akt in cascades downstream from Toll receptor ligands [30].

Actions of SRL on mTOR

Relatively few contacts link the intracellular peptide immunophilin FKBP12 to SRL, which shows a similar conformation to free drug; but this binding is essential for the drug to associate with mTOR. SRL C8–C27, which serves as the FKBP12 "binding domain," involves an association of Ileu-56 with the C23 carbonyl, of Tyr-82 hydroxyl with the C16 carbonyl, and of Asp-37 COOH with the C14 hydroxyl group. The "effector" region of SRL binding to mTOR includes the solvent-exposed C28–C36 as well as the triene subunit.

The association of SRL with mTOR inhibits protein translation by reducing P70S6k and 4E-BP1 activation of mRNAs with 5′TOP. Further, it blocks phosphorylation and signaling by the 70 kDa S6 protein kinase, but does not affect the rsk-encoded S6 or mitogen-activated kinase [27]. In addition, cell cycle progression from G$_1$ to S is blocked by reduced translation of cyclin-D1, inhibited p27 activation, and decreased retinoblastoma protein (Rb) phosphorylation. SRL blocks IL-2R-dependent signaling of the anti-apoptotic factor bcl-2, but not of c-fos, c-jun, or c-myc genes [29]. Additional effects include blunting production of pro-angiogenic vascular endothelial growth factor and its vascular endothelial cell growth factor 2 (Flk/KDR) receptor on vascular endothelial cells.

In addition to effects on the G_1 build-up during T cell activation, SRL interrupts CD28 costimulation signaling due to blockade of the downregulation of inhibitor kappa B alpha (IκBα), thereby interrupting generation of c-Rel, a transcriptional regulator of lymphokine and lymphokine receptor genes [31].

On a cellular level, SRL, on the one hand, inhibits differentiation of pro-inflammatory Th17 cells; on the other hand, it promotes TGFβ-induced emergence of regulatory CD4+CD25+FoxP3 T cells (Tregs) [32]. These beneficial effects of SRL on Tregs are the opposite of the inhibitory actions produced by calcineurin inhibitors (CNIs) [33]. Furthermore, at least in experimental animals, SRL favors the emergence of noncytotoxic IgG_{2B} anti-donor antibodies, which may afford an additional layer of protection against rejection phenomena [34].

Pharmacokinetics (PK)

Absorption, distribution, metabolism, and elimination

Absorption

The low (~14%) oral bioavailability of SRL was primarily determined in animal studies. This value is consistent with findings inferred, on the one hand, from a brief single-center pharmacokinetic and clinical study of escalating iv doses of an SRL formulation, which contained a dimethylacetamide vehicle, and, on the other hand, from concentrations measured in stable renal allograft recipients prescribed the liquid oral formulation. The limited bioavailability is probably due to the drug's poor aqueous solubility, sensitivity to gastric acid, only partial intestinal absorption, and prominent first-pass hepatic metabolism. The bioavailability is reduced by approximately one-third when SRL is administered to renal transplant recipients 4 h after rather than concomitant with CsA. The beneficial effects of CsA to enhance bioavailability may be due to SRL interactions with the vehicle in the Neoral microemulsion (but not the Sandimmune oil formulation) or to contributions of CsA per se to inhibit intestinal cytochrome (CYP) P450, and P-glycoprotein (PgP), as well as hepatic CYP pathways [35]. Among normal

volunteers, Zimmerman et al. [36] showed similar effects on SRL PK of concomitant prescription with CsA: the C_{max}, t_{max}, and AUC increased by 116%, 92%, and 230% respectively.

EVL displays similar oral bioavailability as SRL in rats [37], suggesting that water solubility is not the major determinant of absorption. Kovarick et al. [38] also observed that concomitant prescription of CsA increased EVL trough values (C_{min})/dose by about 20%. In contrast, a high-fat meal delayed EVL t_{max} by 1.25 h, decreased C_{max} by 60%, and reduced the AUC by 16% among healthy subjects, whereas it changed the respective values by 1.75 h, 53%, and 26% among renal transplant recipients. They suggested that, to minimize longitudinal variability, the drug should be consistently administered with or without food [39].

Distribution

In whole blood, SRL strongly partitions into erythrocytes (RBCs), cells, and tissues; the RBC:plasma ratio is 36:1, with 94.5% of drug in the former site. In human blood, there is no temperature or concentration dependence on the cellular binding of either SRL or EVL, which is greater than that of either CsA or TRL. The partition may be explained by the high content of immunophilins and lipoproteins in formed elements. Drug metabolites, which are more hydrophilic and presumably display less affinity for FKBPs, tend to partition into RBCs to a lesser extent than the parent compound. Less than 2% of drug, an amount similar to that of CsA, circulates in a free state in plasma; the remainder is bound to other constituents, particularly lipoproteins, which constitute 40% of this fraction. The blood/plasma ratios shown by healthy subjects are similar to those of renal transplant recipients treated with single or multiple doses of SRL as monotherapy; however, they are higher than those of individuals concomitantly prescribed CsA, which presumably relates to the hyperlipidemic effects of CNIs, which increase the amount of associated SRL in plasma.

The lipophilic nature of SRL favors an extensive volume of distribution (Vd: 12.4 L/kg; range: 5.6–16.73 L/kg). Extensive tissue retention is due to drug distribution in cell membranes and in association with the widely distributed multiprotein rapamycin-sensitive regulatory complex TorC1.

In rats, the tissue to blood partition coefficient is greater than 100, explaining the long half-life – up to 87 h – that permits once-daily dosing of SRL, but causes a delay in reaching steady-state concentrations, interferes with the correlation between dose and concentration, produces broad variability of inter- and intra-individual drug content in the whole blood matrix, as well as suggests the benefit of the use of a loading dose de novo after transplantation [40]. While this strategy rapidly achieves immunosuppression, it may enhance the adverse reaction of poor healing of surgical wounds.

Metabolism

Initial studies documented that metabolites accounted for 56% of SRL products in C_{min} blood samples [41,42]. Renal transplant patients chronically treated with CsA display primarily hydroxy-, demethyl-, dihydroxy-, and didemethyl-SRL metabolites. To achieve a more refined analysis, Zimmerman and colleagues [43] studied the metabolism of a single oral dose of 40 mg ^{14}C-radiolabeled drug in six healthy male volunteers (Figure 17.3). The assignment of metabolite structures was aided by high-resolution measurements of fragmented anions using negative-ion fast-atom bombardment (FAB)-MS and positive lithiated ions as well as by ESI-MS/MS under a negative- or a positive-ion mode. The major metabolites of parent compound (M^+ NH_4^+; m/z 931.7) were didemethyl- (m/z 903.7) and demethyl- (m/z 917.7) forms. In blood, radioactivity was distributed among hydroxydemethyl- or dihydrometabolites comprising 17%; hydroxy- plus didemethyl-, 13%; hydroxy- plus 7-O-demethyl-, 15%; and 41-O-demethyl-, 12%. Plasma contained low levels of unchanged drug, as well as of seco-sirolimus (the macrolide open-ring form), of 41-O-demethyl sirolimus, and of several monohydroxylated metabolites. Although 39-O-dimethyl SRL comprises only 8.14% of the total metabolites, it contributes 86–127% of the cross-reactivity observed in immunoassays. Children have been shown to generally produce the same major metabolites as adult subjects.

An experimental study by Kuhn et al. [44] clustered the 12 or 13 metabolic sites in SRL or EVL respectively into metabolic groups. For example, Groups 1–4 involve hydrocarbon hydroxylation reactions. Group 1 are hydroxyl reactions at C23–C25 and C45–C46 in both drugs. The hydroxylations at carbon atoms C11, C12, and C14 form Group 2 for both SRL and EVL. Group 5 are O-dealkylation at the cyclohexyl ring of SRL and EVL.

Multiple CYP isoforms have been implicated in SRL biotransformation, including 3A4, 3A5, and 3A9, and, to a minor extent, 2C8 [45]. CYP3A4 conversion of SRL was documented by correlation with nifedipine oxidation, inhibition by triacetyloleandomycin, gestodene, or preincubation with specific antibodies [46]. Analysis of metabolite profiles suggested the ontogeny of CYP2C8 expression during development, based upon the age dependence of generation of piperidine-hydroxyl SRL [47,48]. The apparent oral clearance of SRL correlates with CYP3A5*1/*3 polymorphisms: nonexpressors show lower values (*3/*3 genotype: 14.1 L/h) than expressor genotypes (*1/*3 and *1/*1: 28.3 L/h) [49].

Employing small intestinal microsomes or intestinal mucosa in Ussing chambers, Lampen et al. [50] confirmed that intestinal CYP3A enzymes were responsible for drug metabolism at this site. They observed that greater than 99% of metabolites were actively counter-transported into the lumen. There was an eightfold inter-individual variability of intestinal metabolite formation among 14 patients.

SRL inhibits the action of the multidrug efflux pump PgP 100-fold more weakly than CsA or TRL. The Watkins group [51] showed that secretion of SRL, Seco-SRL, and dihydro-SRL by CYP3A4-expressing Caco-2 cell monolayers was inhibited by zosuquidar trihydrochloride, a PgP blocker.

The major metabolite of EVL, a monohydroxyl form, shows an AUC nearly half of that of the parent compound. The overall content of EVL metabolites is threefold lower than that of SRL presumably due to the presence of the hydroxyethyl group [52]. For example, the generation of 39-O-demethylation is slowed by a factor of about 15-fold in EVL biotransformation, probably because 39-O-demethylation, which involves initial H

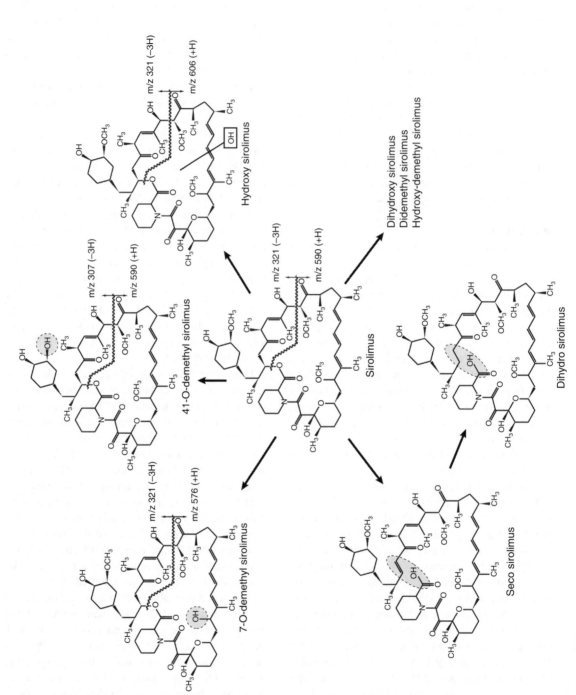

Figure 17.3 Metabolic pathways of sirolimus metabolism. Reprinted with permission from Leung *et al.* [43].

abstraction at C52 (k: 254 pmol mg^{-1} L^{-1} min) is almost completely blocked in EVL.

Overall, the immunosuppressive potency of SRL metabolites appears to be several-fold lower than that of parent compound [41].

Elimination

Zimmerman's team [43] showed that the majority of administered radioactive SRL (91.0±18.0%) was recovered from feces, presumably representing the contribution of biliary secretion and intestinal metabolism, since there was little unchanged drug. Only 2.2±0.9% of administered radioactivity was in urine. In a variety of studies, the elimination $t_{1/2}$ values were approximately 60h (range: 35–95h) and oral CL=6.93 mL/(min kg). Kaplan *et al.* [53] observed that patients who displayed high CsA clearance values on paired iv and oral PK profiles pretransplantation displayed significantly lower mean post-transplant SRL C_{min} values, documenting the impact of inter-individual differences in CYP and PgP on SRL PK.

Subjects with mild (Child-Pugh A, $n=13$) or moderate (Child-Pugh B, $n=5$) hepatic impairment showed decreased oral dose clearance; namely, −31.8% and −36.0% respectively. Severe hepatic impairment (Child-Pugh C) produced an even greater decrease in CL/F to −67% with a 210% increase in AUC [54].

Drug PK

Parameter values

A study of ascending doses of 0.5–6.5 mg/m^2 per 12h of SRL in the liquid formulation in 40 stable renal transplant patients receiving maintenance CsA+prednisone (Pred) treatment showed dose-proportionate exposure with a four- to five-fold intersubject variability. Using an HPLC–MS method, the analysis showed a modest correlation ($r=0.59$) between SRL dose and C_{max} or AUC concentrations, but a good correlation ($r=0.85$) between C_{min} and AUC [18]. A subsequent cohort of patients who were treated chronically with SRL–CsA–Pred revealed a 40% inter-individual variability and confirmed a poor correlation of dose to C_{min} or AUC ($r=0.11$ and $r=0.56$ respectively), but a good one between C_{min} and AUC ($r=0.89$) [40].

Drug disposition was later examined among subjects treated with SRL in the absence of CsA. Brattstrom *et al.* [55] administered single oral doses (0.3–8 mg/m^2) of SRL to healthy male volunteers revealing dose proportionalities of AUC and C_{max} with $t_{1/2}$ of 82±12h, CL/F of 278±117 mL/(h kg), and Vss/F of 23±10 L/kg. The pharmacokinetic curves after oral SRL administration showed a multicompartment distribution with two or three exponential phases of decay from peak concentrations. The PK parameters over the range of therapeutic doses did not show dose dependence. Some of these subjects were included in the summary by Jusko's group [56] of SRL pharmacokinetics among three populations of normal subjects from Germany, the UK, and Sweden. The 36 patients each received single oral doses of 3, 5, 10 or 15 mg/m^2. Bi-exponential fitting procedures were used to examine data generated by an HPLC–MS method. A nonlinear mixed effect model showed a superior fit to the data. In these normal subjects, the blood/plasma ratio (CV) was 30.9 (48.5%), the terminal half-life was 63h (27.5%), and the apparent oral clearance was 8.9 L/h (38.2%). SRL absorption showed a lag time of 0.27h (35.1%) and a k_a of 2.77h (48.4%; Table 17.2).

Table 17.2 Volunteers treated with sirolimus alone: mean population parameter estimates obtained with the standard two-stage (PCNONLIN) and the nonlinear mixed-effect model (P-Pharm, NMEM) methods, with the use of the bi-exponential function.

Sirolimus parameters	Two-stage method		NMEM method	
	Mean	Interpatient variability (%CV)	Mean	Interpatient variability (%CV)
α (h^{-1})	0.44	63.1	0.28	25.1
β (h^{-1})	0.013	30.1	0.011	27.5
k_a (h^{-1})	6.50	93.0	2.77	48.4
t_{tag} (h)	0.29	51.7	0.27	35.1
B/P ratio	34.4	51.2	30.9	48.5

Modified from Ferron *et al.* [56] and used with permission. α: distribution slope; β: elimination slope; κ_a: absorption rate constant; τ_{tag}: lag time; B/P ratio: blood/plasma ratio.

Table 17.3 EVL pharmacokinetics when prescribed in combination with CsA.

Parameter	EVL dose					
	0.75 mg bid			1.5 mg bid		
	Month 2	Month 3	Month 6	Month 2	Month 3	Month 6
N	116	112	99	122	114	96
C_{min} (ng/mL)	4.6±2.1	4.7±2.4	4.6±2.0	7.5±3.5	8.0±4.3	8.2±4.1
t_{max} (h)	2 (1–5)	2 (1–12)	1 (1–5)	1 (1–5)	1 (1–5)	1 (1–5)
C_{max} (ng/mL)	11.0±4.5	11.2±4.7	10.7±4.3	19.8±7.5	21.0±8.9	21.1±8.9
AUC (ng h/mL)	76±31	78±35	76±31	131±51	137±67	138±55
C_{avg} (ng/mL)	6.3±2.6	6.5±2.9	6.3±2.6	10.9±4.3	11.4±5.6	11.5±4.6
PTF (%)	117±49	114±40	106±37	126±47	131±58	123±51

Reprinted with permission from Kovarik *et al.* [38].
Results are mean values plus/minus standard deviations except for t_{max}, which are medians (ranges). N: number of patients at each visit; C_{min}: trough concentration; t_{max}: time to reach peak exposure; C_{max}: peak exposure; AUC: area under the curve over the dosing interval; C_{avg}: average concentration; PTF: peak–trough fluctuation.

A PK analysis of a group of 22 adult renal transplant recipients treated with an SRL–MMF combination also used the nonlinear mixed effects model (NONMEM). The best correlation, which was observed with a two-compartment open model, revealed first-order elimination to describe the transfer rate constant and Erlang distribution for the apparent volumes of the central and peripheral compartments; namely, mean estimates of 5.25 h, 218 L and 292 L, respectively [49].

Kaplan *et al.* [57] explored limited sampling strategies to estimate SRL AUC. Concentrations measured at 0, 2, and 6 h showed an 85.7% prediction efficacy ($r^2 = 0.98$). Later, Cattaneo *et al.* [58], using two time points within the first 4 h after SRL dosing, reported a robust correlation with body weight and surface area.

Kovarick *et al.* [38] analyzed EVL pharmacokinetics among renal transplant patients treated de novo in combination with CsA and Pred. The C_{min} values were 19–34% lower in the first month compared with months 2–6. The AUC was dose proportionate and stable over time at the two dose levels of 1.5 mg/day and 3.0 mg/day, namely, 77±32 ng/(h mL) and 136±5 ng/(h mL) respectively. Within- and between-patient variability in AUC values were 27% and 31% respectively (Table 17.3).

Using EVL population pharmacokinetics to describe drug disposition in 673 renal transplant patents concomitantly treated with CsA and Pred, they calculated that, for a 44-year-old 71 kg Caucasian man, the absorption rate constant would be 6.07/h, the apparent clearance 8.8 L/h, and the apparent central distribution 11 L. The intraindividual CV for CL was 27% and for Vd it was 31%. Using a nonlinear mixed effects model (NONMEM Version V), the population absorption $t_{1/2}$ was 0.11/h, consistent with a t_{max} at 1–2 h post dose. There was a modest underproportionality in exposure by 10% at the 3.0 mg versus the 1.5 mg daily dose. Studying EVL PK in 731 patients over a 6 month interval, this group [59] showed a 20% underproportionality of C_{min} between subjects prescribed 0.75 versus 1.5 mg/day, but a dose-proportionate AUC.

Impact of demographic features
Ethnicity
In an initial study in stable renal transplant patients wherein SRL was added to a CsA–Pred regimen, black subjects showed greater CL_{po} and t_{max} values, reflecting a reduced rate of absorption and an increased rate of elimination, suggesting the need for larger drug doses [18], an hypothesis which was

supported by the US multicenter trial [59]. However, a subsequent study of 150 renal allograft patients chronically treated with SRL–CsA–Pred failed to observe consistent correlations of observed or dose-adjusted C_{max}, C_{min}, or AUC PK parameters of SRL with ethnicity, gender, age, or body weight, possibly due to the high %CVs of 42.4–82.0% [40]. The higher SRL dose requirement of black patients presumably relates to pharmacodynamic resistance to immunosuppression.

While there were no differences in EVL AUC based on gender, age, or weight, the values were 20% lower among blacks [38]. Lorber *et al.* [60] observed that EVL outcomes showed moderate adverse effects of low C_{min} values among African American subjects (1.7-fold; $p<0.02$) and among all patients experiencing delayed graft function (DGF; 1.5-fold; $p=0.014$).

Pediatric patients

Among stable pediatric renal transplant recipients treated with SRL plus MMF (but no CNI), Schachter *et al.* [61] documented that children also displayed greater apparent SRL clearances, suggesting the need for twice-daily dosing and for rapid adjustments of the administered amount (at least initially), since this property seemed to decrease over time. Furthermore, children show a reduced $t_{1/2}$ of 9.7h (range: 7.1–24.6h) at month 1 and 9.6h (range: 5–17.58h) at month 3. SRL C_{min} correlated with AUC ($r^2=0.84$). There was no relationship between SRL and mycophenolic acid AUC values ($r^2=0.04$). In contrast, the apparent clearance of EVL in children may be similar to or even lower than that of adults [62].

Drug–drug interactions
CNIs

CsA to a much greater extent than TRL decreases the apparent clearance of SRL and EVL, probably related to its more potent effects to block cytochrome P450 isoenzymes. Seeking to minimize this interaction, SRL was administered 4h after CsA in the pivotal trials (spaced); however, simultaneous dosing, which is preferred by patients, shows greater, albeit more variable, concentrations due to the mutual capacity of the two drugs to increase the other's concentration (vide supra).

Furthermore, a study in rats revealed that concomitant administration of CsA and SRL produced large, dose-dependent increases in CsA content in hepatic and renal tissues, which were disproportionately greater than those in blood. CsA exerted a similar, albeit less profound, effect on SRL tissue content [63]. Despite these pharmacokinetic interactions, a detailed matrix of whole blood concentration-outcome results evaluated by median effect analysis documented pharmacodynamic synergy in a rat transplantation model [64].

Hariharan *et al.* [65] observed a 30% decrease in TRL exposure (C_{min} and AUC) when that immunosuppressant was prescribed in combination with SRL, suggesting an underlying saturable mechanism in the drug interaction, possibly FKBP12. Kuypers *et al.* [66] examined the PK parameters among a small set of patients treated with SRL–TRL de novo. They observed a good correlation of SRL C_{min} and AUC with an effect of TRL to reduce SRL absorption de novo. In contrast to CsA, SRL reduced the correlation of TRL C_{min} and AUC by 22±0.73%. The PK changes were more pronounced for recipients on a reduced dose of TRL plus a higher dose of SRL than for those on a low dose of SRL in combination with a standard dose of TRL. The latter cohort required greater SRL doses to maintain constant drug exposure (Table 17.4).

In contrast, mean EVL C_{min} values observed serially during 1.5mg/day treatment seemed to show no difference whether the drug was co-administered with CsA, using C_{min} values targeted at months 1–2 versus months 3–6 at 185±121ng/mL versus 144±69ng/mL respectively among a full dose or 107±70ng/mL versus 85±48ng/mL respectively among a reduced-dose cohort [67]. However, owing to the extensive overlap of concentrations, this conclusion cannot be regarded as robust. TRL shows little impact on EVL exposure, nor does EVL display an effect on TRL [68].

Mycophenolic acid analogs and steroids

Low doses of SRL failed to affect MMF exposure [69]. Indeed, co-administration of SRL engenders higher exposure to mycophenolic acid than CsA treatment, owing to the profound effects of this CNI to alter hepatic metabolism and biliary

Table 17.4 EVL pharmacokinetics when prescribed in combination with TRL.

Parameter	Baseline (full-dose TRL without EVL)	Period 1 (full-dose TRL with EVL)	Period 2 (reduced-dose TRL with EVL)
TRL			
C_0 (ng/mL)	7.9±3.9	8.4±4.0	4.0±1.7
t_{max} (h)	2 (1–2)	2 (1–5)	2 (1–2)
C_{max} (ng/mL)	17.7±6.3	16.5±9.6	10.4±4.8
AUC (ng h/mL)	132±56	134±70	72±28
PTF (%)	92±56	69±30	99±30
EVL			
C_0 (ng/mL)	—	3.3±1.2	3.0±1.1
t_{max} (h)	—	1 (1–2)	1 (1–5)
C_{max} (ng/mL)	—	10.4±5.1	8.2±1.3
AUC (ng h/mL)	—	58±2.0	49±10
PTF (%)	—	139±38	133±44

Reprinted with permission from Kuypers *et al.* [66].
Values are mean plus/minus standard deviations except for t_{max}, which are medians (ranges). C_0: trough concentration; t_{max}: time to peak concentration; C_{max}: peak concentration; AUC: area under the concentration-time curve over the dose interval; PTF: peak–trough fluctuation.

secretion. Routine clinical monitoring of renal transplant patients treated with SRL, MMF, and steroid showed CL/F values of SRL of 12.5 L/h that were inversely related to age, but not bilirubin, time after renal transplantation, albumin, weight, gender, or hematocrit (Table 17.5) [49]. Dansirikul *et al.* [70] explored a two-compartment model to analyze SRL C_{min} concentrations using Bayesian forecasting models with whole blood sampling times of 0, 1, and 3 h. They were able to predict the AUC with a −2.1 % bias (−22.2 to +25.9 %).

A study of 40 stable patients to whom SRL was added to a CsA–Pred regimen revealed only a slight effect to decrease prednisolone elimination [71].

Other drugs

Interactions have been documented with other CYP 450 3A substrates: ketoconazole and diltiazem to increase SRL concentrations versus rifampicin, nifedipine, and possibly St. John's wort to decrease SRL concentrations [23].

Kovarik *et al.* [72] employed an open-label, randomized, crossover design in 24 healthy male volunteers who received 2 mg EVL without or with 20 mg atorvastatin or 20 mg pravastatin. On the one hand, the concomitant therapies reduced EVL C_{max} by 9 % and 10 % as well as AUC by 5 % and 6 % respectively. On the other hand, EVL increased atorvastatin C_{max} by 11 % with no effect on AUC, and decreased pravastatin values by 10 % and 5 % respectively. Patients concomitantly receiving erythromycin or azithromycin displayed 19 % reduced EVL clearance. There was no effect of calcium channel blockers, dihydropyridines, diltiazem, verapamil, quinolones, or trimethoprim-sulfamethoxazole on EVL concentrations. Using a CYP inhibitory classification system based on the fold-increase in EVL AUC by a drug, Kovarik *et al.* [73] classified ketoconazole as strong (≥ 5), erythromycin, verapamil, and CsA as moderate (>2), and atorvastatin as weak (≤ 2).

Pharmacodynamic assays

In a preliminary study, extracts of peripheral blood mononuclear cells from SRL–CsA–Pred-treated patients were assayed for inhibition of S6 kinase

Table 17.5 Sirolimus pharmacokinetic parameters, inter-individual variability (IIV) and inter-occasion variability (IOV) (covariate-free models)among patients simultaneously treated with mycophenolate mofetil and steroid.

Parameter	Population mean		IIV		IOV	
	Estimate	SE	Estimate (%)	95 % CI	Estimate (%)	95 % CI
Covariate-free model where each profile is regarded as belonging to a different individual[a]						
k_{tr} (h⁻¹)	5.26	0.26	43	37, 48		
Q/F (L/h)	38.2	5.66	75	31, 103		
V_1/F (L)	219	15.4	53	39, 64		
V_2/F (L)	273	28.5	11.5	0, 44		
CL/F (L/h)	15.9	1.3	58.1	44, 70		
Covariate-free model with IOV[b]						
k_{tr} (h⁻¹)	5.18	0.58	4.5E-05	0, 23	42.5	27.5, 53.5
Q/F (L/h)	38.2	18.9	84	0, 147		
V_1/F (L)	211	42.1	23.6	0, 75	45.9	18.7, 62.2
V_2/F (L)	306	75.5	43.47	0, 105		
CL/F (L/h)	17	3.5	47.9	0, 109	32.5	17.5, 42.6

Modified from Djebli et al. [49] and used with permission.

CL/F: apparent oral clearance; k_{tr}: transfer rate constant; Q/F: intercompartment rate constant; SE: standard error; CI: confidence interval; V_1/F: apparent volume of the central compartment after oral administration; V_2/F: apparent volume of the peripheral compartment after oral administration.

[a]Objective function value 4328 (proportional error: 5.7 %; additive error: 3.1 µg/L).

[b]Objective function value 4293 (proportional error: 5.1 %; additive error: 3.3 µg/L).

activity due to SRL blockade of mTOR using the index of incorporation of gamma ³²P-ATP into proteins [74]. More recently, Tanaka et al. [75] examined pharmacodynamic effects of EVL to inhibit S6k1 activity in peripheral blood mononuclear cells of cancer patients. A radioreceptor assay has been reported to be a pharmacodynamic test. A solid-phase system was employed to measure the competition between tritiated-dihydroFK506 and SRL to bind immunophilins isolated from immune cells [76–78].

Clinical effects

Immunosuppressive efficacy

A Phase II dose-escalation trial [79] documented the efficacy of SRL when prescribed in combination with CsA and steroid to reduce the 1 year rate of acute rejection episodes (AREs) among renal transplant recipients to 7 %. Using full therapeutic doses of CsA and Pred in combination with SRL versus

Aza [59] or versus placebo [80], two Phase III blinded pivotal randomized controlled trials (RCTs) demonstrated superior prophylaxis of ARE to a 14 % rate versus 25 % or 30 %. The benefit was durable at 2 years [81]. Using median effect analyses, synergistic immunosuppressive interactions between SRL and CsA were documented in a series of in vitro [82] and in vivo [83] studies in experimental animals, as well as from the whole blood concentrations derived from the 1295 patients in the pivotal Phase III trials [84]. Thus, in 1999, SRL was FDA approved for de novo treatment of renal transplant recipients in combination with CsA. Two subsequent Phase II open-label, multicenter, concentration-controlled clinical studies reported that patients treated with combinations of SRL and TRL rather than CsA showed 10 % rates of AREs within 6 months [85,86], suggesting that similar benefits could be achieved with this CNI.

Three strategies have sought to overcome the inferior renal function among patients treated with CsA–SRL combinations in the pivotal RCT. First, the possibility that a TRL–SRL regimen would mitigate the renal dysfunction was explored in a Phase IV RCT. However, 1 year estimates of glomerular filtration rates (GFRs) among patients at increased risk for DGF (and consequently impaired long-term function) failed to show any difference between subjects treated with moderately reduced exposures of TRL versus CsA in combination with SRL. Indeed, the TRL group experienced more severe grades of AREs [87]. A second strategy markedly reduces CsA exposure de novo. After a preliminary Phase II RCT showed the benefit of slightly reduced CsA doses [88], a sequential exploration of de novo CsA exposures reduced by 50 %, 66 %, or 80 % revealed an improved GFR at 4 years among a variegated population of renal transplant recipients who were generally high-risk subjects [89]. Although there was little observed benefit of this strategy on graft and patient survivals at 5 years, the improved prediction of the renal function among the 80 % reduced exposure was realized by the 10 year outcomes [90].

A third SRL treatment strategy excludes CNI co-administration entirely. Early de novo studies that coupled SRL with adjunctive Aza or MMF plus steroid showed high 35 % or 28 % rates of AREs respectively [91,92]. In a single-center study of patients at low immunologic risk, the addition of basiliximab induction to an SRL–MMF–Pred regimen benefited renal transplant function compared with a CsA–MMF–Pred regimen [93]. However, subsequent multicenter trials in variegated populations of recipients failed to confirm this finding. One RCT comparing SRL versus CsA [94] in combination with MMF and steroid had to be abandoned due to the excess incidence of AREs. Another experience comparing SRL versus TRL [95] failed to show a benefit of a CNI-free strategy de novo. The failure of the first RCT has been related to most patients in the experimental arm not achieving therapeutic (20–30 ng/mL) concentrations of SRL within the first 6 months. Intensifying the SRL-based immunosuppressive regimen with an induction course using polyclonal antilymphocyte antibody yielded little benefit to reduce the occurrence of AREs among subjects treated with a CNI-free regimen [96].

Alternate uses of SRL include induction treatment together with basiliximab to postpone inception of CNI therapy until resolution of impaired function de novo [97], therapeutic rescue from seemingly irreversible antilymphocyte antibody-resistant AREs [98], and facilitation of early steroid withdrawal at 3–90 days depending on the intensity of the concomitant drug regimen and the perceived rejection risk: for example, a low probability among elderly, non-presensitized Caucasian or Hispanic, or matched living donor versus a high one among black, presensitized, or retransplant recipients [99]. In another setting, Benito et al. [100] observed favorable effects of SRL to treat steroid-refractory acute graft-versus-host disease.

In summary, judicious addition of modest amounts of CsA to an SRL-based regimen de novo minimizes the risk of an ARE among a variegated array of responders [101]. However, de novo SRL therapy must be employed cautiously among patients who are obese or who receive an organ likely to display initial dysfunction. Prudent clinical application restricts a CNI-free, SRL-based therapy de novo to subjects perceived to be weak immune responders.

The observation of impaired kidney transplant function among patients treated de novo and chronically with a CsA–SRL regimen in both pivotal trials led to a Phase IV RCT. The Rapamune Maintenance Regimen (RMR) study compared the courses of subjects who had experienced benign post-transplant courses up to 3 months, the major risk period for an ARE. At this time they either entirely discontinued CsA versus continued with full doses of CsA [102]. The superior renal function among the CNI-discontinued arm documented the efficacy of an SRL–Pred regimen since there was only a slight and insignificant increase in AREs after CNI withdrawal. However, the study has been criticized owing to the known effects of a full-dose regimen to cause renal dysfunction.

The success of the RMR led to a conversion RCT that examined the benefits for patients experiencing graft dysfunction of a switch at 6–130 months post-transplantation from a CNI- to an SRL-based regimen versus continuation of the CNI (generally in combination with MMF and Pred). While patients with measured GFR values of 20–40 mL/min failed to show improvement, those with GFR >40 mL/min showed increases to 62.6 ($n=370$) versus 59.9 mL/min ($n=201$; $p=0.009$), with similar rates of acute rejection episodes (7.8 % versus 6.5 %, respectively). However, subjects in the conversion group displayed significant increases in urinary protein/creatinine ratios [103]. This experience suggested that the conversion strategy may not be safe among patients displaying ≥800 mg/day proteinuria or a GFR ≤40 mL/min [104].

In the Spare the Nephron trial, 100 patients were converted from a CNI to SRL between 1 and 6 months (mean: 117 days) post-transplant, while remaining on MMF and steroid. There was a 26 % improvement in measured GFR among the converted cohort versus 11 % among the CNI maintenance cohort, with similar 7 % incidences of AREs [105]. Thus, conversion from a CNI to SRL may be recommended for subjects experiencing benign clinical courses at 3 months for weak immune responders and possibly after 12 months [106] with caution for stronger responders or patients who had experienced previous reversible AREs.

Unfortunately, the experience with SRL has not been as favorable in transplant settings other than cardiac grafts. Keogh et al. [107] showed reduction in AREs and prevention of coronary artery disease at 2 years using the combination of SRL and CsA with steroid. In liver transplantation, the SRL arm in an RCT showed greater incidences of mortality, graft loss, and hepatic artery thromboses than with CNI treatment. Although a single-center experience with hepatic grafts using an SRL–TRL regimen de novo has been reported to be favorable [108], the FDA issued a black-box warning about prescribing the combination de novo. In lung transplantation, de novo SRL therapy was associated with an excessive rate of bronchial anastomotic dehiscences, which also warranted a black-box warning. However, liver, lung, or cardiac transplant recipients who suffer renal dysfunction, which is usually due to CNI therapy, frequently show significant benefits following conversion to an SRL-based regimen [109, 110], although early conversions were associated with AREs in the Heart Save the Nephron trial.

The development of EVL benefited, but paradoxically suffered, from earlier experiences with SRL. Using an isobologram methodology to analyze experimental animal data, Schuurman et al. [111] reported EVL to display weaker antirejection potency than SRL, but immunosuppressive synergy with CsA. After a preliminary ascending-dose Phase I safety study in stable renal transplant recipients [112] and a Phase II ascending-dose investigation [113], an RCT [114] compared 1.5 or 3 mg of EVL prescribed de novo in divided daily doses (due to the shorter drug half-life than SRL) versus a standard MMF regimen both in conjunction with full doses of CsA plus steroids. Although the 12 month incidences of biopsy-proven AREs (BPARs) were similar, patients in the EVL arm displayed lower mean GFR values: 49.3 mL/min versus 56.9 mL/min respectively.

A series of concentration-controlled RCTs showed EVL C_{min} values of 8–12 ng/mL combined with CsA C_2 of 150–300 ng/mL plus steroids to achieve better death-censored graft survivals than 3–8 ng/mL with CsA C_2 values of 350–500 ng/mL plus steroids, but there were no significant differences in either creatinine clearance or the rate of BPAR [115]. Although these observations were not deemed sufficient by the FDA, the drug was approved by the European Union Registry.

In addition to implementing a rapid tapering of CsA C_2 targets, subsequent trials sought to refine the regimen by the addition of basiliximab induction treatment. This strategy achieved BPAR rates of 14.3 % with improved estimated GFR (eGFR) values of 68 mL/min at 12 months [116,117]. A parallel RCT employing basiliximab induction with EVL (1.5 mg) plus reduced exposure to TRL ($C_0=4$–7 ng/mL) in combination with steroids reported a BPAR rate of 14 % and a mean eGFR of 75 mL/min, suggesting similar effectiveness of TRL as CsA in combination with EVL [118].

The further development of EVL has contrasted with that of SRL. On the one hand, only anecdotal experiences have been reported describing benefits of conversion from a CNI to an EVL-based regimen or from SRL to EVL [119]. On the other hand, EVL has shown considerable benefit in other transplantations. Levy et al. [120] documented the efficacy of an EVL–CNI combination in liver transplantation. Eisen *et al.* [121] demonstrated that addition of EVL versus MMF to a CsA-based regimen reduced the incidences of both BPAR and coronary vascular disease within 2 years after heart transplantation. In 2011, EVL was also approved by the FDA.

Antineoplastic effects

The first evidence of an anticancer effect in transplantation recipients was a retrospective examination of clinical courses of renal transplant patients treated for up to 10 years with SRL in combination with CsA. This analysis demonstrated reduced incidences of post-transplant lymphoproliferative disease (PTLD) or renal cell carcinomas (RCCs) [122, 123]. This observation was confirmed by a retrospective examination of data reported by American transplant centers to the United Network for Organ Sharing (UNOS): there were reduced incidences of nonskin and skin neoplasms among renal transplant patients treated with SRL-based or SRL–CNI regimens compared with those not receiving SRL [124]. Further support for this effect was obtained by subsequent retrospective analyses of the results of Phase II and III outcomes [125]. However, the strongest evidence of a beneficial antineoplastic action of mTOR inhibitors was obtained from the CONVERT RCT. Within 2 years after randomization, 11 % of subjects who continued on CsA versus 3.8 % who were converted to SRL-based maintenance therapy developed a malignancy, an effect particularly evident for skin tumors (7.7 % versus 2.2 %, $p = 0.01$) [126].

The benefits of SRL have been related to its antiproliferative effects as well as to its capacity to block activation pathways via mTOR, particularly those related to idiopathic inactivation of PTEN, as occurs in 50 % of brain, 29 % of metastatic prostate, and some endometrial cancers [127]. Furthermore, SRL has been shown to dampen production of vascular endothelial growth factor (VEGF) and to disrupt signal transduction via its receptor, effects that are critical for tumor vascularization and growth [128].

Among renal transplant patients, SRL treatment has successfully reversed PTLD, and particularly Kaposi sarcoma [129]. Furthermore, a subsequent study showed the benefit of temsirolimus to forestall metastatic RCC among nontransplant patients [130], consistent with observations in an animal model [131] and leading to FDA approval for this indication. Anecdotal experiences have suggested the potential utility of SRL treatment for a variety of other neoplasms in renal and nonrenal transplant recipients.

Mitigation of vasculopathy

Morris *et al.* [132] documented that SRL pretreatment mitigated vascular lesions induced by balloon catheter injury. Subsequently, Ikonen *et al.* [133] noted that SRL stabilized and possibly reversed immuno-obliterative lesions in cardiac allografts as detected by intravascular ultrasound in a subhuman primate model. These findings were confirmed using de novo treatment of cardiac transplant patients with SRL by Mancini *et al.* [134] or EVL by Eisen *et al.* [121]. In addition, Raichlin *et al.* [135] reported beneficial effects of conversion from a CNI to SRL regimen at about 4 years after cardiac transplantation. Intravascular ultrasound measurements showed stabilization of cardiac lesions as opposed to the progression observed among subjects maintained on their previous regimens. The effects on endovascular proliferation were harnessed to control re-stenosis after angioplasty by the development of the Cypher [136] and the Xience cardiac stents impregnated with SRL or EVL respectively. The efficacy of drug-impregnated stents was greater than that of either bare metal [137] or paclitaxel-eluting stents [138]. However, Seitou *et al.* [139] observed a higher incidence and greater serum levels of cardiac biomarkers (troponin-1), creatine kinase isoenzyme MB, and creatine kinase after implantation of the Cypher versus a bare metal stent. Angiogenesis also has been studied in a rabbit corneal model: SRL inhibited cell proliferation and migration as well as expression of VEGF [140]. Although the cardiac findings suggest that mTOR inhibitors exert effects that block the immuno-obliterative reactions that characterize chronic processes mediating graft loss, there is no robust evidence that this drug class retards chronic obliterative processes in human renal transplantation.

Adverse effects of mTOR inhibitors

There is little difference in the spectrum of side effects encountered with SRL versus EVL treatment. The most prominent set of adverse reactions are hyperlipidemias [141]. As opposed to augmented synthesis, SRL impairs catabolism of circulating lipoproteins due to inhibition of the activities of tissue lipases, at least in part due to augmented levels of apolipoprotein C, an inhibitor of these enzymes [142]. While the effect most prominently related to SRL is hypertriglyceridemia, the concomitant hypercholesterolemic reactions are exaggerated by simultaneous combination with a CNI. A head-to-head comparison of SRL in combination with TRL versus CsA showed no significant difference in the degree of hyperlipidemias [87]. Countermeasure therapy using fibrates and statins achieves reasonable control of hypertriglyceridemia and hypercholesterolemia respectively. Indeed, with judicious treatment, human renal transplant patients showed no evidence of an impact of the hyperlipidemia on the occurrence or outcome of cardiac events at least at 4 years [143] and at 10 years [90].

The second major group of adverse reactions relates to inhibition of growth factor signaling, particularly hematopoetic triggers for erythrocyte, leukocyte, and thrombocyte differentiation and proliferation within the bone marrow [144]. Anecdotal experience suggests that erythropoietic and myeloid colony-stimulating factors and IL-11 may be therapeutically useful.

Formulation and possibly compound-based issues can produce gastrointestinal distress, including diarrhea, in a limited subset of subjects. These side effects on the bone marrow and gastrointestinal tract tend to be dose dependent and exacerbated by MMF.

The nature of the renal dysfunction has been explored by two avenues. On the one hand, a study in a rat model showed mutual effects of CsA and of SRL to augment each other's toxicities [145]. This analysis suggested that the effect of SRL to augment CNI nephrotoxicity was apparently due to an increase in intra-renal concentrations. On the other hand, SRL actions to inhibit growth factor signaling and cell proliferation have been cited as a cause of prolongation of DGF. This phenomenon, which was originally reported using an in situ model of native kidneys undergoing an ischemic insult [146], was also observed using a rat renal transplant model [147]. However, both studies employed at least 10-fold supra-therapeutic drug doses. In the clinical arena, delayed resolution of DGF has been particularly observed among subjects concomitantly treated with TRL [148, 149], whereas it was not evident upon retrospective evaluation of patients in the pivotal RCT who received SRL in combination with full doses of CsA, albeit it has been claimed by a single-center study [150].

In the periphery, SRL inhibits actions of fibroblast growth factors, predisposing to defects in wound healing, including bacterial infections and herniae [151]. As yet undefined alterations, presumably in response to cytokine inhibition may cause fluid leakage from injured vascular endothelial barriers, engendering lymphoceles [152] and occasionally diuretic-refractory edema. Less well documented toxicities include an increased frequency of drug-induced type II diabetes mellitus [153] and of an idiopathic, hypoxemic form of interstitial pneumonitis [154], which may be related to the onset of bronchiolitis obliterans organizing pneumonia occasionally observed among cardiac transplant recipients switched from a CNI to SRL [155].

The side effect of proteinuria appears more frequently among patients undergoing conversion from a CNI- to an SRL-based regimen for chronically deteriorating renal function as opposed to those subjects treated de novo with SRL. This toxicity may be at least partially reversible with angiotensin-converting or receptor-blocking agents. While it may partially relate to the absence of CNI-driven afferent arteriolar vasoconstriction, it more likely reflects a blockade of signals necessary to maintain glomerular capillary integrity, for observations among patients treated for pure glomerular immune diseases suggest a distinct primary toxicity of SRL at this site.

Serkova and Christians [156] described a metonomic evaluation of the metabolic effects of supra-therapeutic exposures to SRL versus EVL to exacerbate adverse reactions after 6 days of

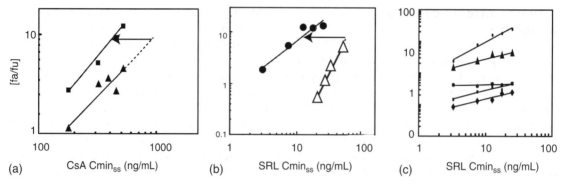

Figure 17.4 Median effect analyses of outcomes of 1295 patients enrolled in pivotal trials. (a) C_{min} of CsA among subjects treated with SRL (closed squares) versus without SRL (closed triangles). (b) Concentrations of SRL among subjects treated in combination with CsA (open dots) versus without it (open triangles), the last data having been derived from a Phase II RCT. (c) The median effect plots of rejection prophylaxis (closed circles) versus the toxicities of hypercholesterolemia (closed triangles), renal function (Nankivell estimates of glomerular filtration rate; closed double diamonds), hypertriglyceridemia (closed rectangles), and thrombocytopenia (closed diamonds). Reprinted with permission from Kahan and Kramer [84].

treatment of rats with 10 mg/kg CsA. The base therapy with the CNI caused significant increases in blood glucose, hydroxybutyrate, creatine, creatinine, trimethylamine N-oxide, and cholesterol, as well as decreases in glutathione. These changes were exacerbated by SRL at a dose of 3 mg/kg, which is 40-fold above the therapeutic amount, but apparently partially mitigated by the same dose of EVL. These findings expanded their previous observations that SRL inhibited cytosolic glycolysis in the brain by increasing the intrinsic dysfunctions caused by CsA. They claimed that these events were dampened by EVL treatment. Exploration of the relevance of these phenomena awaits a study employing drug exposures within the therapeutic range.

SRL treatment engenders an increased incidence of bouts of bacterial and fungal pneumonia [122], possibly related to defective IL-8 actions or to impaired oxidative burst activity [157]. In contrast, despite its enhanced potency, the SRL–CsA combination has been associated with low incidences of BK virus [158] and cytomegalovirus infections [59].

In aggregate, the pleiotropic array of adverse reactions displayed by mTOR inhibitors demonstrates the pivotal role of this kinase in critical pathways of cellular physiology.

Therapeutic drug monitoring: pharmacokinetic/ pharmacodynamic correlations

A median effect analysis linearized concentration-effect data from both Phase III blinded pivotal trials, which included 1295 renal transplant recipients treated with full doses of CsA plus SRL (2 or 5 mg) versus Aza or placebo. SRL concentrations correlated with indicators of efficacy versus toxicity (Figure 17.4) [84]. The model showed that addition of SRL permitted a 2.5-fold decrease in the amount of CsA necessary to render either 50 % or 90 % of recipients free from an ARE (panel A). For the latter metric, CsA C_{min} without SRL extrapolated to 509 ng/mL ($r = 0.906$), but with SRL = 231 ng/mL ($r = 0.956$). Conversely, addition of CsA reduced the C_{min} concentration of SRL that achieved 90 % of patients free of an ARE by fivefold (panel B). The SRL C_{min} to achieve 90 % of recipients free of AREs extrapolated to 61.5 ng/mL ($r = 0.909$) without CsA versus 13.5 ng/mL ($r = 0.957$) with CsA. Furthermore, the analysis revealed a concentration dependence of hypercholesterolemia, hypertriglyceridemia, and thrombocytopenia but not renal dysfunction. Figure 17.5 shows the kinetic–dynamic

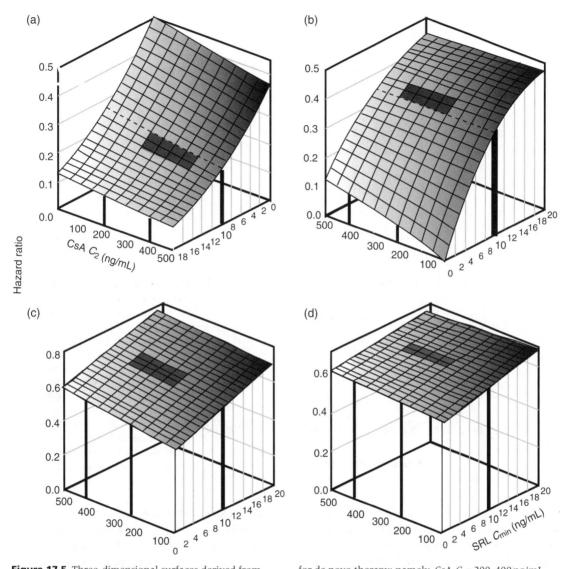

Figure 17.5 Three-dimensional surfaces derived from clinical concentration data showing the hazard ratios of occurrences of clinical events in relation to CsA values at 2 h after dosing (C_2) and SRL C_{min} estimates. The shaded area shows the region of recommended concentrations for de novo therapy; namely, CsA $C_2 = 200$–400 ng/mL and SRL $C_{min} = 10$–12 ng/mL. (a) Prophylaxis of AREs. (b) Nankivell estimates of glomerular filtration < 50 mL/min. (c) Hypercholesterolemia > 240 mg/dL. (d) Hypertriglyceridemia > 250 mg/dL.

outcomes of recipients treated with varying doses of CsA or of SRL. The data yielded the hypothesis that the optimal combination of the drugs de novo that minimizes the occurrence of AREs or renal dysfunction is CsA $C_2 = 200$–400 ng/mL (depending on immune responder status) and SRL

$C_{min} = 10$–12 ng/mL. Receiver operating characteristic functions (Figure 17.6) [40] showed robust correlations of C_{min} and, particularly, AUC values with the occurrence (panel A) and severity of AREs within the first month as well as the risk of graft loss (panel B). In contrast, CsA C_{min}, C_2, or AUC

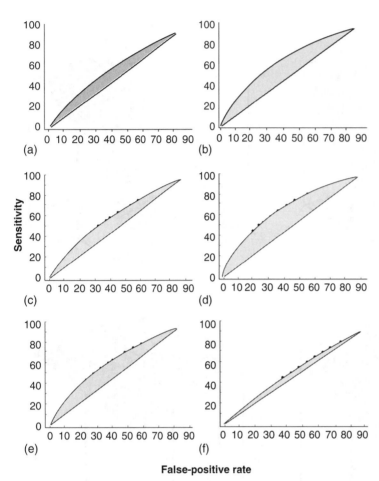

Figure 17.6 Receiver operating characteristic functions that predict occurrence of therapeutic versus toxic effects of SRL. Prediction of an acute rejection episode based upon dose-corrected values of (a) C_{min} and (b) AUC. In contrast, the other sections show the risks of development of (c) thrombocytopenia (<100 000/mm³), (d) leukopenia (<4000/mm³), (e) hypertriglyceridemia (>400 mg/dL), and (f) hypercholesterolemia (>240 mg/dL). Reprinted with permission from Kahan *et al.* [40].

values among patients treated with SRL-based regimens failed to show a significant relationship to these events. For example, the SRL C_{min} levels among patients undergoing Banff 0/1 grade (11.26±7.87 ng/mL) were significantly higher than those among subjects experiencing grade 2/3 acute rejection episodes (4.63±3.68 ng/mL; $p = 0.03$). In addition, the SRL C_{min} values for the presence versus absence of adverse reactions were generally significant: thrombocytopenia (13.7±10.0 versus 9.5±5.5 ng/mL; $p = 0.028$), leukopenia (14.6±9.3 versus 9.2±5.5 ng/mL; $p = 0.008$), hypertriglyceridemia (11.0±7.3 versus 8.4±4.7 ng/mL; $p = 0.04$), but not hypercholesterolemia (13.1±6.8 versus 9.5±5.5 ng/mL). The lack

of an effect on hypercholesterolemia was probably due to the contributions of CsA to the last form of toxicity. The sensitivity, specificity, and predictive values of the receiver operating characteristic analyses are shown in Table 17.6. The recommendations for SRL target concentrations from a variety of studies as updated from the summary by Mahalati and Kahan [15] are summarized in Table 17.7.

Lorber *et al.* [102] demonstrated similar efficacy of EVL C_{min} values of 3–8 or >8 ng/mL as opposed to <3 ng/mL to achieve ARE prophylaxis among renal transplant recipients treated with regimens including CsA and steroid (Figure 17.7a). An EVL dose-escalation (0.75–10 mg daily) study in

Table 17.6 Sensitivity, specificity, and predictive values of last-observed sirolimus concentration measurements when prescribed with full exposure to cyclosporine.

Complication	Cut-off sirolimus, $C_{ss/min}$ (ng/mL)	Sensitivity (%)	Specificity (%)	Positive predictive value (%)	Negative predictive value (%)
Acute rejection	<5	21.43	80.34	11.54	89.52
Cholesterol >400 mg/dL	>13	NC[a]	77.37	0.00	100.0
Triglycerides >300 mg/dL	>11	45.12	92.00	94.87	33.82
Platelets <100 000 mm³	>14	43.75	62.02	46.67	80.22
WBC <4000 mm³	>15	41.03	82.47	48.48	77.67

Reprinted with permission from Kahan et al. [40].
[a]Could not be calculated.

Table 17.7 Recommended sirolimus trough concentrations with respect to acute rejection prophylaxis for 1 year when the drug is prescribed in combination with other immunosuppressive agents.

Concomitant immunosuppressants with sirolimus	No. in sample	Organ	Recipient group	Sirolimus target concentration (μg/L)	Acute rejection rate (%)
Prednisone+azathioprine	41	Kidney	All	30	41.0
Prednisone+mycophenolate mofetil	40	Kidney	All	30	27.5
Prednisone+cyclosporine	150	Kidney	All	5–15	10.5
Prednisone+transient 80% ↓ CsA+induction Ab	256	Kidney	All	10±2	15.0
Prednisone+basiliximab+MMF (no CNI)	60	Kidney	Weak	10–20	10.0
Prednisone+TRL	32	Liver, kidney/pancreas	All	6–12	9.0

stable renal transplant patients also receiving CsA and Pred showed a relationship between drug exposure and the onset of thrombocytopenia. Table 17.8 shows the relation to toxicity parameters of EVL C_{min} as well as CsA C_{min} values over time among the EVL versus MMF cohorts. Table 17.9 describes these relations as a function of quintiles of EVL concentrations. Figure 17.8a shows the median effect relationships documenting a narrow therapeutic window between efficacy and hypertriglyceridemia.

Starling et al. [161] confirmed that the target concentration range of 3–8 ng/mL EVL showed optimal effects on AREs among heart transplant patients treated with 40% reduced doses of CsA

(Figure 17.7b). They used the receiver operating characteristic to show a correlation between C_{min} and graft loss among 434 patients, showing a positive predictive value of 94% and a negative predictive value of 97% (OR=0.852 [95% CI=0.743–0.997]; Figure 17.7c). Figure 17.8a shows the median effect analysis of concentrations derived from this cohort of transplant patients, again documenting a narrow therapeutic window.

Kovarik et al. [159] evaluated PK in lung transplant recipients treated with 3 mg EVL daily in divided doses de novo followed by adjustments to achieve a median C_{min} value of 6.6 ng/mL (10–90% CI=2.8–11.8 ng/mL). Median effect analyses showed linear relations of C_{min}

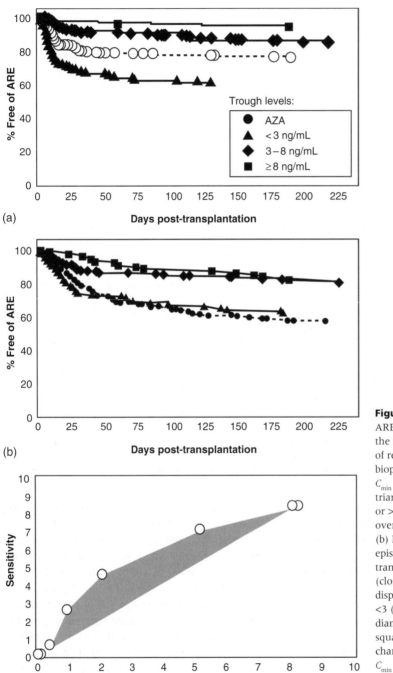

(a)

(b)

(c)

Figure 17.7 EVL C_{min} impact on AREs. (a) Kaplan–Meier plots over the first 6 months of the percentage of renal transplant patients free from biopsy-proven acute rejection for EVL C_{min} concentrations of <3 (closed triangles), 3–8 (closed diamonds), or >8 ng/mL (closed squares), with overall results (open circles) [60]. (b) Freedom from an acute rejection episode over 6 months among a heart transplant cohort treated with Aza (closed circles) versus EVL that displayed average C_{min} levels of <3 (closed triangles), 3–8 (closed diamonds), or >8 ng/mL (closed squares). (c) Operator receiving characteristic function relating EVL C_{min} to the occurrence of graft loss. Reprinted with permission from Kovarik *et al.* [159].

Table 17.8 Drug concentrations and laboratory parameters among renal transplant recipients treated with an EVL–CsA–steroid regimen.

Parameter	Treatment	Baseline	Day 1	Week 1	Week 2	Month 1	Month 2	Month 3	Month 6
Drug trough levels									
EVL (ng/mL)	EVL	—	—	5.4±3.7	5.1±3.4	5.4±3.3	6.1±3.7	6.5±4.5	6.2±3.6
Cyclosporine (ng/mL)	EVL	—	—	246±153	255±160	253±196	219±128	203±136	172±130
	MMF	—	—	232±156	264±191	236±128	207±110	191±89	173±72
Lipids									
Cholesterol (mmol/L)	EVL	4.4±1.2	4.3±1.1	5.3±1.2[a]	6.1±1.4[a]	7.0±1.8[a]	7.3±1.8[a]	7.0±1.7[a]	6.6±1.6[a]
	MMF	4.4±1.1	4.3±1.0	4.9±1.1	5.6±1.2	6.2±1.3	6.2±1.4	6.0±1.3	5.9±1.2
Triglycerides (mmol/L)	EVL	1.4±0.9	1.5±0.8	2.3±1.2[b]	2.5±1.5[a]	2.7±1.6[a]	3.2±2.0[a]	3.2±1.9[a]	3.0±1.8[a]
	MMF	1.5±1.2	1.6±1.0	2.2±1.2	2.2±1.3	2.1±1.1	2.4±1.4	2.3±1.3	2.3±1.3
Hematology									
Leukocytes (10⁹/L)	EVL	10.7±4.3	11.8±4.3	8.8±3.1[a]	9.0±3.2[a]	7.1±2.5[a]	7.7±2.5	7.5±2.5	7.4±2.4
	MMF	10.9±4.4	11.7±4.4	10.5±3.6	12.0±4.1	8.3±3.0	8.0±2.8	7.4±2.7	7.5±2.9
Platelets (10⁹/L)	EVL	213±72	195±63	232±81[a]	224±96[a]	229±88	231±88[a]	233±83[a]	233±79[b]
	MMF	207±63	195±62	250±86	261±99	237±93	244±84	247±90	244±73

Reprinted with permission from Kovarik *et al.* [160].
[a]$p < 0.01$ compared with MMF arm.
[b]$p < 0.05$ compared with MMF arm.

Table 17.9 Percentage of patients in exposure groups with efficacy and safety responses.

Response	MMF	EVL C_{min} quintile (ng/mL)				
		1.0–3.4	3.5–4.5	4.6–5.7	5.8–7.7	7.8–15.0
Freedom from acute rejection	77.0	67.6	81.3	85.6	81.3	91.4
Hypercholesterolemia (>6.5 mmol/L)	59.9	75.5	79.9	85.6	87.1	80.6
Hypertriglyceridemia (>2.9 mmol/L)	47.1	59.0	60.4	71.9	74.1	77.0
Leukocytopenia (<4×10⁹/L)	17.8	16.5	10.8	11.5	19.4	15.1
Thrombocytopenia (<100×10⁹/L)	7.3	10.1	9.4	7.2	13.7	17.3

Reprinted with permission from Kovarik *et al.* [160].
MMF: $n = 357$ patients; EVL C_{min} quintiles: $n = 139$ patients per quintile (total, 695 patients).

values to increased cholesterol and higher triglyceride as well as transiently decreased platelet counts, but not freedom from a change in forced expiratory volume in 1 s (FEV_1) or bronchoobliterative syndrome (Figure 17.8b).

In conclusion, the SRL and EVL data show robust correlations of freedom from renal transplant AREs with C_{min} values. Furthermore, there was a robust association with heart transplant loss, but little association with the occurrence of

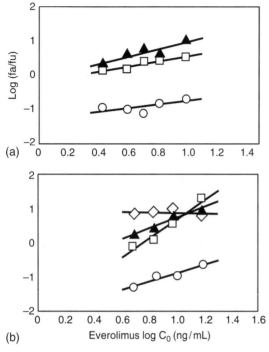

(a)

(b) Everolimus log C_0 (ng/mL)

Figure 17.8 Median-effect plots showing the fraction of patients affected/unaffected (fa/fu) with respect to a given response versus the EVL C_{min} and the associated regression line. The concentration points are plotted at the median value in each exposure quintile. Responses are freedom from AREs (closed diamonds) versus occurrence of hypertriglyceridemia (open squares) and thrombocytopenia (open circles). (a) Relationships for renal transplant recipients treated de novo with EVL plus CsA and steroid. (b) Responses are freedom from >15% decrease in FEV_1 with bronchiolitis obliterans syndrome (open diamond), hypercholesterolemia (closed diamonds), hypertriglyceridemia (open squares), and thrombocytopenia (open circles). Reprinted with permission from Kovarik *et al.* [159].

bronchoobliterative syndrome. The therapeutic windows between efficacy and toxicities tended to be narrow for hyperlipidemia but broader for thrombocytopenia among all transplant recipients. Owing to inter- and intra-individual variabilities, therapeutic drug monitoring appears to be a useful tool to avoid AREs, particularly early after transplantation, although hyperlipidemia seems inextricably tied to drug therapy with this class of agents.

References

1 Sehgal SN, Molnar-Kimber K, Ocain TD, Weichman BM. Rapamycin: a novel immunosuppressive macrolide. *Med Res Rev* 1994;14:1–22.

2 Raymond E, Alexandre J, Faivre S *et al.* Safety and pharmacokinetics of escalated doses of weekly intravenous infusion of CCI-779, a novel mTOR inhibitor, in patients with cancer. *J Clin Oncol* 2004;22:2336–2347.

3 Choi J, Chen J, Schreiber SL, Clardy J. Structure of the FKBP12–rapamycin complex interacting with the binding domain of human FRAP. *Science* 1996;273:239–242.

4 Rizzieri DA, Feldman E, Dipersio JF *et al.* A phase 2 clinical trial of deforolimus (AP23573, MK-8669), a novel mammalian target of rapamycin inhibitor, in patients with relapsed or refractory hematologic malignancies. *Clin Cancer Res* 2008;14:2756–2762.

5 Chen YW, Smith ML, Sheets M *et al.* Zotarolimus, a novel sirolimus analogue with potent anti-proliferative activity on coronary smooth muscle cells and reduced potential for systemic immunosuppression. *J Cardiovasc Pharmacol* 2007;49:228–235.

6 McMillin DW, Ooi M, Delmore J *et al.* Antimyeloma activity of the orally bioavailable dual phosphatidylinositol 3-kinase/mammalian target of rapamycin inhibitor NVP-BEZ235. *Cancer Res* 2009;69:5835–5842.

7 Deore V, Yewalkar N, Bhatia D *et al.* Synthesis and therapeutic evaluation of pyridyl based novel mTOR inhibitors. *Bioorg Med Chem Lett* 2009;19:2949–2952.

8 Wagner R, Mollison KW, Liu L *et al.* Rapamycin analogs with reduced systemic exposure. *Bioorg Med Chem Lett* 2005;15:5340–5343.

9 Kelly PA, Napoli K, Kahan BD. Conversion from liquid to solid rapamycin formulations in stable renal allograft transplant recipients . *Biopharm Drug Dispos* 1999;20:249–253.

10 Mathew TH, Van Buren C, Kahan BD *et al.* A comparative study of sirolimus tablet versus oral solution for prophylaxis of acute renal allograft rejection. *J Clin Pharmacol* 2006;46:76–87.

11 Buech G, Bertelmann E, Pleyer U *et al.* Formulation of sirolimus eye drops and corneal permeation studies. *J Ocul Pharmacol Ther* 2007;23:292–303.

12 Yanez JA, Forrest ML, Ohgami Y *et al.* Pharmacometrics and delivery of novel nanoformulated PEG-b-poly(ε-caprolactone) micelles of rapamycin. *Cancer Chemother Pharmacol* 2008;61:133–144.

13 Budde K, Neumayer HH, Lehne G *et al.* Tolerability and steady-state pharmacokinetics of everolimus in

maintenance renal transplant patients. *Nephrol Dial Transplant* 2004;19:2606–2614.

14 Kovarik JM, Noe A, Berthier S *et al*. Clinical development of an everolimus pediatric formulation: relative bioavailability, food effect, and steady-state pharmacokinetics. *J Clin Pharmacol* 2003;43:141–147.

15 Mahalati K, Kahan BD. Clinical pharmacokinetics of sirolimus. *Clin Pharmacokinet* 2001;40:573–585.

16 Napoli KL, Kahan BD. Sample clean-up and high-performance liquid chromatographic techniques for measurement of whole blood rapamycin concentrations. *J Chromatogr B Biomed Appl* 1994;654:111–120.

17 Napoli KL, Kahan BD. Routine clinical monitoring of sirolimus (rapamycin) whole-blood concentrations by HPLC with ultraviolet detection. *Clin Chem* 1996;42:1943–1948.

18 Zimmerman JJ, Kahan BD. Pharmacokinetics of sirolimus in stable renal transplant patients after multiple oral dose administration. *J Clin Pharmacol* 1997; 37:405–415.

19 Christians U, Jacobsen W, Serkova N *et al*. Automated, fast and sensitive quantification of drugs in blood by liquid chromatography–mass spectrometry with on-line extraction: immunosuppressants. *J Chromatogr B Biomed Sci Appl* 2000;748:41–53.

20 Vidal C, Kirchner GI, Wunsch G, Sewing KF. Automated simultaneous quantification of the immunosuppressants 40-*O*-(2-hydroxyethyl) rapamycin and cyclosporine in blood with electrospray-mass spectrometric detection. *Clin Chem* 1998;44:1275–1282.

21 Zhang J, Todd Reimer M, Alexander NE *et al*. Method development and validation for zotarolimus concentration determination in stented swine arteries by liquid chromatography/tandem mass spectrometry detection. *Rapid Commun Mass Spectrom* 2006;20:3427–3434.

22 Deters M, Kirchner G, Resch K, Kaever V. Simultaneous quantification of sirolimus, everolimus, tacrolimus and cyclosporine by liquid chromatography–mass spectrometry (LC–MS). *Clin Chem Lab Med* 2002;40:285–292.

23 Napoli KL, Taylor PJ. From beach to bedside: history of the development of sirolimus. *Ther Drug Monit* 2001;23:559–586.

24 Salm P, Taylor PJ, Pillans PI. Analytical performance of microparticle enzyme immunoassay and HPLC–tandem mass spectrometry in the determination of sirolimus in whole blood. *Clin Chem* 1999;45: 2278–2280.

25 Holt DW, Moreton M, Laamanen K, Johnston A. A microparticle enzyme immunoassay to measure sirolimus. *Transplant Proc* 2005;37:182–184.

26 Hwang M, Perez CA, Moretti L, Lu B. The mTOR signaling network: insights from its role during embryonic development. *Curr Med Chem* 2008;15:1192–1208.

27 Chung J, Kuo CJ, Crabtree GR, Blenis J. Rapamycin–FKBP specifically blocks growth-dependent activation of and signaling by the 70 kd S6 protein kinases. *Cell* 1992;69:1227–1236.

28 Brown EJ, Schreiber SL. A signaling pathway to translational control. *Cell* 1996;86:517–520.

29 Miyazaki T, Liu ZJ, Kawahara A *et al*. Three distinct IL-2 signaling pathways mediated by bcl-2, c-myc, and lck cooperate in hematopoietic cell proliferation. *Cell* 1995;81:223–231.

30 Saemann MD, Haidinger M, Hecking M *et al*. The multifunctional role of mTOR in innate immunity: implications for transplant immunity. *Am J Transplant* 2009;9:2655–2661.

31 Lai JH, Tan TH. CD28 signaling causes a sustained down-regulation of I kappa B alpha which can be prevented by the immunosuppressant rapamycin. *J Biol Chem* 1994;269:30077–30080.

32 Kopf H, de la Rosa GM, Howard OM, Chen X. Rapamycin inhibits differentiation of Th17 cells and promotes generation of FoxP3+ T regulatory cells. *Int Immunopharmacol* 2007;7:1819–1824.

33 Demirkiran A, Hendrikx TK, Baan CC, van der Laan LJ. Impact of immunosuppressive drugs on CD4+CD25+ FOXP3+ regulatory T cells: does in vitro evidence translate to the clinical setting? *Transplantation* 2008;85:783–789.

34 Ferraresso M, Tian L, Ghobrial R *et al*. Rapamycin inhibits production of cytotoxic but not noncytotoxic antibodies and preferentially activates T helper 2 cells that mediate long-term survival of heart allografts in rats. *J Immunol* 1994;153:3307–3318.

35 Kaplan B, Meier-Kriesche HU, Napoli KL, Kahan BD. The effects of relative timing of sirolimus and cyclosporine microemulsion formulation coadministration on the pharmacokinetics of each agent. *Clin Pharmacol Ther* 1998;63:48–53.

36 Zimmerman JJ, Harper D, Getsy J, Jusko WJ. Pharmacokinetic interactions between sirolimus and microemulsion cyclosporine when orally administered jointly and 4 hours apart in healthy volunteers. *J Clin Pharmacol* 2003;43:1168–1176.

37 Crowe A, Bruelisauer A, Duerr L *et al*. Absorption and intestinal metabolism of SDZ-RAD and rapamycin in rats. *Drug Metab Dispos* 1999;27:627–632.

38 Kovarik JM, Kaplan B, Silva HT *et al*. Pharmacokinetics of an everolimus–cyclosporine immunosuppressive regimen over the first 6 months after kidney transplantation. *Am J Transplant* 2003;3:606–613.

39 Kovarik JM, Hartmann S, Figueiredo J *et al*. Effect of food on everolimus absorption: quantification in healthy subjects and a confirmatory screening in patients with renal transplants. *Pharmacotherapy* 2002;22:154–159.

40 Kahan BD, Napoli KL, Kelly PA *et al*. Therapeutic drug monitoring of sirolimus: correlations with efficacy and toxicity. *Clin Transplant* 2000;14:97–109.

41 Christians U, Sattler M, Schiebel HMA *et al*. Isolation of two immunosuppressive metabolites after in vitro metabolism of rapamycin. *Drug Metab Dispos* 1992; 20:186–191.

42 Streit F, Christians U, Schiebel HM *et al*. Sensitive and specific quantification of sirolimus (rapamycin) and its metabolites in blood of kidney graft recipients by HPLC/electrospray-mass spectrometry. *Clin Chem* 1996; 42:1417–1425.

43 Leung LY, Lim HK, Abell MW, Zimmerman JJ. Pharmacokinetics and metabolic disposition of sirolimus in healthy male volunteers after a single oral dose. *Ther Drug Monit* 2006;28:51–61.

44 Kuhn B, Jacobsen W, Christians U *et al*. Metabolism of sirolimus and its derivative everolimus by cytochrome P450 3A4: insights from docking, molecular dynamics, and quantum chemical calculations. *J Med Chem* 2001;44:2027–2034.

45 Kelly PA, Wang H, Napoli KL *et al*. Metabolism of cyclosporine by cytochromes P450 3A9 and 3A4. *Eur J Drug Metab Pharmacokinet* 1999;24:321–328.

46 Sattler M, Guengerich FP, Yun CH *et al*. Cytochrome P-450 3A enzymes are responsible for biotransformation of FK506 and rapamycin in man and rat. *Drug Metab Dispos* 1992;20:753–761.

47 Filler G, Bendrick-Peart J, Christians U. Pharmacokinetics of mycophenolate mofetil and sirolimus in children. *Ther Drug Monit* 2008;30:138–142.

48 Filler G, Bendrick-Peart J, Strom T *et al*. Characterization of sirolimus metabolites in pediatric solid organ transplant recipients. *Pediatr Transplant* 2009;13:44–53.

49 Djebli N, Rousseau A, Hoizey G *et al*. Sirolimus population pharmacokinetic/pharmacogenetic analysis and Bayesian modelling in kidney transplant recipients. *Clin Pharmacokinet* 2006;45:1135–1148.

50 Lampen A, Zhang Y, Hackbarth I *et al*. Metabolism and transport of the macrolide immunosuppressant sirolimus in the small intestine. *J Pharmacol Exp Ther* 1998;285:1104–1112.

51 Paine MF, Leung LY, Watkins PB. New insights into drug absorption: studies with sirolimus. *Ther Drug Monit* 2004;26:463–467.

52 Kirchner GI, Winkler M, Mueller L *et al*. Pharmacokinetics of SDZ RAD and cyclosporin including their metabolites in seven kidney graft patients after the first dose of SDZ RAD. *Br J Clin Pharmacol* 2000;50:449–454.

53 Kaplan B, Meier-Kriesche HU, Napoli KL, Kahan BD. Correlation between pretransplantation test dose cyclosporine pharmacokinetic profiles and posttransplantation sirolimus blood levels in renal transplant recipients. *Ther Drug Monit* 1999;21:44–49.

54 Zimmerman JJ, Patat A, Parks V *et al*. Pharmacokinetics of sirolimus (rapamycin) in subjects with severe hepatic impairment. *J Clin Pharmacol* 2008;48: 285–292.

55 Brattstrom C, Sawe J, Jansson B *et al*. Pharmacokinetics and safety of single oral doses of sirolimus (rapamycin) in healthy male volunteers. *Ther Drug Monit* 2000;22:537–544.

56 Ferron GM, Mishina EV, Zimmerman JJ, Jusko WJ. Population pharmacokinetics of sirolimus in kidney transplant patients. *Clin Pharmacol Ther* 1997;61: 416–428.

57 Kaplan B, Meier-Kriesche HU, Napoli K, Kahan BD. A limited sampling strategy for estimating sirolimus area-under-the-concentration curve. *Clin Chem* 1997;43: 539–540.

58 Cattaneo D, Cortinovis M, Baldelli S *et al*. Limited sampling strategies for the estimation of sirolimus daily exposure in kidney transplant recipients on a calcineurin inhibitor-free regimen. *J Clin Pharmacol* 2009;49:773–781.

59 Kahan BD. Efficacy of sirolimus compared with azathioprine for reduction of acute renal allograft rejection: a randomised multicentre study. The Rapamune US Study Group. *Lancet* 2000;356:194–202.

60 Lorber MI, Ponticelli C, Whelchel J *et al*. Therapeutic drug monitoring for everolimus in kidney transplantation using 12-month exposure, efficacy, and safety data. *Clin Transplant* 2005;19:145–152.

61 Schachter AD, Meyers KE, Spaneas LD *et al*. Short sirolimus half-life in pediatric renal transplant recipients on a calcineurin inhibitor-free protocol. *Pediatr Transplant* 2004;8:171–177.

62 Hoyer PF, Ettenger R, Kovarik JM *et al*. Everolimus in pediatric de nova renal transplant patients. *Transplantation* 2003;75:2082–2085.

63 Napoli KL, Wang ME, Stepkowski SM, Kahan BD. Relative tissue distributions of cyclosporine and sirolimus after concomitant peroral administration to the rat: evidence for pharmacokinetic interactions. *Ther Drug Monit* 1998;20:123–133.

64 Stepkowski SM, Napoli KL, Wang ME *et al.* Effects of the pharmacokinetic interaction between orally administered sirolimus and cyclosporine on the synergistic prolongation of heart allograft survival in rats. *Transplantation* 1996;62:986–994.

65 Hariharan S, Filo RS, Tomlanovich SJ *et al.* Tacrolimus/sirolimus pharmacokinetic interaction study (Abstract 1074). *Am J Transplant* 2001;1:S406.

66 Kuypers DR, Claes K, Evenepoel P *et al.* Long-term pharmacokinetic study of the novel combination of tacrolimus and sirolimus in de novo renal allograft recipients. *Ther Drug Monit* 2003;25:447–451.

67 Curtis J, Nashan B, Kovarik JM *et al.* RAD (everolimus) pharmacokinetics are unaltered with full-dose versus reduced-dose cyclosporine [Abstract #951218]. *Am J Transplant* 2001;1(Suppl 1):299.

68 Kovarik JM, Curtis JJ, Hricik DE *et al.* Differential pharmacokinetic interaction of tacrolimus and cyclosporine on everolimus. *Transplant Proc* 2006;38:3456–3458.

69 Grinyo JM, Ekberg H, Mamelok RD *et al.* The pharmacokinetics of mycophenolate mofetil in renal transplant recipients receiving standard-dose or low-dose cyclosporine, low-dose tacrolimus or low-dose sirolimus: the Symphony pharmacokinetic substudy. *Nephrol Dial Transplant* 2009;24:2269–2276.

70 Dansirikul C, Morris RG, Tett SE, Duffull SB. A Bayesian approach for population pharmacokinetic modelling of sirolimus. *Br J Clin Pharmacol* 2006;62:420–434.

71 Jusko WJ, Ferron GM, Mis SM *et al.* Pharmacokinetics of prednisolone during administration of sirolimus in patients with renal transplants. *J Clin Pharmacol* 1996;36:1100–1106.

72 Kovarik JM, Hartmann S, Hubert M *et al.* Pharmacokinetic and pharmacodynamic assessments of HMG-CoA reductase inhibitors when coadministered with everolimus. *J Clin Pharmacol* 2002;42:222–228.

73 Kovarik JM, Beyer D, Schmouder RL. Everolimus drug interactions: application of a classification system for clinical decision making. *Biopharm Drug Dispos* 2006;27:421–426.

74 Gallant HL, Yatscoff RW. P70 S6 kinase assay: a pharmacodynamic monitoring strategy for rapamycin; assay development. *Transplant Proc* 1996;28:3058–3061.

75 Tanaka C, O'Reilly T, Kovarik JM *et al.* Identifying optimal biologic doses of everolimus (RAD001) in patients with cancer based on the modeling of preclinical and clinical pharmacokinetic and pharmacodynamic data. *J Clin Oncol* 2008;26:1596–1602.

76 Davis DL, Murthy JN, Napoli KL *et al.* Comparison of steady-state trough sirolimus samples by HPLC and a radioreceptor assay. *Clin Biochem* 2000;33:31–36.

77 Goodyear N, Napoli KL, Murthy JN *et al.* Radioreceptor assay for sirolimus. *Clin Biochem* 1996;29:457–460.

78 Goodyear N, Napoli KL, Murthy JN *et al.* Radioreceptor assay for sirolimus in patients with decreased platelet counts. *Clin Biochem* 1997;30:539–543.

79 Kahan BD, Podbielski J, Napoli KL *et al.* Immunosuppressive effects and safety of a sirolimus/cyclosporine combination regimen for renal transplantation. *Transplantation* 1998;66:1040–1046.

80 MacDonald AS. A worldwide, phase III, randomized, controlled, safety and efficacy study of a sirolimus/cyclosporine regimen for prevention of acute rejection in recipients of primary mismatched renal allografts. *Transplantation* 2001;71:271–280.

81 Kahan BD. Two-year results of multicenter phase III trials on the effect of the addition of sirolimus to cyclosporine-based immunosuppressive regimens in renal transplantation. *Transplant Proc* 2003;35:37S–51S.

82 Kahan BD, Gibbons S, Tejpal N *et al.* Synergistic interactions of cyclosporine and rapamycin to inhibit immune performances of normal human peripheral blood lymphocytes in vitro. *Transplantation* 1991;51:232–239.

83 Stepkowski SM, Chen H, Daloze P, Kahan BD. Rapamycin, a potent immunosuppressive drug for vascularized heart, kidney, and small bowel transplantation in the rat. *Transplantation* 1991;51:22–26.

84 Kahan BD, Kramer WG. Median effect analysis of efficacy versus adverse effects of immunosuppressants. *Clin Pharmacol Ther* 2001;70:74–81.

85 Paczek L, Bechstein W, Wramner L *et al.* A phase II; open-label; concentration-controlled, randomized 6-month study of standard-dose tacrolimus+sirolimus+coricosteriods compared to reduced-dose tacrolimus+sirolimus+corticosteroids in renal allograft recipients (Abstract 170). *Transplantation* 2002;74:70.

86 Wlodarczyk Z, van Hooff JP, Vanrenterghem Y *et al.* Tacrolimus in combination with various dosages of rapamycin in renal recipients: safety and efficacy of the first 6-month multicenter randomized trial (Abstract 554). *Transplantation* 2002;74:187.

87 Gaber AO, Kahan BD, Van Buren C *et al.* Comparison of sirolimus plus tacrolimus versus sirolimus plus cyclosporine in high-risk renal allograft recipients: results from an open-label, randomized trial. *Transplantation* 2008;86:1187–1195.

88 Kahan BD, Julian BA, Pescovitz MD *et al.* Sirolimus reduces the incidence of acute rejection episodes

despite lower cyclosporine doses in Caucasian recipients of mismatched primary renal allografts: a phase II trial. *Rapamune Study Group. Transplantation* 1999;68:1526–1532.

89 Kahan BD, Benavides C, Schoenberg L *et al.* Benefits on renal transplant function from 83% reduced de novo cyclosporine exposure in combination with sirolimus. *Clin Nephrol* 2011;73:344–353.

90 Plisczynski J, Kahan BD. Better actual graft and patient survivals among patients treated with 80% reduced cyclosporine exposure versus those receiving full cyclosporine exposure with and without concomitant sirolimus. *Transplant Proc* 2011;43(10):in press.

91 Groth CG, Backman L, Morales JM *et al.* Sirolimus (rapamycin)-based therapy in human renal transplantation: similar efficacy and different toxicity compared with cyclosporine. Sirolimus European Renal Transplant Study Group. *Transplantation* 1999;67:1036–1042.

92 Kreis H, Cisterne JM, Land W *et al.* Sirolimus in association with mycophenolate mofetil induction for the prevention of acute graft rejection in renal allograft recipients. *Transplantation* 2000;69:1252–1260.

93 Flechner SM, Goldfarb D, Modlin C *et al.* Kidney transplantation without calcineurin inhibitor drugs: a prospective, randomized trial of sirolimus versus cyclosporine. *Transplantation* 2002;74:1070–1076.

94 Flechner S, Glyda MJ, Steinberg S *et al.* A randomized, open-label study to compare the safety and efficacy of two different sirolimus (SRL) regimens with a tacrolimus (Tac) and mycophenolate mofetil (MMF) regimen in de novo renal allograft recipients: renal function results from the ORION study (Abstract). *Am J Transplant* 2007;7:440.

95 Larson TS, Dean PG, Stegall MD *et al.* Complete avoidance of calcineurin inhibitors in renal transplantation: a randomized trial comparing sirolimus and tacrolimus. *Am J Transplant* 2006;6:514–522.

96 Buchler M, Caillard S, Barbier S *et al.* Sirolimus versus cyclosporine in kidney recipients receiving thymoglobulin, mycophenolate mofetil and a 6-month course of steroids. *Am J Transplant* 2007;7:2522–2531.

97 Hong JC, Kahan BD. A calcineurin antagonist-free induction strategy for immunosuppression in cadaveric kidney transplant recipients at risk for delayed graft function. *Transplantation* 2001;71:1320–1328.

98 Hong JC, Kahan BD. Sirolimus rescue therapy for refractory rejection in renal transplantation. *Transplantation* 2001;71:1579–1584.

99 Mahalati K, Kahan BD. Sirolimus permits steroid withdrawal from a cyclosporine regimen. *Transplant Proc* 2001;33:1270.

100 Benito AI, Furlong T, Martin PJ *et al.* Sirolimus (rapamycin) for the treatment of steroid-refractory acute graft-versus-host disease. *Transplantation* 2001;72: 1924–1929.

101 Podder H, Podbielski J, Hussein I *et al.* Sirolimus improves the two-year outcome of renal allografts in African-American patients. *Transpl Int* 2001;14: 135–142.

102 Johnson RW, Kreis H, Oberbauer R *et al.* Sirolimus allows early cyclosporine withdrawal in renal transplantation resulting in improved renal function and lower blood pressure. *Transplantation* 2001;72: 777–786.

103 Letavernier E, Peraldi MN, Pariente A *et al.* Proteinuria following a switch from calcineurin inhibitors to sirolimus. *Transplantation* 2005;80: 1198–1203.

104 Diekmann F, Budde K, Oppenheimer F *et al.* Predictors of success in conversion from calcineurin inhibitor to sirolimus in chronic allograft dysfunction. *Am J Transplant* 2004;4:1869–1875.

105 Weir MR, Mulgaonkar S, Chan L *et al.* Mycophenolate mofetil-based immunosuppression with sirolimus in renal transplantation: a randomized, controlled Spare-the-Nephron trial. *Kidney Int* 2011;79: 897–907.

106 Mulay AV, Cockfield S, Stryker R *et al.* Conversion from calcineurin inhibitors to sirolimus for chronic renal allograft dysfunction: a systematic review of the evidence. *Transplantation* 2006; 82:1153–1162.

107 Keogh A, Richardson M, Ruygrok P *et al.* Sirolimus in de novo heart transplant recipients reduces acute rejection and prevents coronary artery disease at 2 years: a randomized clinical trial. *Circulation* 2004;110:2694–2700.

108 Trotter JF. Sirolimus in liver transplantation. *Transplant Proc* 2003;35:193S–200S.

109 Cabezon S, Lage E, Hinojosa R *et al.* Sirolimus improves renal function in cardiac transplantation. *Transplant Proc* 2005;37:1546–1547.

110 Snell GI, Levvey BJ, Chin W *et al.* Sirolimus allows renal recovery in lung and heart transplant recipients with chronic renal impairment. *J Heart Lung Transplant* 2002;21:540–546.

111 Schuurman HJ, Cottens S, Fuchs S *et al.* SDZ RAD, a new rapamycin derivative: synergism with cyclosporine. *Transplantation* 1997;64:32–35.

112 Kahan BD, Wong RL, Carter C *et al.* A phase I study of a 4-week course of SDZ-RAD (RAD) quiescent cyclosporine–prednisone-treated renal transplant recipients. *Transplantation* 1999;68:1100–1106.

113 Kahan BD, Kaplan B, Lorber MI *et al*. RAD in de novo renal transplantation: comparison of three doses on the incidence and severity of acute rejection. *Transplantation* 2001;71:1400–1406.

114 Lorber MI, Mulgaonkar S, Butt KM *et al*. Everolimus versus mycophenolate mofetil in the prevention of rejection in de novo renal transplant recipients: a 3-year randomized, multicenter, phase III study. *Transplantation* 2005;80:244–252.

115 Nashan B, Curtis J, Ponticelli C *et al*. Everolimus and reduced-exposure cyclosporine in de novo renal-transplant recipients: a three-year phase II, randomized, multicenter, open-label study. *Transplantation* 2004;78:1332–1340.

116 Salvadori M, Scolari MP, Bertoni E *et al*. Everolimus with very low-exposure cyclosporine a in de novo kidney transplantation: a multicenter, randomized, controlled trial. *Transplantation* 2009;88:1194–1202.

117 Vitko S, Tedesco H, Eris J *et al*. Everolimus with optimized cyclosporine dosing in renal transplant recipients: 6-month safety and efficacy results of two randomized studies. *Am J Transplant* 2004;4: 626–635.

118 Chan L, Greenstein S, Hardy MA *et al*. Multicenter, randomized study of the use of everolimus with tacrolimus after renal transplantation demonstrates its effectiveness. *Transplantation* 2008;85:821–826.

119 Kamar N, Jaafar A, Esposito L *et al*. Conversion from sirolimus to everolimus in maintenance renal transplant recipients within a calcineurin inhibitor-free regimen: results of a 6-month pilot study. *Clin Nephrol* 2008;70:118–125.

120 Levy G, Schmidli H, Punch J *et al*. Safety, tolerability, and efficacy of everolimus in de novo liver transplant recipients: 12- and 36-month results. *Liver Transpl* 2006;12:1640–1648.

121 Eisen HJ, Tuzcu EM, Dorent R *et al*. Everolimus for the prevention of allograft rejection and vasculopathy in cardiac-transplant recipients. *N Engl J Med* 2003;349:847–858.

122 Kahan BD, Knight R, Schoenberg L *et al*. Ten years of sirolimus therapy for human renal transplantation: the University of Texas at Houston experience. *Transplant Proc* 2003;35:25S–34S.

123 Kahan BD, Yakupoglu YK, Schoenberg L *et al*. Low incidence of malignancy among sirolimus/cyclosporine-treated renal transplant recipients. *Transplantation* 2005;80:749–758.

124 Kauffman HM, Cherikh WS, Cheng Y *et al*. Maintenance immunosuppression with target-of-rapamycin inhibitors is associated with a reduced incidence of de novo malignancies. *Transplantation* 2005;80:883–889.

125 Mathew T, Kreis H, Friend P. Two-year incidence of malignancy in sirolimus-treated renal transplant recipients: results from five multicenter studies. *Clin Transplant* 2004;18:446–449.

126 Campistol JM, Eris J, Oberbauer R *et al*. Sirolimus therapy after early cyclosporine withdrawal reduces the risk for cancer in adult renal transplantation. *J Am Soc Nephrol* 2006;17:581–589.

127 Hosoi H, Dilling MB, Shikata T *et al*. Rapamycin causes poorly reversible inhibition of mTOR and induces p53-independent apoptosis in human rhabdomyosarcoma cells. *Cancer Res* 1999;59:886–894.

128 Guba M, von Breitenbuch P, Steinbauer M *et al*. Rapamycin inhibits primary and metastatic tumor growth by antiangiogenesis: involvement of vascular endothelial growth factor. *Nat Med* 2002;8:128–135.

129 Stallone G, Schena A, Infante B *et al*. Sirolimus for Kaposi's sarcoma in renal-transplant recipients. *N Engl J Med* 2005;352:1317–1323.

130 Hudes G, Carducci M, Tomczak P *et al*. Temsirolimus, interferon alfa, or both for advanced renal-cell carcinoma. *N Engl J Med* 2007;356:2271–2281.

131 Luan FL, Hojo M, Maluccio M *et al*. Rapamycin blocks tumor progression: unlinking immunosuppression from antitumor efficacy. *Transplantation* 2002;73:1565–1572.

132 Morris RE, Cao W, Huang X *et al*. Rapamycin (sirolimus) inhibits vascular smooth muscle DNA synthesis in vitro and suppresses narrowing in arterial allografts and in balloon-injured carotid arteries: evidence that rapamycin antagonizes growth factor action on immune and nonimmune cells. *Transplant Proc* 1995;27:430–431.

133 Ikonen TS, Gummert JF, Hayase M *et al*. Sirolimus (rapamycin) halts and reverses progression of allograft vascular disease in non-human primates. *Transplantation* 2000;70:969–975.

134 Mancini D, Pinney S, Burkhoff D *et al*. Use of rapamycin slows progression of cardiac transplantation vasculopathy. *Circulation* 2003;108:48–53.

135 Raichlin E, Bae JH, Khalpey Z *et al*. Conversion to sirolimus as primary immunosuppression attenuates the progression of allograft vasculopathy after cardiac transplantation. *Circulation* 2007;116: 2726–2733.

136 Moses JW, Leon MB, Popma JJ *et al*. Sirolimus-eluting stents versus standard stents in patients with stenosis in a native coronary artery. *N Engl J Med* 2003;349:1315–1323.

137 Onuma Y, Kukreja N, Piazza N *et al.* The everolimus-eluting stent in real-world patients: 6-month follow-up of the X-SEARCH (Xience V Stent Evaluated at Rotterdam Cardiac Hospital) registry. *J Am Coll Cardiol* 2009;54:269–276.

138 Stone GW, Midei M, Newman W *et al.* Randomized comparison of everolimus-eluting and paclitaxel-eluting stents: two-year clinical follow-up from the Clinical Evaluation of the Xience V Everolimus Eluting Coronary Stent System in the Treatment of Patients with de novo Native Coronary Artery Lesions (SPIRIT) III trial. *Circulation* 2009;119:680–686.

139 Seitou T, Murakami M, Komatsubara I *et al.* Higher incidence and serum levels of minor cardiac biomarker elevation in sirolimus-eluting stent (Cypher) than bare metal stent implantations. *Coron Artery Dis* 2008;19:63–69.

140 Kwon YS, Kim JC. Inhibition of corneal neovascularization by rapamycin. *Exp Mol Med* 2006;38:173–179.

141 Morrisett JD, Abdel-Fattah G, Hoogeveen R *et al.* Effects of sirolimus on plasma lipids, lipoprotein levels, and fatty acid metabolism in renal transplant patients. *J Lipid Res* 2002;43:1170–1180.

142 Hoogeveen RC, Ballantyne CM, Pownall HJ *et al.* Effect of sirolimus on the metabolism of apoB100-containing lipoproteins in renal transplant patients. *Transplantation* 2001;72:1244–1250.

143 Chueh SC, Kahan BD. Dyslipidemia in renal transplant recipients treated with a sirolimus and cyclosporine-based immunosuppressive regimen: incidence, risk factors, progression, and prognosis. *Transplantation* 2003;76:375–382.

144 Hong JC, Kahan BD. Sirolimus-induced thrombocytopenia and leukopenia in renal transplant recipients: risk factors, incidence, progression, and management. *Transplantation* 2000;69:2085–2090.

145 Podder H, Stepkowski SM, Napoli KL *et al.* Pharmacokinetic interactions augment toxicities of sirolimus/cyclosporine combinations. *J Am Soc Nephrol* 2001;12:1059–1071.

146 Lieberthal W, Fuhro R, Andry CC *et al.* Rapamycin impairs recovery from acute renal failure: role of cell-cycle arrest and apoptosis of tubular cells. *Am J Physiol Renal Physiol* 2001;281:F693–F706.

147 Fuller TF, Freise CE, Serkova N *et al.* Sirolimus delays recovery of rat kidney transplants after ischemia–reperfusion injury. *Transplantation* 2003;76:1594–1599.

148 McTaggart RA, Tomlanovich S, Bostrom A *et al.* Comparison of outcomes after delayed graft function: sirolimus-based versus other calcineurin-inhibitor sparing induction immunosuppression regimens. *Transplantation* 2004;78:475–480.

149 Smith KD, Wrenshall LE, Nicosia RF *et al.* Delayed graft function and cast nephropathy associated with tacrolimus plus rapamycin use. *J Am Soc Nephrol* 2003;14:1037–1045.

150 Stallone G, Di Paolo S, Schena A *et al.* Addition of sirolimus to cyclosporine delays the recovery from delayed graft function but does not affect 1-year graft function. *J Am Soc Nephrol* 2004;15:228–233.

151 Benavides C, Mahmoud KH, Knight R *et al.* Rabbit antithymocyte globulin: a postoperative risk factor for sirolimus-treated renal transplant patients? *Transplant Proc* 2005;37:822–826.

152 Langer RM, Kahan BD. Incidence, therapy, and consequences of lymphocele after sirolimus–cyclosporine–prednisone immunosuppression in renal transplant recipients. *Transplantation* 2002;74:804–808.

153 Johnston O, Rose CL, Webster AC, Gill JS. Sirolimus is associated with new-onset diabetes in kidney transplant recipients. *J Am Soc Nephrol* 2008;19:1411–1418.

154 Morelon E, Stern M, Israel-Biet D *et al.* Characteristics of sirolimus-associated interstitial pneumonitis in renal transplant patients. *Transplantation* 2001;72:787–790.

155 Lindenfeld JA, Simon SF, Zamora MR *et al.* BOOP is common in cardiac transplant recipients switched from a calcineurin inhibitor to sirolimus. *Am J Transplant* 2005;5:1392–1396.

156 Serkova NJ, Christians U. Biomarkers for toxicodynamic monitoring of immunosuppressants: NMR-based quantitative metabonomics of the blood. *Ther Drug Monit* 2005;27:733–737.

157 Gee I, Trull AK, Charman SC, Alexander GJ. Sirolimus inhibits oxidative burst activity in transplant recipients. *Transplantation* 2003;76:1766–1768.

158 Benavides CA, Pollard VB, Mauiyyedi S *et al.* BK virus-associated nephropathy in sirolimus-treated renal transplant patients: incidence, course, and clinical outcomes. *Transplantation* 2007;84:83–88.

159 Kovarik JM, Snell GI, Valentine V *et al.* Everolimus in pulmonary transplantation: pharmacokinetics and exposure–response relationships. *J Heart Lung Transplant* 2006;25:440–446.

160 Kovarik JM, Tedesco H, Pascual J *et al.* Everolimus therapeutic concentration range defined from a prospective trial with reduced-exposure cyclosporine in de novo kidney transplantation. *Ther Drug Monit* 2004;26:499–505.

161 Starling RC, Hare JM, Hauptman P *et al.* Therapeutic drug monitoring for everolimus in heart transplant recipients based on exposure–effect modeling. *Am J Transplant* 2004;4:2126–2131.

CHAPTER 18

Inhibitors Targeting JAK3[*]

Gary Chan[1] and Paul S. Changelian[2]

[1]Pfizer, Groton, CT, USA
[2]Lycera Corporation, Plymouth, MI, USA

Introduction

Recent advances in the understanding of the immune response have identified select cytokines to be crucial mediators of the response to alloantigens through their effects on the development, homeostasis, and function of immune cells. The protein tyrosine kinase Janus kinase 3 (JAK3) is a vital component of the intracellular signaling cascade downstream from the corresponding cytokine receptors. As a result, JAK3 has emerged as an attractive target for developing selective inhibitory agents to treat a variety of immune-related diseases. The attention paid to JAK3 as a drug development target by pharmaceutical companies is evidenced by the growing number of publications on JAK3 inhibition, as well as the increasing number of JAK or JAK3 inhibitors that are currently under development. This chapter will describe the current status of agents that target inhibition of JAK3 and will focus on data relating to prevention of allograft rejection.

Mechanism of action

JAK/STAT pathway

The intact allogeneic immune response requires recognition of the alloantigen by the T cell receptor (TCR) (signal 1), costimulation (signal 2), and the autocrine or paracrine effects of select cytokines (signal 3) to alter gene expression in the nucleus. Cytokines are essential for lymphocyte activation, differentiation, and function. Cytokines bind to cognate cytokine receptors located on the cell membrane. Type I and Type II cytokine receptors lack intrinsic kinase activity. Therefore, they rely on the noncovalent association of protein kinases to relay signals to the cell interior. Using adenosine triphosphate (ATP) or guanosine triphosphate (GTP), these kinases phosphorylate the associated receptor and additional substrates to initiate the signaling cascade [1].

The Janus kinases (JAKs) are a small family of cytoplasmic, nonreceptor protein tyrosine kinases that relay the effects of cytokines, growth factors, and hormones from the external environment to the nucleus in a variety of cells, including immune cells. There are four members in the JAK family: JAK1, JAK2, JAK3, and Tyk2. Each JAK consists of approximately 1000 amino acids and has a molecular weight of approximately 120–140 kDa. JAK3 is exclusively associated with the common gamma chain (γc) subunit of the receptors for the IL-2 family of cytokines, which consist of interleukin (IL)-2, -4, -7, -9, -15, and -21. These cytokines are crucial to the development, survival, activation, and differentiation of NK cells, and T and B lymphocytes (Table 18.1), and thus exert diverse effects on both the innate and adaptive immune responses.

The JAKs are constitutively associated with the cytoplasmic domain of receptors. Some receptors (e.g., erythropoietin receptor, IL-3 receptor) require only a single member of the JAK family (JAK2) to

[*]Conflict of interest statement: G. Chan is a Pfizer employee.

Immunotherapy in Transplantation: Principles and Practice, First Edition. Edited by Bruce Kaplan, Gilbert J. Burckart and Fadi G. Lakkis.
© 2012 Blackwell Publishing Ltd. Published 2012 by Blackwell Publishing Ltd.

Table 18.1 Functions of cytokine receptors sharing the γc subunit.

Cytokine receptor	Functions
IL-2R	Stimulate the proliferation and differentiation of helper and cytotoxic T cells, B cells and NK cells
	Regulate peripheral self-tolerance
	Stimulate the development of regulatory T cells
	Stimulate the apoptosis of antigen-activated T cells
IL-4R	Induce the differentiation of naive helper T cell (T_H0) to the T_H2 subset
	Inhibit T_H1 differentiation
	Induce immunoglobulin class switching in B cells to IgE
IL-7R	Stimulate the development of pluripotent hematopoietic stem cells into lymphoid progenitor cells
	Promote the development, proliferation and survival of T, B, and NK cells
IL-9R	Stimulate intrathymic T cell development
	Regulate lung eosinophilia and serum IgE levels
	Promote protective immunity to intestinal nematodes
	Regulate goblet cell hyperplasia and mucus production
IL-15R	Promote the proliferation, cytotoxicity and cytokine production of NK cells and regulate NK–macrophage interaction
	Promote the development, homeostasis and activation of dendritic epidermal T cells, intestinal intraepithelial lymphocytes and NK-T cells
IL-21R	Enhance primary T cell response and effector T cell differentiation
	Enhance B cell function after interaction between T and B cells
	Regulate expansion of NK cells
	Induce proinflammatory T_H17 cells

Table 18.2 JAKs and STATs involved in the downstream signaling of the IL-2 family of cytokines (IL-2, -4, -7, -9, -15, and -21). Receptors of these cytokines share a common component, the γc, and at least a ligand-specific component known as the α-chain. The receptors for IL-2 and IL-15 also include a third component, the β-chain. JAK1 and JAK3 are associated with the intracellular domains of the receptors. Downstream signal transduction is mediated through the STAT proteins.

Cytokine	Cytokine receptor subunits	JAKs associated with the cytokine receptor	STATs activated by the JAKs
IL-2	α, β, γ	JAK1 and JAK3	STAT3, STAT5a, and STAT5b
IL-4	α, γ	JAK1 and JAK3	STAT5a, STAT5b, and STAT6
IL-7	α, γ	JAK1 and JAK3	STAT3, STAT5a, and STAT5b
IL-9	α, γ	JAK1 and JAK3	STAT3, STAT5a, and STAT5b
IL-15	α, β, γ	JAK1 and JAK3	STAT3, STAT5a, and STAT5b
IL-21	α, γ	JAK1 and JAK3	STAT1, STAT3, STAT5a, and STAT5b

be associated with their corresponding cytoplasmic domains. In contrast, most cytokine receptors utilize two distinct members of the JAK family. For example, both JAK3 and JAK1 are implicated in signaling from the IL-2 family of cytokines. The key substrates for phosphorylation following binding of a cytokine to its receptor and JAK activation are proteins called the signal transducers and activators of transcription (STATs) (Table 18.2). The STATs are latent transcription factors which travel to the nucleus and induce cytokine-specific transcription following phosphorylation on a single tyrosine residue. Among the IL-2 family of cytokine receptors, the receptors for IL-2, -7, -9, -15, and -21 primarily signal through STAT5, while the IL-4 receptor mainly activates STAT6 [2].

The JAK/STAT pathway is not the only signaling mechanism between the cell membrane and the nucleus. Additional secondary (nonobligatory) pathways include the Ras–Raf–MAP kinase pathway, and a pathway involving phosphatidyl inositol 3-kinase, protein kinase B and p70 S6 kinase [3]. Current evidence suggests that JAKs also participate in these additional intracellular signaling pathways, though the precise roles of the JAKs, and particularly JAK3, are not clear.

The steps thought to be involved in signaling through the JAK/STAT pathway are shown in Figure 18.1. Binding of a cytokine to its receptor results in oligomerization of the receptor subunits, which in turn leads to activation of receptor-associated JAKs through phosphorylation. Once activated, the JAKs phosphorylate tyrosine residues on the intracellular domain of the receptor, thereby creating docking sites for signaling proteins that possess an Src homology 2 (SH2) domain, such as STATs.

The STATs exist latently in the cytoplasm as monomers, and are inactive as transcription factors in the absence of specific interaction with and stimulation by cytokine receptors [4]. Upon docking of STATs at the cytokine receptor, they undergo phosphorylation and then dissociate, as bivalent STAT dimerization via their SH2 domains is favored over monovalent association with the receptor. The dimerized STATs (as either monodimers or heterodimers) translocate to the nucleus and bind DNA at sequences known as gamma interferon activated site (GAS) motifs. These STAT-binding elements are located in the promoter region of various target genes, such as genes for cyclin D2, the anti-apoptotic proteins Bcl-2 and Bcl-x, and various cytokines and chemokines. The STATs cooperate with other transcription factors and/or coactivators to regulate transcription of target genes required for cell proliferation, differentiation, and progress from G_1 to S phase [3]. Subsequently, the STAT signals are terminated by dephosphorylation by tyrosine phosphatases or proteasome-mediated degradation [3].

Multiple control mechanisms operate along the JAK/STAT pathway to afford orderly intracellular signaling. Negative regulators of JAKs include the suppressor of cytokine signaling (SOCS) proteins, e.g., SOCS1, SOC2, SOC3, and cytokine-inducible SH2 domain protein (CIS), which interfere with JAK-catalyzed phosphorylation of STATs and mediate degradation of the JAKs by the ubiquitin–proteasome pathway [5]. Protein tyrosine phosphatases (PTPs), e.g., SHP1, SHP2, PTP1, and CD45, can also dephosphorylate activated JAKs [6]. The constitutive and inducible expression of these regulators in aggregate determines the time-course and strength of signal transduction in the cell [4].

The architecture of the JAKs consists of seven distinct JAK homology domains (JH1–JH7), with the catalytic domain JH1 located at the carboxyl terminus. The JH1 domain serves to bind the ATP donor and the protein substrate, and transfer the phosphate from ATP to the protein substrate [7]. Juxtapositioned to JH1, and characteristic of the JAKs, is the catalytically inactive pseudokinase domain JH2, which is believed to be a negative regulator of JH1. The coexistence of a kinase and an inactive pseudokinase domain confers the nomenclature of Janus to this family of tyrosine kinases after the two-faced Roman deity [8]. An SH2-like segment exists in the JH3–JH4 domains. An SH2 domain typically binds phosphotyrosine residues, although the ligand corresponding to the SH2 domain in JAK3 is unknown at this time. JH6–JH7 represents the FERM (4.1, ezrin, radixin, moesin) domain that binds to the intracellular component of the cytokine receptor and positively regulates kinase activity [9].

Physiological role of JAK3

JAK3 was identified in the search for a genetic basis of severe combined immunodeficiency disease

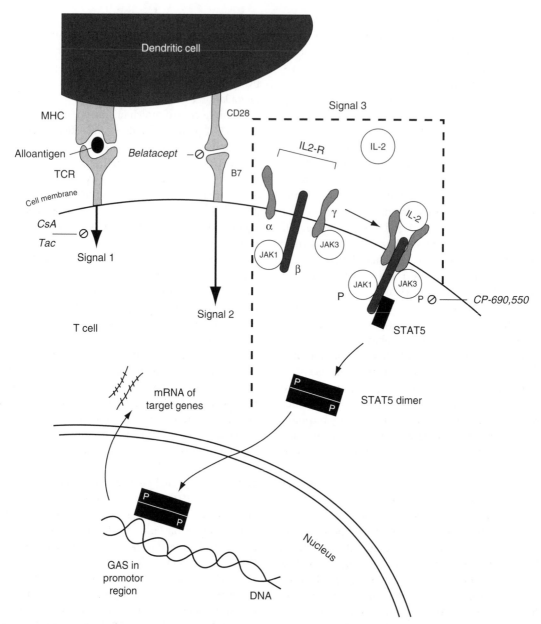

Figure 18.1 Steps involved in the JAK–STAT signaling pathway downstream of the IL-2 family cytokine receptors in T cells. IL-2 is shown as the prototype cytokine of the IL-2 family.

(SCID). The gene for JAK3 is located on chromosome 19p13.1. A key role of JAK3 in cytokine signaling is illustrated in cases of inherited immunodeficiency in which loss-of-function mutations affecting γc-JAK3 interaction or JAK3

kinase activity result in a dysfunctional immune response. In humans, mutations of the γc gene result in X-linked SCID, which accounts for approximately 50% of SCID cases [10]. An additional 7–14% of SCID cases are autosomal recessive SCID attributable to loss-of-function mutations of the JAK3 gene [10]. Each of these mutations results in an identical T⁻NK⁻B⁺ phenotype, in which the numbers of circulating T lymphocytes and NK cells are decreased. B cell number was normal or increased, but the function of circulating B cells was impaired. The genetic basis for these SCID phenotypes has been recapitulated by gene knockout experiments. In JAK3 knockout mice, lymphoid cell development is deficient, resulting in a SCID phenotype defective in circulating numbers of T, B, and NK cells, but the animals do not manifest disorders outside the immune system [9]. These observations confirm that JAK3 plays an obligatory role in the function of the innate and adaptive immune systems.

The nonredundant nature of JAK3-mediated signaling is further illustrated by disruption of steps proximal or distal to JAK3. Treatment of mice with transplanted pancreatic islets with anti-γc monoclonal antibodies resulted in prolonged islet survival [11]. Distal to the γc-associated JAK3, STAT5 is activated as part of the JAK/STAT parthway. In double knockout mice deficient of the closely related STAT5a and STAT5b, there is a decrease in NK and B cell numbers, and decreased proliferative response of lymphocytes to TCR activation [2]. This provides further evidence of the essential role of the JAK/STAT pathway to intact immune function.

JAK3 as a therapeutic target

The importance of JAK3 as a therapeutic target is clearly reflected in the large number of investigational JAK3 inhibitors that are currently in development. The appeal of JAK3 as a target for development of selective immunomodulatory agents lies in the relevance of the JAK/STAT pathway to the immune response and the restricted distribution of JAK3.

Observations from knockout mice and SCID patients confirm the crucial and nonredundant role played by JAK3 in the immune response. The corollary follows that inhibition of JAK3 would have a potent suppressive effect on both the innate and adaptive immune response. Contrary to other members of the JAK family (JAK1, JAK2, and Tyk2), which are present ubiquitously in mammals,

JAK3 is exclusively associated with γc and is thus selectively confined to lympho-hematopoietic cells. JAK3 is expressed constitutively in NK cells and thymocytes but is absent in resting T and B cells. Expression is induced upon activation in T and B lymphocytes and monocytes. Expression of JAK3 has been reported in endothelium and vascular smooth muscle cells [2], but the function of JAK3 in these cell types appears to be redundant. This restricted distribution of JAK3 suggests that the effect of JAK3 inhibition could theoretically be limited to the lymphoid cells. Further evidence of functional restriction is provided by SCID patients, whose abnormality is restricted to the immune system, and gene therapy of X-linked SCID, e.g., replacement of the mutated γc gene, is curative.

A challenge in developing kinase inhibitors, including inhibitors for JAK3, lies in the degree of selectivity required for such inhibition. The vast majority of kinase inhibitors discovered through screening and combinatorial chemistry are ATP-competitive molecules [12]. This has allowed identification of very potent inhibitors. However, with over 500 kinases in the human kinome which all utilize ATP as the key substrate, selectivity is a challenge. Theoretically, non-ATP-competitive kinase inhibitors could be more selective than ATP-competitive inhibitors. However, efficient screening for such non-ATP-competitive molecules is challenging, since the mechanism of their binding to kinases is unknown. A high degree of selectivity or even absolute selectivity was initially considered essential for the development of kinase inhibitors. It is now increasingly recognized that kinase inhibitors of only moderate selectivity can prove clinically useful with an acceptable risk/benefit ratio [13].

It is not clear what degree of selectivity is necessary for inhibitors that target JAK3. As all members of the JAK family are involved with diverse receptors that play some role in the immune system, the efficacy of a JAK inhibitor can be expected be enhanced by intra-family cross-reactivity. In contrast, JAK2 is also involved in the production of red blood cells and platelets (via the erythropoietin and thrombopoietin receptors respectively). Thus, some selectivity is certainly required. The acceptable degree of selectivity will ultimately be defined by in

Compound name	Structure
AG-490	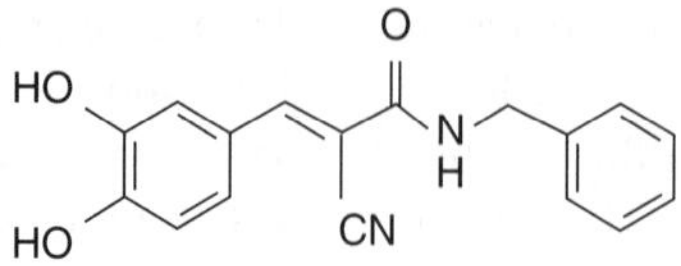
WHI-P131	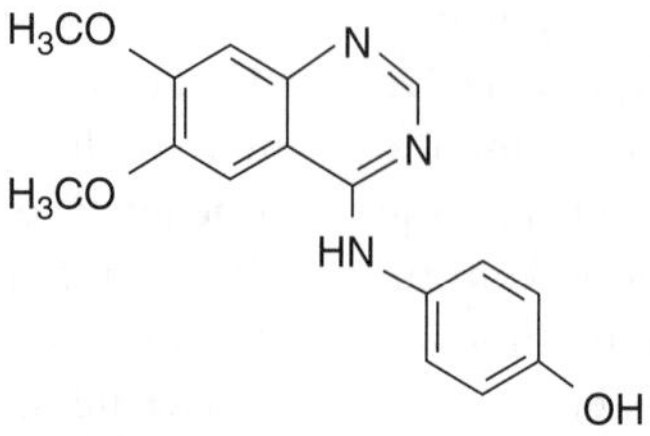
WHI-P154	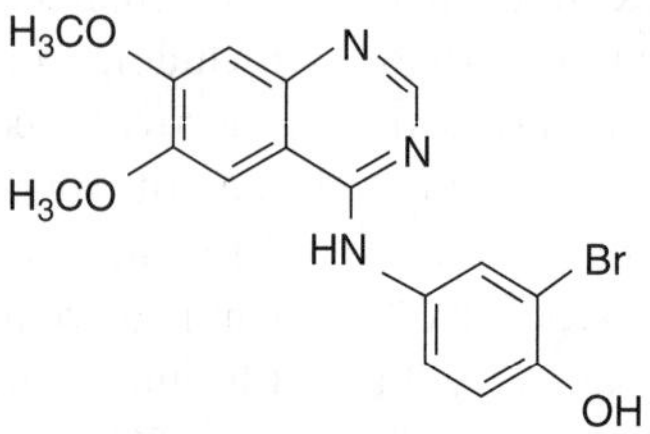
PNU156804	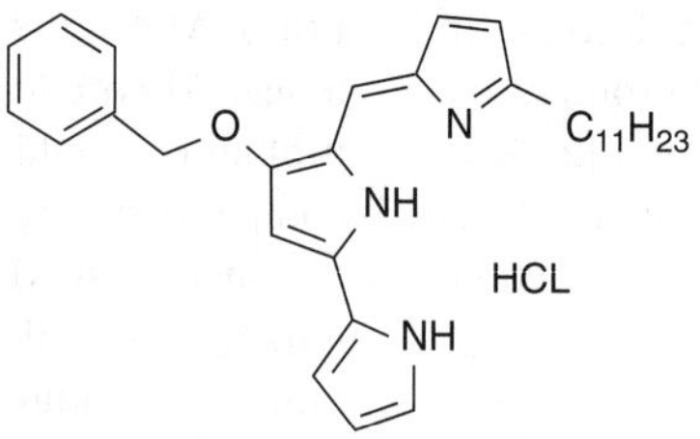
CP-690,550	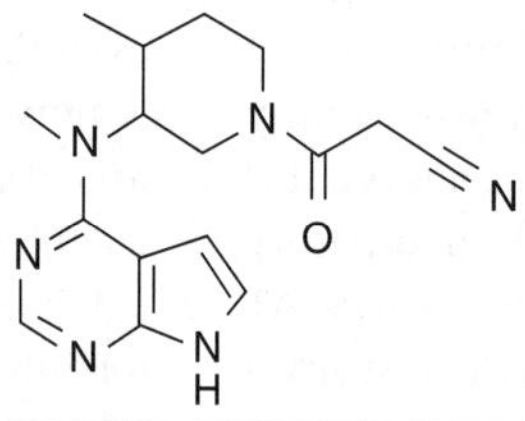
NC1153	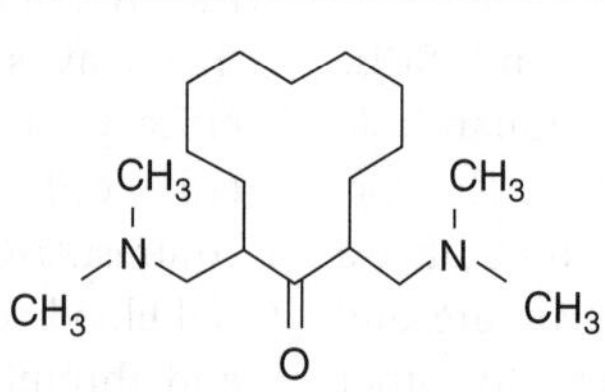

Figure 18.2 Chemical structures of investigational compounds that target JAK3 inhibition.

vivo studies. A therapeutic window can be defined by comparing the drug exposures at which therapeutic efficacy is observed with those at which deleterious effects (e.g., infections, suppression of erythropoiesis) occur.

Current efforts in developing JAK3 inhibitors have focused on the JH1 kinase domain. The multidomain architecture of JAK3 and the connected functionality of the different domains raise the possibility of alternative approaches. Theoretically, inhibitors that act on the JH2 domain may also be effective in downregulating the kinase activity of JH1. Alternatively, binding of JAK3 to the γc subunit of the cytokine receptor may be disrupted. The feasibility of this approach has been demonstrated through observation of the effects of FERM domain mutations in human subjects [14]. However, acceptable small molecules inhibiting the binding of JAK3 to the receptor have not yet been found. The same is also true for the inhibition of STAT protein binding at the GAS site on the chromosomes.

Individual inhibitors targeting JAK3

Prior to the recent resolution of the crystal structure of the JAK3 kinase domain [15], JAK3 inhibitors were discovered using conventional kinase or cell-based assays. Several small molecules have been identified as inhibitors of JAK3, and their activity in vitro and in animal transplant models has been extensively published. More recent data indicate that some of these agents have low potency for inhibiting JAK3 and significant cross-reactivity for other members within the JAK family and non-JAK kinases. Although the pharmacological effects reported for these relatively nonselective JAK3 inhibitors are not in dispute, these data must be interpreted with caution given the uncertainty regarding the extent to which the demonstrated effects could directly be attributable to inhibition of JAK3 or JAKs.

The chemical structures of these investigational agents are shown in Figure 18.2. A summary of the developmental status of these agents is presented in Table 18.3. This section will focus on data relating to

transplantation rather than autoimmune diseases, for which some of these agents are also being developed. Compounds for which only in vitro data on JAK3 inhibition are available will not be addressed in this chapter.

AG-490, WHI-P131, WHI-P154, PNU156804

AG-490 belongs structurally to the tyrphostin family and was first synthesized in the early 1990s. AG-490 was initially found to be a JAK2 inhibitor and shown to be cytotoxic to acute lymphoblastic leukemia cells [16]. For its time, this was a significant development supporting kinase inhibition as a viable target for drug development. Subsequently, AG-490 was demonstrated to inhibit JAK3-dependent IL-2-induced T cell proliferation with an IC_{50} of 25 μM [17]. Inhibition of JAK3 autophosphorylation and activation of STAT5a/b by AG-490 were also reported [18]. In a heterotopic heart allograft model in rats, intravenous AG-490 prolonged allograft survival in monotherapy was synergistic with the signal 1 inhibitor cyclosporine but demonstrated only additive effect when combined with sirolimus [19]. Nonetheless, more recent evidence indicates that AG-490 is neither potent nor selective for either JAK2 or JAK3 [20, 21].

The dimethoxyquinazoline compounds WHI-P131 (also known as JANEX1) and WHI-P154 were purported to be JAK3 inhibitors with IC_{50} of 9 μM and 28 μM respectively in JAK3-dependent cell proliferation assays [22]. Initial analyses suggested that WHI-P131 did not inhibit other kinases, such as JAK1, JAK2, Syk, BTK, or LYN, even at concentrations as high as 350 μM [23]. WHI-P131 was effective in attenuating the severity of acute GVHD after bone marrow transplantation in mice [24], preventing autoimmune diabetes in nonobese diabetic mice [25], and prolonging murine islet allograft survival [22]. However, recent kinase panel testing has revealed that both these molecules are in fact potent inhibitors of epidermal growth factor (EGF) receptor kinase, with very little or no activity against the JAK family [20, 21]. The data published using these compounds should be interpreted with these findings in mind. The cellular

Table 18.3 Status of development of investigational compounds targeting JAK3 inhibition. This table focuses on transplant-related data and includes only data published in manuscripts or abstracts.[a]

	Rodent transplant models		Primate transplant model	Clinical trials		
	Monotherapy	Combination with CNI		Phase I studies	Phase II transplant studies	Phase II nontransplant studies
AG-490	Heart transplants in rats	Synergistic	—	—	—	—
WHI-P131	aGvHD after bone marrow transplants in rats; islet transplants in rats	—	—	—	—	—
WHI-P154	—	—	—	—	—	—
PNU156804	Heart transplants in rats	Synergistic	—	—	—	—
CP-690,550	Heart transplants in mice; neonatal heart-to-pinna transplants in mice	Synergistic	Kidney transplants in cynomolgus monkeys	Stable kidney transplant patients, various clinical pharmacology studies, completed	De novo kidney transplant patients, ongoing	Patients with various autoimmune disorders, ongoing
R348	Heart transplants in rats	Synergistic	—	—	—	—
NC1153	Kidney transplants in rats; spleen transplants in rats	Synergistic	—	—	—	—

[a]aGVHD: acute graft-versus-host disease; CNI: calcineurin inhibitor.

effects previously reported for WHI-P131, e.g., its ability to stabilize mast cells, inhibit glioblastoma cell proliferation, and block platelet aggregation, may not be attributable to its activity on JAK3 [5].

PNU156804 is an undecylprodigiosin analog that was initially reported to inhibit the activation of nuclear factor-κB and adaptor protein-1 transcription factors [26]. Subsequently, it was shown to block IL-2-induced T cell proliferation (IC$_{50}$ ~7.5 μM), JAK3 autophosphorylation, and IL-2-mediated phosphorylation of STAT5a and STAT5b [27]. PNU156804 inhibits JAK3-dependent T cell proliferation induced by IL-2, IL-4, IL-7, and IL-15 and was at least twofold less potent in inhibiting JAK2-induced Nb2-11c cell growth. PNU156804 does not seem to affect signal 1 events, such as the activity of Lck or ZAP70, or expression of IL-2Rα.

When administered orally, PNU156804 extended the survival of heterotopic heart allografts in rats and demonstrated synergism with cyclosporine, but only additive activity with sirolimus [27]. Owing to myelosuppressive activity, further development of PNU156804 was not pursued [22].

CP-690,550

Among the inhibitors that target JAK3, CP-690,550 is currently the only one undergoing clinical trials in organ transplantation. Phase II/III trials are ongoing for prevention of acute renal allograft rejection and treatment of a variety of autoimmune disorders (e.g., rheumatoid arthritis, psoriasis, Crohn's disease, ulcerative colitis, dry eye). This review will focus on data relating to organ transplantation.

History and chemical structure

CP-690,550 was identified through a screening and synthesis program designed to optimize JAK3 inhibitory activity based on inhibition of the JH1 catalytic domain of JAK3 fused to glutathione S-transferase. A lead compound CP-352,664 was initially identified from screening several thousand candidates for JAK3 inhibitory activity. This was followed by extensive chemical modifications to improve the kinase-inhibitory activity, resulting in the synthesis of CP-690,550, a substituted piperidine linked to a deazapurine [28]. Two chiral centers exist in CP-690,550, with the (3R,4R)-isomer being the primary stereoisomer accounting for JAK3 inhibition [29].

Potency and selectivity

CP-690,550 is a potent inhibitor of JAK3 with an IC_{50} of 1 nM in purified enzyme assays, and an IC_{50} of 11 nM in a cell-based assay of IL-2-induced T cell blast proliferation [28]. CP-690,550 demonstrates cross-species activity in inhibiting the mix lymphocyte reactions of murine, monkey, or human cells. Cellular assays using YT cells confirmed that IL-2-induced phosphorylation of JAK3 and STATs was blocked by CP-690,550 [28].

CP-690,550 is highly selective for the JAK family of kinases, with IC_{50} of >3000 nM for a panel of 30 other kinases, including the signal-1-related Lck [28]. The selectivity for the JAK family was further confirmed using a panel of 354 kinases and KINOMEscan technology [29]. A separate study evaluating a panel of 317 kinases also found only limited cross-reactivity with kinases outside of the JAK family [30]. In cellular assays, CP-690,550 lacked significant inhibitory activity against TCR signaling or serum-induced fibroblast proliferation [28].

Within the JAK family, the potency of CP-690,550 was initially reported to be 20-fold and 112-fold lower for JAK2 and JAK1 respectively based on in vitro kinase assays [28]. Subsequent studies using alternative kinase assay formats have reported negligible differences in potencies for JAK1, JAK2, and JAK3 [29,31]. Despite the apparent similarity in in vitro potency for JAK2 and JAK3, functional selectivity for JAK3 was demonstrated in cellular

assays. An initial study found an approximately 30-fold selectivity for JAK3 over JAK2, with an IC_{50} of 11 nM for the JAK3-mediated IL-2-induced T cell proliferation compared with an IC_{50} of 324 nM for the JAK2-mediated GM-CSF-induced proliferation of HUO3 cells [28]. In a separate study using the TF1 cellular assay, a 10-fold selectivity in favor of JAK3 over JAK2 was demonstrated by comparing IC_{50} values of CP-690,550 in IL-4-induced proliferation (80 nM) versus IL-3-induced proliferation (800 nM) [31]. A separate study also reported selective JAK3 inhibition by CP-690,550 over JAK2 by evaluating the phosphorylation of STAT4 in IL-12-stimulated cells [29]. In contrast to the relatively low potency in inhibiting wild-type JAK2, CP-690,550 demonstrates enhanced inhibitory activity against the mutated JAK2, $JAK2^{v617F}$, found in the erythroid progenitor cells in polycythemia vera patients [32].

When IL-2-induced increase in phosphorylated STAT5 levels was measured in immune cells derived from healthy subjects, CP-690,550 had significantly higher IC_{50} in $CD4^+CD25^{high}FoxP3^+$ T cells (136 ng/mL) than in $CD4^+CD25^{-/dim}$ T cells (58 ng/mL) [33]. This demonstrates that CP-690,550 preferentially inhibits the function of effector T cells but spares regulatory T cells (Tregs). In addition, the suppressive activity of the Tregs was unaltered by in vitro incubation with CP-690,550.

Nonclinical transplant models

CP-690,550 has been shown to be effective in preventing acute allograft rejection in several experimental models of transplantation in rodents and nonhuman primates.

In a heterotopic cardiac allograft model in mice, CP-690,550 treatment prolonged mean survival time of the allograft to >60 days from 12 days in control animals [28]. RNA analysis showed that CP-690,550 treatment was associated with decreased gene expression of Fas ligand, granzyme B, interferon-inducible protein 10 (IP-10), monkine induced by interferons (MIG), and RANTES [28]. CP-690,550 was also evaluated in a model of neonatal hearts transplanted to ear pinnae in MHC-mismatched mice [34]. CP-690,550 monotherapy prolonged allograft survival compared with vehicle. Synergism with cyclosporine was demonstrated without evidence of altered exposure of either compound [34].

The immunosuppressive efficacy of CP-690,550 was also evaluated in mixed leukocyte reaction (MLR)-mismatched, ABO-compatible cynomolgus monkeys that received life-supporting renal transplants. CP-690,550 monotherapy significantly prolonged mean survival time to 53±7 days (mean±SEM) compared with 7±1 days in vehicle-treated control animals and delayed the onset of acute rejection [35]. Combination of CP-690,550 and mycophenolate mofetil (MMF) significantly extended mean survival time compared with MMF treatment alone (60±10 days versus 23±1 days) but did not further improve survival time or graft pathology compared with CP-690,550 monotherapy [36]. Higher CP-690,550 exposures were associated with longer survival times. In particular, a strong positive correlation between early (day 3) drug exposure and survival was found. With either CP-690,550 monotherapy or combination therapy with MMF, subclinical or overt acute rejection eventually developed in most of the treated animals [35, 36], suggesting that combination with additional immunosuppressants may be required to optimize outcomes. Persistent anemia was observed among the 10 animals receiving monotherapy with high CP-690,550 exposure (12 h area under the curve AUC_{0-12} >550 ng h/mL), and two of these animals developed polyoma-virus-associated nephropathy [35]. The combination of CP-690,550 and MMF was associated with reduced reticulocyte counts compared with CP-690,550 monotherapy, suggesting that the combination may have more adverse impact on erythropoiesis. Notably, none of the animals manifested nephrotoxicty, neurotoxicity, or overt metabolic derangement. CP-690, 550 monotherapy was associated with significant reductions in the number of NK, CD4+, and CD8+ cells, but the percentage of CD8+ effector memory T cells appeared unaffected [37]. In comparison, a progressive decrease in NK cell count was observed during combination treatment, whereas CD4+, CD8+ T cell and B cell numbers were unchanged. It is not clear why the effects on immune cells in primate recipients of renal allografts are somewhat different from earlier findings in nontransplanted cynomolgus monkeys in which CP-690,550 treatment resulted in reduced effector memory CD8+ and NK cell numbers [38].

In a heterotopic aorta transplant model in rats, CP-690,550 reduced allograft vasculopathy as demonstrated by a 51 % reduction in intimal hyperplasia compared with the untreated control group [39]. In addition, donor-specific IgG production was decreased in the CP-690,550-treated animals. In a tracheal transplant model in rats, CP-690,550 ameliorated obliterative bronchiolitis by significantly reducing airway obliteration compared with the untreated control group, and eliminating the loss of epithelia coverage [40]. These treatment effects were associated with reduced lymphocyte and macrophage infiltration of the trachea allograft and increased expression of TGFβ3, a cytokine with antifibrotic properties [41].

Clinical pharmacology
Pharmacokinetics

Following oral administration of radiolabeled CP-690,550, plasma total radioactivity peaked approximately 1 h post-dose, and >80 % of the radioactivity was recovered in the urine, suggesting rapid and extensive oral absorption. It was estimated that total body clearance consisted of approximately 30 % renal excretion of unchanged drug and approximately 70 % hepatic metabolism [42].

The pharmacokinetics of CP-690,550 was evaluated in 14 de novo renal allograft recipients following administration of 15 mg twice daily (BID) and 30 mg BID in combination with MMF [43]. The absorption on day 1 post-transplant was decreased with variable times to peak plasma concentration (T_{max}). By post-transplant day 3, the pharmacokinetic profile was similar to that in healthy volunteers with consistent absorption (median T_{max} 1–2 h) and rapid elimination (mean $T_{1/2}$ 3.5 h). Mean 12 h AUC values on day 3 post-transplant increased in a dose-proportional manner from 15 mg BID to 30 mg BID (678 ng h/mL and 1141 ng h/mL respectively) and were similar to the steady-state 12 h AUC values observed in stable renal transplant patients. Over a 6 month period, geometric mean trough concentrations of CP-690,550 were 17 ng/mL and 32 ng/mL for the 15 mg and 30 mg BID doses respectively and were highly variable, with coefficients of variation of approximately 100%. Concentrations at 4h post-dose showed higher correlation with AUC_{0-t} ($r=0.92$) than trough concentrations ($r=0.63$) [43].

Renal excretion of unchanged drug partly accounts for CP-690,550 elimination. In patients with mild, moderate, and severe renal impairment the AUC values were elevated by 37%, 43%, and 123% respectively, relative to subjects with normal renal function [44]. Among end-stage renal disease patients, the AUC was 40% higher on nondialysis days than that in healthy volunteers.

Drug–drug interactions
Co-administration of CP-690,550 and MMF in stable renal transplant patients did not result in clinically relevant pharmacokinetic interaction between the two agents [45]. On the other hand, co-administration of cyclosporine or tacrolimus appeared to moderately increase CP-690,550 exposure without alterations in the post-treatment cyclosporine or tacrolimus trough concentrations [45]. The magnitude of this potential interaction between calcineurin inhibitors and CP-690,550 requires confirmation in more formal pharmacokinetic evaluations.

Hepatic metabolism of CP-690,550 is mediated by CYP3A4 and CYP2C19. Therefore, CP-690,550 pharmacokinetics is expected to be affected by CYP3A4 inhibitors. When CP-690,550 was co-administered with the moderately potent CYP3A4 and CYP2C19 inhibitor fluconazole in healthy volunteers, the CP-690,550 AUC increased by 79% and C_{max} increased by 27% [46].

Effect on renal function and QT interval
The effect of 14 day treatment with CP-690,550 15 mg BID on renal function was evaluated in 34 healthy volunteers in a placebo-controlled study [47]. Glomerular filtration rate (GFR) was measured by iohexol serum clearance, effective renal plasma flow (ERPF) by *para*-aminohippuric acid urinary clearance, and creatinine clearance by 24h urine collection. Results of this study showed that CP-690,550 had no effect on GFR, ERPF, or creatinine secretion in healthy volunteers.

The effect of CP-690,550 on QTc interval was evaluated using concentration–response analysis of pooled data obtained from a single-dose study in 94 healthy subjects and a multiple-dose study in 58 psoriatic patients [48]. No clinically relevant changes in Fridericia correction QTc interval were found.

Clinical trials: Phase I transplant study
The short-term safety and tolerability of co-administration of CP-690,550 and MMF were established in stable renal allograft recipients in a randomized, dose-escalation, placebo-controlled Phase I study [45]. Six patients received CP-690,550 5 mg BID, six patients received 15 mg BID, ten patients received 30 mg BID, and six patients received placebo, each for 29 days. All 28 patients received MMF concomitantly. The majority of patients randomized to CP-690,550 5 mg BID and 15 mg BID also received concomitant calcineurin inhibitors (either cyclosporine or tacrolimus), whereas patients assigned 30 mg BID did not to avoid overimmunosuppression. There were no deaths, malignancies, systemic opportunistic infections, or acute rejection episodes during the study. In the CP-690,550-treated patients, the most common adverse effects were infection and gastrointestinal disorders. The overall incidence of these adverse events was comparable to that in the placebo patients. Most infections were mild or moderate in severity. However, there appeared to be a preponderance of severe infections in the CP-690,550 15 mg and 30 mg BID groups. These observations confirm the in vivo potency of CP-690,550 as an immunosuppressive agent.

Compared with pretreatment baseline, a mean decrease in hemoglobin of 11% was observed among the patients receiving CP-690,550 15 mg and 30 mg BID [45]. This may represent an off-target inhibitory effect of CP-690,550 on JAK2 when co-administered with MMF. There were no changes in the numbers of neutrophils, total lymphocytes, or platelets. There were also no clinically meaningful changes in clinical chemistry, vital signs, or electrocardiograms from baseline.

Clinical trials: Phase II transplant studies
In a pilot multicenter Phase IIA study, relatively low rates of acute renal allograft rejection were achieved

with CP-690,550 in a calcineurin-inhibitor-free regimen. In this proof-of-concept study, 61 de novo renal allograft recipients were randomized to CP-690,550 15 mg BID (CP15, $N=20$), CP-690,550 30 mg BID (CP30, $N=20$), or standard-dose tacrolimus ($N=21$) [49]. Immunologically high-risk recipients were excluded and 75% of the study subjects were living-related donor recipients. All patients also received IL-2R antagonist induction, concomitant MMF, and corticosteroid taper. CP-690,550 dose was reduced after the first 6 months. In the CP30 group, BK virus nephropathy developed in 4 of 20 patients, prompting the implementation of a protocol amendment to discontinue MMF in this group. The 6 month biopsy-proven acute rejection (BPAR) rates were 1/20 in CP15, 4/20 in CP30, and 1/21 in the tacrolimus control group. No new CP-690,550-treated patients developed acute rejection between 6 and 12 months so that the 12 month BPAR rates were 1/20 in CP15, 4/20 in CP30, and 2/21 in the control group. The paradoxically higher BPAR rate at the higher CP-690,550 dose level (CP30) than in CP15 may be due to the small sample size in each of the three groups.

Through 12 months post-transplant, the most common adverse events observed in this study were in gastrointestinal disorders and infections [49]. Gastrointestinal disorders occurred at similar rates in all three treatment groups. Clinically significant infections occurred more frequently in CP30 than in the tacrolimus group. Although four patients in CP30 developed BK virus nephropathy while receiving concomitant MMF, there had been no new cases of BK virus nephropathy after MMF was discontinued. More patients developed cytomegalovirus diseases in 6 months in the CP-690,550 groups (2/20 in CP15, 4/20 in CP30) than in the tacrolimus control group (0/21). In addition, between 6 and 12 months, herpes zoster infection developed in five patients (four in CP15 and one in the tacrolimus control group). GFR estimated by the Nankivell equation exceeded 70 mL/min in all three groups at 6 and 12 months. Compared with the control group, the two CP-690,550 groups showed a trend toward more frequent anemia and neutropenia in the first 6 months, but there was no apparent difference between the CP-690,550

groups and the control group in hemoglobin concentration or neutrophil counts by 12 months. Within 12 months post-transplant, total cholesterol, low- and high-density lipoprotein cholesterol, and triglycerides increased by 34–44% in the CP-690,550 groups compared with the tacrolimus control group.

These results support the clinical relevance of JAK or JAK3 inhibition as a target for immunosuppressive drug development. However, co-administration of CP-690,550 30 mg BID with MMF was overimmunosuppressive. Further dose-finding appears warranted from the results of this pilot study. Phase IIB evaluations of CP-690,550 in combination with MMF are ongoing.

Clinical trials: nontransplant studies

CP-690,550 has been evaluated in clinical trials in patients with autoimmune diseases – i.e., psoriasis and rheumatoid arthritis. The results of these studies provide further support of the immunomodulatory effects of CP-690,550.

In a double-blind, dose-escalation Phase I study, 59 patients with active psoriatic lesions received one of six CP-690,550 dose levels (5, 10, 20, 30, or 50 mg BID or 60 mg once daily) or placebo for 14 days. There was a statistically significant improvement in the severity of the index psoriasis lesion for all CP-690,550 doses compared with the placebo group except for 5 mg BID [50]. In addition, the expression of K16 (a keratinocyte growth activation marker) had completely or mostly normalized in three of four biopsies obtained after 14-day treatment with CP-690,550 30 mg BID. Phase IIB studies of CP-690,550 in psoriasis patients are ongoing.

In three double-blind placebo-controlled Phase II studies, CP-690,550 was evaluated in a total of 1157 patients with active rheumatoid arthritis. A Phase IIA study ($N=264$) assessed CP-690,550 doses of 5 mg to 30 mg BID for 6 weeks [51]. By week 6, all CP-690,550 doses were statistically improved compared with placebo in the American College of Rheumatology 20% improvement criteria (ACR20). The most common adverse events reported were headache and nausea. The two Phase IIB studies ($N=509$ and 384) assessed doses of 1 mg to 15 mg BID and 20 mg once daily for 12 weeks with and without concomitant methotrexate [52, 53]. At the end of 12 weeks, patients who were randomized to CP-690,550 1 mg BID, 3 mg BID, 20 mg QD or placebo and did not achieve adequate response were reassigned to 5 mg BID for another 12 weeks. Compared with placebo, ACR20 rate was significantly higher than placebo at week 12 for all CP-690,550 dose groups except 1 mg BID [52, 53]. The improvements in ACR20 were associated with improvements in pain, physical functioning, and quality of life [54]. With co-administration of CP-690,550 and methotrexate, the most common adverse events were headache, nausea, and increased hepatic aminotransferases [52]. When CP-690,550 was administered as monotherapy, the most common adverse events were urinary tract infection, diarrhea, bronchitis, and headache [53]. There were dose-dependent increases in serum lipids and decreases in hemoglobin and neutrophil count.

Effect on immune parameters in clinical transplant studies

The effect of CP-690,550 on peripheral immune parameters was evaluated in a subgroup of eight stable renal transplant patients in the aforementioned Phase I study [55]. All eight subjects were at least 6 years post-transplant and received CP-690,550 30 mg BID in combination with MMF and corticosteroids. CP-690,550 treatment was associated with a 65 % mean reduction of peripheral NK cell (CD3$^-$CD16$^+$CD56$^+$) count from pretreatment baseline. This observation is consistent with the role played by IL-15 and IL-21, members of the JAK3-dependent IL-2 cytokine family, in the homeostasis of NK cells. CP-690,550 treatment also resulted in a 100 % mean increase in the peripheral B lymphocyte count, which was not associated with changes in IgG, IgA, and IgM levels. A significant effect of CP-690,550 on the peripheral regulatory T cell count was observed, with numbers of CD4+CD25$^{bright+}$ cells reduced by 38 %. This observation can be explained by the dependence of the survival of Tregs on the IL-2 family of cytokines. In contrast, no significant changes were observed in CD3$^+$, CD3$^+$CD4$^+$, and CD3$^+$CD8$^+$ T cell counts during

CP-690,550 treatment. Similar to the observations made on immune cells derived from healthy subjects, the regulatory capacity of the residual CD4$^+$CD25$^{bright+}$ cells in these renal transplant patients remain intact. Reconstitution of CD25$^{bright+}$ cells to responder CD25$^{-/dim}$ cells resulted in similar dose-dependent inhibition of proliferation before and during CP-690,550 treatment [55]. In addition, in the presence of CP-690,550, the interferon-γ production capacity of peripheral blood mononuclear cells was reduced by 39 %.

An inhibitory effect of CP-690,550 on the phosphorylation of STAT5 was also demonstrated ex vivo in the same subgroup of stable renal transplant patients. Incubation with patient serum collected after 29 days of CP-690,550 treatment reduced IL-2-induced STAT5 phosphorylation by a median of 20 % in patient CD3$^+$ cells ($p<0.05$), by 37 % in CD3$^+$CD4$^+$ (helper) T cells ($p<0.05$), and by 34 % in CD3$^+$CD8$^+$ (cytotoxic) T cells ($p<0.01$) [56]. The reduction in lymphocyte STAT5 phosphorylation was associated with reduced expression of the target genes SOCS3 by 57 % ($p<0.05$) and IFNγ by 27 % ($p<0.05$). Expression of FoxP3, Fas ligand, and granzyme B were also reduced, albeit to a lesser extent.

In de novo renal transplant patients, treatment with CP-690,550 15 mg and 30 mg BID was associated with a reduction in circulating CD3$^-$CD56$^+$ (NK) cell counts by 67–77 % in 12 months compared with the tacrolimus control group [49]. However, no discernable association between NK cell counts and opportunistic viral infections was apparent. There was no difference in circulating T cell and B cell counts between the CP-690,550 groups and the tacrolimus group.

NC1153

NC1153 is a Mannich base identified through an extensive screening program for compounds with similar structure to AG-490. Screening was performed for 200 000 small molecules in the National Cancer Institute Drug Discovery Program, and the nine compounds identified were tested for inhibitory activity on IL-2-induced lymphocyte proliferation [57]. NC1153 inhibited the activity of purified JAK3 enzyme with an IC$_{50}$ of approximately 2.5–5.0 μM. In IL-2-responsive YT cells, NC1153 inhibited phosphorylation of JAK3 with a similar IC_{50} of 2.5 μM, and also reduced phosphorylation of STAT5a and STAT5b. NC1153 was reported to show >40-fold selectivity for JAK3 over JAK2 using the prolactin-dependent T lymphoma cell line Nb2-11c assay, and did not affect the activity of the signal 1 enzymes Lck or ZAP70, or IL-2Rα production [22].

Extensive preclinical evaluations of NC1153 in rodents have been published. Treatment with NC1153 orally for 90 days in a rat MHC/non-MHC-mismatched renal allograft model achieved survival of >200 days in 75% of treated animals. Further extension of the treatment duration by 90 days produced long-term graft acceptance and appeared to confer tolerance, with acceptance of donor but not third-party cardiac allografts by the treated animals [57]. Therapeutic synergism between NC1153 and cyclosporine was also demonstrated in the rat allograft model. In a spleen transplant model in rats, NC1153 treatment prevented rejection and reduced the number of graft infiltration cells [57].

NC1153 had no effect on renal function, lipid metabolism or bone marrow in rats. In a salt-deprived rate model, NC1153 alone did not result in changes in renal function or histopathology, and did not exacerbate the adverse functional or histopathological effects of cyclosporine [57]. In rats fed with a high-fat diet, NC1153 treatment was not associated with elevated serum total cholesterol, low-density lipoprotein cholesterol or, triglycerides. Treatment of rats with NC1153 had no apparent adverse effects on hemoglobin levels or femoral bone marrow cellularity [57].

In vitro assays suggest that NC1153 did not compete with substrates for CYP3A4 or 1A2 but would interact with 2D6 and 2C19.

Clinical trials with NC1153 have not been published. No ongoing clinical trials are listed in www.clinicalTrials.gov.

R348

R348 is an orally active JAK3 inhibitor that also inhibits the signal-1-related spleen tyrokine kinase (Syk). R348 is metabolized by the intestine to its active metabolite R333. After oral administration of R348 in rats, blood levels of R333 were 10–15 times higher than those of R348 through 24h post-dose

[58]. In vitro cell culture assays demonstrated the IC_{50} for JAK3-dependent IL-2-driven T cell proliferation to be 0.18 μM, compared with an IC_{50} of 0.84 μM for the JAK2-dependent EPO CHEP Hb cell line [59].

In a heterotopic cardiac transplant model in rats, R348 preserved graft function and reduced graft infiltration, rejection scores, and intragraft expression of inflammatory cytokines [59]. Oral administration of R348 achieved similar cardiac allograft survival to therapeutically dosed tacrolimus or sirolimus. Synergism was demonstrated when R348 was combined with tacrolimus. In a heterotopic trachea allograft model in rats, administration of R348 attenuated the development of chronic airway allograft rejection [58]. R348 reduced airway luminal obliteration to 16–21% compared with 100% in untreated controls, and preserved the physiological epithelial coverage in the allograft. In addition, R348 significantly suppressed peritracheal graft infiltrating cells and donor-specific IgG level [58].

The immunomodulatory effect of R348 has also been evaluated in a nontransplant preclinical model. In mice with T-cell-dependent spontaneous psoriasiform skin disease, R348 resulted in a marked attenuation of skin lesion, and histology analyses showed reductions of epidermal and dermal lesion severity and decreased CD4[+] T cell infiltration [60].

Phase I clinical trials on R348 have not been reported.

Summary

JAK3 plays a vital role in the intracellular signaling cascade downstream of select cytokine receptors in immune cells. Inhibition of JAK3 is expected to result in potent immunosuppression, and thus JAK3 appears to be a rational pharmaceutical target. Nonclinical and clinical data relating to transplantation have become available for several molecules targeting inhibition of JAK3. Clinical trials on CP-690,550 in calcineurin-inhibitor-free regimens have provided preliminary evidence that JAK3 inhibition is a promising approach to prevent acute allograft rejection. However, dose-limiting adverse events, such as opportunistic viral infections and hematological aberrations, have been observed. Further evaluations of this class of agents are warranted to ascertain the dose/concentration range for individual agents and the combination regimens that optimize clinical efficacy and minimize adverse effects.

References

1 Ghoreschi K, Laurence A, O'Shea JJ. Janus kinases in immune cell signaling. *Immunol Rev* 2009;228:273–287.

2 Paukku K, Silvennoinen O. STATs as critical mediators of signal transduction and transcription: lesions learned from STAT5. *Cytokine Gr Factors Rev* 2004;15:435–455.

3 Lin JX, Leonard WJ. The role of Stat5a and Stat5b in signaling by IL-2 family cytokines. *Oncogene* 2000; 19:2566–2576.

4 Aaronson DS, Horvath CM. A road map for those who don't know JAK–STAT. *Science* 2002;296:1653–1655.

5 Thompson JE. JAK protein kinase inhibitors. *Drug News Perspect* 2005;18:305–310.

6 Shuai K, Liu B. Regulation of JAK–STAT signalling in the immune system. *Nat Rev* 2003;3:900–911.

7 Pesu M, Laurence A, Kishore N *et al.* Therapeutic targeting of Janus kinases. *Immunol Rev* 2008;223: 132–142.

8 Wilks AF. The JAK kinases: not just another kinase drug discovery target. *Semin Cell Dev Biol* 2008;19:319–328.

9 Yamaoka K, Saharinen P, Pesu M *et al.* The Janus kinases (Jaks). *Genome Biol* 2004;5:253–258.

10 O'Shea JJ, Husa M, Li D *et al.* Jak3 and the pathogenesis of severe combined immunodeficiency. *Mol Immunol* 2004;41:727–737.

11 Li XC, Ima A, Li Y *et al.* Blocking the common gamma chain of cytokine receptors induces T cell apoptosis and long term islet allograft survival. *J Immunol* 2000;164:1193–1199.

12 Luo C, Laaja P. Inhibitors of JAKs/STATs and the kinases: a possible new cluster of drugs. *Drug Dis Today* 2004;9:268–275.

13 Ghoreschi K, Laurence, O'Shea J. Selectivity and therapeutic inhibition of kinases: to be or not to be? *Nat Immunol* 2009;10:356–360.

14 Zhou Y, Chen M, Cusack NA *et al.* Unexpected effects of FERM domain mutations on catalytic activity of Jak3: structural implication for Janus kinases. *Mol Cell* 2001;8:959–969.

15 Boggon TJ, Li Y, Manley PW, Eck MJ. Crystal structure of the Jak3 kinase domain in complex with a staurosporine analog. *Blood* 2005;106:996–1002.

16 Meydan N, Grunberger T, Dadi H *et al.* Inhibition of acute lymphoblastic leukaemia by a Jak-2 inhibitor. *Nature* 1996;379:645–648.

17 Wang LH, Kirken RA, Erwin RA *et al.* JAK3, STAT and MAPK signaling pathways as novel molecular targets for the tyrphostin AG-490 regulation of IL-2-mediated T cell response. *J Immunol* 1999;162:3897–3904.

18 Kirken RA, Erwin RA, Taub D *et al.* Tyrphostin AG-490 inhibits cytokine-mediated JAK3/STAT5a/b signal transduction and cellular proliferation of antigen-activated human T cells. *J Leukoc Biol* 1999;65: 891–899.

19 Behbod F, Erwin-Cohen RA, Wang ME *et al.* Concomitant inhibition of Janus kinase 3 and calcineurin-dependent signaling pathways synergistically prolongs the survival of rat heart allografts. *J Immunol* 2001;166:3724–3732.

20 Burns C, Wilks A, Su S. JAK kinase inhibitors. *Drug Dis Today* 2004;9:694–695.

21 Changelian PS, Moshinsky D, Kuhn CF *et al.* The specificity of JAK3 kinase inhibitors. *Blood* 2008;111: 2155–2157.

22 Podder H, Kahan BD. Janus kinase 3: a novel target for selective transplant immunosuppression. *Expert Opin Ther Targets* 2004;8:613–629.

23 Sudbeck EA, Liu-XP, Narla RK *et al.* Structure-based design of specific inhibitors of Janus kinase 3 as apoptosis-inducing antileukemic agents. *Clin Cancer Res* 1999;5:1569–1582.

24 Uckun FM, Roers BA, Waurzyniak B *et al.* Janus kinase 3 inhibitor WHI-P131/JANEX-1 prevents graft-versus-host disease but spares the graft-versus-leukemia function of the bone marrow allografts in a murine bone marrow transplantation model. *Blood* 2002;99: 4192–4199.

25 Cetkovic-Cvrlje M, Dragt AL, Vassilev A *et al.* Targeting JAK3 with JAKEX-1 for prevention of autoimmune type 1 diabetes in NOD mice. *Clin Immunol* 2003;106: 213–225.

26 Mortellaro A, Songia S, Gnocchi P *et al.* New immunosuppressive drug PNU156804 blocks IL-2-dependent proliferation and NF-κB and AP-1 activation. *J Immunol* 1999;162:7102–7109.

27 Stepkowski SM, Erwin-Cohen RA, Behbod F *et al.* Selective inhibitor of Janus tyrosine kinase 3, PNU156804, prolongs allograft survival and acts synergistically with cyclosporine but additively with rapamycin. *Blood* 2002;99:680–689.

28 Changelian PS, Flanagan ME, Ball DJ *et al*. Prevention of organ allograft rejection by a specific Janus kinase 3 inhibitor. *Science* 2003;302:875–878.

29 Jiang JK, Ghoreschi K, Deflorian F *et al*. Examining the chirality, conformation and selective kinase inhibition of 3-((3*R*,4*R*)-4-methyl-3-(methyl(7*H*-pyrrolo[2,3-*d*]pyrimidin-4-yl)amino)piperidin-1-yl)-3-oxopropane-nitrile (CP-690,550). *J Med Chem* 2008;51:8012–8018.

30 Karaman MW, Herrgard S, Treiber DK *et al*. A quantitative analysis of kinase inhibitor selectivity. *Nat Biotechnol* 2008;26:127–132.

31 Clark MP, George KM, Bookland RG *et al*. Development of new pyrrolopyrimidine-based inhibitors of Janus kinase 3 (JAK3). *Bioorg Med Chem Lett* 2007;17:1250–1253.

32 Manshouri T, Quintás-Cardama A, Nussenzveig RH *et al*. The JAK kinase inhibitor CP-690,550 suppresses the growth of human polycythemia vera cells carrying the JAK2v617F mutation. *Cancer Sci* 2008;99:1265–1273.

33 Sewgobind V, Quaedackers M, van der Laan L *et al*. The Jak inhibitor CP-690,550 inhibits effector T cells but does not affect the function of human CD4+CD25^bright^FoxP3+ regulatory T cells. *Am J Transplant* 2009;9(Suppl 2);381 [abstract].

34 Kudlacz E, Perry B, Sawyer P *et al*. The novel JAK-3 inhibitor CP-690550 is a potent immunosuppressive agent in various murine models. *Am J Transplant* 2004;4:51–57.

35 Borie DC, Changelian PC, Larson MJ *et al*. Immunosuppression by the JAK3 inhibitor CP-690,550 delays rejection and significantly prolongs kidney allograft survival in nonhuman primates. *Transplantation* 2005;79:791–801.

36 Borie DC, Larson MJ, Flores MG *et al*. Combined use of the JAK3 inhibitor CP-690,550 with mycophenolate mofetil to prevent kidney allograft rejection in nonhuman primates. *Transplantation* 2005;80:1756–1764.

37 Paniagua R, Si MS, Flores MG *et al*. Effects of JAK3 inhibition with CP-690,550 on immune cell populations and their functions in nonhuman primate recipients of kidney allografts. *Transplantation* 2005;80:1283–1292.

38 Conkyln M, Andresen C, Changelian P *et al*. The JAK3 inhibitor CP-690550 selectively reduces NK and CD8+ cell numbers in cynomolgus monkey blood following chronic oral dosing. *J Leukoc Biol* 2004;76:1248–1255.

39 Rousvoal G, Si MS, Lau M *et al*. Janus kinase 3 inhibition with CP-690,550 prevents allograft vasculopathy. *Transpl Int* 2006;19:1014–1021.

40 Rousvocal G, Zhang S, Berry G *et al*. JAK3 inhibition with CP-690,550 prevents obliterative bronchiolitis in a rat tracheal transplant model. *Transplantation* 2004;78:46 [abstract].

41 Zhang S, Lau M, Berry G *et al*. Prevention of obliterative bronchiolitis by Jak3 inhibition with CP-690,550 is accompanied by a distinct growth factor gene expression profile. *Transplantation* 2004;78:557 [abstract].

42 Prakash C, Lin J, Chan G *et al*. Metabolism, pharmacokinetics and excretion of a Janus kinase-3 inhibitor, CP-690,550 in healthy male volunteers. *AAPS J* 2008;10(S2):abstract 2492.

43 Krishnaswami S, Busque S, Leventhal J *et al*. Pharmacokinetic profile of CP-690,550 in de novo renal allograft recipients. *Transplantation* 2008;86(Suppl 2):414 [abstract].

44 Chow V, Krishnaswami S, Boy M *et al*. Pharmacokinetics of CP-690,550, a Janus kinase inhibitor, in subjects with impaired renal function. *Clin Pharmacol Ther* 2009;85:S63 [abstract].

45 Van Gurp E, Weimar E, Gaston R *et al*. Phase 1 dose-escalation study of CP-690,550 in stable renal allograft recipients: Preliminary findings of safety, tolerability, effects on lymphocyte subsets and pharmacokinetics. *Am J Transplant* 2008;8:1711–1718.

46 Chow V, Ni G, LaBadie R *et al*. An open label study to estimate the effect of fluconazole on the pharmacokinetics of CP-690,550 in healthy adult subjects. *Clin Pharmacol Ther* 2008;83:S36 [abstract].

47 Lawendy N, Krishnaswami S, Wang R *et al*. Effect of CP-690,550, an orally active Janus kinase inhibitor, on renal function in healthy adult volunteers. *J Clin Pharmacol* 2009;49:423–429.

48 Krishnaswami S, Gupta P, French J *et al*. The effect of CP-690,550, a Janus kinase inhibitor, on QTc interval and blood pressure: a concentration-response analysis of Phase 1 data. *Transplantation* 2008;86(suppl 2):414 [abstract].

49 Busque S, Leventhal J, Brennan DC *et al*. Calcineurin-inhibitor-free immunosuppression based on the JAK inhibitor CP-690,550: a pilot study in de novo kidney allograft recipients. *Am J Transplant* 2009;9:1936–1945.

50 Boy MG, Wang C, Wilkinson BE *et al*. (2009) Double-blind, placebo-controlled, dose-escalation study to evaluate the pharmacologic effect of CP-690,550 in patients with psoriasis. *J Invest Dermatol* 2009;129(9):2299–2302.

51 Kremer JM, Bloom BJ, Breedveld FC *et al*. The safety and efficacy of a JAK inhibitor in patients with active rheumatoid arthritis: results of a double-blind, placebo-controlled Phase IIa trial of three dosage levels of CP-690,550 versus placebo. *Arthritis Rheum* 2009;60:1895–1905.

52 Kremer J, Cohen S, Wilkinson B *et al*. The oral Jak inhibitor CP-690,550 in combination with methotrexate is

efficacious, safe and well tolerated in patients with active rheumatoid arthritis with an inadequate response to methotrexate alone. *Am Coll Rheumatol* 2008;28:L13 [abstract].

53 Kanik K, Fleischmann R, Cutolo M *et al*. Phase 2b dose ranging monotherapy study of the oral JAK inhibitor CP-690,550 or adalimumab vs placebo in patients with active rheumatoid arthritis with an inadequate response to DMARDs. *Ann Rheum Dis* 2009;68(Suppl 3):123 [abstract].

54 Wallenstein G, Kanik K, Wilkinson B *et al*. Results of two phase IIb studies of the oral JAK inhibitor CP-690,550 and its effects on pain, physical functioning, and health-related quality of life (HRQOL). *Ann Rheum Dis* 2009;68(Suppl 3):587 [abstract].

55 Van Gurp EAFJ, Schoordijk-Verschoor W, Klepper M *et al*. The effect of the JAK inhibitor CP-690,550 on peripheral immune parameters in stable kidney allograft patients. *Transplantation* 2009;87:79–86.

56 Quaedackers ME, Mol W, Korevaar SS *et al*. Monitoring of the immunomodulatory effect of CP-690,550 by analysis of the JAK/STAT pathway in kidney transplant patients. *Transplantation* 2009;88(8):1002–1009.

57 Stepkowski SM, Kao J, Wang ME *et al*. The Mannich base NC1153 promotes long-term allograft survival and spares the recipient from multiple toxicities. *J Immunol* 2005;175:4236–4246.

58 Velotta JB, Deuse T, Haddad M *et al*.. A novel JAK3 inhibitor, R348, attenuates chronic airway allograft rejection. *Transplantation* 2009;87:653–659.

59 Deuse T, Velotta JB, Hoyt G *et al*. Novel immunosuppression: R348, a JAK3- and Syk-inhibitor attenuates acute cardiac allograft rejection. *Transplantation* 2008;85:885–892.

60 Chang BY, Zhao F, He X *et al*. JAK3 inhibition significantly attenuates psoriasiform skin inflammation in CD18 mutant PL/J mice. *J Immunol* 2009;183:2183–2192.

CHAPTER 19
Cyclophosphamide

John J. Curtis
University of Alabama at Birmingham, Birmingham, AL, USA

Introduction

Cyclophosphamide is the generic name for an anticancer drug that is toxic to human cells both abnormal and normal. As standard chemotherapy, oncologists represent cyclophosphamide with the letter C in the acronym CHOP (cyclophosphamide, doxorubicin, vincristine, and prednisone). Besides destroying human cells, cyclophosphamide inhibits the immune system in a fairly nonspecific fashion and, thus, has been used in various diseases felt to be related to immunity. This includes solid organ transplantation. In addition to cancer and organ transplantation, cyclophosphamide has been used in rheumatoid arthritis, lupus, nephrotic syndrome, multiple sclerosis, and vasculitis (especially Wegener's). These are mostly nonapproved uses, and both effectiveness and safety are debated.

History

Norbert Brock, a pharmacist working with chemists Arnold and Bourseaux at the small German pharmaceutical company ASTA Werke AG, developed cyclophosphamide in 1958 [1]. Brock's work was remarkable in that it attempted to develop a prodrug that would not be toxic until it was metabolized to active form in cancer cells. He tried nearly 1000 analogs of nitrogen-mustard-like alkylating agents until he developed cyclophosphamide [2]. Nitrogen mustard, created as early as 1822, but first employed

as a chemical warfare agent in 1917 during World War I, caused severe skin blisters (and eventually cancer) and was effective in clearing a battlefield of soldiers, whose wounds were so severe as to assure they would not return to battle. It is ironic that this agent would eventually be used as an effective treatment for cancer. The most dramatic historical event involving nitrogen mustard occurred during World War II when a US supply ship, in the 1943 battle of Bali, was hit in an air raid, exploded, and released its supply of nitrogen mustard. There were large numbers of causalities of both civilians and army troops, but the observation was made that white blood cells were markedly decreased in those unprotected soldiers. Medical workers' observation [3] of this leukopenia prompted early attempts to use the agent to treat Hodgkin's lymphoma [4].

It was Brock who was awarded the Charles F. Kettering Prize by General Motors for cancer research in 1995, however, who found the analog that had a good therapeutic index and that has served as a cornerstone for cancer therapy for nearly half a century, especially lymphoma and leukemia. Unfortunately, cyclophosphamide did not prove to be as specific as Brock had hoped, since it was not metabolized to its active form only in the cancer cells. The liver metabolizes cyclophosphamide quickly to its active metabolites [5]. Yet, cyclophosphamide does have a relatively good therapeutic index, as will be discussed later.

By 1963, cyclophosphamide was given to kidney transplant patients [6, 7], but not with great

Immunotherapy in Transplantation: Principles and Practice, First Edition. Edited by Bruce Kaplan, Gilbert J. Burckart and Fadi G. Lakkis.
© 2012 Blackwell Publishing Ltd. Published 2012 by Blackwell Publishing Ltd.

enthusiasm until a report by Starzl *et al.* in 1971 [8]. Starzl *et al.* suggested that the drug had been overlooked and that it was especially effective in triple drug regimes replacing azathioprine and used with prednisone and antithymocyte globulin (ATG). They noted six patients who had liver dysfunction, which they attributed to azathioprine. They had improved liver enzymes after conversion to cyclophosphamide. This was, of course, long before hepatitis C was recognized and it is possible that azathioprine liver toxicity (and more recently cyclosporine liver toxicity) was overestimated in the era before the recognition of widespread hepatitis C among kidney failure patients [9]. Nonetheless, Starzl *et al.*'s optimistic review of cyclophosphamide use in kidney transplantation in the *Lancet* was followed by reports by Berlyne and Danovitch [10] and others of adverse effects.

Despite Starzl *et al.*'s early enthusiasm, cyclophosphamide remained a drug that most groups only used when azathioprine (a purine synthesis inhibitor that inhibited the proliferation of white blood cells) was believed to need replacement. As newer drugs like mycophenolate mofetil replaced azathioprine [11], cyclophosphamide use became even less common. Transplant units went from triple drug regimes of ATG, prednisone, and azathioprine to cyclosporine, prednisone, and mycophenolate mofetil with cyclophosphamide left mostly on the sidelines. In their early *Lancet* paper, however, Starzl *et al.* quoted the work of Santos *et al.* [12], who used cyclophosphamide for preparation for bone marrow transplant and could create donor chimerism. They also speculated about its ability to eliminate stimulated clones of lymphocytes in an early effort towards tolerance. Starzl *et al.* saw that perhaps cyclophosphamide might eventually be used in a fashion differently than azathioprine.

Chemistry/structure

Cyclophosphamide is chemically *N,N*-bis-(2-chloroethyl)-*N,O*-propylene phosphoric acid ester diamine monohydrate. It is a cyclic phosphamide mustard that is an alkylating agent but as a prodrug is inactive. It is soluble in body fluids and can be widely distributed in the human. It is metabolized by the liver and eliminated by the kidney.

Mechanism of action

Cyclophosphamide as a prodrug must be metabolized in the liver to ifosfamise mustard, phosphoramide mustard, and acrolein. This metabolism is by the cytochrome P450 system and is required for therapeutic activity [13]. Phosphoramide mustard is the DNA binding metabolite creating cross-links and DNA strand lesions [14]. These cytostatic effects are most effective in rapidly reproducing and proliferating of sensitive white blood cells; however, cyclophosphamide also appears to exhibit immunomodulatory effects. Maguire and coworkers demonstrated that cyclophosphamide potentiated delayed hypersensitivity [15] and cyclophosphamide has been shown to increase antibody production [16]. Neither of these effects would seem to help kidney transplant patients. However, cyclophosphamide, in addition to its general cytostatic effects, inhibits (in an irreversible fashion) the proliferative response of lymphocytes to interleukin-2 [17]. Thus, both general cytostatic effects on rapidly proliferating lymphocytes and perhaps important immunomodulatory effects on immune cell communication systems are important features of this drug's mechanism of action.

Pharmacokinetics and pharmacodynamics

As noted, cyclophosphamide is a prodrug and is converted to its active and toxic metabolites in the liver. The prodrug can be taken orally and is well absorbed and free of cytotoxicity until bioactivated in the liver. There are two major pathways for liver metabolism: the cytochrome P450 pathway, which handles most of the oxidative metabolism, and an alternative pathway involves a CYP3A4-mediated *N*-dechloroethylation, which handles less than 10 % of the dose [18].

Because the prodrug is inactive it is the pharmacokinetics of the cytotoxic metabolites that are of interest, but these have been difficult to define. The activities of the metabolites are not well predicted by the doses of the parent compound [19]. Less than 30 % of the prodrug is excreted in the urine and the rest excreted as metabolites. There is tremendous variability between individual patients in metabolism of cyclophosphamide [20]. Carboxyethylphosphoramide mustard is the metabolite most associated with alkylating DNA; acrolein is a metabolite believed to be responsible for hemorrhagic cystitis. The therapeutic index of cyclophosphamide was believed to be better than other alkylating agents (chlorambucil, melphalan). Recent studies suggest that this has not been well established [21]. Alkylating agents used in cancer therapy have poor such ratios between cancer cells and normal cells destruction.

Therapeutic drug monitoring

Like azathioprine, the early users of cyclophosphamide relied on monitoring of the total white blood cell count and any other signs of toxicity, such as hematuria, to monitor the use of the drug. Even later, when it was possible to monitor cyclophosphamide in the blood, it was of little use because of tremendous intra-patient variability and lack of correlation with the prodrug and metabolite levels. More recently, monitoring of the metabolite carboxyethylphosphoramide has been employed [22] with some success; and as more-sophisticated methods of monitoring the various metabolites of cyclophosphamide become more widespread, its employment in organ transplantation may become more rational with fewer adverse events.

Pharmacogenomic considerations

The genetic contribution to metabolism of cyclophosphamide has been investigated primarily in mouse models and demonstrated that a number of genes can influence especially the CYP3A4-mediated pathway [23, 24]. Application of such considerations has been employed mostly in cyclophosphamide use in cancer therapy [25]. As with more recent use of monitoring of metabolites, the emergence of pharmacogenomic tools may pave a path for the return of more routine use of cyclophosphamide in solid organ transplantation and possibly improve the therapeutic index.

Clinical efficacy/safety

Cyclophosphamide, developed more than a half century ago, did not undergo some of the more current preclinical safety and effectiveness testing. Yet, this drug has remained a cornerstone in the armature of clinical oncologists for the treatment of cancers (usually in combination with other drugs). Cyclophosphamide has Food and Drug Administration (FDA) approval for treatment of breast cancer, many forms of leukemia, Hodgkin lymphoma, multiple myeloma, mycosis fungoides, neuroblastoma, non-Hodgkin lymphoma ovarian cancer, and retinoblastoma.

Despite the early predication of Starzl *et al.* that cyclophosphamide was an overlooked drug that would gain wider use in kidney transplantation and despite the clinical observations that it was as effective as azathioprine in preventing acute rejection, cyclophosphamide has not assumed a prominent role in the routine clinical regimens of transplant physicians (except bone marrow transplantation). It is, however, used in several routine settings, such as efforts to prevent recurrent glomerulonephritis [26–28] and patients with vasculitis [29]. Cyclophosphamide is sometimes used as a substitute for other, more accepted agents when patients cannot tolerate them.

More experimental protocols have used cyclophosphamide to condition patients for such procedures as ABO-incompatible transplants [30, 31] and Wegener's granulomatosis [32]. Other protocols that focus on antibody-mediated rejection, highly sensitized patients, and/or creation of tolerance and xenografts [33] have employed cyclophosphamide [34–37].

Cyclophosphamide as a potent cytotoxic agent is used in such experimental protocols with a rationale that dates back to the work of Santos *et al.*, who felt that new clones of lymphocytes that might begin to have active proliferation in response to foreign antigen stimulation would be especially sensitive to a powerful agent such as cyclophosphamide. The more recent recognition of the importance of antibody-mediated rejection in late allograft failure along with advances in drug metabolite monitoring and pharmacogenomic advances may yet prove Starzl *et al.*'s 1971 prophecy [8] about the use of cyclophosphamide correct – just delayed. As opposed to the current drugs that transplant physicians employ in routine protocols, cyclophosphamide is very cost effective.

Major reasons for transplant physicians' reluctance for routine use of cyclophosphamide concern the drug's safety profile. While bone marrow suppression with leukopenia and thrombocytopenia was seen with azathioprine, transplant clinicians found the issue more marked with cyclophosphamide. The drug was also associated with reduced fertility or infertility among young transplant patients [38]. Hemorrhagic cystitis and transitional cell carcinoma of the bladder, while not common, are disastrous complications. Cyclophosphamide patients were also noted to have late leukemia and other cancers after successful transplantation. Mensa (Na salt of methyl-ethylsulfonate) can be given to protect the bladder from the toxic effects of cyclophosphamide [39].

In higher does cyclophosphamide has been reported to result in kidney toxicity [40], liver toxicity [20], and heart toxicity [41]. Perhaps better ability to monitor and determine individual patient's dosage requirements can help to decrease the long list of problems reported with cyclophosphamide, but it is little wonder that transplant physicians have been reluctant to incorporate this drug into routine regimens when seemingly safer agents are available.

The role of B cells and antibody-mediated rejection [42] is receiving renewed attention in clinical transplantation [43]. It is possible that long-term allograft failure will be significantly improved as our understanding of both the mechanisms of antibody-mediated rejection and its treatment is better understood [44]. In the shift of research attention towards treatment of B-cell-mediated antibody, cyclophosphamide, which has been believed to be more toxic to B cells than T cells [45], may make a comeback in the future of transplant physicians' routine regimens.

References

1 Brock N. Oxazaphosphorine cytostatics: past–present–future. Seventh Cain Memorial Award lecture. *Cancer Res* 1989;49(1):1–7.

2 Brock N. The history of the oxazaphosphorine cytostatics. *Cancer* 1996;78(3):542–547.

3 Trethewie ER. Wartime research on nitrogen mustard. *Nature* 1979;282(5735):128.

4 Lichtman MA. Battling the hematol ogical malignancies: the 200 years' war. *Oncologist* 2008;13(2):126–138.

5 McDonald GB, Slattery JT, Bouvier ME *et al.* Cyclophosphamide metabolism, liver toxicity, and mortality following hematopoietic stem cell transplantation. *Blood* 2003;101(5):2043–2048.

6 Goodwin WE, Kaufman JJ, Mims MM *et al.* Human renal transplantation. I. Clinical experiences with six cases of renal homotransplantation. *J Urol* 1963;89:13–24.

7 Parsons FM, Fox M, Anderson CK *et al.* Cyclophosphamide in renal homotransplantation. *Br J Urol* 1966;38(6):673–676.

8 Starzl TE, Halgrimson CG, Penn I *et al.* Cyclophosphamide and human organ transplantation. *Lancet* 1971;2(7715):70–74.

9 Roth D, Zucker K, Cirocco R *et al.* The impact of hepatitis C virus infection on renal allograft recipients. *Kidney Int* 1994;45(1):238–244.

10 Berlyne GM, Danovitch GM. Cyclophosphamide for immunosuppression in renal transplantation. *Lancet* 1971;2(7730):924–925.

11 Ciancio G, Burke GW, Miller J. Current treatment practice in immunosuppression. *Expert Opin Pharmacother* 2000;1(7):1307–1330.

12 Santos GW, Sensenbrenner LL, Burke PJ *et al.* Marrow transplanation in man following cyclophosphamide. *Transplant Proc* 1971;3(1):400–404.

13 Chen L, Waxman DJ. Cytochrome P450 gene-directed enzyme prodrug therapy (GDEPT) for cancer. *Curr Pharm Des* 2002;8(15):1405–1416.

14 Hengstler JG, Hengst A, Fuchs J *et al.* Induction of DNA crosslinks and DNA strand lesions by cyclophosphamide after activation by cytochrome P450 2B1. *Mutat Res* 1997;373(2):215–223.

15 Maguire HC, Jr, Chase MW. Exaggerated delayed-type hypersensitivity to simple chemical allergens in the guinea pig. *J Invest Dermatol* 1967;49(5):460–468.

16 Berd D, Maguire HC, Jr, Mastrangelo MJ. Potentiation of human cell-mediated and humoral immunity by low-dose cyclophosphamide. *Cancer Res* 1984;44(11): 5439–5443.

17 Issels RD, Meier TH, Muller E *et al.* Ifosfamide induced stress response in human lymphocytes. *Mol Aspects Med* 1993;14(3):281–286.

18 Pass GJ, Carrie D, Boylan M *et al.* Role of hepatic cytochrome p450s in the pharmacokinetics and toxicity of cyclophosphamide: studies with the hepatic cytochrome p450 reductase null mouse. *Cancer Res* 2005;65(10):4211–4217.

19 Moore MJ. Clinical pharmacokinetics of cyclophosphamide. *Clin Pharmacokinet* 1991;20(3):194–208.

20 McDonald GB, McCune JS, Batchelder A *et al.* Metabolism-based cyclophosphamide dosing for hematopoietic cell transplant. *Clin Pharmacol Ther* 2005; 78(3):298–308.

21 Bosanquet AG, Bell PB. Ex vivo therapeutic index by drug sensitivity assay using fresh human normal and tumor cells. *J Exp Ther Oncol* 2004;4(2):145–154.

22 McCune JS, Batchelder A, Guthrie KA *et al.* Personalized dosing of cyclophosphamide in the total body irradiation–cyclophosphamide conditioning regimen: a phase II trial in patients with hematologic malignancy. *Clin Pharmacol Ther* 2009;85(6):615–622.

23 Watters JW, Kloss EF, Link DC *et al.* A mouse-based strategy for cyclophosphamide pharmacogenomic discovery. *J Appl Physiol* 2003;95(4):1352–1360.

24 Emmenegger U, Shaked Y, Man S *et al.* Pharmacodynamic and pharmacokinetic study of chronic low-dose metronomic cyclophosphamide therapy in mice. *Mol Cancer Ther* 2007;6(8):2280–2289.

25 Liedtke C, Wang J, Tordai A *et al.* Clinical evaluation of chemotherapy response predictors developed from breast cancer cell lines. *Breast Cancer Res Treat* 2009;121(2):301–309.

26 Saleem MA, Ramanan AV, Rees L. Recurrent focal segmental glomerulosclerosis in grafts treated with plasma exchange and increased immunosuppression. *Pediatr Nephrol* 2000;14(5):361–364.

27 Lien YH, Scott K. Long-term cyclophosphamide treatment for recurrent type I membranoproliferative glomerulonephritis after transplantation. *Am J Kidney Dis* 2000;35(3):539–543.

28 Cheong HI, Han HW, Park HW *et al.* Early recurrent nephrotic syndrome after renal transplantation in children with focal segmental glomerulosclerosis. *Nephrol Dial Transplant* 2000;15(1):78–81.

29 Stratta P, Marcuccio C, Campo A *et al.* Improvement in relative survival of patients with vasculitis: study of

101 cases compared to the general population. *Int J Immunopathol Pharmacol* 2008;21(3):631–642.

30 Tyden G, Kumlien G, Genberg H *et al.* ABO incompatible kidney transplantations without splenectomy, using antigen-specific immunoadsorption and rituximab. *Am J Transplant* 2005;5(1):145–148.

31 Shishido S, Asanuma H, Tajima E *et al.* ABO-incompatible living-donor kidney transplantation in . *Transplantation* 2001;72(6):1037–1042.

32 Riccieri V, Valesini G. Treatment of Wegener's granulomatosis. *Reumatismo* 2004;56(2):69–76.

33 Zaidi A, Schmoeckel M, Bhatti F *et al.* Life-supporting pig-to-primate renal xenotransplantation using genetically modified donors. *Transplantation* 1998;65(12): 1584–1590.

34 Grauhan O, Knosalla C, Ewert R *et al.* Plasmapheresis and cyclophosphamide in the treatment of humoral rejection after heart transplantation. *J Heart Lung Transplant* 2001;20(3):316–321.

35 Mapara MY, Pelot M, Zhao G *et al.* Induction of stable long-term mixed hematopoietic chimerism following nonmyeloablative conditioning with T cell-depleting antibodies, cyclophosphamide, and thymic irradiation leads to donor-specific in vitro and in vivo tolerance. *Biol Blood Marrow Transplant* 2001;7(12):646–655.

36 Lam TT, Hausen B, Hook L *et al.* The effect of soluble complement receptor type 1 on acute humoral xenograft rejection in hDAF-transgenic pig-to-primate life-supporting kidney xenografts. *Xenotransplantation* 2005;12(1):20–29.

37 Snanoudj R, Beaudreuil S, Arzouk N *et al.* Immunological strategies targeting B cells in organ grafting. *Transplantation* 2005;79(3 Suppl):S33–S36.

38 Von der Weid NX. Adult life after surviving lymphoma in childhood. *Support Care Cancer* 2008;16(4):339–345.

39 Takamoto S, Sakura N, Namera A, Yashiki M. Monitoring of urinary acrolein concentration in patients receiving cyclophosphamide and ifosfamide. *J Chromatogr B Anal Technol Biomed Life Sci* 2004 25;806(1):59–63.

40 Beyzadeoglu M, Arpaci F, Surenkok S *et al.* Acute renal toxicity of 2 conditioning regimens in patients undergoing autologous peripheral blood stem-cell transplantation. Total body irradiation–cyclophosphamide versus ifosfamide, carboplatin, etoposide. *Saudi Med J* 2008;29(6):832–836.

41 Morandi P, Ruffini PA, Benvenuto GM *et al.* Cardiac toxicity of high-dose chemotherapy. *Bone Marrow Transplant* 2005;35(4):323–334.

42 Uber WE, Self SE, Van Bakel AB, Pereira NL. Acute antibody-mediated rejection following heart transplantation. *Am J Transplant* 2007;7(9):2064–2074.

43 Fehr T, Rusi B, Fischer A *et al*. Rituximab and intravenous immunoglobulin treatment of chronic antibody-mediated kidney allograft rejection. *Transplantation* 2009;87(12):1837–1841.

44 Womer KL, Kaplan B. Recent developments in kidney transplantation – a critical assessment. *Am J Transplant* 2009;9(6):1265–1271.

45 Wilmer JL, Erexson GL, Kligerman AD. Sister chromatid exchange induction in mouse B- and T-lymphocytes exposed to cyclophosphamide in vitro and in vivo. *Cancer Res* 1984;44(3):880–884.

CHAPTER 20

Application of Antisense Technology in Medicine

Beata Mierzejewska and Stanislaw M. Stepkowski

University of Toledo College of Medicine, Toledo, OH, USA

Introduction: an antisense technology

The concept of antisense technology stems from the understanding of deoxyribonucleic acid (DNA) and ribonucleic acid (RNA) structures and functions. The first potential for DNA oligonucleotides to act as a therapeutic antisense was noted in 1978 by Zamecnik and Stephenson, who used a complementary DNA sequence to inhibit Rous sarcoma viral replication in cell cultures [1]. Next, multiple developments established antisense as a powerful tool to validate gene targets and for therapeutic purposes. From the theoretical perspective, an antisense approach may cure, or at least alleviate, any disease by intervening with expression of the targeted gene or genes; e.g., viral infection, cancer growth, or inflammatory process. While extremely elegant in its concept, antisense technology proved to be challenging in practical applications. Despite these challenges, there are now over 100 ongoing clinical trials with antisense oligonucleotides designed to inhibit different messenger RNAs (mRNAs) to treat orphan diseases, cancers, and inflammatory diseases. The antisense technology investigated in experimental and clinical transplantation showed very promising results. This chapter is conceived to inform about the newest progress in antisense technology, both experimental and clinical endeavors, including organ and cell transplantation.

Screening for active antisense oligonucleotides in cell cultures has been simplified by the availability of large volume oligonucleotide synthesizers and high-throughput RNA quantitation methods with robotic sample handling. The vast majority of antisense oligonucleotides in development use an RNase H-dependent mechanism to cleave mRNA in an mRNA–DNA antisense heteroduplex [2]. Following cleaving of the targeted RNA strand, the intact DNA strand (antisense oligonucleotide) may again bind to another "free" targeted RNA strand. There are two human RNase H enzymes, with RNase H1 active as a single enzyme and RNase H2 active as a heterotrimeric enzyme [2]. RNase H1 binds the RNA–DNA heteroduplex through an RNA binding domain located on the N-terminus of the protein, cleaving the RNA at 7 to 10 nucleotides from the 5'-end of the RNA (that is one helical turn).

Antisense oligonucleotides may also work through an RNA interference mechanism by inducing a cleavage of the targeted RNA through an RNase-like enzyme, Argonaute 2 [3, 4]. Furthermore, small interfering (si)RNA oligonucleotides that work through the RNA interference mechanism mimic functions of endogenous small RNAs physiologically present in cells to regulate expression of the targeted genes. Antisense oligonucleotides can also modulate RNA function without causing degradation, such as blocking protein translation or promoting alternative splicing [5–8].

Immunotherapy in Transplantation: Principles and Practice, First Edition. Edited by Bruce Kaplan, Gilbert J. Burckart and Fadi G. Lakkis.

The last decade has experienced dramatic developments in the understanding of RNA functions in cells, and that included some unforeseen surprises [9]. The central dogma about RNA established three principle functions as mRNAs, transfer (t)RNAs, and ribosomal (r)RNAs. The RNAs are transcribed from DNA by RNA polymerase and changed into the mRNAs, which are moved from the nucleus to the ribosomes to be translated into proteins. While DNA has two intercoiled strands, mRNA contains a single strand and it is built from adenine (A), guanine (G), cytosine (C), and uracil (U). Noncoding tRNA and rRNA help in the process of protein translation: tRNA is a short, 80 nucleotides carrier of a particular amino acid to the polypeptide chain in the ribosome; and four different rRNAs form with proteins called nucleoproteins or ribosomes. However, most RNAs are first encoded by much longer precursors from which large RNA fragments must be processed out to remove noncoding sequences. These noncoding RNAs regulate often the rate at which genes are transcribed and translated; thus, they are natural regulatory RNAs. Subsequently, a family of small nuclear RNAs (snRNAs) emerged as playing an important role in splicing processes by binding to the splice donor and acceptor sites. Such small RNAs (20–25 nucleotides) may interfere with the expression of a specific gene. Even more recently, a new family of microRNAs were identified to control translation of targeted mRNAs, by acting as natural antisense oligonucleotides [10]; they may block mRNA by speeding its breakdown. The microRNAs are on average only 22 nucleotides long and are post-transcriptional regulators binding to a complementary sequence of mRNA. It is estimated that the human genome may encode as many as 1000 microRNAs which target almost 60 % of human genes. These recent observations extended the established dogma that RNAs are only involved in creating proteins and suggest that they have important regulatory functions in cells.

Another coding-independent activity of RNA emerged by identification of RNA-mediated diseases caused by the appearance of two-to-six nucleotide repetitive sequences [11]. The most characterized RNA-mediated diseases include X-associated tremor ataxia syndrome, spino-cerebellar ataxia 8, Huntington's-like disease, and types 1 and 2 neuromuscular myotonic dystrophies. For example, the type 1 myotonic dystrophy was found to be caused by a repeated cytotide–thymidine–guanidine (CTG) sequence in the 3′-untranslated region of the dystrophia myotonica-protein kinase (DMK) gene. In effect, the DMK RNAs with 80–3000 trinucleotide CTG repeats fail to leave the nucleus and, therefore, form the multiple nuclear foci [11]. In other examples, pathological changes were caused by microRNAs binding to the encoded proteins and blocking their transcription, thereby resulting in permanent changes [12, 13].

We define antisense oligonucleotides as those with 8 to 50 nucleotides in length, which bind to targeted mRNA through Watson–Crick base pairing, resulting in a selective functional modulation of targeted mRNA when measured by its protein level. The antisense interference includes mRNA degradation by endogenous enzymes (like RNase H, Argonaute 2) or a functional mRNA blockade without its degradation. Because of this definition, antisense activity does not include oligonucleotides forming double-stranded DNAs, or triple helix structures with DNA, or binding directly to proteins.

The actual binding of antisense oligonucleotides to mRNA includes specific hydrogen bonding of matching bases to targeted RNA strand; hydrophobic interactions resulting from base shape complementarity and coaxial base stacking. Targeted RNAs differ in size from smaller than 20 nucleotides in length to hundreds of thousands or even millions of nucleotides in length. Similar to proteins, RNAs folding into complex three-dimensional structures with a primary structure (the nucleotide sequence) and a secondary structure (the RNA folding and interacting with itself) limit accessibility of antisense to RNA binding sites [14]. Consequently, a number of antisense sequences need to be pretested to identify easily accessible locations on RNAs.

While each cell may contain 100 million RNA molecules, the number of targeted RNA transcripts may range from one copy to 1 million copies for mRNAs or even 10 million copies for snRNAs.

Therefore, it is remarkable that antisense oligonucleotides localize targeted mRNAs with a very high degree of fidelity [9, 15]. Some RNA binding proteins may enhance the hybridization of oligonucleotides to RNAs [11, 16].

Natural DNAs and RNAs are unstable in cells and tissue fluids as they are cleaved at the phosphodiester linkages by ubiquitously expressed nucleases.

Because of this, "natural" synthetic DNA fragments cannot be used as therapeutic agents; they are degraded before reaching their mRNA targets. In addition, synthetic "natural" DNA fragments are rapidly excreted by kidneys. A real breakthrough in widely applied antisense drug designs came with PS-containing oligonucleotides (Figure 20.1). In particular, PS-modified oligonucleotides have one

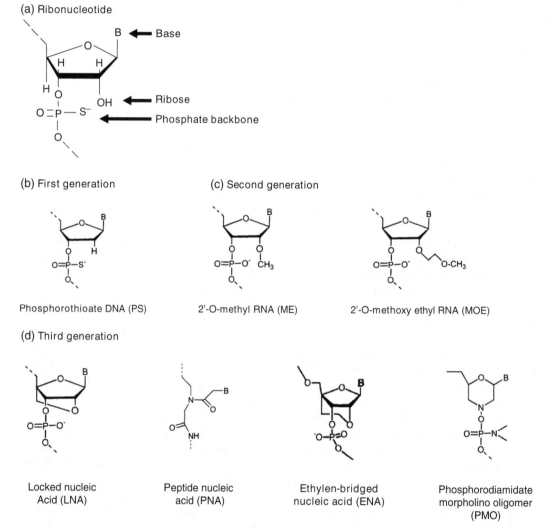

Figure 20.1 Antisense oligonucleotides and their chemical modifications. (a) Sites for chemical modifications of ribonucleotides, as base denotes one of the nucleotides: adenine, guanine, cytosine, or thymine. (b) First generation of DNA modification with phosphorotioate. (c) Second generation of modifications included 2′-O-methyl and 2-O-methoxy ethyl RNAs. (d) Third generation of modifications included locked nucleic acid (LNA), peptide nucleic acid (PNS), ethylene-bridged nucleic acid (ENA), and phosphorodiamidate morpholino oligomer (PMO).

of the nonbridging phosphate oxygen atoms replaced with a sulfur atom. This change introduced several new properties [17], namely significantly increased stability to nucleolytic degradation [18] and improved pharmacokinetics by increasing binding to plasma proteins and preventing rapid renal excretion. However, since antisense oligonucleotides target different mRNAs, their individual pharmacology may be quiet diverse; therefore, each antisense oligonucleotide must be individually examined in vivo.

In the most common design, antisense oligonucleotides are synthetic 20–25-base-long single-strand DNAs with PS modifications hybridizing to a complementary mRNA. In 1998, Isis Pharmaceuticals received approval for the first antisense PS-oligonucleotide, Vitravene (Fomivirsen), registered by the Food and Drug Administration (FDA) for retinitis caused by cytomegalovirus infection, which occurred predominantly in AIDS patients. In addition, various chemistries have been proposed for antisense oligonucleotides to overcome the unstable nature of a single-strand phosphodiester DNA (Figure 20.1). In a ribonucleotide structure, a purine (adenine or guanine in both DNA and RNA) or pyrimidine (cytosine and thymine in DNA or uracil in RNA) base is linked to a ribose sugar and one, two, or three phosphate groups (Figure 20.1a). Several chemical modifications have been developed to improve antisense activities, including first-generation PS-oligonucleotide (Figure 20.1b), newer generation 2′-O-methyl phosphorothioate (ME), 2′-O-methoxy ethyl (MOE) (Figure 20.1c), bicyclic-locked nucleic acid (LNA), peptide nucleic acid (PNA), ethylene-bridged nucleic acid (ENA), phosphorodiamidate morpholino oligomer (PMO: morpholino), and peptide-linked PMO (PPMO) (Figure 20.1d).

Development of appropriate antisense requires consideration of several of their characteristics such as the chemical specificity, affinity, nuclease resistance, stability, safety, and ease of synthesis. Among these different modifications, selectively ME-modified PS-oligonucleotide is the most promising design because of its superior antisense properties. Searches for new technological approaches are still underway. Idera Pharmaceuticals has recently announced the creation of a novel class of compounds which are called gene-silencing oligonucleotides containing two 3′-ends complementary to target mRNA [19]. Both oligoribonucleotide and oligodeoxynucleotide with PS-backbone consist of two identical segments complementary to the targeted mRNA which are expected to attach to its 5′-ends, thereby leaving two accessible 3′-ends. It was already found that 19-mer long oligoribonucleotide and oligodeoxynucleotide provide accessible 3′-ends which are conductive for efficacy of gene-silencing effects; three tested genes (MyD88, TLR9, and VEGF) were inhibited more by gene-silencing technique than by antisense PS-oligonucleotides [19].

The sequencing of the human genome has generated enormous opportunities for antisense technology to develop a gene-targeted medical intervention [20]. However, there are several aspects that need to be addressed during antisense development. First of all, the selection and validation of a targeted gene or genes (functional signaling pathway) in the context of the molecular environment; for example, a protein kinase targeted by antisense oligonucleotide may regulate cell proliferation in one cell type or production and secretion of cytokines in another cell type. Alternatively spliced transcripts like Bcl-xL and Bcl-xS may encode functionally antagonistic proteins, thus switching onto opposite effects [21]. It is important to determine whether an alteration in gene expression is causing the disease or rather it is the disease's effect. Second, the identification of a sequence within mRNA which will be accessible and support RNase H cleavage remains somewhat empirical, as it needs to be pretested from a number of choices. Third, it is necessary to demonstrate that selected antisense oligonucleotide results in selective gene knock-out in human cells and it is therapeutic in an animal disease model. Fourth, pharmacokinetic studies in animals are used to adjust the chemical backbone modifications. Fifth, the final phase of a clinical trial selects doses and the frequency of therapies. Additional technical aspects of antisense oligonucleotides as a therapeutic platform have recently been reviewed by Bennett and Swayze [22].

Development of antisense for different therapeutic indications

Cholesterol therapy

Cholesterol is one of the most extensively studied molecules with intriguing chemical properties, as it possesses a hydroxyl group allowing it to be oriented towards lipid–water interfaces. Physiologically, cholesterol is a structural component of cell membranes, as well as serving as a precursor of steroid hormones, a precursor of vitamin D, and a precursor of bile in the liver. Besides these obvious benefits, cholesterol participates in pathological processes involved in formation of coronary athero-sclerotic plaques, as pure cholesterol crystals form components in these lesions. This "bad cholesterol" in atherosclerotic plaques is derived from circulating lipoproteins, primarily low-density lipoprotein (LDL), but also very-low-density lipoprotein (VLDL), and intermediate-density lipoprotein (IDL). In contrast, high-density lipoprotein (HDL) or "good cholesterol" removes "bad cholesterol" from peripheral tissues, including the arterial wall, delivering it to the liver for elimination in the form of bile acids as a reverse cholesterol transport. Thus, pathogenic dyslipidemias (e.g., hypercholesterolemia, hyperlipidemia, and hypertriglyceridemia) are expressed as disequilibrium between pro-atherogenic apolipoprotein B (apoB)-containing lipoproteins and anti-atherogenic HDL, resulting in enhanced arterial cholesterol deposition. As apoB comprises VLDL, IDL, and LDL, targeting apoB mRNA has combined impact on atherogenic disorders, even in the most severe genetically-regulated disease; e.g., familial hypercholesterolemia. The apoB protein levels reliably reflect the total burden of atherogenic lipoproteins and have strong prognostic values for cardiovascular events, even exceeding the predictive value of LDL-cholesterol (LDL-c). ISIS Pharmaceuticals is currently developing mipomersen, an antisense oligonucleotide targeting apoB. At present, mipomersen has reached the Phase III clinical trial in patients with severe hyperlipidemia who are resistant to statins.

In preclinical development, animals exposed to antisense-mediated reduction of apoB mRNA had reduced levels of apoB protein and LDL-c in blood plasma [23]. The mouse-specific apoB antisense (147764) was tested in models of hyperlipidemia, such as mice fed high-fat diets or mice deficient for apolipoprotein E gene (apoE) or LDL receptor gene (LDLr) [23]. In mice on a Western-style high-fat diet, therapy with apoB antisense correlated with a reduction of liver apoB-100 mRNA and protein contents, as well as with lower serum apoB-100 levels. The hepatic apoB mRNA reduction of up to 88 % coincided with a commensurate reduction of plasma LDL-c levels. Similarly, when exposed twice a week to 147764 antisense, apoE-deficient mice and LDLr-deficient mice reduced their hepatic apoB mRNA by 75 % and their LDL-c by 40–62 %. Human apoB transgene-expressing LDLr-deficient mice, treated with mipomersen (human 301012 antisense; 50 mg/kg per week) for 14 weeks, had significantly reduced human apoB mRNA (89 %) and serum apoB protein levels (68 %) with attenuation of aortic sinus plaques (76 %). Work in monkeys confirmed lack of general side effects when treated with apoB antisense, as confirmed by the lack of effects on the expression of unrelated liver enzymes (acyl-CoA cholesterol acyltransferase, MTP, and 3-hydroxy-3-methyl-glutaryl-CoA reductase). Based on these findings, mipomersen was introduced into multiple safety and efficacy Phases I–III clinical trials. First, a double-blinded and placebo-controlled dose-escalation study was completed in 36 volunteers with mild dyslipidemia [24]. Subcutaneous dosing of 50–400 mg mipomersen by three alternate-day infusions reduced apoB (14–50 %) and LDL-c (4–44 %) without serious side effects, with an exception of occasional erythema at the injection site.

The Phase II trial conducted in patients with mild hypercholesterolemia [25] and treated for 3 months with escalating mipomersen doses (50, 100, 200, and 300 mg/week) lowered apoB-100 by 22–61 % and LDL-c by 12–62 % [25]. The reductions in triglyceride by 43–46 % in patients treated with 200 or 300 mg/week mipomersen was achieved without any alteration of a "good" HDL-c. Most importantly, 200 or 300 mg/week mipomersen combined with standard statin therapy (simvastatin or atorvastatin) in patients that had LDL-c levels above 2.6 mmol/L (100 mg/dL) lowered their apoB-100 levels by

24–52 % and their LDL-c levels by 30–51 %. Based on different mechanisms of action by statins and antisense, these drugs proffer different clinical approaches as a monotherapy or a combined therapy, especially because the pharmacokinetic studies of mipomersen revealed no effect on the efficacy or half-life of statins.

The Phase III positive data reported at the American Heart Association annual meeting in May 2009 evaluated mipomersen in patients with homozygous familial hypercholesterolemia (FH). This severe genetic disorder causes extremely high cholesterol levels, resulting in an early onset of heart disease. Mipomersen was administered once weekly by subcutaneous injection in a randomized double-blinded and placebo-controlled study which enrolled 51 homozygous FH patients. International patients on 200 mg/week mipomersen for 26 weeks reduced LDL-c by 25 % compared with only 3 % in placebo controls ($p < 0.001$). Commensurate with these endpoints was reduction of apoB, total cholesterol, and non-HDL cholesterol (all $p < 0.001$). Although patients were on maximally tolerated statins, their average LDL-c baseline levels were greater than 400 mg/dL, confirming a very challenging patient population. This mipomersen study was completed in 28 out of 34 patients, while the most common side effects included injection-site reactions, flu-like symptoms, and elevations in liver transaminases [25].

The results of Phase III studies of mipomersen in patients who had high cholesterol levels while on lipid-lowering therapy were presented in 2011 at the American College of Cardiology meeting. In patients with severe heterozygous familial hypercholesterolemia, mipomersen reduced LDL-c by 36 % compared with 13 % elevation in a placebo group ($p < 0.001$). As in previous studies, adverse events included flu-like symptoms and elevations in liver transaminases. The double-blind and placebo-controlled trial was performed in 58 patients on lipid-lowering medications with LDL-c levels ≥300 mg/dL or with LDL-c levels ≥200 mg/dL but suffering from coronary heart disease. Patients received 200 mg s.c. injections of mipomersen or placebo once a week for 26 weeks. The average LDL-c of 276 mg/dL dropped 36 % to

175 mg/dL. In the other group, 158 patients with hypercholesterolemia (LDL-c ≥100 mg/dL) and high risk of developing coronary heart disease treated with statins were treated for 26 weeks with 200 mg mipomersen. These patients' LDL-c of 123 mg/dL decreased 37 % to 75 mg/dL, confirming efficacy for high-risk patients. Consequently, Genzyme and Isis Pharmaceuticals have completed the four Phase III studies and are preparing the filings for marketing approval of mipomersen in the USA and the European Union. Similar findings were reported in two publications [26, 27]. Mipomersen seems an attractive alternative for the therapy of hypercholesterolemia in transplant patients treated with immunosuppressive drugs.

Cancer therapy

The biggest problems of standard anticancer therapies are their side effect profiles, with patients experiencing life-threatening complications and the devastating drug-resistant mutations among cancer cells. In contradistinction, an antisense technology with its very selective targeting of mRNA provides a unique strategy for blocking resistant cancer cells with maximum efficacy and minimum side effects. An antisense strategy also may be used to target proteins responsible for development of resistance to drugs. During the last 20 years, a number of reports have described different therapeutic targets for a variety of tumors [28]. At the present time, the antisense therapy has been investigated in oncology with multiple different antisense oligonucleotides in more than 65 clinical trials, including clusterin, X-linked inhibitor of apoptosis (XIAP), heat shock protein 27 (Hsp27), survivin, B cell lymphoma 2 (Bcl-2), and tumor growth factor β2 (TGFβ2; Table 20.1). These and other targets have been implicated in the development and growth of different types of cancer wherein a common thread seems to be anti-apoptotic signaling and/or unregulated cellular proliferation [28]. Considering their importance in cancer development and survival, these molecules are targeted in multiple clinical trials for different cancer types (Table 20.1).

One of the most important targets of drug-resistance in cancers is Bcl-2 protein. Bcl-2 belongs

Table 20.1 Antisense oligonucleotides in clinical trials.

Name	Target molecule	Clinical development	
OGX-011 (custirsen)	Clusterin	Phase I/II	Non-small-cell lung cancer (with GEM/CIS or CARB); hormone refractory prostate cancer (with docetaxel/pred or mitoxantrone/pred)
		Phase I	Metastatic or locally recurrent solid tumors (with docetaxel)
		Phase II/III	Prior to prostatectomy in localized prostate cancer (with neoadjuvant hormone therapy); locally advanced or metastatic breast cancer (with docetaxel); recurrent or metastatic prostate cancer that did not respond to previous hormone therapy (with docetaxel)
OGX-427	Heat shock protein 27	Phase I/II	Prostate, ovarian, non-small-cell lung, breast, bladder cancers (with docetaxel)
LY2181308	Survivin	Phase II	Hormone refractory prostate cancer (with docetaxel); relapsed or refractory acute myeloid leukemia
		Phase I/II	Hepatocellular carcinoma
Genasense (oblimersen, G3139)	Bcl-2	Phase III	Melanoma (with dacarbazine); chronic lymphocytic leukemia (with fludarabine and cyclophosphamide); myeloma (with dexamethasone); acute myeloid leukemia (with cytarabine and daunorubicin); non-small-cell lung cancer (with docetaxel)
		Phase II	Small-cell lung cancer (with carboplatin and etoposide); acute myeloid leukemia (with gemtuzumab); hormone refractory prostate cancer (with docetaxel); non-Hodgkin lymphoma (with rituximab); chronic myeloid leukemia (with imatinib); gastrointestinal stromal tumor (with imatinib); liver cancer (with doxorubicin); renal cancer (with interferon); myeloma (with thalidomide and dexamethasone); Merkel-cell carcinoma
		Phase I/II	Colorectal cancer (with FOLFOX or irinotecan); Breast cancer (with doxorubicin and docetaxel); Oesophageal cancer (with cisplatin and fluorouracil); Non-Hodgkin lymphoma (with RICE or R-CHOP); small-cell lung cancer (with paclitaxel); melanoma (with albumin-bound paclitaxel and temozolomide); Waldenstrom's macroglobulinemia
SPC2996		Phase I/II	Relapsed or refractory chronic lymphocytic leukemia
Trabedersen (A12009)	TGFβ2	Phase III	Recurrent or refractory anaplastic astrocytoma
		Phase I/II	Advanced tumors known to overproduce TGFβ2; colorectal cancer; advanced pancreatic cancer

to a family of genes producing proteins localized in the outer mitochondrial membrane, which regulate their permeabilization with either pro-apoptotic (Bax, BAD, Bak, and Bok) or anti-apoptotic (Bcl-2, Bcl-xL, and Bcl-w) proteins. As Bcl-2 is an anti-apoptotic protein, its overexpression in large numbers of cancers is linked to the resistance to anticancer treatments. The antisense PS-oligonucleotide Genasense (oblimersen, G3139), designed to target the initiation codon region of Bcl-2 mRNA, inhibited Bcl-2 mRNA and protein expression in tumor cell lines. After oblimersen binds to the first six codons of Bcl-2 mRNA forming a DNA–RNA complex, the resulting duplexes are subsequently cleaved enzymatically, preventing Bcl-2 mRNA translation. Oblimersen was developed by Genta for reducing the amount of Bcl-2 protein in cancer cells to enhance the effectiveness of conventional anticancer treatments (Table 20.1). Recently, Genta has reported results from randomized Phase III trials of oblimersen in four different indications: malignant melanoma, chronic lymphocytic leukemia (CLL), multiple myeloma, and acute myeloid leukemia.

First, oblimersen was investigated in a Phase I trial to assess the safety and tolerability when given with carboplatin and paclitaxel chemotherapy [29]. Patients with advanced malignancies received therapies comprised of G3139 (intravenous (iv) infusion days 1–7) combined with carboplatin and paclitaxel, which were repeated as 3-week cycles in the dose-escalation cohorts. Out of 42 patients evaluated for primary toxicities in dose-escalating groups, hematologic problems (myelosuppression and thrombocytopenia) were observed at a maximum dose of 7 mg/kg/day G3139 combined with carboplatin at area under the curve of 6, and paclitaxel (175 mg/m^2). When treated patients underwent tumor biopsies, they had an increased intra-tumor G3139 level that coincided with a decreased intra-tumor Bcl-2 expression. In another Phase I trial, the effects of Bcl-2 downregulation by oblimersen was tested in breast tumor biopsies [30]. As Bcl-2 protein expression conferred with the resistance to chemotherapy, this chemo-sensitizing drug may provide new treatment options. Consequently, workers investigated oblimersen to downregulate Bcl-2 protein translation and to enhance the antitumor effects of subtherapeutic doses of docetaxel. The Phase I trial examined administration of escalating doses of oblimersen (3–7 mg/kg/day) as a continuous infusion (days 1–7) in combination with docetaxel, doxorubicin, and cyclophosphamide in women with advanced breast cancers. Read-outs of Bcl-2 mRNAs had diminished values in 2 of 13 patients. Another study explored whether a combination of oblimersen with temozolomide and abraxane may act synergistically *in vitro* in melanoma cell lines [31]. As the results of Bcl-2 antisense and dacarbazine were encouraging, patients with melanoma were enrolled in the Phase I/II trial. Observation of 18 treated patients suggested that the combined triple-drug therapy with Bcl-2 antisense was synergistic in advanced melanoma patients. Biomarker analysis supported the rationale that Bcl-2 antisense therapy had an impact on apoptotic signaling pathways in melanoma cells from metastatic tumors. In Phase II

trial, escalated doses of Bcl-2 antisense were used prior to a docetaxel therapy in patients with the castration-resistant prostate cancer [32]. Results confirmed that prostate-specific antigen (PSA) decreased in 46 % and 37 % of patients treated with docetaxel and docetaxel/oblimersen, respectively.

Application of oblimersen also was explored with docetaxel (Phase I/II) in patients with hormone-refractory prostate cancer [33]. The decreased PSA values observed in 52 % of patients treated with oblimersen were much better than in 33 % of patients treated only with docetaxel. These promising anti-tumor activities promoted further ongoing clinical trials. The 5-year Phase III survival trial was conducted for a relapsed or refractory CLL treated with fludarabine and cyclophosphamide standard therapy without or with oblimersen. In a group with fludarabine-sensitive disease, patients with maximum benefit with oblimersen were observed for the 5-year survival and they showed a 50 % reduction in the risk of death ($P<0.004$). Thus, in relapsed/refractory leukemia, oblimersen and fludarabine offered a significant survival benefit. Although Genta Inc. filed for the FDA registration for oblimersen, their application was unsuccessful for both melanoma and CLL. There was also another antisense PS-oligonucleotide SPC2996 targeting Bcl-2 mRNA [34]. Patients with CLL were treated with 6 doses and examined by microarray. The therapy induced an upregulation of 466 genes related to immune response and apoptotic regulatory molecules causing a 50 % reduction of circulating lymphocytes in 5 out of 18 patients.

Histone deacetylase inhibitors (HDI) belong to one of the most promising class of anti-cancer compounds [35]. To express genes, cells must coil and uncoil DNA around histones done with the assistance of histone acetylases (HATs) and histone deacetylases (HDACs). While HATs acetylate the lysine residues in histones leading to less compact chromatin, HDACs remove the acetyl groups from the lysine residues leading to the condensed and silenced chromatin. The microarray analysis of HDI-treated cancer cell lines revealed that clusterin (a stress-induced cytoprotective chaperone protein with potent pro-survival functions) was always over-expressed in cancerous cells [36]. In contrast, blockade of clusterin protein enhanced cytochrome C-dependent mitochondrial apoptosis even in HDI-resistant cancer cells. One of the recently developed OGX-011 antisense (Custirsen), a PS-oligodeoxynucleotide with chimera-like ME modifications, is complementary to clusterin mRNA (Table 20.1). Anti-clusterin activity of OGX-011 increased sensitivity of cancer cells to chemo- and radio-therapies. Indeed, mice injected with neuroblastoma xenografts treated with a combination of OGX-011 and HDI compound (valproate) inhibited growth of tumors. Since over-expression of clusterin rendered cancer cells resistant to apoptosis and growth arrest, therapy with OGX-011 may offer a unique approach of sensitizing resistant cancer cells to a standard anti-cancer therapy. To address these questions, clusterin expression was evaluated in prostate cancer cells treated with docetaxel, while the impact of clusterin inhibition by OGX-011 was evaluated in reversing the docetaxel resistance in androgen-independent human prostate cancer cells [37]. When a PC-3 human prostate cancer cell line was repeatedly exposed *in vitro* to docetaxel chemotherapy, a docetaxel-resistant PC-3dR cell subline was created. The PC-3dR cells had an elevated clusterin level that was much higher than those observed in the "non-resistant" prostate cancer specimens. When treatment with OGX-011 antisense decreased clusterin levels in PC-3dR cells, they became *in vitro* sensitive to docetaxel and mitoxantrone, as confirmed by the increased apoptotic rates in PC-3dR cells. Similarly, the *in vivo* growth of PC-3dR xenografts in nude mice was synergistically inhibited by exposure to OGX-011 in combination with paclitaxel or mitoxantrone by 76% and 44%, respectively. Since mismatched clusterin antisense oligonucleotides were ineffective in parallel control experiments, clusterin regulates resistance to apoptosis in tumor cells and its inhibition improves the cytotoxic chemotherapy in docetaxel refractory cells. Thus, HDIs combined with clustering antisense oligonucleotides may provide a novel approach for therapy eliminating drug-resistant cancer cells [38].

Based on these promising preclinical results, the Phase I clinical study was undertaken to determine the biologically-effective dose of OGX-011 [39].

High-risk patients with prostate cancer were treated with weekly infusions of OGX-011 (40 to 640 mg/dose) in combination with androgen blockade and followed by prostatectomy. The OGX-011 therapy decreased clusterin expression by 90% in prostate cancer cells, and that led to the Phase II clinical trial in patients with an advanced metastatic castrate-resistant prostate cancer [40]. Based on the overall 23.8 months survival observed in patients treated with OGX-011 plus docetaxel compared to 16.9 months for patients treated with docetaxel alone, addition of OGX-011 therapy improved the overall survival by 61%.

Another Phase II study with OGX-011 was conducted in patients with a hormone-refractory prostate cancer who relapsed after docetaxel therapy. In this clinical trial, OGX-011 combined with docetaxel and prednisone appeared superior to OGX-011 combined with mitoxantrone and prednisone in both efficacy and safety. There is an ongoing Phase III study to evaluate docetaxel/prednisone with or without OGX-011 in patients treated already with docetaxel protocol. The combined OGX-011 and docetaxel therapy was also evaluated for a metastatic breast cancer in Phase I/II study [41]. Women with measurable metastatic breast cancer were treated with a docetaxel regimen and three 640 mg/dose loading doses of OGX-011 delivered intravenously were followed by weekly OGX-011 and docetaxel (75 mg/m^2 over 3 weeks). The median duration of stable disease was 9.3 months and the median time to progression was 8 months (95% confidence interval; ranging from 5.62 to 9.43 months). While combination of OGX-011 and docetaxel was well tolerated, there was not enough evidence to proceed to the next clinical stage. A randomized clinical study in castrate resistant prostate cancer reported a 7 month improvement in survival after docetaxel/custirsen therapy of 23.8 months versus 16.9 months after docetaxel-alone therapy [42]. The Phase III clinical trial began in 2010.

Similar hopes are expected by therapy with the MOE-modified PS oligonucleotide OGX-427 targeting Hsp27 (Table 20.1). Similar to clusterin, Hsp27 is an important cell-survival protein overproduced in response to many cancer treatments, including chemotherapy, as well as hormone ablation and radiation therapies. Furthermore, elevated Hsp27 expression was observed in prostate, breast, ovarian, bladder, renal, pancreatic, multiple myeloma, non-small-cell lung, and liver cancers. Extensive studies correlated an increased Hsp27 level to accelerated cancer progression, resistance to anticancer treatment, and short survival.

Functionally, as cytoprotective chaperone, Hsp27 is phosphoactivated in response to stress, preventing an aggregation of stress-responsive proteins, leading to their degradation. Recent evidence supports the notion that Hsp27 regulates tumor progression and is involved in the development of drug resistance in various tumors. The impact of Hsp27 downregulation by siRNA and OGX-427 was examined in a UMUC-3 bladder carcinoma cell line [43]. Although overexpression of Hsp27 increased growth of UMUC-3 cells and their resistance to paclitaxel (anticancer drug), both OGX-427 and Hsp27 siRNA decreased Hsp27 protein and mRNA levels by more than 90%. Even more promising, an exposure to OGX-427 or Hsp27 siRNA induced apoptosis and enhanced sensitivity to paclitaxel in UMUC-3 cells. In an in vivo model, OGX-427 dramatically inhibited UMUC-3 tumor growth in mice and enhanced sensitivity to paclitaxel when compared with control oligo-nucleotides. Again, inhibition of Hsp27 may increase efficacy of drugs by neutralizing development of resistance in tumor cells, or at least in bladder cancer, as concluded by other two independent studies [44].

The purpose of the Phase I/II study was to evaluate OGX-427 alone and in combination with docetaxel [45]. Eligible patients had different phases of metastatic cancers, including breast, ovarian, prostate, non-small-cell lung, or bladder cancers. These patients obtained weekly OGX-427 therapy after three loading infusions at the escalated five dose levels ranging from 200 to 1000 mg/dose. All doses were well tolerated, with the toxicity consisting of only infusion site reactions and transient thromboplastin time changes. Declining tumor markers in blood during monotherapy suggested an anticancer activity of OGX-427. Based on these positive observations, OncoGenex initiated the

clinical trial (August 2009) for bladder cancer patients with intra-bladder administration of OGX-427.

Another novel oncology target is survivin, which belongs to the family of apoptosis inhibitors and blocks function of caspases mediating apoptosis [46]. Interestingly, while survivin is expressed in most human cancer cells, it is completely absent in fully differentiated normal cells. Survivin localizes to the mitotic spindle of cancer cells, interacting with tubulin during mitosis, and it is linked to vital pathways of cancer cells, namely the "anticancer" p53 tumor suppressor protein and Wnt involved in embriogenesis and cancer cells. Thus, overexpression of survivin in tumors coincides with the tumor resistance to apoptosis, thereby contributing to their immortality even in the presence of death stimuli [47]. The importance of survivin is emphasized by the fact that another antisense oligonucleotide (SPC3042) has been tested for clinical application [48]. The most optimal cancer therapy would be a fine balance between effective killings of cancer cells with no damage to the surrounding healthy tissue. Survivin represents an excellent target, as it is functionally exclusive in cancer cells (Table 20.1). It was shown that the downregulation of survivin with SPC3042 antisense led to cell-cycle arrest, cancer-cell apoptosis, and downregulation of Bcl-2. Treatment with SPC3042 sensitized prostate cancer cells to Taxol treatment in vitro and in vivo. Downregulation of survivin mRNA and protein by PS/MOE-modified oligonucleotides (LY2181308) resulted in an increased apoptosis of an A549 tumor cell line. Since normal cells do not express survivin, LY2181308 should produce fewer side effects compared with traditional chemotherapy [49]. In preclinical study, survivin was examined as a possible radiation resistance factor in colorectal cancer. Indeed, survivin mRNA levels in patients with rectal cancer predicted their tumor responses after neoadjuvant radiochemotherapy, whereas an inhibition of survivin by antisense oligonucleotides enhanced radiation responses [50]. When SW480 colorectal carcinoma cells were transfected with LY2181308 and irradiated with escalating doses ranging from 0 to 8 Gy, antisense therapy increased the percentage of apoptotic cells. Treatment of nude mice with fast-growing SW480 xenografts by the same survivin antisense significantly decreased tumor growth and increased sensitivity to irradiation. Survivin appeared to be a molecular target improving sensitivity to radiotherapy in patients with rectal cancer. Because of these promising results, LY2181308 is currently evaluated for multiple cancers in Phase II clinical studies in patients with relapsed or refractory acute myeloid leukemia and hormone refractory prostate cancer.

Duchenne muscular dystrophy

Duchenne muscular dystrophy (DMD) is the most common childhood neuromuscular X-recessive disorder, with the incidence rate as high as one of 3500 newborn boys. DMD is caused by the absence of dystrophin protein as a consequence of different mutations in the dystrophin gene (DMD gene), resulting in nonfunctional dystrophin proteins [51]. Since dystrophin is required for muscle fiber membrane stability during contraction, its loss leads to permanent muscle fiber damage. After attempts at regeneration, damaged muscle fibers are replaced by adipose and fibrotic tissues. The loss of muscle function leads in the majority of patients to wheelchair dependency before the age of 13 and premature death before the age of 30. While several therapeutic strategies of DMD have been investigated, including adenovirus vector expressing dystrophin, stem cells, or bone marrow stromal cells transplantation, no effective treatment has been established. In recent years, an exon-skipping strategy by antisense oligonucleotides has been tried to restore dystrophin expression at the sarcolemma [52]. The antisense 2'-O-methyl and morpholinos oligonucleotides are designed individually for the mutated DMD mRNA to change its splicing pattern and promoting functional translation. Although exon skipping is not a cure for DMD disease, such an approach slows down the fast-progressing DMD into the much milder form of Becker dystrophy.

In practical terms, antisense deoxynucleotides are designed to attach themselves precisely to the matching pre-mRNA sequence inside the exon to be spliced out at its border regions. Such interfering with the splicing machinery causes exon skipping to get the protein back to frame, allowing for productive translation of the remaining DMD mRNA. In the mdx mouse (DMD model), intramuscular injection with antisense oligonucleotides targeting exon 23 resulted in its skipping, and dystrophin restoration for 90 days was confirmed by the functional improvement [53]. The proof of concept was recently reproduced in four DMD patients who were injected locally in the tibialis anterior muscle with an antisense targeting exon 51 (PRO051). Dystrophin expression was restored in the majority of muscle fibers at significant levels (17% and 35%) in the absence of adverse effects. Consequently, clinical trials are being conducted in the UK using phosphorodiamidate morpholino oligomers targeting exon 51 (PMO, AVI 4658) [54]. In the clinical protocol, 0.09 mg in two patients and 0.9 mg in five patients of AVI-4658 in 900 µL saline were injected to extensor digitorum brevis (EDB) muscle. The results showed a biopsy-proven increased dystrophin expression in all treated EDB muscles [55]. In the areas adjacent to the site of injection, 44–79% of myofibers displayed increased expression of dystrophin. Even more encouraging were results with PRO051, which was administered weekly by subcutaneous injections for 5 weeks at doses of 0.5, 2, 4, or 6 mg/kg [56]. PRO051 induced detectable exon 51-skipping effects at 2 mg/kg with new dystrophin expression between 60 and 100% of muscle fibers in 10 out of 12 patients, which increased up to 15.6% of the expression in healthy muscles; after a 12 weeks extension phase there was an improvement in the 6 min walk test by 35.2±28.7 m from the baseline of 384±121 m. Thus, local, but most importantly systemic, antisense therapy showed efficacy in patients with DMD.

To improve therapy, several different chemistries were investigated for effective systemic delivery. Biodistribution studies in mice revealed that uptake of antisense was better by dystrophic than healthy muscle, as dystrophic fibers are "leaky"; systemic treatment (iv, intraperitoneal (ip), or subcutaneous injections) with 2'-O-methyl phosphorothioate or PMO antisense resulted in the body-wide exon-skipping restoration of dystrophin and significant functional improvement [57]. The encouraging results described above with PRO051 and AVI4658 did not address another difficult challenge that had been observed in heart muscle: mouse studies revealed that the exon skipping and dystrophin levels were much lower or even nonexistent in hearts. While local injection of antisense into the ventricle wall resulted in local exon skipping, the dystrophin expression levels were much lower than in skeletal muscles. This was probably because access to heart muscle fibers seems more difficult than to damage-affected skeletal muscle fibers. Arginine-rich peptides attached to PMO antisense greatly improved uptake by skeletal and heart muscles. These improved antisense RNAs are under investigation for human application. To achieve more permanent exon skipping, an "antisense gene" may be introduced with viral vectors. These antisense genes were modified U7 or U1 small nuclear ribonucleoprotein (snRNP) genes. Indeed, long-term (18 months) exon skipping and dystrophin restoration with improved muscle morphology was observed in the skeletal and heart muscles of mdx mice treated with viral vectors containing modified snRNP genes [58, 59].

In summary, the use of antisense oligonucleotides and other approaches to modulate splicing has been developed during the last decade. Although recent experiments have focused mainly on antisense-mediated exon skipping, an even more promising snRNA method is under development for DMD disease. As proof-of-concept for these different approaches has been obtained, the DMD exon-skipping approach needs to be mutation specific and thus clinical trials are very unique, because in the entire method there is not one universal antisense sequence for approval by the FDA for final clinical application [60].

Antisense in transplantation

Application of antisense technology in transplantation showed its great potential for a variety of targets. One of the most comprehensive developments for antisense application has been targeting of intercellular adhesion molecule-1 (ICAM-1). The ICAM-1 molecule is expressed at low levels on endothelial cells and leukocytes [61]. In response to pro-inflammatory cytokines (IL-1, TNF, and IFNγ) the expression of ICAM-1 is significantly increased on endothelial cells and leukocytes. ICAM-1 expressed on endothelial cells binds circulating leukocytes through interactions with β-2 integrins, namely LFA-1 (CD11a) and macrophage antigen-1 (MAC-1), thereby facilitating emigration of leukocytes out of the vasculature [62]. Because ICAM-1-mediated migration of leukocytes into allografts promotes rejection, we performed extensive preclinical and clinical studies on whether its inhibition may have immunosuppressive effects. The PS-modified antisense oligodeoxynucleotide (IP-3082), specific for mouse ICAM-1 mRNA, inhibited ICAM-1 mRNA and protein but not VCAM-1 mRNA and VCAM-1 protein in mouse endothelial cells [63]. Following in vitro selection, we performed in vivo analysis with IP-3082. While untreated mice acutely rejected heart allografts (a mean survival time (MST) of 7.7 ± 1.4 days), the iv therapy of 5 or 10 mg/kg IP-3082 delivered for only 7 days by osmotic infusion pump prolonged the survival of heart allografts to 14.1 ± 2.7 days and 15.3 ± 5.8 days respectively (both $p < 0.01$). While addition of 7-day anti-LFA-1 monoclonal antibody (mAb) therapy (50 μg/day; ip) prolonged allograft survival to 14.1 ± 2.7 days, the addition of 5 mg/kg IP-3082 induced donor-specific transplantation tolerance (>150 days). We also documented that in mice IP-3082 may interact synergistically with antilymphocyte serum, rapamycin, or brequinar, but not with cyclosporine (CsA). This study proffered evidence that ICAM-1 antisense therapy works in vivo as a selective gene-targeted immunosuppression in transplantation [63].

The initial success with mouse ICAM-1 antisense oligonucleotide inspired more studies, including the first ever oral application for therapeutic purpose. To select the best rat antisense, 10 PS-oligonucleotides were tested matching different regions of rat ICAM-1 mRNA [64]. One of them, PS-9125, hybridized to the 3′-end of mRNA and inhibited the expression of ICAM-1 protein by 90 % in rat endothelial cells. Furthermore, 10 mg/kg PS-9125 infused intravenously by a 7-day osmotic pump prolonged heart allograft survival to

16.8±3.5 days ($p<0.01$) in comparison with those treated with the scrambled PS-12140 oligonucleotides (9.0±1.0 days; NS). In the same rat model, 4 mg/kg CsA alone prolonged the MST to 14.8±0.8 days, whereas in combination of 10 mg/kg PS-9125 acted synergistically, extending survivals to 21.2±4.7 days ($p<0.001$) with the combination index (CI) value of 0.5 confirming the benefit of two-drug therapy (CI<1 shows synergism). When the same therapy was continued to 14 days, 10 mg/kg PS-9125 extended survivals of kidney allografts to 50.4±21.6 days and when combined with 1 mg/kg CsA to 90 days ($p<0.001$; CI=0.1). Even perfusion of kidney allograft with PS-9125 (20 mg/2 mL) prior grafting prolonged recipient survivals to 35.0±2.0 days, compared with only 10.0±2.0 days in recipients treated with the scrambled PS-12140. These multiple approaches showed that antisense ICAM-1 PS-oligonucleotides specifically inhibit ICAM-1 protein expression and block allograft rejection. Combination therapy showed that ICAM-1 antisense acted synergistically with CsA to prolong the survival of rat kidney allografts.

Meanwhile, other studies supported our observations that the ICAM-1-dependent mechanism of graft infiltration by leukocytes is involved in allograft rejection and ischemic–reperfusion (I/R) injury [65, 64]. It also became obvious that while addition of PS groups to natural PD antisense oligodeoxynucleotides prevented their hydrolysis by nucleases in vivo, such modifications allowed an RNase-dependent elimination of targeted ICAM-1 mRNA [65]. To further improve antisense function, 2′-methoxyethyl (ME) groups were attached to selected nucleotides at the 3′-end because ME groups block RNase activity. Such "wing" ME groups attached to PS- or PD/PS-oligonucleotides were tested both in vitro and in vivo [66]. To confirm the site for human target selection on human ICAM-1 mRNA (15839), we designed rat antisense to hybridize the same site on rat ICAM-1 mRNA (17470). To show the impact of ME modification, an identical rat oligonucleotide was made without ME groups (117725). In vitro, rat ME/PS-oligonucleotide (17470; IC_{50} of 156 nM) was twofold more effective than two PS oligonucleotides (117725; IC_{50} of 250 nM and

PS-9125; IC_{50} of 335 nM) in inhibiting ICAM-1 mRNA expression in rat endothelial cells. In vivo, an iv infusion of 10 mg/kg 17470 was also twofold more effective than 10 mg/kg PS-9125 in extending survivals of kidney allografts. Because an oral formulation had 10–15 % bioavailability, an oral gavage with 50, 75, or 100 mg/kg IP-17470 documented similar twofold improvement in kidney allograft survivals in comparison with IP-9125. Because oral gavage with mismatched 100 mg/kg ME-modified human ICAM-1 oligonucleotide (15839) was ineffective in rats (10.2±2.5 days; NS), ME-modifications improved effectiveness in vivo. Furthermore, the pharmacokinetic study produced threefold higher exposures in liver and kidneys for ME-modified PS oligonucleotide [66]. The same study showed that inhibition of ICAM-1 protein expression at the graft site prevented CsA-induced nephrotoxicity. Overall, we accumulated evidence that the ME-modification of PS oligonucleotides significantly improves their affinity, extends their half-life, and increases their resistance to nucleases.

As ICAM-1–LFA-1 interaction seems important for I/R injury, we explored PS-9125 to improve kidney function after kidney graft perfusion prior transplantation. An ex vivo perfusion of grafts with PS-9125 (suspended in Euro-Collins solution) prolonged the survival of kidney allografts in rats [64], so we examined whether perfusion of kidneys with PS-9125 may prevent an I/R injury [67]. When kidneys were perfused ex situ with 2 mL of Euro-Collins solution containing PS-9125 followed by a 30 min cold and 30 min warm ischemia, the glomerular filtration rate values were increased by 60 % with decreased blood creatinine levels. These results correlated with reduced expression of ICAM-1 protein and mRNA. Thus, perfusion of grafts with ICAM-1 antisense oligonucleotide specifically reduces intragraft ICAM-1 protein expression and prevents I/R injury. Similar observations were reported by other investigators who worked with different ICAM-1 antisense oligonucleotides [68].

To confirm these very promising results obtained in rodents, we have compared human (ISIS-2302) and cynomolgus monkey (IP-17878) antisense PS-oligodeoxynucleotide targeting the 3′-untranslated region of ICAM-1 mRNA. Despite that their sequences differ at one nucleotide (G → A), they both specifically inhibited the expression of ICAM-1 mRNA and protein expression in monkey aortic endothelial cells; two scrambled controls were ineffective. The oligonucleotides at the doses of 5.0 mg/kg were infused iv by a 2 h daily infusion in two different experimental protocols. In the first protocol, the high responder cynomolgus monkey recipients of kidney allografts (as defined by the mixed lymphocyte culture (MLC) index of 50–225) were treated from the day of transplantation with monkey antisense oligonucleotide and CsA adjusted to a 24 h trough blood level of 200–600 ng/mL. In the second protocol, the low-responder recipients (MLC index of 12–25) were treated with CsA adjusted to 200–600 ng/mL for the first 30 days, which was then lowered to 100–200 ng/mL and withdrawn 15 days later; human oligonucleotide therapy was applied daily between days 31 and 90 postgrafting. Untreated cynomolgus recipients rejected kidney allografts at an MST of 8.5 ± 1.1 days ($n=4$). Although daily intramuscular administration of CsA (adjusted to 200–600 ng/mL) in high responders prolonged the survival of kidney allografts to 17.2 ± 16.4 days ($n=3$), the addition of monkey ICAM-1 oligonucleotide extended survivals to 43.0 ± 17.5 days ($n=4$). In the second protocol, low-responder recipients ($n=3$) treated with decreasing CsA doses and human ICAM-1 oligonucleotide (ISIS-2302) maintained good kidney transplant function for more than 2 years postgrafting. All three recipients permanently accepted donor, but not third-party (<10 days), skin allografts, documenting induction of tolerance. In conclusion, monkey or human ICAM-1 antisense oligonucleotide inhibited ICAM-1 protein expression in vitro and blocked kidney allograft rejection in cynomolgus monkeys.

These results culminated in the design of a clinical trial for prevention of kidney allograft rejection. An antisense PS-oligonucleotide (ISIS-2302) targeting ICAM-1 was evaluated in combination with CsA and prednisone (Pred) in a first Phase I safety and pharmacokinetic study and then in a Phase II assessment of prophylaxis of acute rejection episodes in deceased donor renal allografts. Both trials were double blinded and placebo controlled, including 17 stable long-term transplant recipients in Phase I and 39 de novo transplanted patients in Phase II. Each study compared the outcomes of eight alternate-day iv infusions of four ISIS-2302 doses (0.05, 0.5, 1, or 2 mg/kg) versus placebo. Patients were followed for only 34 days in Phase I or for 6 months in Phase II, while all transplants were observed for 3 years. First of all, therapy with ISIS-2302 produced no evidence of toxicity, but a significant and dose-related increase in activated partial thromboplastin time was accompanied by a trend toward a decreased platelet count. Therapy with ISIS-2302 did not alter the pharmacokinetic behavior of CsA, and at 6 months the rates of acute rejection episodes were 38.1 % in the ISIS-2302 group versus 20.0 % in the placebo group. Three-year graft survivals were similar and the mean creatinine levels at 1, 2, and 3 years for all ISIS dose groups versus placebo over 3 years showed no significant differences. Based on this study, ISIS-2302 did not evoke side effects and produced slightly improved renal function. However, in this pilot study, it did not further reduce the rate of acute rejection episodes or increase graft survival compared with a concentration-controlled CsA–Pred regimen [69].

We also explored a variety of additional antisense target molecules as possible immunosuppressants. One of the most investigated molecules in immunology is interleukin-2 (IL-2), as this cytokine seems critical for T cell clonal expansion. While IL-2 knockout mice reject allografts at a similar tempo as normal mice [70], this may be explained by the redundant utilization of the other common γ-chain cytokines, such as IL-4, IL-7, IL-9, IL-13, and IL-15 [71]. It is also possible that T cells in IL-2 knockout mice are selecting T cells biased for their response to available cytokines. Therefore, we performed gene therapy with IL-2-specific antisense oligonucleotides to prevent allograft rejection and to examine the T cell functions [72]. The PS oligonucleotide with MOE "wing" modifications (17359) was selected to block IL-2 mRNA in a mouse T cell lymphoma cell line, and tested in vivo to inhibit heart allograft rejection alone or in combination with sirolimus (SRL). While untreated mouse recipients rejected heart allografts (8.2±0.8 days), 20 mg/kg 17359 IL-2 antisense oligonucleotides prolonged survivals (17.3±63.6 days; $p > 0.001$). Although 2 mg/kg SRL alone extended survivals to 22.6±4.4 days, the combination of 20 mg/kg 17359 with SRL produced much better results (53.3±10.1 days). Compared with rejectors, RT-PCR analysis showed reduced expression of IL-2 (by 90%), but not of IL-4, IL-7, IL-9, or IL-15 on postgrafting days 2 (graft only) and 5 (graft and spleen) in recipients treated with 17359 alone or in combination with SRL. Purified splenic T cells stimulated with donor alloantigens displayed a reduction of proliferative response in both therapeutic groups (day 2 by 75% and day 5 by 50%). In conclusion, selective inhibition of IL-2 gene expression reduces clonal expansion of alloantigen-specific T cells, and thereby extended the survival of heart allografts [72].

Another target molecule considered for transplantation was targeting C-raf kinase [73]. After T cell receptor (TCR) engagement by alloantigen, the TCR signal is transduced by CD3 ($\gamma\delta\epsilon\epsilon\zeta\zeta$) chains in association with the Fyn, Lck, and ZAP70 kinase network, leading to the initiation of the Ras/Raf/Mek mitogen-activated protein (MAP) kinase cascade [74]. In addition to TCR signaling, CD28/B7 signal also utilizes the MAP kinase pathway to stabilize and increase the production of cytokines via the CD28 response element present in the IL-2 promoter. Finally, the binding of cytokines to cytokine receptors initiates differential activation of Janus tyrosine kinase (JAK)/ signal transducers and activators of transcription (STAT) signals also requiring participation of MAP kinase pathways. Thus, all three activation signals necessary for T cell proliferation and differentiation use the Ras/Raf/Mek MAP kinase cascade. The Raf family of genes (A-raf, B-raf, C-raf, D-Raf, and Ce-raf) encodes serine/threonine (Ser/Thr) protein kinases [71]. After identifying an antisense PS-oligodeoxynucleotide, IP-11061, to block the expression of rat C-raf mRNA and protein [75], we designed three oligonucleotides with an identical antisense sequence but with different chemical modifications. In particular, one is uniform PS groups alone; the second is the same PS backbone but with ME attached to the first and last five nucleotides; and the third is a mixed PS/PD backbone and ME modifications on the first and last five nucleotides. In vitro, both PS/ ME-modified C-raf antisense oligonucleotides were at least fivefold more effective than PS-modified C-raf antisense oligo in blocking C-raf mRNA expression in two cell lines. Similarly, each of the C-raf antisense PS/ME-oligonucleotides produced better heart allograft survival rates than did C-raf PS-oligonucleotide. Although the combination of C-raf antisense PS-oligonucleotide with SRL acted synergistically to extend heart allograft survival, the synergistic effect was potentiated by C-raf ME-modified oligonucleotides. These results again confirmed that ME-attachments to antisense oligonucleotides improve their in vivo activity [73].

Very important application for antisense intervention could be coronary vasculopathy (CAV), a phenomenon that is associated with heart diseases and also with chronic rejection in heart allografts. While CAV requires angioplasty, stenting, or even bypass grafting, these interventions are not practical treatments for patients with heart allografts. Because of these limitations, antisense targeting the transcripts of CAV-related genes may have therapeutic applications for heart transplants [76]. For example, when investigators applied antisense for cdk2 kinase (as this enzyme is important in cell transition through the G_1/S phase), they prevented or at least reduced CAV in experimental cardiac allografts [77–79]. In another experimental effort, targeting by antisense of proliferating cell nuclear antigen (PCNA), a nuclear protein required for DNA synthesis and transition through both the G_1/S and G_2/M phases [80], limited neointimal formation in heart allografts [81]. Furthermore, antisense targeting apoptosis by reducing Bcl-x expression suppressed CAV. Alternative technology of transfection with double-stranded DNA "decoys" has also been reported as a useful method for gene therapy of CAV targeting the transcription factor E2F (regulating multiple cell-cycle regulatory genes), nuclear factor-κB (NF-κB) (coordinating transcription of multiple inflammatory genes). More studies need to be conducted in other transplant models to explore the clinical utility for prevention of CAV.

Conclusions

Because of its unique mechanism of action, antisense technology proffers an exceptionally attractive method to target individual genes. While multiple experimental and some clinical efforts proved that antisense oligonucleotides selectively block gene functions leading to significant expected changes, development of clinical drugs met several challenges (design, in vitro validation, in vivo activity, pharmacology, toxicology, and clinical trials). Each of these technological phases presents complex problems, which limited the pipeline of clinical drugs to only two approved by the FDA. Despite these difficulties, there are currently over 100 ongoing clinical trials with antisense in different phases in cancer, metabolic, and inflammatory diseases. The vitality of antisense technology stems from the dramatic progress of most advanced chemistries, as well as from the development of oral, intranasal, and subcutaneous applications allowing only weekly dosing schedules. Persistent efforts produced antisense such as mipomersen for hyperlipidemia, a drug used in combination with statins in patients with exceptionally pro-atherogenic problems who have resistance to statins. Cancer therapies have developed very promising methods to overcome the expression of cancer survival genes censurable for resistance to standard drugs and irradiation treatments, with OGX-011 preventing expression of clusterin, OGX-427 of Hsp27, LY2181308 of surviving, and oblimersen of Bcl-2. A very elegant approach was developed for some orphan diseases, such as DMD, allowing an individually selected antisense for mutations in each patient to overcome the blockade in expression of muscle cell molecules. All these efforts are providing a completely new dimension to medical therapy by intervention with individual genes. Transplantation may benefit either indirectly by therapies for other applications than immunosuppression, or by developing completely new drugs that may contribute to induction of permanent graft acceptance.

Glossary

Antisense oligonucleotide is a single strand of DNA or RNA complementary to a chosen sequence. Natural antisense RNA prevents protein translation by binding to certain messenger RNA strands. Antisense DNA targets a complementary (coding or non-) RNA. The DNA–RNA hybrid may be degraded by the enzyme RNase H type I/II or by Argonaute-2.

siRNA, small interfering RNA (or short interfering RNA or silencing RNA), is a class of double-stranded RNA molecules, which are 20–25 nucleotides in length, which interfere in the expression of a specific gene. First discovered by David Baulcombe *et al.* at the Sainsbury Laboratory in Norwich, England, during research on post-transcriptional gene silencing in plants. Synthetic siRNAs are able to interfere with RNA in mammalian cells.

snRNA, small nuclear RNA is present in the nucleus of all eukaryotic cells. The snRNA transcribed by RNA polymerase II or RNA polymerase III is involved in RNA splicing (removal of introns), regulation of transcription factors (7SK RNA), regulation of RNA polymerase II (B2 RNA), and maintaining the telomeres. They are always associated with specific proteins, and the complexes are referred to as small nuclear ribonucleoproteins (snRNPs) or sometimes as snurps. These elements are rich in uridine content.

tRNA, transfer RNA, is usually about 74–95 nucleotides in length. It transfers a specific active amino acid to a polypeptide chain at the ribosomal site of protein synthesis. Each type of tRNA attaches one type of amino acid at its 3′ terminal site. It contains a three-base region called the anticodon that matches the base pair of the corresponding three base codons of mRNA.

rRNA, ribosomal RNA, is located in the ribosome, which is the protein manufacturing machinery of all living cells. The rRNA is decoding mRNA into amino acids and interact with the tRNAs during translation. Specific tRNA carrying each amino acid brings it the appropriate mRNA codon.

mRNA, messenger ribonucleic acid is a molecule of RNA encoding a sequence for a protein product. The mRNA is transcribed from a DNA template, and carries coding information to the sites of protein synthesis: the ribosomes. Here, the nucleic acid polymer is translated into a polymer of amino acids: a protein. In mRNA as in DNA, genetic information is encoded in the sequence of nucleotides arranged into codons consisting of three bases each. Each codon encodes for a specific amino acid, except the stop codons that terminate protein synthesis.

References

1 Zamecnik PC, Stephenson ML. Inhibition of Rous sarcoma virus replication and cell transformation by a specific oligodeoxynucleotide. *Proc Natl Acad Sci U S A* 1978;75(1):280–284.

2 Cerritelli SM, Crouch RJ. Ribonuclease H: the enzymes in eukaryotes. *FEBS J* 2009;276(6):1494–1505.

3 Elbashir SM, Harborth J, Lendeckel W *et al*. Duplexes of 21-nucleotide RNAs mediate RNA interference in cultured mammalian cells. *Nature* 2001;411(6836):494–498.

4 Liu J, Carmell MA, Rivas FV *et al*. Argonaute2 is the catalytic engine of mammalian RNAi. *Science* 2004;305(5689):1437–1441.

5 Bill BR, Petzold AM, Clark KJ *et al*. A primer for morpholino use in zebrafish. *Zebrafish* 2009;6(1):69–77.

6 Vickers TA, Koo S, Bennett CF *et al*. Efficient reduction of target RNAs by small interfering RNA and RNase H-dependent antisense agents. *A comparative analysis*. *J Biol Chem* 2003;278(9):7108–7118.

7 Allerson CR, Sioufi N, Jarres R *et al*. Fully 2′-modified oligonucleotide duplexes with improved in vitro potency and stability compared to unmodified small interfering RNA. *J Med Chem* 2005;48(4):901–904.

8 Birmingham A, Anderson E, Sullivan K *et al*. A protocol for designing siRNAs with high functionality and specificity. *Nat Protoc* 2007;2(9):2068–2078.

9 Sharp PA. The centrality of RNA. *Cell* 2009;136(4):577–580.

10 Carthew RW, Sontheimer EJ. Origins and mechanisms of miRNAs and siRNAs. *Cell* 2009;136(4):642–655.

11 Cooper TA, Wan L, Dreyfuss G. RNA and disease. *Cell* 2009;136(4):777–793.

12 He L, Thomson JM, Hemann MT *et al*. A microRNA polycistron as a potential human oncogene. *Nature* 2005;435(7043):828–833.

13 Wang G, van der Walt JM, Mayhew G *et al*. Variation in the miRNA-433 binding site of FGF20 confers risk for Parkinson disease by overexpression of α-synuclein. *Am J Hum Genet* 2008;82:283–289.

14 Batey RT, Rambo RP, Doudna JA. Tertiary motifs in RNA structure and folding. *Angew Chem Int Ed Engl* 1999;38(16):2326–2343.

15 Monia BP, Johnston JF, Ecker DJ *et al*. Selective inhibition of mutant Ha-ras mRNA expression by antisense oligonucleotides. *J Biol Chem* 1992;267(28):19954–19962.

16 Pontius BW, Berg P. Renaturation of complementary DNA strands mediated by purified mammalian heterogeneous nuclear ribonucleoprotein A1 protein: implications for a mechanism for rapid molecular assembly. *Proc Natl Acad Sci U S A* 1990;87(21):8403–8407.

17 Eckstein F. Phosphorothioate oligodeoxynucleotides: what is their origin and what is unique about them? *Antisense Nucleic Acid Drug Dev* 2000;10(2):117–121.

18 Stein CA, Subasinghe C, Shinozuka K, Cohen JS. Physicochemical properties of phosphorothioate oligodeoxynucleotides. *Nucleic Acids Res* 1988;16(8):3209–3221.

19 Bhagat L, Putta MR, Wang D *et al*. Novel oligonucleotides containing two 3′-ends complementary to target mRNA show optimal gene-silencing activity. *J Med Chem* 2011;54(8):3027–3036.

20 Dean NM. Functional genomics and target validation approaches using antisense oligonucleotide technology. *Curr Opin Biotechnol* 2001;12(6):622–625.

21 Taylor JK, Zhang QQ, Wyatt JR, Dean NM. Induction of endogenous Bcl-xS through the control of Bcl-x pre-mRNA splicing by antisense oligonucleotides. *Nat Biotechnol* 1999;17(11):1097–1100.

22 Bennett CF, Swayze EE. RNA targeting therapeutics: molecular mechanisms of antisense oligonucleotides as a therapeutic platform. *Annu Rev Pharmacol Toxicol* 2010;50:259–293.

23 Crooke RM, Graham MJ, Lemonidis KM *et al*. An apolipoprotein B antisense oligonucleotide lowers LDL cholesterol in hyperlipidemic mice without causing hepatic steatosis. *J Lipid Res* 2005;46(5):872–884.

24 Kastelein JJ, Wedel MK, Baker BF *et al*. Potent reduction of apolipoprotein B and low-density lipoprotein cholesterol by short-term administration of an antisense inhibitor of apolipoprotein B. *Circulation* 2006;114(16):1729–1735.

25 Akdim F, Stroes ES, Kastelein JJ. Antisense apolipoprotein B therapy: where do we stand? *Curr Opin Lipidol* 2007;18(4):397–400.

26 Raal FJ, Santos RD, Blom DJ *et al.* Mipomersen, an apolipoprotein B synthesis inhibitor, for lowering of LDL cholesterol concentrations in patients with homozygous familial hypercholesterolaemia: a randomised, double-blind, placebo-controlled trial. *Lancet* 2010; 375(9719):998–1006.

27 Visser ME, Kastelein JJ, Stroes ES. Apolipoprotein B synthesis inhibition: results from clinical trials. *Curr Opin Lipidol* 2010;21(4):319–323.

28 Call JA, Eckhardt SG, Camidge DR. Targeted manipulation of apoptosis in cancer treatment. *Lancet Oncol* 2008;9(10):1002–1011.

29 Liu G, Kolesar J, McNeel DG *et al.* A Phase I pharmacokinetic and pharmacodynamic correlative study of the antisense Bcl-2 oligonucleotide g3139, in combination with carboplatin and paclitaxel, in patients with advanced solid tumors. *Clin Cancer Res* 2008;14(9): 2732–2739.

30 Rom J, von Minckwitz G, Marmé F *et al.* Phase I study of apoptosis gene modulation with oblimersen within preoperative chemotherapy in patients with primary breast cancer. *Ann Oncol* 2009;20:1829–1835.

31 Pavlick AC, Ott P, Escalon J *et al.* Survival of advanced melanoma patients with normal LDH treated with oblimersen, temozolomide, and nab-paclitaxel. *J Clin Oncol* 2009;27:(Suppl):abstract 9080.

32 Sternberg CN, Dumez H, Van PH *et al.* Docetaxel plus oblimersen sodium (Bcl-2 antisense oligonucleotide): an EORTC multicenter, randomized Phase II study in patients with castration-resistant prostate cancer. *Ann Oncol* 2009;20(7):1264–1269.

33 Tolcher AW, Chi K, Kuhn J *et al.* A Phase II, pharmacokinetic, and biological correlative study of oblimersen sodium and docetaxel in patients with hormone-refractory prostate cancer. *Clin Cancer Res* 2005;11(10):3854–3861.

34 Durig J, Duhrsen U, Klein-Hitpass L *et al.* The novel antisense Bcl-2 inhibitor SPC2996 causes rapid leukemic cell clearance and immune activation in chronic lymphocytic leukemia. *Leukemia* 2011;25(4):638–647.

35 Drummond DC, Noble CO, Kirpotin DB *et al.* Clinical development of histone deacetylase inhibitors as anticancer agents. *Annu Rev Pharmacol Toxicol* 2005;45: 495–528.

36 Chi KN, Zoubeidi A, Gleave ME. Custirsen (OGX-011): a second-generation antisense inhibitor of clusterin for the treatment of cancer. *Expert Opin Investig Drugs* 2008;17(12):1955–1962.

37 Sowery RD, Hadaschik BA, So AI *et al.* Clusterin knockdown using the antisense oligonucleotide OGX-011 re-sensitizes docetaxel-refractory prostate

cancer PC-3 cells to chemotherapy. *BJU Int* 2008; 102(3):389–397.

38 Liu T, Liu PY, Tee AE *et al.* Over-expression of clusterin is a resistance factor to the anti-cancer effect of histone deacetylase inhibitors. *Eur J Cancer* 2009;45(10): 1846–1854.

39 Chi KN, Eisenhauer E, Fazli L *et al.* A Phase I pharmacokinetic and pharmacodynamic study of OGX-011, a 2′-methoxyethyl antisense oligonucleotide to clusterin, in patients with localized prostate cancer. *J Natl Cancer Inst* 2005;97(17):1287–1296.

40 Chi KN, Hotte SJ, Yu E *et al.* Mature results of a randomized Phase II study of OGX-011 in combination with docetaxel/prednisone versus docetaxel/prednisone in patients with metastatic castration-resistant prostate cancer. *J Clin Oncol* 2009;27(Suppl): abstract 5012.

41 Chia S, Dent S, Ellard S *et al.* Phase II trial of OGX-011 in combination with docetaxel in metastatic breast cancer. *Clin Cancer Res* 2009;15(2):708–713.

42 Zoubeidi A, Chi K, Gleave M. Targeting the cytoprotective chaperone, clusterin, for treatment of advanced cancer. *Clin Cancer Res* 2010;16(4):1088–1093.

43 Kamada M, So A, Muramaki M *et al.* Hsp27 knockdown using nucleotide-based therapies inhibit tumor growth and enhance chemotherapy in human bladder cancer cells. *Mol Cancer Ther* 2007;6(1):299–308.

44 Hadaschik BA, Jackson J, Fazli L, Zoubeidi A, Burt HM, Gleave ME *et al.* Intravesically administered antisense oligonucleotides targeting heat-shock protein-27 inhibit the growth of non-muscle-invasive bladder cancer. *BJU Int* 2008 Aug 5;102(5):610–6.

45 Hotte S, Yu EY, Hirte HW *et al.* OGX-427, a 2′methoxyethyl antisense ologonucleotide (ASO), against HSP27: results of a first-in-human trial. *J Clin Oncol* 2009; 27(Suppl):abstract 3506.

46 Sah NK, Khan Z, Khan GJ, Bisen PS. Structural, functional and therapeutic biology of survivin. *Cancer Lett* 2006;244(2):164–171.

47 Huynh T, Walchli S, Sioud M. Transcriptional targeting of small interfering RNAs into cancer cells. *Biochem Biophys Res Commun* 2006;350(4):854–859.

48 Hansen JB, Fisker N, Westergaard M *et al.* SPC3042: a proapoptotic survivin inhibitor. *Mol Cancer Ther* 2008; 7(9):2736–2745.

49 Mita AC, Mita MM, Nawrocki ST, Giles FJ. Survivin: key regulator of mitosis and apoptosis and novel target for cancer therapeutics. *Clin Cancer Res* 2008;14(16): 5000–5005.

50 Rodel F, Frey B, Leitmann W *et al.* Survivin antisense oligonucleotides effectively radiosensitize colorectal cancer cells in both tissue culture and murine

xenograft models. *Int J Radiat Oncol Biol Phys* 2008; 71(1):247–255.

51 Aartsma-Rus A, van Ommen GJ. Progress in therapeutic antisense applications for neuromuscular disorders. *Eur J Hum Genet* 2009;18(2):146–153.

52 Aartsma-Rus A, Fokkema I, Verschuuren J *et al.* Theoretic applicability of antisense-mediated exon skipping for Duchenne muscular dystrophy mutations. *Hum Mutat* 2009;30(3):293–299.

53 Lu QL, Mann CJ, Lou F *et al.* Functional amounts of dystrophin produced by skipping the mutated exon in the mdx dystrophic mouse. *Nat Med* 2003;9(8):1009–1014.

54 Muntoni F, Bushby KD, van Ommen G. 149th ENMC International Workshop and 1st TREAT-NMD Workshop on: "Planning Phase I/II Clinical Trials Using Systemically Delivered Antisense Oligonucleotides in Duchenne Muscular Dystrophy". *Neuromuscul Disord* 2008;18(3): 268–275.

55 Kinali M, Arechavala-Gomeza V, Feng L *et al.* Local restoration of dystrophin expression with the morpholino oligomer AVI-4658 in Duchenne muscular dystrophy: a single-blind, placebo-controlled, dose-escalation, proof-of-concept study. *Lancet Neurol* 2009;8(10):918–928.

56 Goemans NM, Tulinius M, van den Akker JT *et al.* Systemic administration of PRO051 in Duchenne's muscular dystrophy. *N Engl J Med* 2011;364(16): 1513–1522.

57 Alter J, Lou F, Rabinowitz A *et al.* Systemic delivery of morpholino oligonucleotide restores dystrophin expression bodywide and improves dystrophic pathology. *Nat Med* 2006;12(2):175–177.

58 Denti MA, Incitti T, Sthandier O *et al.* Long-term benefit of adeno-associated virus/antisense-mediated exon skipping in dystrophic mice. *Hum Gene Ther* 2008; 19(6):601–608.

59 Goyenvalle A, Vulin A, Fougerousse F *et al.* Rescue of dystrophic muscle through U7 snRNA-mediated exon skipping. *Science* 2004;306(5702):1796–1799.

60 Nakamura A, Takeda S. Exon-skipping therapy for Duchenne muscular dystrophy. *Neuropathology* 2009; 29(4):494–501.

61 Rothlein R, Dustin ML, Marlin SD, Springer TA. A human intercellular adhesion molecule (ICAM-1) distinct from LFA-1. *J Immunol* 1986;137(4):1270–1274.

62 Marlin SD, Springer TA. Purified intercellular adhesion molecule-1 (ICAM-1) is a ligand for lymphocyte function-associated antigen 1 (LFA-1). *Cell* 1987;51(5): 813–819.

63 Stepkowski SM, Tu Y, Condon TP, Bennett CF. Blocking of heart allograft rejection by intercellular adhesion molecule-1 antisense oligonucleotides alone or in combination with other immunosuppressive modalities. *J Immunol* 1994;153(11):5336–5346.

64 Stepkowski SM, Wang ME, Condon TP *et al.* Protection against allograft rejection with intercellular adhesion molecule-1 antisense oligodeoxynucleotides. *Transplantation* 1998;66(6):699–707.

65 Stepkowski SM. Development of antisense oligodeoxynucleotides for transplantation. *Curr Opin Mol Ther* 2000;2(3):304–317.

66 Chen W, Langer RM, Janczewska S *et al.* Methoxyethyl-modified intercellular adhesion molecule-1 antisense phosphorothiateoligonucleotides inhibit allograft rejection, ischemic-reperfusion injury, and cyclosporine-induced nephrotoxicity. *Transplantation* 2005;79(4):401–408.

67 Chen W, Bennett CF, Wang ME *et al.* Perfusion of kidneys with unformulated "naked" intercellular adhesion molecule-1 antisense oligodeoxynucleotides prevents ischemic/reperfusion injury. *Transplantation* 1999;68(6):880–887.

68 Dragun D, Lukitsch I, Tullius SG *et al.* Inhibition of intercellular adhesion molecule-1 with antisense deoxynucleotides prolongs renal isograft survival in the rat. *Kidney Int* 1998;54(6):2113–2122.

69 Kahan BD, Stepkowski S, Kilic M *et al.* Phase I and Phase II safety and efficacy trial of intercellular adhesion molecule-1 antisense oligodeoxynucleotide (ISIS 2302) for the prevention of acute allograft rejection. *Transplantation* 2004;78(6):858–863.

70 Huber C, Irschick E. Cytokines in the regulation of allograft rejection. *Bibl Cardiol* 1988;(43):103–110.

71 Leonard WJ, O'Shea JJ. Jaks and STATs: biological implications. *Annu Rev Immunol* 1998;16:293–322.

72 Qu X, Kirken RA, Tian L *et al.* Selective inhibition of IL-2 gene expression by IL-2 antisense oligonucleotides blocks heart allograft rejection. *Transplantation* 2001;72(5):915–923.

73 Stepkowski SM, Qu X, Wang ME *et al.* Inhibition of C-raf expression by antisense oligonucleotides extends heart allograft survival in rats. *Transplantation* 2000; 70(4):656–661.

74 Weiss A. T cell antigen receptor signal transduction: a tale of tails and cytoplasmic protein-tyrosine kinases. *Cell* 1993;73(2):209–212.

75 Cioffi CL, Garay M, Johnston JF *et al.* Selective inhibition of A-Raf and C-Raf mRNA expression by antisense oligodeoxynucleotides in rat vascular smooth muscle cells: role of A-Raf and C-Raf in serum-induced proliferation. *Mol Pharmacol* 1997;51(3):383–389.

76 Morishita R. Perspective in progress of cardiovascular gene therapy. *J Pharmacol Sci* 2004;95(1):1–8.

77 Suzuki JI, Isobe M, Morishita R, Nagai R. Characteristics of chronic rejection in heart transplantation. *Circ J* 2010;74(2):233–239.

78 Tsai LH, Harlow E, Meyerson M. Isolation of the human cdk2 gene that encodes the cyclin A- and adenovirus E1A-associated p33 kinase. *Nature* 1991;353(6340): 174–177.

79 Suzuki J, Isobe M, Morishita R *et al.* Prevention of graft coronary arteriosclerosis by antisense cdk2 kinase oligonucleotide. *Nat Med* 1997;3(8):900–903.

80 Morishita R, Gibbons GH, Ellison KE *et al.* Single intraluminal delivery of antisense cdc2 kinase and proliferating-cell nuclear antigen oligonucleotides results in chronic inhibition of neointimal hyperplasia. *Proc Natl Acad Sci U S A* 1993;90(18): 8474–8478.

81 Suzuki J, Isobe M, Morishita R *et al.* Prevention of cardiac allograft arteriosclerosis using antisense proliferating-cell nuclear antigen oligonucleotide. *Transplantation* 2000;70(2):398–400.

CHAPTER 21

The Role of Ganciclovir in Transplantation

Lyndsey J. Bowman[1] *and Daniel C. Brennan*[2]

[1]Barnes-Jewish Hospital, St. Louis, MO, USA
[2]Washington University in St. Louis, St. Louis, MO, USA

Introduction

A deeper understanding of the immune system, coupled with advancements in immunosuppressive protocols, has led to a substantial reduction in the incidence of acute rejection following transplantation [1]. Despite an overall increase in graft survival, the true success of transplantation depends on multiple factors, including the incidence of infection. Thus, the primary objective of immunosuppressive agents is to provide a balance of preserving allograft function, while minimizing associated adverse effects and maintaining host defense mechanisms against infection and malignancy.

Virologic infections are common post-transplantation and negatively impact graft survival. Cytomegalovirus (CMV) is the most prominent of these viral infections, and the direct and indirect effects of CMV on patient and allograft outcomes have been well described [2–5]. With the advent of more potent immunosuppression and increased transplant allograft longevity, CMV continues to be a major cause of morbidity and mortality in transplant recipients.

In the USA, nearly 60 % of persons aged 6 years or older have previously been exposed to CMV [6]. CMV seroprevalence also increases with age, with over 90 % of individuals 80 years of age and older having been exposed to CMV [6]. Thus, the majority of transplant donors and recipients are not CMV naive. As a result, the lack of preventative strategies against CMV has resulted in the development of CMV infection in 40–100 % of transplant recipients within the first 100 days post-transplant [7]. Through the development and use of potent antivirals as prophylaxis, along with the heightened awareness of CMV infection through advanced and routine monitoring with a preemptive approach, the incidence of symptomatic CMV post-transplant has greatly declined [8]. The utilization of these preventative strategies against CMV infection and disease has led to successful minimization of the direct effects of CMV, such as allograft dysfunction and failure [8].

History

Ganciclovir (Cytovene®, Roche Pharm US, Inc.) was first approved for the treatment of CMV retinitis in 1989 [9]. Ganciclovir subsequently gained Food and Drug Administration (FDA) approval for prevention of CMV post-transplantation. Over 20 years after its initial approval for use, both intravenous (IV) and oral ganciclovir are used in the treatment and prophylaxis of various types of CMV infections today. Furthermore, based on its potent antiviral activity, ganciclovir serves as an effective agent for use in the treatment and prevention of other herpes viruses.

Immunotherapy in Transplantation: Principles and Practice, First Edition. Edited by Bruce Kaplan, Gilbert J. Burckart and Fadi G. Lakkis.
© 2012 Blackwell Publishing Ltd. Published 2012 by Blackwell Publishing Ltd.

Chemistry/structure

Ganciclovir is a cyclic analog of guanosine, the endogenous purine nucleoside. Based on its chemical structure, ganciclovir is also known as DHPG or 9-[(1,3-dihydroxy-2-propoxy)methyl]guanine (Plate 21.1a).

Valganciclovir (Valcyte®, Roche Pharm US, Inc.) is the hydrochloride salt of the L-valyl ester, or prodrug, of ganciclovir [10]. Valganciclovir is a mixture of two diastereomers that are converted to ganciclovir by gastrointestinal (GI) and hepatic esterases. The chemical name for valganciclovir is L-valine, 2-[(2-amino-1,6-dihydro-6-oxo-9*H*-purin-9-yl)methoxy]-3-hydroxypropyl ester, monohydrochloride (Plate 21.1b).

Mechanism of action

Ganciclovir is a nucleoside analog that inhibits viral DNA synthesis by several pathways (Figure 21.1). Through intracellular phosphorylation of ganciclovir to ganciclovir triphosphate, it acts as a competitive inhibitor of deoxyguanosine triphosphate to inhibit viral DNA synthesis [11]. In vivo, ganciclovir exerts its antiviral activity against cells infected with CMV and herpes simplex virus (HSV).

In HSV-infected cells, ganciclovir is first converted to the monophosphate form by a viral thymidine kinase [11]. Monophosphate ganciclovir is further phosphorylated to the triphosphate version via cellular enzymes. CMV does not have a viral thymidine kinase. In CMV-infected cells, ganciclovir is phosphorylated through a separate enzyme homologue with protein kinase activity, produced by the CMV UL97 gene [12].

Pharmacokinetics

The pharmacokinetics of ganciclovir have been extensively evaluated in various populations and a summary may be found in Table 21.1. Ganciclovir exerts its antiviral activity when administered intravenously, orally, and via intravitreal implantation.

Absorption and distribution

Oral absorption of ganciclovir is delayed, with a time to peak concentration T_{max} ranging between 2 and 14h, depending on the type of transplanted organ and the conditions under which the medication is administered [13–16]. Absorption of ganciclovir is also erratic and incomplete, with a mean bioavailability of 4.5% (±1%) under fasting conditions [17]. The rate and extent of ganciclovir absorption is greatly affected by food, particularly meals high in fat [15]. An open-label, randomized, crossover study was conducted in patients who were seropositive for both human immunodeficiency virus (HIV) and CMV. On days 4 and 8, of an 8-day treatment course of ganciclovir dosed at 1000 mg orally every 8 h, patients were randomized to receive the

Figure 21.1 Ganciclovir (GCV) is converted to ganciclovir monophosphate (GCV-MP) by a viral kinase (UL97 of CMV or the thymidine kinase of herpes simplex virus). Cellular kinases catalyze the formation of ganciclovir triphosphate (GCV-TP), which competitively inhibits the binding of deoxyguanosine triphosphate (dGTP) to DNA polymerase resulting in the inhibition of viral DNA synthesis. GCV-TP is also incorporated into viral DNA and serves as a poor substrate for DNA chain elongation, thereby inhibiting viral DNA synthesis by a second route.

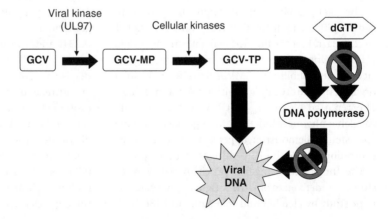

Table 21.1 Ganciclovir pharmacokinetic parameters following oral and intravenous ganciclovir administration. Values reported as mean plus/minus SD.

Parameter	Ganciclovir	
	Oral[a]	IV[b]
C_{max} (μg/mL)	2.12–4.8	9
C_{min} (μg/mL)	0.78–1.15	0.57–2.65
AUC_{0-24} (μg h/mL) fasting	15.4±4.3	21.4±3.1
T_{max} (h)	1.8–14	0.97±0.08
F (%)	4.5 (±1)[c]	N/A
$t_{1/2}$ (h)[d]	4.4±0.6	3.3±0.3
Renal elimination (% of systemic clearance)		91±11

C_{max}: maximum observed concentration; C_{min}: minimum observed concentration; AUC: area under the curve; T_{max}: time to maximum observed concentration; F: absolute bioavailability; $t_{1/2}$: half-life.
[a] 1000 mg orally three times daily.
[b] 5 mg/kg IV every 12 h.
[c] Under fasting conditions, bioavailability increases in the fed state.
[d] Normal renal function, $t_{1/2}$ increases significantly with renal impairment.

morning dose after either an overnight fast or after a 600-calorie, high-fat breakfast. While T_{max} was significantly prolonged after a high-fat breakfast from 1.8 h in the fasting state to 3 h in the fed state, area under the curve (AUC) and the peak concentration C_{max} were significantly higher. A mean increase AUC by approximately 22 % and an increase in C_{max} by 15 % were observed following high-fat food consumption.

The ganciclovir concentration necessary to achieve 50 % viral inhibition (IC_{50}) ranges from 0.1 to 2.8 μg/mL according to available in vitro data [18, 19]. One study by Boivin et al. determined ganciclovir susceptibility to CMV isolates from 42 solid organ transplant recipients with CMV viremia [20]. The reported mean IC_{50} to CMV was 0.4 μg/mL. Available pharmacokinetic data of ganciclovir have consistently demonstrated peak and trough concentrations above the IC_{50} with varying dosages.

The therapeutic range of ganciclovir in various studies is derived from the original pharmacokinetic study by Fletcher and colleagues in 1986 [21].

This study was conducted in six nonsolid organ transplant patients receiving 2.5 mg/kg or 5 mg/kg every 8 or 12 h for CMV pneumonitis or retinitis. The reported peak and trough concentrations of ganciclovir, with the 2.5 mg/kg dose, were 4.75–6.2 μg/mL and <0.25–0.63 μg/mL respectively.

The pharmacokinetic literature evaluating ganciclovir for the treatment and prophylaxis of CMV following solid organ transplantation varies widely in regard to peak and trough drug concentrations [4, 13, 22, 23]. The mean peak and trough plasma concentrations following IV dosing of ganciclovir at 5 mg/kg every 12 h in three separated studies conducted in solid organ transplant recipients were found to be approximately 9 μg/mL and a trough range of 0.57 to 2.65 μg/mL [4, 13]. Two studies with the objective to evaluate plasma peak and trough concentrations following oral administration of ganciclovir 1000 mg three times daily have reported concentrations of 2.12–4.8 μg/mL and 0.78–1.15 μg/mL respectively [13, 23]. Despite published literature supplying us with ranges for AUC, peak, and trough concentrations of ganciclovir, none of these studies was able to define a correlation between drug concentrations and efficacy or toxicity of ganciclovir treatment [4, 13, 22, 23]. Therefore, there is not an immediate role for routine clinical pharmacokinetic monitoring of ganciclovir therapy.

The disposition of IV ganciclovir is described by a two-compartment model and exhibits bi-exponential decay [13, 21, 24]. Results of more recent studies are consistent with the initial pharmacokinetics studies conducted in the late 1980s. In patients exhibiting normal renal function, ganciclovir has a mean distribution half-life $t_{1/2}$ of 0.23 h and a terminal $t_{1/2}$ of 2.53 h [21]. Despite a serum $t_{1/2}$ of less than 5 h, ganciclovir triphosphate persists in CMV-infected cells for several days, with an intracellular $t_{1/2}$ of 16.5 h. Minimal plasma protein binding exists with ganciclovir and is reported to be 1–2 % [9]. Ganciclovir is extensively distributed throughout the body, with a steady-state volume of distribution (VDss) of approximately 0.75 L/kg [13, 16, 25]. A large volume of distribution is often arbitrarily defined as greater than 0.7–1 L/kg; thus, ganciclovir exhibits a relatively large volume of distribution. Ganciclovir also penetrates the blood–brain barrier, which was demonstrated by cerebrospinal fluid concentrations of ganciclovir 24–67 % of correlating serum concentrations [21].

Metabolism and excretion

The primary means of ganciclovir elimination is via renal excretion through glomerular filtration and active tubular secretion [13, 26]. In patients with normal renal function, 91.3 ± 5 % of IV ganciclovir is recovered unchanged in the urine, with renal elimination accounting for 91 ± 11 % of the systemic clearance of ganciclovir [9].

The terminal $t_{1/2}$ of ganciclovir is significantly prolonged (11.5 ± 3.9 h) in patients with renal insufficiency, necessitating renal dosage adjustments based on a predicted creatinine clearance (CrCl) calculated from the Cockcroft–Gault (C–G) equation [9, 24, 27]. The correlation between CrCl and the clearance of ganciclovir has been assessed [13, 21]. From these pharmacokinetic studies, corresponding equations have been developed to predict the average clearance of ganciclovir from CrCl in various degrees of renal insufficiency. While these analyses demonstrate a strong correlation between ganciclovir clearance and CrCl, one such study evaluating this relationship in four renal transplant recipients demonstrated that ganciclovir clearance was consistently greater than CrCl, indicating the involvement of tubular secretion of ganciclovir [13]. This discrepancy was evident irrespective of whether the C–G equation or measured CrCl was used. While this study provides useful pharmacokinetic information, the limited number of study patients restricts the clinical application for the prospective dosing of ganciclovir.

The effects of hemodialysis (HD) on ganciclovir clearance have been assessed in various pharmacokinetic analyses [24, 26, 28]. The plasma concentration of ganciclovir is decreased approximately 50 % following a 4 h HD session, thus necessitating dosage post-HD. Currently, no data exist to guide the appropriate use of ganciclovir during peritoneal dialysis.

Ganciclovir has a low molecular weight of 255, is hydrophilic with a water solubility of 2.6 mg/mL, and has an extremely low protein binding of 1–2 %

[9]. Ganciclovir's given characteristics are consistent with the degree in which it is removed from the plasma during continuous venovenous HD (CVVHD) and continuous venovenous hemodiafiltration (CVVHDF). The effects of CVVHD on ganciclovir at a dose of 5 mg/kg IV every 48 h was studied in two small studies [29, 30]. Boulieu *et al.* specifically analyzed the pharmacokinetics of ganciclovir in three heart transplant patients undergoing CVVHD [29]. The mean elimination $t_{1/2}$ of ganciclovir under CVVHD was 18.9 h, with a mean clearance of 0.42 mL/(min kg). At steady state, the clearance of ultrafiltration was 12.9 mL/min and the average fraction of removal of the administered dose during CVVHD was 89.7 ± 10.6 %. A case report by Gando *et al.* demonstrated the efficiency of ganciclovir removal during CVVHDF [30]. Pharmacokinetic parameters of ganciclovir were determined on day 3 of drug administration based on a 5 mg/kg dosage given over a 60 min period under CVVHDF. Samples from the arterial and venous blood catheters, and from the ultradiafiltrate, were collected over 12 h after the start of the infusion. The elimination $t_{1/2}$ of ganciclovir in this patient was 12.6 h, with a total clearance of 0.55 mL/(min kg). The mean hemodiafiltration clearance was 29.6 mL/min. The differences between CVVHD and CVVHDF in regard to solute removal should be considered when evaluating the differences in observed pharmacokinetic parameters of ganciclovir during continuous renal replacement therapy. CVVHDF combines both diffusion and convection for solute removal, while CVVHD uses convection alone based on a pressure gradient [31]. Based on the low molecular weight and low protein binding of ganciclovir, the differing mechanisms between CVVHD and CVVHDF may explain the shorter elimination $t_{1/2}$ and greater plasma clearance of ganciclovir during CVVHDF.

Pharmacodynamics

Drug–drug Interactions

Ganciclovir exhibits a minimal drug interaction profile as it is not metabolized through the cytochrome P450 system or by P-glycoprotein, and is minimally protein bound. Few formal drug interaction studies have been conducted with ganciclovir; however, recommendations against the concurrent use of ganciclovir with various agents have been expressed. The use of ganciclovir in combination with probenecid should be done cautiously or avoided if possible. Owing to competition for renal tubular secretion, a greater than 50 % increase in AUC and 20 % decrease in renal clearance of ganciclovir increases the risk of ganciclovir toxicity [32].

The use of ganciclovir in combination with two different antiretrovirals has resulted in altered pharmacokinetic profiles of one or both of the agents involved. One open-label crossover drug interaction study demonstrated an increase in didanosine AUC by 87.3 to 124 % when given immediately after or 2 h before ganciclovir [33]. An elevation in didanosine C_{max} was also seen. No significant effects on the steady-state pharmacokinetics of ganciclovir were observed. Variations in the pharmacokinetic profiles have also been studied for the combination of oral ganciclovir and zidovudine [32]. The use of these agents together resulted in a lower AUC for ganciclovir, but an increase in zidovudine AUC by approximately 20 %. Despite a speculative offset in toxicity due to the altered levels of each agent, the co-administration of ganciclovir and zidovudine may exacerbate neutropenia and anemia.

Manufacturer-derived recommendations for the use of ganciclovir in combination with other agents are from observations and known characteristics of ganciclovir [9]. Generalized seizures have been described in patients receiving ganciclovir along with imipenem and cilastatin and should be avoided if possible. Owing to the potential for synergistic renal impairment, caution should be exercised with the use of ganciclovir with other nephrotoxins such as amphotericin B, aminoglycosides, cisplatin, and calcineurin inhibitors.

Clinical efficacy
Treatment of CMV Infections
CMV retinitis
Ganciclovir is used for the prevention and treatment of various CMV infections, yet it holds an FDA-approved indication for treatment only for CMV retinitis in immunocompromised individuals. Published literature demonstrating the efficacy of ganciclovir for the treatment of CMV retinitis dates back to the mid 1980s; however, the lack of maintenance therapy resulted in significant relapse rates post-drug discontinuation [34]. The efficacy of both induction and maintenance therapy with IV ganciclovir was later established when studied in 314 immunocompromised patients with CMV [35]. Specifically, the 108 patients with CMV retinitis in this cohort had a favorable clinical response rate of 84 % when treated with IV ganciclovir at 5 mg/kg twice daily for 14 days. Maintenance therapy with IV ganciclovir delayed the time to relapse by over 50 days, with a median time to relapse of retinitis of 105 days in patients receiving maintenance treatment as compared to 47 days in those who did not receive maintenance therapy. A separate prospective, randomized, multicenter study was conducted in acquired immunodeficiency syndrome (AIDS) patients with concomitant CMV retinitis to demonstrate the safety and efficacy of IV ganciclovir for the treatment of CMV retinitis [36].

Oral ganciclovir dosed at 1000 mg three times a day, or 500 mg six times a day as an alternative, may be used as a maintenance regimen following induction therapy for the treatment of CMV retinitis [9, 37]. Evidence supporting the oral use of ganciclovir was shown primarily during three separate trials evaluating the efficacy of oral ganciclovir as an alternative to IV maintenance therapy for CMV retinitis. Oral ganciclovir was shown to effectively slow the time to progression of CMV retinitis in all three studies. The difference in the mean time to progression in the IV and the oral form (IV-oral) ranged between 5 and 12 days.

The addition of the valine ester moiety to ganciclovir, as valganciclovir, led to a 10-fold increase in oral bioavailability compared with ganciclovir [14]. In March of 2001, valganciclovir was granted FDA approval for the treatment of CMV retinitis in patients with AIDS [38]. Oral valganciclovir dosed at 900 mg twice daily has been shown to be equally as effective at ganciclovir 5 mg/kg IV twice daily for the treatment of CMV retinitis [39]. A randomized controlled trial comparing valganciclovir 900 mg twice daily for 3 weeks, followed by 900 mg daily for 1 week and ganciclovir 5 mg/kg IV twice daily for 3 weeks, with 5 mg/kg IV daily maintenance for 1 week was conducted in 160 AIDS patients with known CMV retinitis. The primary endpoint was the progression of CMV retinitis in each treatment arm. Both treatment arms were effective at preventing the progression of CMV retinitis, with approximately 10 % of patients in both treatment groups demonstrating progression at 4 weeks.

Finally, local therapy with intraocular ganciclovir implants and intravitreal injections of ganciclovir have also been successful in treating CMV retinitis. The ganciclovir implant (Vitrasert®, Bausch & Lomb) is highly successful at preventing the progression of CMV retinitis, and was found to be significantly more effective than IV ganciclovir at slowing this progression [40]. Despite a greater decline in the progression of CMV retinitis, the implantation alone was unsuccessful at preventing extraocular CMV infections or infection in the contralateral eye. Combination therapy with ganciclovir IV or oral valganciclovir in conjunction with the intravitreal implant of ganciclovir should be considered and clinical judgment employed depending on the severity of such infection.

Other CMV infections: GI, pulmonary, nervous system

Despite a specific FDA-approved indication and little primary literature supporting its use, ganciclovir has been used successfully and continues to be used for the treatment of various CMV infections in various populations. The Centers for Disease Control and Prevention (CDC) released practice guidelines in March 2009 for the prevention and treatment of opportunistic infections, including CMV infection and disease, in HIV-infected persons [41]. These recommendations may be extrapolated in some instances to the transplant population, in which data are even more sparse.

The first adequately powered study comparing IV ganciclovir with oral valganciclovir for the treatment of CMV disease was conducted by Asberg *et al.* and became an important addition to the transplant infectious diseases literature in 2007 [42]. In this international trial, 321 solid organ transplant patients with CMV disease were randomized to receive valganciclovir 900 mg twice daily or ganciclovir 5 mg/kg IV twice daily each for 21 days, followed by valganciclovir 900 mg once daily for an additional 28 days of therapy. As determined by investigators, treatment success at 21 days was 77.4 % for valganciclovir and 80.3 % for ganciclovir. The authors concluded that oral valganciclovir is not inferior to IV ganciclovir for the treatment of CMV disease in solid organ transplant recipients.

Preventative strategies against CMV

Currently, two strategies using ganciclovir or valganciclovir for the prevention of CMV are employed. Prophylactic antiviral therapy uses administration of ganciclovir or valganciclovir to patients immediately post-transplantation based on pre-transplant serologic status of the donor and recipient for a defined time period. The second tactic in the prevention of CMV is the preemptive approach. This approach initiates antiviral therapy in response to evidence of CMV infection as indicated by defined laboratory or clinical triggers. Patients are monitored at regular intervals for early identification of CMV replication prior to the onset of clinical symptoms with a goal to prevent progression of asymptomatic infection into CMV disease. Each approach to the prevention of CMV disease has its advantages and disadvantages, and the use of either strategy varies significantly between organ groups and transplant centers. Several randomized trials and meta-analyses have been conducted to compare these strategies [7, 8, 43].

One meta-analysis conducted by Strippoli *et al.* in 2006 identified 10 randomized controlled trials, consisting of 476 solid organ transplant recipients, evaluating the safety and efficacy of the preemptive approach in preventing CMV disease [43]. Of the included trials, six were preemptive versus placebo or standard of care (treatment of CMV disease once it occurred), three were preemptive versus antiviral prophylaxis, and one compared IV versus oral preemptive strategies. While there was no significant difference in the incidence of acute rejection or all-cause mortality, the preemptive approach significantly reduced the incidence of CMV disease when compared with placebo or standard of care (RR 0.29, 95 % CI 0.11–0.8). Trials evaluating discrepancies between preemptive and prophylaxis approaches in preventing various outcomes demonstrated no significant differences between the two groups in terms of acute rejection, all-cause mortality, or CMV disease. Finally, the one trial comparing IV and oral therapies was conducted solely in liver transplant patients and also showed no differences in the incidence of CMV disease or all-cause mortality.

A separate meta-analysis evaluated 17 trials (1980 solid organ transplant recipients) to determine the efficacy of prophylaxis and preemptive strategies in preventing the direct and indirect effects of CMV [8]. Eleven trials (1582 kidney, heart, and liver transplant recipients) were assessed for prophylaxis against CMV, while six trials (398 kidney and liver transplant recipients) were selected for the preemptive analysis. Despite the limitations of this meta-analysis, such as moderately sized studies that did not assess all outcomes compared, both prophylactic and preemptive strategies effectively reduced the incidence of CMV disease and acute rejection. A decrease in the occurrence of bacterial and fungal infections, as well as death, was only demonstrated in the prophylaxis group. Although a difference in these indirect outcomes was observed between the prophylaxis and preemptive studies, the small number of patients in the preemptive trials makes it extremely difficult to provide meaningful assessments regarding the impact of preemptive therapy on indirect outcomes of CMV, such as concomitant infections and mortality.

Oral and IV ganciclovir

Multiple studies have been conducted specifically evaluating the utilization of both IV and oral ganciclovir for the prevention of CMV in solid organ transplant recipients. All of the studies comparing IV or oral ganciclovir with placebo demonstrate significantly lower incidences of CMV infection and disease. Given the successful results with the use of oral ganciclovir, coupled with its convenient administration, IV ganciclovir is seldom utilized for the prevention of CMV in solid organ transplant recipients. Furthermore, the shortcomings of oral

ganciclovir with its poor bioavailability have essentially been replaced in the transplant arena by its prodrug, valganciclovir.

The optimal duration of prophylaxis is unknown. Doyle *et al.* compared 12 versus 24 weeks of CMV prophylaxis with oral ganciclovir in high-risk (donor seropositive and recipient seronegative) renal transplant patients [44]. The 24-week regimen demonstrated a significant decrease in the development of CMV infection (7 % versus 31 %, $p \leq 0.01$) and delayed graft function (29 % versus 45 %, $p=0.04$) compared with prophylaxis for 12 weeks. These results suggest that a longer course of prophylaxis course may be warranted in patients at increased risk for CMV.

Valganciclovir

Valganciclovir was granted FDA approval in September 2003 for the prevention of CMV disease in a select group of patients [45]. Valganciclovir is indicated for prophylaxis against CMV disease in kidney, kidney–pancreas, and heart transplant patients who are CMV seronegative and receive an organ from a CMV seropositive donor. The safety and efficacy of oral valganciclovir was demonstrated in a prospective, randomized, double-blind, double-dummy study comparing valganciclovir 900 mg daily with oral ganciclovir 1000 mg three times a day in high-risk (donor CMV seropositive into recipient seronegative) solid organ transplant recipients (PV 16000 study) [46]. The 364 patients included in this analysis were initiated on one of the above prophylactic regimens within 10 days of transplantation and continued for 100 days. The primary efficacy endpoint of the proportion of patients developing CMV disease during the first 6 months post-transplant was similar between the valganciclovir and the oral ganciclovir groups, with committee-defined CMV disease occurring in 12.1 % and 15.2 % of patients respectively. The safety profile was similar between groups, but with a trend toward an increase in neutropenia with valganciclovir (8.2 % valganciclovir, 3.2 % ganciclovir). This study did not include lung transplant recipients, and an FDA-mandated retrospective evaluation of this data suggested an increase in the incidence of invasive CMV disease with the use of valganciclovir in liver transplant recipients. In relation to these findings, valganciclovir is not FDA approved for use in liver transplant patients and the safety and efficacy of its use in lung transplant recipients has not been established. Despite these results and lack of abundant literature for its use in these populations, valganciclovir is consistently used in clinical practice for all solid organ transplant recipients.

Late-onset CMV disease typically occurs within 3 months following the discontinuation of a 3 month prophylaxis regimen. Given the direct and indirect effects of CMV disease, a recent multicenter, double-blind, placebo-controlled trial was undertaken by Humar *et al.* to assess the safety and efficacy of 200 days versus 100 days of valganciclovir prophylaxis for the prevention of CMV disease in 326 high-risk kidney allograft recipients (IMPACT trial) [47]. The primary efficacy endpoint was the incidence of CMV disease (CMV syndrome or CMV tissue invasive disease) up to 1 year post-transplant, which occurred in 16.1% of the 200-day versus 36.8% of the 100-day group ($p<0.0001$). This statistically significant difference was evident at 6 and 9 months post-transplant. The 200-day group also demonstrated a lower incidence of CMV viremia and a longer time to onset of viremia, both of which were statistically significant. The incidence of acute rejection and impaired renal function were similar between groups, as was hematologic and GI adverse effects. While most opportunistic infections occurred within the first 50 days post-transplant, the overall incidence up to 1 year was significantly lower in the 200-day group ($p=0.001$). This should be interpreted cautiously given the imbalance seen early while each group was still receiving therapy. The 2-year follow-up analysis continued to show a significant difference in the incidence of CMV disease, in favor of the 200-day study arm [48]. Important points not assessed in this study, such as economical implications and potential resistance with an extended prophylaxis regimen, have since been evaluated and again support the use of 200 days of valganciclovir in high-risk renal transplant recipients [49, 50].

The FDA approval of valganciclovir 900 mg daily for the prevention of CMV in solid organ transplant recipients was based on the PV 1600 study. A pharmacokinetic crossover study was later performed solely in kidney transplant recipients to determine pharmacokinetic characteristics of IV ganciclovir and oral ganciclovir compared to two different valganciclovir doses [51]. Oral ganciclovir 1000 mg every eight h, IV ganciclovir 2.5 mg/kg every 12 h, and valganciclovir 900 mg daily and 450 mg daily were evaluated. Oral valganciclovir 900 mg daily and IV ganciclovir achieved similar AUC and systemic ganciclovir exposure, which was consistent with results of the PV 16000 study. More importantly for this study, valganciclovir 450 mg daily provided similar systemic exposure of ganciclovir to oral ganciclovir dosed at 1000 mg every 8 h. Given the hematologic toxicity associated with valganciclovir, coupled with previous pharmacokinetic data, studies have suggested that 450 mg daily is effective at preventing CMV and may exhibit less toxicity that the standard 900 mg daily [52–54]. A recent network meta-analysis by Kalil *et al.* compared 12 studies for 900 mg daily and eight for 450 mg daily for the prophylaxis of CMV with a comparator arm (oral ganciclovir, valacyclovir, or preemptive approach) in abdominal organ transplant recipients [55]. The primary finding of this analysis was the equal efficacy for the prevention of CMV disease between 900 mg per day and 450 mg daily. Valganciclovir dosed at 900 mg daily produced three times the amount of leukopenia and a higher incidence of acute rejection compared with the 450 mg dose. A randomized, head-to-head trial would be best to truly assess the risks and benefits of the two valganciclovir dosing schematics. Based on available literature and pharmacokinetic data, it is reasonable to assume that valganciclovir 450 mg daily is a suitable option for the prevention of CMV in abdominal organ transplant recipients.

Safety and tolerability
Hematologic

The adverse effects (AEs) of ganciclovir are predominantly hematologic in nature. The most commonly reported hematologic toxicities associated with ganciclovir include anemia, thrombocytopenia, leukopenia, and neutropenia. The reported incidence of such AEs varies within available literature, and depends heavily on the type of transplant received, the duration of treatment, and the indication for therapy (prophylaxis versus treatment) [7, 42, 46, 56].

The development of anemia with the concurrent use of ganciclovir post-solid organ transplant ranges between 7 and 65 % [42, 56]. Gane *et al.* conducted a randomized, placebo-controlled, multicenter trial in approximately 300 liver transplant recipients [56]. While the incidence of anemia, defined as a hemoglobin less than or equal to 9.5 g/dL, in the ganciclovir group was elevated at 64.7 %, this was not significantly greater than the placebo arm (62.3 %), owing to the high prevalence of anemia to other contributory factors. Thrombocytopenia occurs in approximately 25 % of ganciclovir-treated patients, and is the by-product of multiple pre- and post-transplant etiologies [46, 57].

Ganciclovir is known for its profound bone marrow suppressive effects, most commonly manifested as leukopenia and neutropenia. Leukopenia occurs in 7–35 % of solid organ transplant recipients receiving ganciclovir, with the highest incidence amongst liver transplant recipients [42, 46, 57]. One prospective, randomized study conducted in 219 CMV-seropositive liver transplant recipients demonstrated a 35 % incidence of leukopenia, defined as a white blood cell (WBC) count of less than 3×10^9/L, with the prophylactic use of oral ganciclovir [57]. Of the ganciclovir-treated group, 15 % required discontinuation of the prophylaxis secondary to the leukopenia.

Neutropenia, generally defined as an absolute neutrophil count [13] of less than 500 to 1000/mm³, has been described and associated with ganciclovir in approximately 3–15 % of solid organ transplant cases [7, 46, 56]. While this complication generally occurs early in therapy and is typically dose limiting and reversible with drug discontinuation, neutropenia secondary to ganciclovir therapy can be associated with infection and death. The incidence of neutropenia can be minimized with the concomitant administration of granulocyte colony-stimulating factor (G-CSF) or granulocyte-macrophage colony-stimulating factor (GM-CSF) [58]. Despite a reduction in the incidence of

neutropenia, the lack of long-term, well-controlled studies of G-CSF and GM-CSF in the transplant populations warrants a cautious approach to therapy in transplant recipients.

The hematologic complications associated with ganciclovir therapy are heightened by a multitude of additional factors contributing to such toxicities post-transplantation. Specific agents utilized for induction and maintenance immunosuppression have been associated with various cytopenias. Of the induction agents frequently utilized for solid organ transplantation, alemtuzumab (Campath®) and rabbit antithymocyte globulin (Thymoglobulin®) are the two agents most commonly linked to profound hematologic toxicities [59]. The incidence of anemia, thrombocytopenia, and neutropenia post-alemtuzumab exposure ranges between 12 and 64 %, depending on the specific cytopenia and previous drug exposure [60]. Through massive T cell depletion in blood and peripheral lymphoid tissues through complement-dependent lysis and T cell apoptosis, Thymoglobulin causes profound lymphopenia that remains lower than baseline for at least 1 year post-administration [61]. Furthermore, the incidence of thrombocytopenia associated with Thymoglobulin is close to 40 % [62]. The antimetabolites, mycophenolate mofetil (Cellcept®) and enteric-coated mycophenolate sodium (Myfortic®), utilized as a component of maintenance immunosuppression in the majority of solid organ transplant recipients today, have all been associated with various cytopenias. The high incidence of anemia (20–40 %), thrombocytopenia (20–40 %), and leukopenia (20–45 %) shown with these agents may exacerbate the hematologic toxicities demonstrated with ganciclovir [63, 64]. Furthermore, the use of sulfamethoxazole/trimethoprim is associated with leukopenia, neutropenia, and thrombocytopenia, and thus perpetuates similar effects seen in patients treated with ganciclovir [65].

Presently, the most common indication for ganciclovir is treatment of CMV. Cytomegalovirus directly contributes to blood dyscrasias through viral suppression of the G_1 and S phases of the cell cycle in various human cell lines [66]. The decrease in production of WBCs, red blood cells, and thrombocytes, in addition to the lytic nature of

CMV on these cells lines, further confounds the true hematologic effects of ganciclovir therapy for the treatment of CMV infection and disease.

Nonhematologic

Despite an overabundant increase in hematologic toxicities reported with the use of IV and oral ganciclovir, other nonhematologic AEs have been associated with ganciclovir therapy. While some of these incidences are relatively high, it is important to be mindful of other variables common to these patients that may have contributed to, or exacerbated, such AEs.

Neurologic

Seizure activity has been reported with the use of ganciclovir [67]. Other, less serious central nervous system AEs have been observed with the use of ganciclovir and include dizziness, confusion, headache, insomnia, peripheral neuropathy, and psychosis [9].

Gastrointestinal

GI adverse effects of ganciclovir include anorexia, nausea, vomiting, diarrhea, and abdominal pain [9]. The most prevalent GI complaint is diarrhea, with an observed incidence of ganciclovir-associated diarrhea of over 40 %. Reported GI toxicity does not differ between IV and oral formulations of ganciclovir.

Elevated serum creatinine

The monitoring of renal function is essential with the utilization of ganciclovir. While ganciclovir dosage adjustments are required for impaired renal function, ganciclovir has also been associated with elevations in serum creatinine levels [9]. The exact mechanism in which ganciclovir causes an increase in serum creatinine levels is unknown.

Infertility and teratogenicity

The toxic effects of ganciclovir on the male reproductive system causing inhibition of spermatogenesis and subsequent infertility have been exhibited in preclinical animal studies [9]. Animal models have demonstrated infertility issues in female subjects as well. Although no human data

of this nature exist, it is possible that recommended doses of ganciclovir may cause temporary or permanent infertility in humans based on the extrapolation of data. Dosage comparisons between animals and humans were made based on human AUC values following the administration of a single 5 mg/kg IV dose of ganciclovir. Teratogenicity and carcinogenic effects have also been reported through animal data. Effective contraception in females and barrier contraceptive practices by male patients should be employed during treatment and 90 days post-treatment with ganciclovir. Despite this possibility of infertility and teratogenicity, the benefits associated with the utilization of ganciclovir often outweigh its risks. Furthermore, the data are based purely on animal data and ganciclovir has been safely used in women with AIDS since the late 1980s.

Therapeutic drug monitoring

While the pharmacokinetic parameters of ganciclovir have been defined, routine therapeutic drug monitoring does not seem to have a definitive role in clinical practice. A concise review on the utility of clinical pharmacokinetic monitoring of ganciclovir was developed by Scott *et al.* in 2004 [68]. The review addressed specific issues, such as the ability to measure ganciclovir in human plasma, the relationship between pharmacological response and drug concentrations in the general population and then per specific indication, and if the results of such drug assay would make a significant difference in the clinical decision-making process. The authors concluded that while multiple assays are available to measure plasma concentrations of ganciclovir, no clear correlation between drug concentrations and either efficacy or toxicity of the drug has been established. With the lack of a clear relationship with such drug assays, it would make it difficult to interpret and adjust ganciclovir doses based on drug concentrations. The true therapeutic efficacy of ganciclovir should be evaluated based on clinical response to therapy through patient monitoring and use of CMV PCR testing. While ganciclovir peak and trough concentrations have not been linked to toxicity parameters, such as hematologic AEs, the routine monitoring of complete blood counts is necessary during ganciclovir therapy.

Though more commonly seen in the AIDS patient population, ganciclovir resistance has been reported in the transplant population. The main mechanism of resistance is through the selection of viral mutants that are unable to phosphorylate ganciclovir in infected cells [69]. Mutations in the UL97 protein kinase gene are the most common mutation present in ganciclovir-resistant CMV isolates; however, mutations in the CMV polymerase gene, UL54, have been identified and can lead to resistance to ganciclovir [70]. Specific risk factors for ganciclovir resistance have been identified [71]. These factors include: seronegative recipients of a seropositive donor organ, intense immunosuppressive regimens, prolonged ganciclovir exposure, inadequate ganciclovir plasma concentrations, and high CMV viral load. Valganciclovir seems to be associated with a lower risk of resistance than ganciclovir [20, 46].

Conclusion

Ganciclovir was the first agent to effectively treat and prevent CMV infection and disease in transplant patients and it remains an invaluable therapeutic option for such use today. It is known that the best approach to CMV is prevention; however, the debate over the prophylaxis versus preemptive strategy for prevention with ganciclovir and valganciclovir lingers. While numerous arguments of each strategy focus on proposed advantages and disadvantages, the practical approach is based largely in part upon the transplant center, patient risk factors, and available institutional resources. Given its improved oral bioavailability, and a presumed lower risk of ganciclovir resistance, valganciclovir appears to be a superior alternative to ganciclovir for the prevention of CMV in transplant recipients. The duration of therapy is yet to be fully determined, but in the setting of modern and potent immunosuppressive regimens a prolonged course of therapy (>100 days) is warranted in high-risk individuals. Both IV ganciclovir and oral valganciclovir may be used for the treatment of CMV.

References

1 Hariharan S, Johnson CP, Bresnahan BA *et al.* Improved graft survival after renal transplantation in the United States, 1988 to 1996. *N Engl J Med* 2000;342:605–612.

2 Preiksaitis JK, Brennan DC, Fishman J, Allen U. Canadian Society of Transplantation consensus workshop on cytomegalovirus management in solid organ transplantation final report. *Am J Transplant* 2005; 5:218–227.

3 Rubin RH. The indirect effects of cytomegalovirus infection on the outcome of organ transplantation. *JAMA* 1989;261:3607–9.

4 Fishman JA, Doran MT, Volpicelli SA *et al.* Dosing of intravenous ganciclovir for the prophylaxis and treatment of cytomegalovirus infection in solid organ transplant recipients. *Transplantation* 2000;69:389–394.

5 Snydman DR. Infection in solid organ transplantation. *Transpl Infect Dis* 1999;1:21–28.

6 Staras SA, Dollard SC, Radford KW *et al.* Seroprevalence of cytomegalovirus infection in the United States, 1988–1994. *Clin Infect Dis* 2006;43:1143–1151.

7 Hodson EM, Jones CA, Webster AC *et al.* Antiviral medications to prevent cytomegalovirus disease and early death in recipients of solid-organ transplants: a systematic review of randomised controlled trials. *Lancet* 2005;365:2105–2115.

8 Kalil AC, Levitsky J, Lyden E *et al.* Meta-analysis: the efficacy of strategies to prevent organ disease by cytomegalovirus in solid organ transplant recipients. *Ann Intern Med* 2005;143:870–880.

9 Genentech, Inc. Cytovene®-IV (ganciclovir sodium for injection); 2010. http://www.gene.com/gene/products/information/cytovene/pdf/pi.pdf.

10 Genentech, Inc. Valcyte®, 2010. www.gene.com/gene/products/information/valcyte/pdf/pi.pdf.

11 Martin JC, Dvorak CA, Smee DF *et al.* 9-[(1,3-Dihydroxy-2-propoxy)methyl]guanine: a new potent and selective antiherpes agent. *J Med Chem* 1983;26:759–761.

12 Sullivan V, Talarico CL, Stanat SC *et al.* A protein kinase homologue controls phosphorylation of ganciclovir in human cytomegalovirus-infected cells. *Nature* 1992;358:162–164.

13 Tornatore KM, Garey KW, Saigal N *et al.* Ganciclovir pharmacokinetics and cytokine dynamics in renal transplant recipients with cytomegalovirus infection. *Clin Transplant* 2001;15:297–308.

14 Pescovitz MD, Rabkin J, Merion RM *et al.* Valganciclovir results in improved oral absorption of ganciclovir in liver transplant recipients. *Antimicrob Agents Chemother* 2000;44:2811–2815.

15 Lavelle J, Follansbee S, Trapnell CB *et al.* Effect of food on the relative bioavailability of oral ganciclovir. *J Clin Pharmacol* 1996;36:238–241.

16 Anderson RD, Griffy KG, Jung D *et al.* Ganciclovir absolute bioavailability and steady-state pharmacokinetics after oral administration of two 3000-mg/d dosing regimens in human immunodeficiency virus- and cytomegalovirus-seropositive patients. *Clin Ther* 1995;17:425–432.

17 Spector SA, Busch DF, Follansbee S *et al.* Pharmacokinetic, safety, and antiviral profiles of oral ganciclovir in persons infected with human immunodeficiency virus: a Phase I/II study. AIDS Clinical Trials Group, and Cytomegalovirus Cooperative Study Group. *J Infect Dis* 1995;171:1431–1437.

18 Balfour HH, Jr. Management of cytomegalovirus disease with antiviral drugs. *Rev Infect Dis* 1990;12(Suppl 7):S849–S860.

19 Plotkin SA, Drew WL, Felsenstein D, Hirsch MS. Sensitivity of clinical isolates of human cytomegalovirus to 9-(1,3-dihydroxy-2-propoxymethyl)guanine. *J Infect Dis* 1985;152:833–834.

20 Boivin G, Erice A, Crane DD *et al.* Ganciclovir susceptibilities of cytomegalovirus (CMV) isolates from solid organ transplant recipients with CMV viremia after antiviral prophylaxis. *J Infect Dis* 1993;168:332–335.

21 Fletcher C, Sawchuk R, Chinnock B *et al.* Human pharmacokinetics of the antiviral drug DHPG. *Clin Pharmacol Ther* 1986;40:281–286.

22 Erice A, Jordan MC, Chace BA *et al.* Ganciclovir treatment of cytomegalovirus disease in transplant recipients and other immunocompromised hosts. *JAMA* 1987;257:3082–3087.

23 Snell GI, Kotsimbos TC, Levvey BJ *et al.* Pharmacokinetic assessment of oral ganciclovir in lung transplant recipients with cystic fibrosis. *J Antimicrob Chemother* 2000;45:511–516.

24 Sommadossi JP, Bevan R, Ling T *et al.* Clinical pharmacokinetics of ganciclovir in patients with normal and impaired renal function. *Rev Infect Dis* 1988;10(Suppl 3):S507–S514.

25 Boeckh M, Zaia JA, Jung D *et al.* A study of the pharmacokinetics, antiviral activity, and tolerability of oral ganciclovir for CMV prophylaxis in marrow transplantation. *Biol Blood Marrow Transplant* 1998;4:13–19.

26 Pescovitz MD, Pruett TL, Gonwa T *et al.* Oral ganciclovir dosing in transplant recipients and dialysis patients based on renal function. *Transplantation* 1998;66:1104–1107.

27 Cockcroft DW, Gault MH. Prediction of creatinine clearance from serum creatinine. *Nephron* 1976;16:31–41.

28 Lake KD, Fletcher CV, Love KR *et al.* Ganciclovir pharmacokinetics during renal impairment. *Antimicrob Agents Chemother* 1988;32:1899–1900.

29 Boulieu R, Bastien O, Bleyzac N. Pharmacokinetics of ganciclovir in heart transplant patients undergoing continuous venovenous hemodialysis. *Ther Drug Monit* 1993;15:105–107.

30 Gando S, Kameue T, Nanzaki S *et al.* Pharmacokinetics and clearance of ganciclovir during continuous hemodiafiltration. *Crit Care Med* 1998;26:184–187.

31 John S, Eckardt KU. Renal replacement strategies in the ICU. *Chest* 2007;132:1379–1388.

32 Cimoch PJ, Lavelle J, Pollard R *et al.* Pharmacokinetics of oral ganciclovir alone and in combination with zidovudine, didanosine, and probenecid in HIV-infected subjects. *J Acquir Immune Defic Syndr Hum Retrovirol* 1998;17:227–234.

33 Jung D, Griffy K, Dorr A *et al.* Effect of high-dose oral ganciclovir on didanosine disposition in human immunodeficiency virus (HIV)-positive patients. *J Clin Pharmacol* 1998;38:1057–1062.

34 Collaborative DHPG Treatment Study Group. Treatment of serious cytomegalovirus infections with 9-(1,3-dihydroxy-2-propoxymethyl)guanine in patients with AIDS and other immunodeficiencies. *N Engl J Med* 1986;314:801–805.

35 Buhles WC, Jr, Mastre BJ, Tinker AJ *et al.* Ganciclovir treatment of life- or sight-threatening cytomegalovirus infection: experience in 314 immunocompromised patients. *Rev Infect Dis* 1988;10(Suppl 3):S495–S506.

36 Spector SA, Weingeist T, Pollard RB *et al.* A randomized, controlled study of intravenous ganciclovir therapy for cytomegalovirus peripheral retinitis in patients with AIDS. AIDS Clinical Trials Group and Cytomegalovirus Cooperative Study Group. *J Infect Dis* 1993;168:557–563.

37 Drew WL, Ives D, Lalezari JP *et al.* Oral ganciclovir as maintenance treatment for cytomegalovirus retinitis in patients with AIDS. Syntex Cooperative Oral Ganciclovir Study Group. *N Engl J Med* 1995;333:615–620.

38 US FDA. Approved therapies for the treatment of complications of HIV/AIDS; 2007. http://www.fda.gov/ForConsumers/ByAudience/ForPatientAdvocates/HIVandAIDSActivities/ucm118949.htm (accessed 26 August 2009).

39 Martin DF, Sierra-Madero J, Walmsley S *et al.* A controlled trial of valganciclovir as induction therapy for cytomegalovirus retinitis. *N Engl J Med* 2002;346:1119–1126.

40 Musch DC, Martin DF, Gordon JF *et al.* Treatment of cytomegalovirus retinitis with a sustained-release

ganciclovir implant. The Ganciclovir Implant Study Group. *N Engl J Med* 1997;337:83–90.

41 Department of Health and Human Services, Centers for Disease Control and Prevention. Guidelines for prevention and treatment of opportunistic infections in HIV-infected adults and adolescents. Morbidity and Mortality Weekly Report, March 24, 2009. http://www.cdc.gov/mmwr/pdf/rr/rr58e324.pdf (accessed 26 August 2009).

42 Asberg A, Humar A, Rollag H *et al.* Oral valganciclovir is noninferior to intravenous ganciclovir for the treatment of cytomegalovirus disease in solid organ transplant recipients. *Am J Transplant* 2007;7:2106–2113.

43 Strippoli GF, Hodson EM, Jones C, Craig JC. Preemptive treatment for cytomegalovirus viremia to prevent cytomegalovirus disease in solid organ transplant recipients. *Transplantation* 2006;81:139–145.

44 Doyle AM, Warburton KM, Goral S, Blumberg E, Grossman RA, Bloom RD. 24-week oral ganciclovir prophylaxis in kidney recipients is associated with reduced symptomatic cytomegalovirus disease compared to a 12-week course. *Transplantation* 2006;81:1106–1111.

45 US FDA. Valcyte (valganciclovir HCl tablets) Dear Healthcare Professional Letter, September, 2003. http://www.fda.gov/Safety/MedWatch/SafetyInformation/SafetyAlertsforHumanMedicalProducts/ucm169502.htm (accessed 26 August 2009).

46 Paya C, Humar A, Dominguez E *et al.* Efficacy and safety of valganciclovir vs. oral ganciclovir for prevention of cytomegalovirus disease in solid organ transplant recipients. *Am J Transplant* 2004;4:611–620.

47 Humar A, Lebranchu Y, Vincenti F *et al.* The efficacy and safety of 200 days valganciclovir cytomegalovirus prophylaxis in high-risk kidney transplant recipients. *Am J Transplant* 2010;10:1228–1237.

48 Humar A, Limaye AP, Blumberg EA *et al.* Extended valganciclovir prophylaxis in D+/R− kidney transplant recipients is associated with long-term reduction in cytomegalovirus disease: two-year results of the IMPACT study. *Transplantation* 2010;90:1427–1431.

49 Blumberg EA, Hauser IA, Stanisic S *et al.* Prolonged prophylaxis with valganciclovir is cost effective in reducing posttransplant cytomegalovirus disease within the United States. *Transplantation* 2010;90:1420–1426.

50 Chou S, Marousek G, Boivin G *et al.* Recombinant phenotyping of cytomegalovirus sequence variants detected after 200 or 100 days of valganciclovir prophylaxis. *Transplantation* 2010;90:1409–1413.

51 Chamberlain CE, Penzak SR, Alfaro RM *et al.* Pharmacokinetics of low and maintenance dose valganciclovir in kidney transplant recipients. *Am J Transplant* 2008;8:1297–1302.

52 Gabardi S, Magee CC, Baroletti SA *et al.* Efficacy and safety of low-dose valganciclovir for prevention of cytomegalovirus disease in renal transplant recipients: a single-center, retrospective analysis. *Pharmacotherapy* 2004;24:1323–1330.

53 Park JM, Lake KD, Arenas JD, Fontana RJ. Efficacy and safety of low-dose valganciclovir in the prevention of cytomegalovirus disease in adult liver transplant recipients. *Liver Transpl* 2006;12:112–116.

54 Weng FL, Patel AM, Wanchoo R *et al.* Oral ganciclovir versus low-dose valganciclovir for prevention of cytomegalovirus disease in recipients of kidney and pancreas transplants. *Transplantation* 2007;83:290–296.

55 Kalil AC, Mindru C, Florescu DF. Effectiveness of valganciclovir 900 mg versus 450 mg for cytomegalovirus prophylaxis in transplantation: direct and indirect treatment comparison meta-analysis. *Clin Infect Dis* 2011;52:313–321.

56 Gane E, Saliba F, Valdecasas GJ *et al.* Randomised trial of efficacy and safety of oral ganciclovir in the prevention of cytomegalovirus disease in liver-transplant recipients. The Oral Ganciclovir International Transplantation Study Group [corrected]. *Lancet* 1997;350:1729–1733.

57 Winston DJ, Busuttil RW. Randomized controlled trial of oral ganciclovir versus oral acyclovir after induction with intravenous ganciclovir for long-term prophylaxis of cytomegalovirus disease in cytomegalovirus-seropositive liver transplant recipients. *Transplantation* 2003;75:229–233.

58 Hardy WD. Combined ganciclovir and recombinant human granulocyte-macrophage colony-stimulating factor in the treatment of cytomegalovirus retinitis in AIDS patients. *J Acquir Immune Defic Syndr* 1991;4(Suppl 1):S22–S28.

59 Health Resources and Services Administration. OPTN/SRTR Annual Report, Table 1.9a Immunosuppression use by organ in 2007 and 2008. http://www.ustransplant.org/annual_reports/current/109a_dh.htm (accessed 10 September 2011).

60 http://berlex.bayerhealthcare.com/html/products/pi/Campath_PI.pdf.

61 Brennan DC, Flavin K, Lowell JA *et al.* A randomized, double-blinded comparison of Thymoglobulin versus Atgam for induction immunosuppressive therapy in adult renal transplant recipients. *Transplantation* 1999;67:1011–1018.

62 Genzyme. Thymoglobulin® [Anti-thymocyte Globulin (Rabbit)]; 2008. http://www.thymoglobulin.com/home/thymo_pdf_pi.pdf.

63 Novartis. Myfortic®; 2009. http://www.pharma.us. novartis.com/product/pi/pdf/myfortic.pdf.

64 Genentech, Inc. CellCept®; 2010. http://www.gene. com/gene/products/information/cellcept/pdf/pi.pdf.

65 US FDA. Bactrim™. http://www.accessdata.fda.gov/ drugsatfda_docs/label/2010/017377s067lbl.pdf (accessed 14 September 2011).

66 Mocarski ES, Jr. Immunomodulation by cytomegaloviruses: manipulative strategies beyond evasion. *Trends Microbiol* 2002;10:332–339.

67 Barton TL, Roush MK, Dever LL. Seizures associated with ganciclovir therapy. *Pharmacotherapy* 1992;12:413–415.

68 Scott JC, Partovi N, Ensom MH. Ganciclovir in solid organ transplant recipients: is there a role for clinical pharmacokinetic monitoring? *Ther Drug Monit* 2004;26:68–77.

69 Gilbert C, Boivin G. Human cytomegalovirus resistance to antiviral drugs. *Antimicrob Agents Chemother* 2005;49:873–883.

70 Sullivan V, Biron KK, Talarico C *et al*. A point mutation in the human cytomegalovirus DNA polymerase gene confers resistance to ganciclovir and phosphonylmethoxyalkyl derivatives. *Antimicrob Agents Chemother* 1993;37:19–25.

71 Limaye AP, Corey L, Koelle DM *et al*. Emergence of ganciclovir-resistant cytomegalovirus disease among recipients of solid-organ transplants. *Lancet* 2000;356: 645–649.

CHAPTER 22

Transplantation Immunotherapy with Antithymocyte Globulin (ATG)

John L. Dzuris[1], Christian Bloy[2], Melanie Ruzek[1], and John M. Williams[1]

[1]Genzyme Corporation, Framingham, MA, USA

[2]Genzyme Corporation, Lyon, France

Introduction

In the field of transplantation, reality has long been preceded by art and legend. Thanks to Donatello's chisel and Huguet's brush, the miraculous leg grafts attributed to St. Anthony, St. Cosmas, and St. Damian have fed the imagination of generations.

As early as 1906, in Lyon, Jaboulay attempted to graft goat and pig kidneys into two uremic women. The modern era of renal allotransplantation in humans dates back approximately 50 years, and the initial progress resulted from the work of two teams in particular: Hamburger's in Paris and Merill's in Boston. The use, first, of irradiation techniques, and later of immunosuppressive chemotherapy, enabled these two teams to achieve the first successful renal transplantations from non-monozygotic twins in 1959, then from non-twin related donors in 1962, and finally from cadaveric donors in 1963. During this period, other renal transplantation centers grew throughout the world, and in particular in Lyon, France.

All the results pointed to the necessity of improving the selection of donors as well as the treatment of recipients to prevent rejection. This treatment was, and still remains, based on the establishment of nonspecific and protracted immunosuppression. The first antilymphocyte sera were prepared by Metchnikoff in 1899. During the following decades, several authors reported the immunological changes induced by these sera. Since

that time, although a large number of experimental and clinical observations have ensued, this biological agent has not yet disclosed all its secrets.

Polyclonal antithymocyte globulin (ATG) or antilymphocyte globulin (ALG) reagents can be distinguished from each other by the cells used for the immunization and the animal species from which they are produced. The potency of these preparations is typically enhanced through purification of the gamma immunoglobulin fraction of whole sera of the immunized animal. Clinically significant preparations include rabbit ATG (Thymoglobulin®, Genzyme), horse ATG (Lymphoglobulin®, Genzyme; ATGAM, Pharmacia Upjohn), and rabbit anti-Jurkat T cell line globulin (Fresenius ATG, Fresenius-Biotech). These antibodies are often lumped together under the term ATG in the medical and scientific literature, but while these agents share common functional properties upon administration to patients, including lymphocyte depletion, it should be appreciated that these preparations have distinct characteristics given their origin from different host species and unique immunization protocols. Thymoglobulin may be the most widely studied ATG, and appears the basis for the majority of mechanistic data in the field of polyclonal ATG. Therefore, many of the data presented in this chapter and most discussion of the ATG mechanism of action in this chapter are based on Thymoglobulin.

Thymoglobulin is a purified, pasteurized, gamma immunoglobulin, obtained by immunization of

---

Immunotherapy in Transplantation: Principles and Practice, First Edition. Edited by Bruce Kaplan, Gilbert J. Burckart and Fadi G. Lakkis.
© 2012 Blackwell Publishing Ltd. Published 2012 by Blackwell Publishing Ltd.

rabbits with human thymocytes. The thymocyte cell preparation contains all cellular components of the thymus, including in large majority T cells, with a low quantity of B cells [1, 2]. The resulting polyclonal antibody is an immunosuppressive drug that contains cytotoxic antibodies directed against a broad array of surface antigens expressed on the collective cellular antigen used in its generation.

In most international markets, Thymoglobulin is indicated for the prevention and treatment of solid organ transplant rejection, prevention and treatment of graft-versus-host disease following hematopoietic cell transplantation, and treatment of aplastic anemia. Thymoglobulin, which was first available in Europe in 1984 and later in the USA (1999), has been employed to treat over 100 000 patients

The extensive clinical experience with Thymoglobulin suggests that, in addition to providing benefit in solid organ transplantation [3–6], it may also offer potential in other indications, including autoimmune diseases such as type I diabetes [7]. It is clear that a more complete understanding of the mechanism of action of the drug will facilitate optimization of its use in solid organ transplantation, as well as exploration of the full potential value of the drug in additional disease states.

Mechanism of action

The accepted mechanism by which ATGs, including Thymoglobulin, achieve their immunosuppressive profile is lymphocyte depletion. When used as a short course of treatment for induction therapy in kidney transplantation, peripheral blood lymphocyte depletion with Thymoglobulin can be observed at the typical dose of 1.0 mg/(kg day), but is significantly prolonged at higher dosages [8]. In cynomolgus monkeys, where Thymoglobulin-induced cell depletion can be characterized in both blood and lymphoid tissues, peripheral T cell depletion was observed in both compartments [9]. A rapid T cell depletion is achieved in the peripheral lymphoid tissues, and animals administered human equivalent doses of 1.0 mg/kg and 3.5 mg/kg of Thymoglobulin exhibited a dose-dependent cellular depletion of T cells in the spleen and lymph nodes. B cells and

NK cells were also affected, but only at the highest dose. Overall, clinical studies in renal transplantation have shown Thymoglobulin treatment consistently results in a greater degree of lymphopenia, a longer duration of lymphopenia, and a significantly increased duration of rejection-free graft survival in comparison with another ATG [3, 4].

Several possible mechanisms of ATG action leading to T cell depletion have been put forward. Opsonization with subsequent phagocytosis by macrophages and antibody-dependent cell cytotoxicity (ADCC) are both candidates for mediating lymphocyte depletion after Thymoglobulin treatment. However, the majority of cell depletion is thought to be mediated by complement-dependent lysis (CDC) and T cell activation-induced apoptosis [10]. However it is likely that the entire set of mechanisms by which Thymoglobulin generates prolonged lymphopenia, and thus improved graft survival, have not been elucidated.

Thymoglobulin-induced CDC is reported to occur predominantly in the peripheral blood compartment [11, 12]. This is thought to result as a function of the concentration of complement proteins, which is maximal in the blood. Thymoglobulin concentrations that are attained in the serum during treatment have been shown to efficiently activate human complement, resulting in CDC in clinically relevant models in vitro.

ADCC is primarily dependent on antibody density on the surface of cells rather than on antibody specificity. Thymoglobulin has a diverse number of reactive antibodies, recognizing at least 44 different cell-surface receptors on many different cells that populate the human immune system [1, 13–15]. This diverse reactivity contributes to a dense population of antibody deposited on cell surfaces. Additionally, rabbit antibodies (in contrast to equine antibodies) bind with high affinity to the human Fc receptor [16]. These two factors may be important mechanisms of action of Thymoglobulin in facilitating ADCC-dependent cell depletion.

Thymoglobulin appears to promote apoptosis of pre-activated T cells [12, 17]. In vitro, even at concentrations of 10 µg/mL (maximal plasma concentrations achieved therapeutically are 100–200 µg/mL), apoptosis of 30–40 % of mitogen-activated peripheral blood lymphocytes was achieved with Thymoglobulin treatment, whereas resting lymphocytes were spared. This pro-apoptotic activity is dependent on Fas/Fas ligand interaction and can be inhibited by an anti-Fas monoclonal antibody. The expression of Fas is induced in naive cells by Thymoglobulin, whereas Fas ligand gene and protein expression are induced in both naive and primed T cells. Furthermore, the susceptibility of Thymoglobulin-treated cells to Fas/Fas ligand apoptosis is dependent on interleukin-2 (IL-2). Apoptosis induced by Thymoglobulin can be prevented by cyclosporine and tacrolimus, both of which block IL-2 expression at a transcriptional level, and by SRL, which blocks IL-2 signaling. In vivo data in cynomolgus monkeys confirmed that T cell apoptosis is another key mechanism for the dose-dependent peripheral depletion of lymphocytes induced by Thymoglobulin in vivo [9].

Previous in vitro studies indicated that, in general, ALGs and ATGs could inhibit the proliferation of activated B cells [18]. Subsequently, the same group of investigators reported that apoptosis appeared to be the primary mechanism [19]. The observation that Thymoglobulin may have anti-B cell activity in vitro was recently confirmed by Zand et al. [1]. These investigators reported that Thymoglobulin induces complement-independent apoptosis of naive and activated B cells and plasma cells. This effect appeared to involve the caspase- and cathepsin-mediated apoptosis pathways.

While as discussed above it is clear that cell depletion is a key immunosuppressive mechanism of action for Thymoglobulin, there is a growing body of evidence suggesting that nondepletive effects of Thymoglobulin may also play a pivotal role in suppressing the immune system [10] Modulation of cell-surface molecules or the internalization of the antigen–antibody complexes after binding is one of the major nondepleting functional mechanisms of Thymoglobulin. When surface antigens are bound by Thymoglobulin, antigen is masked or is no longer expressed, and the related pathway is inhibited as long as the antibody is present. Nondepleted T cells in cynomolgus monkeys treated with Thymoglobulin were found to be coated by ATG and functionally altered. Cells

exhibited decreased expression of several membrane receptors (T cell receptor/CD3) and coreceptors (CD2, CD4, CD8), which correlated with hypo-responsiveness in a mixed leukocyte reaction [9]. The down-modulation of these surface antigens occurred not only in the peripheral circulation, but also in the lymph nodes and spleens. In vitro, Thymoglobulin induced the down-modulation of CD2, CD3, CD4, and CD8 with dose-dependent kinetics and magnitude [9].

Modulation of cell-surface adhesion proteins and chemokine receptors also plays a major role in the suppression of the immune response by Thymoglobulin. The ability of antibodies present in thymoglobulin to down-modulate cell-surface adhesion molecules and to inhibit the function of chemokine receptors may be an important factor in decreasing graft cellular infiltration during acute rejection or ischemia–reperfusion injury. Antigen reactivity within Thymoglobulin includes LFA-1, the leukocyte function-associated antigen, an inter-cellular adhesion molecule selectively expressed on lymphocytes [15, 20]. Thymoglobulin also contains antibodies to the leukocyte adhesion receptors ICAM-1, ICAM-2, and ICAM-3, three ligands of LFA-1. The cell-surface expression of LFA-1 is down-modulated in dose-dependent manner on lymphocytes, monocytes, and neutrophils after treatment with as low as 5–10 μg/mL of Thymo-globulin, substantially below the concentration of 80–200 mg/mL achieved in clinical use [11, 12, 15]. The down-modulation of LFA-1 makes it no longer available to contribute to interactions involving these adhesion molecules, such as those between leukocytes and endothelial cells. Similar decreases in cell-surface expression of integrins can be induced by Thymoglobulin. The expression of both the integrins VLA-4, the ligand for VCAM-1, and LPAM-1, the ligand for MadCAM-1, can be decreased by Thymoglobulin [15].

The contribution of decreased adhesion molecule expression induced by Thymoglobulin was demon-strated in a primate model of ischemia–reperfusion [21]. The microcirculation of Thymoglobulin-treated blood infused into the femoral artery of a cynomolgus monkey was observed through an intravital microscope and CDD camera. Blood cells treated with control saline exhibited rolling, increased cell numbers, significant sticking to blood vessel, and decreased blood flow. By comparison, treatment of blood cells with Thymoglobulin significantly prevented these events, exhibiting no clumping or agglutination and helped maintain post-transplant blood flow.

Thymoglobulin also may interfere with the chemotactic signaling process during an immune response. This may be clinically relevant, as chemokines are expressed in damaged tissues and serve to upregulate leukocyte infiltration to the target tissue. Because host immune cell infiltration into transplanted organs is an essential step in the initiation of the cellular rejection process, inhibition of chemotaxis of responder cells by Thymoglobulin-mediated chemokine blockade could contribute to graft survival. Present within Thymoglobulin are antibody reactivities to the chemokine receptors CXCR4, CCR7, and CCR5 expressed on lymphocytes and monocytes [15]. Incubation of lymphocytes with Thymoglobulin in vitro results in the down-modulation of CCR7. Additionally, chemotactic responses analyzed in vitro demonstrated that Thymoglobulin, at a plasma level of 10–25 µg/mL, which is below the maximal concentration achieved in clinical use (100–200 µg/mL), can interfere with monocyte responses to CCL5 and lymphocyte responses to CCL19 and SDF-1 [15, 22].

Binding to many different cell-surface molecules, Thymoglobulin may also interfere with the functional properties of some immune cells. Thymoglobulin was found to inhibit the maturation of immature monocyte-derived dendritic cells (DCs) and allowed the generation of DCs expressing ILT-3, CD123, and CCR6 but not CCR7, and producing indoleamine 2,3-dioxygenase mRNA, a phenotype compatible with tolerogenic DCs [23]. Reduction of solid-organ-graft rejection after Thymoglobulin pretreatment may be caused not only by the substantial in vivo T cell depletion, but also by a significant effect on DCs that are likely oriented towards a tolerogenic phenotype.

Additional evidence that thymoglobulin interferes with immune cell function is the finding that T cells and antigen-presenting cell (APC) interactions can be disrupted. A stable interaction between T cells and professional APC and full T cell stimulation requires a complex molecular rearrangement at the T cell–APC interface. This involves the interaction of adhesion and signaling receptors, and their ligands, on both cells. The microenvironment encompassing this concentration of molecules, named the immunological synapse, facilitates stable and prolonged interactions of T cells with APCs. Recent in vitro findings have shown that Thymoglobulin can inhibit relocalization of the T cell receptor/CD3 complex, adhesion molecules, and cytoskeletal proteins in a concentration- and time-dependent manner [24]. More significantly, peripheral blood T cells treated with Thymoglobulin also were incapable of forming cell–cell conjugates with APCs. The impairment of immunological synapse formation may be another mechanism that may help to understand the functional inactivation of peripheral blood T cells that have escaped depletion after Thymoglobulin treatment.

More recent findings suggest that Thymoglobulin may suppress immune responses, not by down-modulation, but by promoting the induction of immune cells that can regulate immune responses. Regulatory T cells (Tregs) are a specialized subset of T cells shown to play an important role in modulating the immune response to alloantigens and in maintaining tolerance to self [25, 26]. Tregs have been identified in patients with stable renal transplant, where they may function to maintain hyporesponsiveness to alloantigens [27]. Thymoglobulin has been demonstrated to cause significant and sustained expansion of Tregs in vitro [16, 22, 28]. The expansion of the CD4$^+$CD25$^+$Foxp3$^+$ Treg population by Thymoglobulin occurs in a dose-dependent manner. Primarily, CD4$^+$ CD25$^-$ cells were converted to functionally immunosuppressive CD4$^+$CD25$^+$ cells. Less significantly, Thymoglobulin also induced the proliferation of natural CD4$^+$CD25$^+$ T cells. Importantly, the CD4$^+$CD25^{high}Foxp3$^+$ Tregs generated by Thymoglobulin were shown to suppress a direct allo-immune response in a mixed lymphocyte reaction, but did not suppress the memory response to recall antigens [28].

Preclinical studies

Preclinical ATGs

Although several mechanisms of action of Thymoglobulin have been suggested, it is difficult to definitively determine the contribution of these mechanisms in vivo owing to inaccessibility of various immune compartments, concomitant immunosuppression applied to patients receiving Thymoglobulin, and their disease state that could compromise the evaluation. Studies in nonhuman primates with Thymoglobulin have demonstrated depletion of CD4 and CD8 T cells as well as delay of skin and heart transplant rejection [9]. However, Thymoglobulin is less efficacious in nonhuman primates and, thus, may not reflect the full range of activities of an agent generated against human thymocytes. Murine or rat counterpart reagents have also been generated and, in addition to depleting T cells in vivo similar to Thymoglobulin,

are also effective in a variety of transplant and autoimmune disease models (summarized in Table 22.1). Recently, a rabbit anti-mouse thymocyte reagent (mATG) that is prepared analogously to Thymoglobulin has been used for evaluating in vivo effects in normal mice, as well as in models of heart allograft transplantation and graft-versus-host disease (GHVD) [54–56].

In vivo effects of anti-mouse lymphocyte/thymocyte reagents in normal animals

A comprehensive evaluation of the depletive effects of mATG in normal mice showed similar dose response, kinetics of T cell depletion and recovery, and depletion of T cell subsets and other leukocytes compared with Thymoglobulin treatment in patients [55]. CD8 T cells in mice are depleted to a greater extent than CD4 T cells, and binding of mATG to all residual T cells persists up to 21 days. Detectable

Table 22.1 Animal models of transplantation or autoimmunity where anti-thymocyte/lymphocyte reagents are beneficial.[a]

Model	Species	Other agents/procedures used in combination	References
Transplant			
Renal allograft	Rat, dog, primate	Cyclosporine A + azathioprine	[29–32]
Heart allograft	Mouse, rat, dog, primate	Total lymphoid irradiation	[9, 33–36]
Pancreas allograft	Mouse		[37]
Islet allograft	Mouse, dog, pig, primate	Sirolimus, cyclosporine + azathioprine + prednisolone + 15-deoxyspergualin	[38–42]
Skin allograft	Mouse, primate		[9, 43, 44]
Bone marrow allograft	Mouse		[45]
GVHD	Mouse	Total lymphoid irradiation	[46], Genzyme data on file
Autoimmune			
Non-obese diabetic (NOD)	Mouse, rat	Granulocyte-colony stimulating factor (G-CSF)	[47–50], Genzyme data on file
Aplastic anemia	Mouse		[51]
Experimental autoimmune encephalomyelitis (EAE)	Mouse		[52]
Lupus	Mouse	TGFβ1	[53]
Collagen-induced arthritis	Mouse		Genzyme data on file
Experimental autoimmune uveitis	Mouse		Genzyme data on file

[a]Does not include xenotransplantation studies or studies utilizing donor cell infusions, although benefit of Thymoglobulin or other antilymphocytes polyclonal antibodies have been demonstrated in those systems as well.

T cell depletion is observed in all lymphoid organs down to a dose of 1 mg/kg total mATG with the exception of the thymus, where even the highest dose tested (25 mg/kg) showed no evidence of depletion. The lack of mATG depletion of thymocytes in vivo was not unexpected, as there is evidence in the literature suggesting that the thymus is not as accessible to depleting antibodies as other lymphoid organs are [57, 58]. Nonhuman primate studies with Thymoglobulin also showed a lack of depletion in the thymus and decreased binding to thymocytes in vivo [9]. The lack of thymic depletion also explains the rapid repopulation of T cells (begins within 5 days of last treatment) in both our murine studies and patients treated with Thymoglobulin [59].

NK cells, NK T cells, granulocytes, plasma cells, and plasmablasts are also depleted by mATG, but to a lesser degree and more transiently than T cell populations [55]. There was no detectable depletion of B cells or DCs by mATG even though human B cells and DCs have been shown in vitro to be depleted by Thymoglobulin [1, 2, 60, 61]. B cells are depleted in vivo by Thymoglobulin in primates [9] and there is evidence of B cell depletion in patients (M. Zand, personal communication). The lack of B cells and DC depletion in mice with mATG does highlight potential differences between mATG and Thymoglobulin. The NK cell depletion observed with mATG is consistent with the demonstration that human NK cells are bound and undergo apoptosis with Thymoglobulin in vitro [62–64] as well as in vivo depletion in nonhuman primates [9, 65], and more recently in patients following treatment with Thymoglobulin [64]. This depletion of NK cells, however, may be mediated through the rabbit IgG Fc binding to FcRIII expressed by NK cells [64, 66]. NK-T cells, on the other hand, are elevated in Thymoglobulin-treated patients [67] and in mice treated with antithymocyte serum (ATS) in conjunction with total lymphoid irradiation [68, 69]. We have not observed elevations in NK-T cells at any time following mATG administration to normal mice (Genzyme data on file), suggesting that elevations in NK-T cells may be driven by additional factors such as disease state or irradiation.

Thymoglobulin and mATG depletion of T cells also appears to be selective for different T cell subpopulations. In both human and murine systems, memory T cells increase in percentage of total T cells following Thymoglobulin or mATG/ALS treatment [55, 67, 69–73]. Increased Tregs and OX40 expressing regulatory and memory T cells are also seen following mATG or ALS treatment in mice [55, 71, 74]. Possible mechanisms for increased percentages of these populations include sparing, selective proliferation, conversion of residual naive T cells into these cell types, or selective recruitment from nondepleted organs (i.e. thymus). Sparing is supported by the observation that in vitro Thymoglobulin treatment spared human memory T cells following an 8 h culture [70], as well as that both memory and Treg populations begin to predominate within 1 day following mATG in vivo in mice [55]. However, conversion, homeostatic proliferation, or selective proliferation of the nondepleted populations also occur within 1 week following ALS or mATG administration [72, 74]. Thus, it appears that multiple mechanisms are responsible for the predominance of memory and Tregs following mATG/ALS treatment. Memory T cell percentages do increase in patients following Thymoglobulin treatment [67, 69, 73] and can persist for years [73]. However, it has not been conclusively demonstrated that there are increased percentages of Tregs in patients treated with Thymoglobulin [75, 76], but this could be due to lack of accessibility to organs where Tregs accumulate or function, such as lymphoid organs or target tissues.

Regardless of how memory and Tregs emerge following Thymoglobulin, the induction or sparing of regulatory cells would be beneficial for prevention and treatment of organ rejection and graft-versus-host disease (GVHD) given their immunosuppressive properties. Similarly, the predominance of memory T cells following ATG administration may also be beneficial under conditions of allogeneic transplantation. In murine studies, induction of GVHD with purified allogeneic memory T cells shows reduced GVHD compared with naive T cells [77], even when the donor was alloantigen primed [78], and memory CD4 T cells can mediate graft-versus-leukemia without inducing GVHD compared with naive T cells, which induce both [79]. Sparing of memory T cells may also help preserve responses to latent viruses or reinfections and, thus, may be beneficial, both for retaining responses to infections and malignancy while at the same time reducing graft rejection or GVHD.

Effects of anti-mouse lymphocyte/ thymocyte reagents in solid organ transplantation

The efficacy of Thymoglobulin for the prevention of transplant rejection has been demonstrated in clinical studies in humans. [4, 80–85]. Avenues for improving Thymoglobulin treatment regimens may be gained from preclinical studies using mATG in mouse models of transplantation. Such studies have shown that the dosing and timing of administration can significantly affect post-transplantation outcomes.

Graft survival in mice given either no treatment or various doses of mATG at different time points prior to or after graft transplantation was determined. In the absence of mATG treatment, mice rejected heterotopic heart allografts within 7–10 days after transplantation [54]. The administration of mATG (up to 25 mg/kg) on the day of transplantation and at 4 days after transplantation modestly improved graft survival. All mice treated with this dosing regimen rejected transplanted grafts within 15–20 days post-transplantation. Mice administered two injections of a range of doses of mATG within a time window of days 3 to 14 prior to transplantation displayed mATG dose-dependent graft survival rates of 30–55% at 100 days post-transplantation (25 and 30 mg/kg mATG) with no additional therapy [54]. Thus, graft survival in transplanted mice appears to be enhanced when mATG doses are provided early, prior to transplantation, suggesting that the prevention of graft rejection in human transplantation may also be improved with optimization of Thymoglobulin dosing and timing.

Effects of anti-mouse lymphocyte/ thymocyte reagents in GVHD

GVHD is a major complication following allogeneic bone marrow transplantation [86, 87]. Thymoglobulin is effective at preventing GVHD in patients [10, 88, 89] and is approved for this indication in many countries. In addition, murine GVHD studies have shown significant benefit with mATG or ATS treatment [46, 90] (Genzyme data on file).

One well-established murine system has demonstrated that treatment of recipient mice with ATS in combination with total lymphoid irradiation protects against GVHD through regulatory CD1-restricted NK-T cells [90], but can also preserve graft-versus-tumor effects [91]. It was also shown that the IL-4-producing NK-T cells induce Tregs derived from the donor that also participate in suppressing GVHD [92]. This regimen has also been translated to the clinic with matched related and matched unrelated donors using Thymoglobulin and 10 doses of TLI for conditioning followed by mycophenolate mofetil and cyclosporine for maintenance showing an incidence of acute GVHD at 5% [93]. Antitumor activity against the underlying malignancy also appears to be retained in the clinic [94].

In addition to the potential role of NK-T cells, Tregs alone have also been demonstrated to play a prominent role in murine models of GVHD, as adoptive transfer of purified or in-vitro-generated Tregs show protection against GVHD lethality in bone marrow transplant model systems [95–97]. This protection is mediated in part by inhibiting IFNγ production, activation marker expression, and blocking rapid expansion of alloreactive donor T cells after transplantation [98, 99]. Based on the observation that Thymoglobulin induces Tregs in vitro, we tested whether mATG could protect against GVHD lethality in a murine model of acute GVHD via induction of Tregs in vivo. We used a model system where C57BL/6 splenocytes were injected into BALB/c RAG-2 KO mice (lacks T and B cells) so that it is possible to evaluate the fate of the transferred T cells without dilution from developing T cells. We found that treatment with mATG down to doses of 1 mg/kg given twice, 3 days apart, protected mice against acute GVHD after allogeneic cell transfer. Mice treated with mATG showed minimal signs of weight loss for at least 12 weeks following allogeneic cell transfer compared with rapid and progressive weight loss in the IgG-treated mice, as well as reduced splenomegaly, serum pro-inflammatory cytokines, and hepatic pathology. Percentages and numbers of

Tregs in the spleen were increased in the mATG-treated mice and became greater with time. Delayed treatment with mATG in this model also showed benefits with respect to lethality and weight change (Genzyme, data on file).

Because efficacy of mATG in our GVHD model was also coincident with T cell depletion, we attempted to separate T cell depletion from the induction of T regulatory cells and evaluated whether in vitro mATG-generated T regulatory cells could suppress GVHD upon adoptive transfer. We first determined that treatment of mouse splenocytes in combination with exogenous IL-2 with mATG generated functionally suppressive cells in vitro. Adoptive transfer of these cells 1 day prior to the induction of GVHD significantly protected against lethality and weight change, as well as inhibited the expansion of CD8 T cells [56]. Other murine studies have shown that depletion of regulatory cells under conditions of chronic GVHD converts disease to the acute form that is coincident with expansion of CD8[+] cells [100]. These results are consistent with ours and suggest that regulatory cells, including those generated by mATG, may be particularly effective at suppressing CD8 T cell responses. Studies to date in patients, however, have been conflicting with respect to the potential role of regulatory cells in GVHD [101–105].

Collectively, these preclinical studies with murine anti-thymocyte/lymphocyte polyclonal antibodies further our understanding of Thymoglobulin's activities that go beyond T cell depletion, but also highlight the complexity of this effective drug.

Effects in humans

Owing to its use for more 25 years, the clinical experience that follows is a synopsis of the results of more than 125 selected studies published in the literature.

Pharmacokinetics

In the first published study of pharmacokinetics in a single center, blood samples were obtained from 20 kidney transplant recipients who received 1.25 mg/(kg day) of Thymoglobulin for 10 days [29]. These samples' analysis included the measurement of circulating rabbit IgG and antibody to rabbit IgG. In the first 24 h, the half-life was determined to be 44.2 h. After 10 days, the terminal half-life was 13.8 days. The terminal half-life was found to be highly variable, as the elimination is dependent on individual patients' elimination of the foreign protein.

More recently, Regan et al. [106] have evaluated the mean dose of Thymoglobulin in both total rabbit IgG (total Thymoglobulin) and active Thymoglobulin fraction (those rabbit IgGs available for binding to lymphocytes). The active fraction of Thymoglobulin revealed that 7 % of the rabbit IgG is specific for human peripheral blood lymphocytes and 93 % are nonspecific rabbit IgG. The average maximal total Thymoglobulin level ranged from 171 µg/mL for patients receiving 14 doses (1.5 mg/kg per dose) to 66 µg/mL for patients receiving six doses (1.5 mg/kg perdose). A gradual decline in Thymoglobulin was observed following discontinuation of treatment. Although the active Thymoglobulin concentration profiles had a similar general appearance as the total Thymoglobulin concentration profiles, there are some distinct differences. Active fraction of Thymoglobulin disappeared much more rapidly than total Thymoglobulin, with only 12 % of patients demonstrating detectable active Thymoglobulin by day 90 compared with 81 % of patients with detectable total Thymoglobulin at this same time [106]. Sufficient time points were not available in this study to assess the half-life of Thymoglobulin, but the authors estimated a bimodal disappearance of total Thymoglobulin with the initial half-life of 10 days and a final terminal half-life of 30 days. For active Thymoglobulin, the initial half-life was about 10 days, but it was virtually nondetectable after completion of the first phase. Similar results comparing the relationship between active and total Thymoglobulin were obtained by Lowsky et al. [107] in a study of Thymoglobulin in patients receiving hematopoietic stem cell transplantation (v). However, it is difficult to compare the pharmacokinetics of total and active fractions of Thymoglobulin across doses and conditioning regimens since the pharmacokinetics of active Thymoglobulin vary depending on the number of lymphocytes available for Thymoglobulin to bind to. For example, in myeloablative conditioning, or if given "late" in relation to the conditioning regimen for other indications, there may be very few T cells for Thymoglobulin to bind to. This will affect Thymoglobulin elimination and pharmacokinetics. Therefore, the pharmacokinetic profile of Thymoglobulin may be different across different therapeutic uses [106–109].

Apart from duration and dosage, the timing of Thymoglobulin administration, linked with the transplant methodology, may be critical for the efficacy profile. However, monitoring of Thymoglobulin effect has frequently been based on the total fraction of rabbit IgG dosage, and peripheral blood T lymphocyte count, with an objective to maintain CD3 T cell counts below 20/mm^3. The active fraction of Thymoglobulin rather than the total rabbit IgG should probably be measured, in order to lead to a better understanding of the pharmacokinetics and pharmacodynamics of the product.

Pharmacodynamics

Thymoglobulin is a selective immunosuppressive agent (acting on T lymphocytes), but the mechanism of action of Thymoglobulin is probably not yet fully understood. The immune system effects include T cell depletion in blood and lymphoid tissues [3, 4, 110], modulation of leucocytes and endothelial cell interaction [11, 15, 20], induction of apoptosis [10] and induction of DCs [10] and Tregs [28]. Therefore, a multi-action immunosuppression is provided by Thymoglobulin, with probably an important link to the dose ranging.

Clinical efficacy

Since it was first registered in France in 1984, a great deal of information has become available in the published literature on the efficacy of Thymoglobulin for various indications. The clinical use of Thymoglobulin in various types of clinical setting, including the prevention and treatment of rejection in solid organ transplantation, prevention and treatment of GVHD in HSCT, and treatment of aplastic anemia and myelodysplastic syndrome (MDS) is supported by several Phase II and III studies and by published literature.

Solid organ transplantation

The safety and efficacy of Thymoglobulin as either induction therapy or treatment of rejection in solid organ transplantation has been extensively reported in the literature. Among the various types of organ transplant, the most extensively studied is Thymoglobulin as induction therapy and rejection treatment in renal transplantation . In adult renal transplant recipients, Thymoglobulin induction resulted in higher patient and graft survival when considering graft loss from all causes and in lower acute rejection rates at 1 and 5 years post-transplant compared with equine-ATG-treated patients. Thymoglobulin-treated patients also had a lower incidence of CMV infections, fewer serious adverse events, but more frequent early leukopenia than equine-ATG-treated patients [4, 5]. When compared with basiliximab for induction in cadaveric renal transplant recipients, Thymoglobulin induction was associated with a lower incidence of acute allograft rejection, graft loss, and death at 6 and 12 months. The safety results were similar for the two treatments, although there were more infections (other than CMV) in the Thymoglobulin group, while CMV infections were more frequent and more severe in the basiliximab group. In pediatric renal transplant recipients, 93 % of patients who received a full course (2 mg/(kg day) for 5 days) of Thymoglobulin as induction therapy survived through 12 months post-transplant [6].

For rejection treatment in renal transplantation, Thymoglobulin was shown to be at least as effective as equine ATG in reversing acute rejection episodes in adults [3]. Toxicities were generally not dose limiting, and the benefits of antirejection therapy outweigh the negative aspects of adverse events and toxicities. When compared with Muromonab-CD3 (OKT3), treatment of steroid-resistant acute rejection in renal transplant recipients with Thymoglobulin was associated with lower re-rejection rates.

For induction therapy in adult liver transplantation patients, reports in the literature show acute rejection rates to be lower for Thymoglobulin induction than for no antibody induction therapy and graft survival to be similar for both. The acute rejection rates ranged from 6 % to 28 % and graft survival rates ranged from 74 % to 100 % for Thymoglobulin.

In pancreas transplantation (including simultaneous pancreas–kidney transplant, pancreas after kidney transplant, and pancreas transplant alone), Thymoglobulin induction was associated with kidney graft survival rates of 92–100 %, pancreas graft survival rates of 60–100 %, and rejection rates (acute rejection or re-rejection) of 2–80%.

For induction therapy in heart transplantation, Thymoglobulin induction was associated with acute rejection rates ranging from 25 % to 85 % over follow-up periods of 4 months to 5 years, compared with acute rejection rates ranging from 20 % to 92 % for ATG-Fresenius and 69 % for OKT3.

In a prospective, randomized, clinical trial conducted by Hartwig *et al.* [111], 74 lung transplant recipients were randomly assigned to receive either Thymoglobulin or conventional immunosuppression alone (control). Primary immunosuppression following lung transplantation included steroids combined with cyclosporine A (CsA). Overall, there was no difference in graft survival between the Thymoglobulin and control groups at 8 years post-transplant (36 % versus 23 %; $p=0.48$). The Thymoglobulin group had fewer early rejections than the control group did (5 % versus 41 %; $p=0.01$); however, the overall rejection incidence did not differ between the groups (62 % versus 68 %; $p=0.52$).

Vianna *et al.* [112] conducted a retrospective review of 27 adult patients who underwent 29 intestinal transplants (isolated intestinal transplantation, $n=7$; modified multivisceral transplantation, $n=3$; and multivisceral transplantation, $n=19$). All transplant recipients received induction therapy using Thymoglobulin (10 mg/kg total dose) and rituximab (150 mg/m² single dose). Primary immunosuppression following transplantation included steroids and tacrolimus. The 1 year patient and graft survival rate were 81 % and 76 % respectively. Thirteen (48 %) patients experienced 19 episodes of acute rejection. Patients with a multivisceral graft experienced fewer episodes of severe acute rejection (1/19, 5 %) when compared with isolated intestinal transplants and modified multivisceral transplants (7/10, 70 %).

Hematologic indications

The safety and efficacy of Thymoglobulin in the prevention and treatment of GVHD and in the treatment of aplastic anemia and MDS have been studied.

The dosages and times of administration of Thymoglobulin in the prevention of GVHD in HSCT vary widely in the literature. In published reports on the prevention of GVHD with various donor sources and follow-up periods ranging from 5 months to 4.5 years, the rates of acute GVHD (aGVHD; II–IV or III–IV) range from 0 % to 51 % for patients treated with Thymoglobulin compared with 28–63 % in patients who did not receive Thymoglobulin. For the treatment of GVHD, Thymoglobulin was associated with a complete response rate of 38 % in patients with steroid-resistant aGVHD. In patients with moderate to severe GVHD, observed response rates were as high as 80 % with early Thymoglobulin treatment and as low as 38 % with late Thymoglobulin treatment.

In a study by Di Bona *et al.* [113], 77 % of patients with severe aplastic anemia who had not responded to a first course of therapy with either ATG or ALG became transfusion independent after a second course of therapy with Thymoglobulin and G-CSF. In this study, approximately 30 % of patients who were unresponsive to the first course of immunosuppressive therapy achieved either complete or partial remission after a second course with Thymoglobulin and G-CSF [113]. A separate retrospective study reported response rates of 27 % following retreatment with Thymoglobulin in patients who were refractory to antilymphocyte/CsA-based regimens and response rates of 66 % for patients who relapsed after antilymphocyte/CsA-based regimens [114].

In MDS, 15 % of Thymoglobulin-treated patients but none of the control (standard therapy) patients reached the primary endpoint (transfusion and growth-factor independence for at least eight consecutive weeks) at 6 months. However, the incidence of adverse events and infection was higher with Thymoglobulin treatment. A prospective study evaluated the safety and efficacy of either equine ATG or Thymoglobulin in patients with MDS with short duration of refractory anemia. For Thymoglobulin, the complete response (CR) rate was 20% and the good response (GR) rate was 7%. For equine ATG, the CR rate was 5% and the GR rate was 25%. All patients with CR or GR were patients with refractory anemia, and none of the patients reaching CR or GR had disease progression. Safety and survival were comparable in both arms [115].

Safety in humans

Both induction and treatment with Thymoglobulin in graft rejection and GVHD are generally well tolerated. The tolerability profile of Thymoglobulin is generally similar to other immunosuppressive treatments. The most common selected adverse events reported are fever, chills, gastrointestinal disorder, leukopenia, thrombocytopenia, cutaneous rash, and serum sickness. Nevertheless, the immunosuppression also increases the risk of infection, including unusual viral and fungal infection. Viral infections, such as reactivation of cytomegalovirus, herpes simplex, adenovirus and Epstein–Barr virus, occur more frequently. But, the overall incidence of infection associated with Thymoglobulin induction is generally no different from that seen with the different ATG or basiliximab induction.

From the data accumulated through clinical investigations and literature, it can be concluded that the risk/benefit profile of Thymoglobulin is favorable overall and that the therapeutic advantages provided by this therapy outweigh the potential risks associated with this therapy.

Discussion and perspectives

ATGs represent an interesting case study: a single drug that can be considered to deliver a combination therapy. This results from the polyclonal/polyepitope reactive nature of ATG, with antibody specificities that bind and interfere with the function of multiple cell-surface determinants and receptors on key component cells of the immune system (Plate 22.1). These multiple antibody reactivities deliver a set of negative "hits" that collectively serve to down-modulate the immune effector arm. As discussed in this chapter, the functional repertoire of the ATG

Thymoglobulin has been extensively studied; yet, owing to the complex mix of reactivities that it contains, the complete mechanism of action has not been resolved. Not only does the antibody react to over 40 cell-surface determinants and receptors, the functional result of these reactivities is dependent on the concentration of antibody available at any given time. For example, at the time of Thymoglobulin administration, plasma levels of the drug have been reported to reach 100–200 µg/mL [29, 106]. A significant function at that concentration is cytotoxicity led by CDC, while shortly later, when the plasma level of Thymoglobulin has declined to ~10 µg/mL, the function shifts away from CDC, revealing inhibition of chemotaxis and cell--cell interactions [9–12]. All of these functions are immunosuppressive, however, and appear to result from different mechanisms that are in turn driven by the various specific reactivities contained within Thymoglobulin. The cast of immunosuppressive functions mediated by Thymoglobulin includes cytotoxicity (CDC, ADCC, and activation-induced cellular apoptosis). Modulation or merely "coating" of key cell-surface receptors has been shown to block costimulation, antigen recognition, cytokine, and chemokine signals which in turn results in decreased effector cell activation, clonal expansion, chemotaxis, and cell trafficking into target tissues. In addition, reactivities in Thymoglobulin have been shown to directly inhibit delivery of effector signals to target cells (e.g., inhibition of cytotoxicity mediated by CD8 cells, etc.). Finally, the recent finding that ATG can generate Tregs suggests yet another way in which the drug is able to down-modulate immune responses via favoring a mechanism of natural immunoregulation. The variety of mechanisms for immune modulation by Thymoglobulin, including the induction of Tregs, suggests additional applications to autoimmune disease. Extrapolation of the positive effects of Thymoglobulin seen in solid organ transplantation to autoimmune disease has recently involved new-onset diabetes [7]. Briefly, diabetes patients were enrolled in a protocol combining G-CSF mobilized autologous stem cell transplant (HSCT) with Thymoglobulin and cyclophosphamide conditioning. The study is ongoing, but was reported to result in disease reversal and insulin independence for up to

3 years [7]. To our knowledge, this represents the only published demonstration of reversal of diabetes and regaining insulin independence. In a parallel preclinical study, synergism of mATG and G-CSF was demonstrated and resulted in enhanced diabetes reversal in NOD mice [47]. Taken together, the preliminary positive results obtained with mATG and Thymoglobulin preclinically and clinically suggest that the multiple immunomodulatory mechanisms imparted by the polyclonal ATG could serve as proof of concept for new indications that could benefit from the existing drug, as well as allowing use of the multifunctional ATG as a prototype to identify important immunomodulatory mechanisms. Dissection of these distinct antibody reactivities within the polyclonal antibody could then elucidate key targets that could be the focus for new therapeutics that would ultimately offer the ability to tailor chosen aspects of the inflammatory/immune response.

References

1 Zand MS, Vo T, Huggins J et al. Polyclonal rabbit antithymocyte globulin triggers B cell and plasma cell apoptosis by multiple pathways. *Transplantation* 2005;79: 1507–1515.

2 Zand MS, Vo T, Pellegrin T et al. Apoptosis and complement-mediated lysis of myeloma cells by polyclonal rabbit antithymocyte globulin. *Blood* 2006;107: 2895–2903.

3 Gaber AO, First MR, Tesi RJ et al. Results of the double-blind, randomized, multicenter, Phase III clinical trial of Thymoglobulin versus Atgam in the treatment of acute graft rejection episodes after renal transplantation. *Transplantation* 1998;66:29–37.

4 Brennan DC, Flavin K, Lowell A et al. A randomized, double-blinded comparison of Thymoglobulin versus Atgam for induction immunosuppressive therapy in adult renal transplant recipients. *Transplantation* 1999;67:1011–1018.

5 Hardinger KL, Schnitzler MA, Miller B et al. Five-year follow up of thymoglobulin versus ATGAM induction in adult renal transplantation. *Transplantation* 2004;78: 136–141.

6 Brophy PD, Thomas SE, McBryde KD, Bunchman TE. Comparison of polyclonal induction agents in pediatric renal transplantation. *Pediatr Transplant* 2001;5: 174–178.

7 Voltarelli JC, Couri CEB, Straciori ABPI et al. Autologous nonmyeloablative hematopoietic stem cell transplantation in newly diagnosed type I diabetes mellitus. *JAMA* 2007;297:1568–1576.

8 Wong W, Agrawal N, Pascual M et al. Comparison of two dosages of Thymoglobulin used as a short-course for induction in kidney transplantation. *Transpl Int* 2006;19:629–635.

9 Preville X, Flacher M, LeMauff B et al. Mechanism involved in antithymocyte globulin immunosuppressive activity in a nonhuman primate model. *Transplantation* 2001;71:460–468.

10 Mohty M. Mechanisms of action of antithymocyte globulin: T-cell depletion and beyond. *Leukemia* 2007;21:1387–1394.

11 Bonnefoy-Berard N, Revillard JP. Mechanisms of immunosuppression induced by antithymocyte globulins and OKT3. *J Heart Lung Transplant* 1996;15: 435–442.

12 Genestier L, Fournel S, Flacher M. Induction of Fas [Apo-1, CD95]-mediated apoptosis of activated lymphocytes by polyclonal antithymocyte globulins. *Blood* 1998;91:2360–2368.

13 Mueller F. Thymoglobulin: an immunologic review. *Curr Opin Organ Transpl* 2003;8:305–312.

14 Monti P, Allavena P, Di Carlo V et al. Effects of antilymphocytes and anti-thymocytes globulin on human dendritic cells. *Int Immunopharmacol* 2003;3:189–196.

15 Michallet MC, Preville X, Flacher M et al. Functional antibodies to leukocyte adhesion molecules in antithymocyte globulins. *Transplantation* 2003;75:657–662.

16 Feng X, Kajigaya S, Solomou EE et al. Rabbit ATG but not horse ATG promotes expansion of functional CD4+CD25highFOXP3+ regulatory T cells in vitro. *Blood* 2008;111:3675–3683.

17 Michallet MC, Saltel F, Preville X. Cathepsin-B-dependent apoptosis triggered by antithymocyte globulins: a novel mechanism of T-cell depletion. *Blood* 2003;102:3719–3726.

18 Bonnefoy-Berard, N, Flacher M, Revillard JP et al. Antiproliferative effect of antilymphocyte globulins on B cells and B-cell lines. *Blood* 1992;79:2164–2170.

19 Bonnefoy-Berard N, Genestier L, Flacher M. Apoptosis induced by polyclonal antilymphocyte globulins in human B-cell lines. *Blood* 1994;583:1051–1059.

20 Bonnefoy-Berard N, Vincent C, Revillard JP. Antibodies against functional leukocyte surface molecules in polyclonal antilymphocyte and antithymocyte globulins. *Transplantation* 1991;51:669–673.

21 Chappell D, Beiras-Fernandez A, Hammer C et al. In vivo visualization of the effect of polyclonal

antithymocyte globulins on the microcirculation after ischemia/reperfusion in a primate model. *Transplantation* 2006;81:552–558.

22 LaCorcia G, Swistak M, Lawendowski C *et al.* Polyclonal rabbit antithymocyte globulin exhibits consistent immunosuppressive capabilities beyond cell depletion *Transplantation* 2009;87:966–974.

23 Gillet-Hladky S, de Carvalho CM, Bernaud J *et al.* Rabbit antithymocyte globulin inhibits monocyte derived dendritic cells maturation in vitro and polarizes monocyte-derived dendritic cells towards tolerogenic dendritic cells expressing indoleamine 2,3-dioxygenase. *Transplantation* 2006;82:965–974.

24 Haidinger M, Geyeregger R, Poglitsch M *et al.* Antithymocyte globulin impairs T-cell/antigen-presenting cell interaction: disruption of immunological synapse and conjugate formation. *Transplantation* 2007;84:117–121.

25 Wood KJ, Sakaguchi S. Regulatory T cells in transplantation tolerance. *Nat Rev Immunol* 2003;3:199–210.

26 Sakaguchi S, Sakaguchi N. Regulatory T cells in immunologic self-tolerance and autoimmune disease. *Int Rev Immunol* 2005;24:211–226.

27 Salama AD, Najafian N, Clarkson MR *et al.* Regulatory CD25+ T cells in human kidney transplant recipients. *J Am Soc Nephrol* 2003;14:1643–1651.

28 Lopez M, Clarkson MR, Albin M *et al.* A novel mechanism of action for anti-thymocyte globulin: induction of CD4+CD25+Foxp3+ regulatory T cells. *J Am Soc Nephrol* 2006;17:2844–2853.

29 Guttmann RD, Caudrelier P, Alberici G, Touraine J-L. Pharmacokinetics, foreign protein immune response, cytokine release, and lymphocyte subsets in patients receiving thymoglobulin and immunosuppression. *Transplant Proc* 1997;29:24 S–26 S.

30 Mathews KA, Holmberg DL, Miller CW. Kidney transplantation in dogs with naturally occurring end-stage renal disease. *J Am Anim Hosp Assoc* 2000;36:294–301.

31 Block T, Jarck HU, Hammer C *et al.* Analysis of in situ inflammation of allogeneic canine kidney grafts under antilymphocyte globulin treatment. *Eur Surg Res* 1984;16:340–347.

32 Biesecker JL, Fitch FW, Rowley DA *et al.* Cellular and humoral immunity after allogeneic transplantation in the rat. IV. The effect of heterologous antilymphocyte serum on cellular and humoral immunity after allogeneic renal transplantation. *Transplantation* 1973;16:441–450.

33 Mjörnstedt L, Olausson M, Hedman L *et al.* Induction of long-term heart allograft survival in the rat by rabbit ATG. *Int Arch Allergy Appl Immunol* 1984;74:193–199.

34 Strober S, Modry DL, Hoppe RT *et al.* Induction of specific unresponsiveness to heart allografts in mongrel dogs treated with total lymphoid irradiation and antithymocyte globulin. *J Immunol* 1984;132:1013–1018.

35 Judd KP, Allen CR, Jr, Guiberteau MJ *et al.* Prolongation of murine cardiac allografts with antilymphocyte serum. *Transplant Proc* 1969;1:470–473.

36 Ono K, Lindsey ES, DeWitt CW *et al.* Prolongation of rat heart allograft function with heterologous antilymphocyte serum. *Circulation* 1969;39:I27–I29.

37 Purcell LJ, Mottram PL, Mandel TE. Immunosuppressive antibody treatment prolongs graft survival in two murine models of segmental pancreas transplantation. *Immunol Cell Biol* 1993;71:349–352.

38 Hirshberg B, Preston EH, Xu H *et al.* Rabbit antithymocyte globulin induction and sirolimus monotherapy supports prolonged islet allograft function in a nonhuman primate islet transplantation model. *Transplantation* 2003;76:55–60.

39 Mellert J, Hering BJ, Liu X *et al.* Successful islet auto- and allotransplantation in diabetic pigs. *Transplantation* 1998;66:200–204.

40 Falqui L, Finke EH, Cael JC. Marked prolongation of human islet xenograft survival [human-to-mouse] by low-temperature culture and temporary immunosuppression with human and mouse anti-lymphocyte sera. *Transplantation* 1991;51:1322–1324.

41 Kaufman DB, Morel P, Field MJ *et al.* Extended survival of purified canine islet allografts with heterologous antilymphocyte globulin. *Transplant Proc* 1991;23:761–763.

42 Gotoh M, Porter J, Monaco AP, Maki T. Induction of antigen-specific unresponsiveness to pancreatic islet allografts by antilymphocyte serum. *Transplantation* 1988;45:429–433.

43 Kobayashi K, Hricko GM, Reisner GS *et al.* The monkey skin graft model as an assay of human antilymphocyte globulin. *Transplantation* 1972;14:698–704.

44 Sharma K, Grone M, Sampson D *et al.* Immunosuppressive effects of antimacrophage serum and antithymocyte serum on mouse skin allografts. *J Med* 1972;3:199–211.

45 Riches AC, Thomas DB. The effects of antilymphocyte sera on bone marrow allograft rejection. *Exp Hematol* 1975;3:169–180.

46 Lan F, Zeng D, Higuchi M, Huie P. Predominance of NK1.1+TCRab+ or DX5+TCRab+ T cells in mice conditioned with fractionated lymphoid irradiation protects against graft-versus-host disease: "natural suppressor" cells. *J Immunol* 2001;167:2087–2096.

47 Parker MJ, Xue S, Alexander JJ et al. Immune depletion with cellular mobilization imparts immunoregulation and reverses autoimmune diabetes in NOD mice. *Diabetes* 2009; 58(10):2277–2284.

48 Simon G, Parker M, Ramiya V et al. Murine antithymocyte globulin therapy alters disease progression in NOD mice by a time-dependent induction of immunoregulation. *Diabetes* 2008;57:405–414.

49 Ogawa N, Minamimura K, Kodaka T et al. Short administration of polyclonal anti-T cell antibody [ALS] in NOD mice with extensive insulitis prevents subsequent development of autoimmune diabetes. *J Autoimmun* 2006;26:225–231.

50 Maki T, Ichikawa T, Blanco R et al. Long-term abrogation of autoimmune diabetes in nonobese diabetic mice by immunotherapy with anti-lymphocyte serum. *Proc Natl Acad Sci U S A* 1992;89:3434–3438.

51 Bloom ML, Wolk AG, Simon-Stoos KL et al. A mouse model of lymphocyte infusion-induced bone marrow failure. *Exp Hematol* 2004;32(12):1163–1172.

52 Chung DT, Korn T, Richard J et al. Anti-thymocyte globulin (ATG) prevents autoimmune encephalomyelitis by expanding myelin antigen-specific Foxp3+ regulatory T cells. *Int Immunol* 2007;19:1003–1010.

53 Kaplan J, Woodworth L, Smith K et al. Therapeutic benefit of treatment with anti-thymocyte globulin and latent TGF-β1 in the MRL/lpr lupus mouse model. *Lupus* 2008;17:822–831.

54 Ruzek M, Dzuris JL, Gao L et al. Selected mechanistic studies and future directions for Thymoglobulin. *Transplantation* 2007;84(11 Suppl):S27–S34.

55 Ruzek MC, Neff KS, Luong M. (2009) In vivo characterization of rabbit anti-mouse thymocyte globulin: a surrogate for rabbit anti-human thymocyte globulin. *Transplantation* 88: 170–179.

56 Ruzek MC, Waire JS, Hopkins D et al. Characterization of in vitro antimurine thymocyte globulin-induced regulatory T cells that inhibit graft-versus-host disease in vivo. *Blood* 2008;111:1726–1734.

57 Ghobrial RRM, Boublik M, Winn HJ et al. In vivo use of monoclonal antibodies against murine T cell antigens. *Clin Immunol Immunopathol* 1989;52:486–506.

58 Le Gros GS, Prestidge RL, Watson JD. In vivo modulation of thymus-derived lymphocytes with monoclonal antibodies in mice. I. Effect of anti-Thy-1 antibody on the tissue distribution of lymphocytes. *Immunology* 1983;50:537–546.

59 Muller TF, Grebe SO, Reckzeh B. Short- and long-term effects of polyclonal antibodies. *Transplant Proc* 1999;31:12S–15S.

60 Ayuk FA, Atassi N, Schuch G et al. Complement-dependent and complement-independent cytotoxicity of polyclonal antithymocyte globulins in chronic lymphocytic leukemia. *Leuk Res* 2008;32:1200–1206.

61 Monti P, Allavena P, Di Carlo V, Piemonti L. Effects of anti-lymphocytes and anti-thymocytes globulin on human dendritic cells. *Int Immunopharmacol* 2003;3:189–196.

62 Penack O, Fischer L, Stroux A et al. Serotherapy with thymoglobulin and alemtuzumab differentially influences frequency and function of natural killer cells after allogeneic stem cell transplantation. *Bone Marrow Transplant* 2008;41:377–383.

63 Penack O, Fischer L, Gentilini C et al. The type of ATG matters – natural killer cells are influenced differently by Thymoglobulin, Lymphoglobulin and ATG-Fresenius. *Transpl Immunol* 2007;18:85–87.

64 Stauch D, Dernier A, Marchese ES et al. Targeting of natural killer cells by rabbit antithymocyte globulin and Campath-1H: Similar effects independent of specificity. *PLoS One* 2009;4(3):e4709.

65 Kawai T, Wee SL, Bazin H et al. Association of natural killer cell depletion with induction of mixed chimerism and allograft tolerance in non-human primates. *Transplantation* 2000;70:368–374.

66 Dalle J-H, Dardari R, Menezes J et al. Binding of Thymoglobulin to natural killer cells leads to cell activation and interferon-γ production. *Transplantation* 2009;87:473–481.

67 Klaus G, Mostert K, Reckzeh B. Phenotypic changes in lymphocyte subpopulations in pediatric renal-transplant patients after T-cell depletion. *Transplantation* 2003;76:1719–1724.

68 Huang Y, Parker M, Xia C et al. Rabbit polyclonal mouse antithymocyte globulin administration alters dendritic cell profile and function in NOD mice to suppress diabetogenic responses. *J Immunol* 2009;182:4608–4615.

69 Novitsky N, Davison GM, Hale G et al. Immune reconstitution at 6 months following T-cell depleted hematopoietic stem cell transplantation is predictive for treatment outcome. *Transplantation* 2002;74:1551–1559.

70 Pearl JP, Parris J, Hale DA et al. Immunocompetent T-cells with a memory-like phenotype are the dominant cell type following antibody-mediated T-cell depletion. *Am J Tranplant* 2005;5:465–474.

71 Kroemer A, Xiao X, Vu MD et al. OX40 controls functionally different T cell subsets and their resistance to depletion therapy. *J Immunol* 2007;179:5584–5591.

72 Minamimura K, Sato K, Yagita H. Strategies to induce marked prolongation of secondary skin allograft survival

in alloantigen-primed mice. *Am J Transplant* 2008;8: 761–772.

73 Muller, TF, Grebe SO, Neuman MC *et al*. Persistent long-term changes in lymphocyte subsets induced by polyclonal antibodies. *Transplantation* 1997;64: 1432–1437.

74 Minamimura K, Gao W, Maki T. CD4⁺ regulatory T cells are spared from deletion by antilymphocyte serum, a polyclonal anti-T cell antibody. *J Immunol* 2006;176:4125–4132.

75 Bestard O, Cruzado JM, Mestre M *et al*. Achieving donor-specific hyporesponsiveness is associated with FOXP3⁺ regulatory T cell recruitment in human renal allograft infiltrates. *J Immunol* 2007;179:4901–4909.

76 Sewgobind VDK, Kho MML, van der Laan LJW *et al*. The effect of rabbit anti-thymocyte globulin induction therapy on regulatory T cells in kidney transplant patients. *Nephrol Dial Transplant* 2009;24:1635–1644.

77 Anderson BE, McNiff J, Yan J. Memory CD4⁺ T cells do not induce graft-versus-host disease. *J Clin Invest* 2003;112:101–108.

78 Dutt, S, Tseng D, Ermann J *et al*. Naive and memory T cells induce different types of graft-versus-host disease. *J Immunol* 2007;179:6547–6554.

79 Zheng H, Matte-Martone C, Li H *et al*. Effector memory CD4⁺ T cells mediate graft-versus-leukemia without inducing graft-versus-host disease. *Blood* 2008;111: 2476–2484.

80 Agha IA, Rueda J, Alvarez *et al*. Short course induction immunosuppression with Thymoglobulin for renal transplant recipients. *Transplantation* 2002;73: 473–475.

81 Matas AJ, Dandaswamy R, GIllingham KJ *et al*. Prednisone-free maintenance immunosuppression – a 5-year experience. *Am J Transplant* 2005;5: 2473–2478.

82 Eason J, Nair S, Cohen AJ *et al*. Steroid-free liver transplantation using rabbit antithymocyte globulin and early tacrolimus monotherapy. *Transplantation* 2003;75:1396–1399.

83 Tector AJ, Fridell JA, Mangus RS *et al*. Promising early results with immunosuppression using rabbit anti-thymocyte globulin and steroids with delayed introduction of tacrolimus in adult liver transplant recipients. *Liver Transplant* 2004;10:404–407.

84 Friese CE, Kang SM, Feng S *et al*. Experience with steroid-free maintenance immunosuppression in simultaneous pancreas-kidney transplantation. *Transplant Proc* 2004;36:1067–1068.

85 Tan M, Cantarovich M, Mangel R *et al*. Reduced dose Thymoglobulin, tacrolimus, and mofetil mycophenolate results in excellent solitary pancreas transplantation outcomes. *Clin Transplant* 2002;16:414–418.

86 Klingebiel T, PG Schlegel. GVHD: overview on pathophysiology, incidence, clinical and biological features. *Bone Marrow Transplant* 1998;21(Suppl 2):S45–S49.

87 Deeg HJ, Storb R. Graft-versus-host disease: pathophysiological and clinical aspects. *Annu Rev Med* 1984;35:11–24.

88 Bacigalupo A, Lamparelli T, Barisione G. Thymoglobulin prevents chronic graft-versus-host disease, chronic lung dysfunction and late transplant-related mortality: long-term follow-up of a randomized trial in patients undergoing unrelated donor transplantation. *Biol Blood Marrow Transplant* 2006;12:560–565.

89 Toor A, Rodriguez T, Bauml M. Feasibility of conditioning with thymoglobulin and reduced intensity TBI to reduce acute GVHD in recipients of allogeneic SCT. *Bone Marrow Transplant* 2008;42:723–731.

90 Lan F, Zeng D, Higuchi M. Host conditioning with total lymphoid irradiation and antithymocyte globulin prevents graft-versus-host disease: the role of CD1-reactive natural killer T cells. *Biol Blood Marrow Transplant* 2003;9:355–363.

91 Pillai AB, George TI, Dutt S. Host NKT cells can prevent graft-versus-host disease and permit graft antitumor activity after bone marrow transplantation. *J Immunol* 2007;178:6242–6251.

92 Pillai AB, George TI, Dutt S *et al*. Host natural killer T cells induce an interleukin-4-dependent expansion of donor CD4⁺CD25⁺Foxp3⁺ T regulatory cells that protects against graft-versus-host disease. *Blood* 2009; 113:4458–4467.

93 Lowsky R, Takahashi T, Liu YP. Protective conditioning for acute graft-versus-host disease. *N Engl J Med* 2005;353:1321–1331.

94 Kohrt HE, Turnbull BB, Heydari K. TLI and ATG conditioning with low risk of graft-versus-host disease retains antitumor reactions after allogeneic hematopoietic cell transplantation from related and unrelated donors. *Blood* 2009;114:1099–1109.

95 Cohen JL, Trenado A, Vasey D. CD4⁺CD25⁺ immunoregulatory T cells: new therapeutics for graft-versus-host disease. *J Exp Med* 2002;196:401–406.

96 Hoffmann P, Ermann J, Edinger M. Donor-type CD4⁺CD25⁺ regulatory T cells suppress lethal acute graft-versus-host disease after allogenic bone marrow transplantation. *J Exp Med* 2002;196:389–399.

97 Taylor PA, Lees CJ, Blazar BR. The infusion of ex vivo activated and expanded CD4⁺CD25⁺ immune regulatory cells inhibits graft-versus-host disease lethality. *Blood* 2002;99:3493–3499.

98 Trenado A, Sudres M, Tang Q *et al.* Ex vivo-expanded CD4+CD25+ immunoregulatory T cells prevent graft-versus-host-disease by inhibiting activation/differentiation of pathogenic T cells. *J Immunol* 2006;176: 1266–1273.

99 Edinger M, Hoffman P, Ermann J *et al.* CD4+CD25+ regulatory T cells preserve graft-versus-tumor activity while inhibiting graft-versus-host disease after bone marrow transplantation. *Nat Med* 2003;9:1144–1150.

100 Kim J, Kim HJ, Choi WS. Maintenance of CD8+ T cell anergy by CD4+CD25+ regulatory T cells in chronic graft-versus-host disease. *Exp Mol Med* 2006;38: 494–501.

101 Schneider M, Munder M, Karakhanova S. The initial phase of graft-versus-host disease is associated with a decrease of CD4+CD25+ regulatory T cells in the peripheral blood of patients after allogeneic stem cell transplantation. *Clin Lab Haem* 2006;28:382–390.

102 Zhai Z, Sun Z, Li Q. Correlation of the CD4+CD25high T-regulatory cells in recipients and their corresponding donors to acute GVHD. *Transpl Int* 2007;20: 440–446.

103 Clark FJ, Gregg R, Piper K. Chronic graft-versus-host disease is associated with increased numbers of peripheral blood CD4+CD25high regulatory T cells. *Blood* 2004;103:2410–2416.

104 Miura Y, Thoburn CJ, Bright EC. Association of Foxp3 regulatory gene expression with graft-verus-host disease. *Blood* 2004;104:2187–2193.

105 Arimoto K, Kadowaki N, Ishikawa T *et al.* FOXP3 expression in peripheral blood rapidly recovers and lack correlation with the occurrence of graft-versus-host disease after allogeneic stem cell transplantation. *Int J Hematol* 2007;85:154–162.

106 Regan JF, Lyonnais C, Campbell K. Total and active thymoglobulin levels: effects of dose and sensitization on serum concentrations. *Transpl Immunol* 2001;9:29–36.

107 Lowsky R, Takahashi T, Liu YP *et al.* Protective conditioning for acute graft-versus-host disease. *N Engl J Med* 2005;353:1321–1331.

108 Seidel MG, Fritsch G, Matthes-Martin S *et al.* Antithymocyte globulin pharmacokinetics in pediatric patients after hematopoietic stem cell transplantation. *J Pediatr Hematol Oncol* 2005;27:532–536.

109 Waller EK, Langston AA, Lonial S *et al.* Pharmacokinetics and pharmacodynamics of anti-thymocyte globulin in recipients of partially HLA-matched blood hematopoietic progenitor cell transplantation. *Biol Blood Marrow Transplant* 2003;9:460–471.

110 Starzl TE, Murase N, Abu-Elmagd K *et al.* Tolerogenic immunosuppression for organ transplantation. *Lancet* 2003;361:1502–1510.

111 Hartwig M, Snyder L, Appel JZ *et al.* Rabbit anti-thymocyte globulin induction therapy does not prolong survival after lung transplantation. *J Heart Lung Transplant* 2008;27:547–553.

112 Vianna R, Mangus R, Fridell J *et al.* Induction immunosuppression with thymoglobulin and rituximab in intestinal and multivisceral transplantation. *Transplantation* 2008;85:1290–1293.

113 Di Bona E, Rodeghiero F, Bruno B *et al.* Rabbit antithymocyte globulin [r-ATG] plus cyclosporine and granulocyte colony stimulating factor is an effective treatment for aplastic anaemia patients unresponsive to a first course of intensive immunosuppressive therapy. *Br J Haematol* 1999;107:330–334.

114 Scheinberg P, Nunez O, Young NS. Retreatment with rabbit anti-thymocyte globulin and ciclosporin for patients with relapsed or refractory severe aplastic anaemia. *Br J Haematol* 2006;133:622–627.

115 Stadler M, Germing U, Kliche KO *et al.* A prospective, randomized, Phase II study of horse antithymocyte globulin vs rabbit antithymocyte globulin as immune-modulating therapy in patients with low-risk myelodysplastic syndromes. *Leukemia* 2004;18:460–465.

CHAPTER 23

The Role of Alemtuzumab in Solid Organ Transplantation

Avinash Agarwal, David Bruno, and Stuart J. Knechtle

Department of Surgery and the Emory Transplant Center, Emory University, Atlanta, GA, USA

Introduction

In the past two decades the field of organ transplantation has witnessed unparalleled advances in short-term patient and graft survival [1]. Much of this success can be attributed to the development of potent immunosuppressive agents, including brief courses of lymphocyte-depleting antibodies [2]. The result has been a marked reduction in graft loss due to acute rejection [1, 3] and an unprecedented variety of effective immunosuppressive agents available to clinicians [4–6]. Indeed, no fewer than 30 combinations of immunosuppressive drugs are reportedly used clinically in North America [3]. Perhaps the use of more potent induction antibodies and more potent maintenance immunosuppression in organ transplantation has been permitted by the simultaneous development of more potent anti-infective agents, particularly antiviral prophylaxis, monitoring, and treatment.

Unfortunately, despite exceptional success in early graft and patient survival, late results remained plagued by excessive patient morbidity and mortality [1]. Importantly, the immunosuppressive agents responsible for admirable early transplant results are not benign and their chronic administration is associated with significant immunosuppression-related complications. Notably, herpesvirus reactivation, post-transplant diabetes mellitus, and cardiovascular disease have been shown to shorten the lives of chronically immunosuppressed patients despite excellent allograft function. In particular, lymphocyte-depleting antibody therapies used for induction have been shown to increase infectious and malignant morbidities, especially when paired with standard multidrug immunosuppressive regimens [7–14]. Thus, there is growing interest in the development of strategies that reduce dependence of chronic immunosuppression without sacrificing the freedom from acute rejection now typical of modern transplant regimens.

Immunosuppressive regimens can be fundamentally divided into induction, maintenance, or rescue therapies. Induction therapy is characterized by an intense prophylactic therapy initiated at the time of transplantation based on the tenet that powerful immunosuppression is required early to prevent acute rejection. Over time, the risk of rejection diminishes and, therefore, induction therapy is replaced by maintenance regimens. These are often of less potency and adapted to an individual's needs and pharmacological responses. Rescue therapy is similar to induction therapy, in that it represents an aggressive yet brief course of immunosuppression designed to reverse established rejection episodes.

As evidenced by the many regimens in routine clinical use, every transplant center develops its preferred immunosuppression regimens based on institutional and anecdotal experiences. Despite these differences, the principle of induction therapy is time honored and commonly employed. Strategies may include high doses of maintenance agents

Immunotherapy in Transplantation: Principles and Practice, First Edition. Edited by Bruce Kaplan, Gilbert J. Burckart and Fadi G. Lakkis.
© 2012 Blackwell Publishing Ltd. Published 2012 by Blackwell Publishing Ltd.

(bolus glucocorticosteroids or intravenous calcineurin inhibitors (CNIs)), or specific induction drugs such as antibody therapy. The use of antibody induction therapy has been steadily growing in the USA and exceeds 50% of patients for all organs except liver [2, 15]. Many of these specialized induction agents have been studied in randomized trials and have proved to be efficacious in combination with standard maintenance immunosuppression. No agent has yet to distinguish its superiority in the clinical setting. These agents, when considered collectively, have been shown to reduce the incidence of early acute rejection in renal allograft recipients, with the greatest advantage in those who are at high risk of rejection [16, 17]. The role of antibody induction therapy in cardiac transplantation is unclear and there is limited evidence showing any benefit in liver transplantation [18]. In the setting of simultaneous kidney–pancreas transplantation, there is modest evidence of their efficacy in reducing acute rejection [19, 20].

Specific induction antibody therapy can be divided into T-cell-depleting agents or nondepletion therapies based on whether their use leads to bulk reduction of peripheral lymphocytes. Examples of nondepleting antibody therapies include the CD25-specific antibodies. Both daclizumab and basiliximab have been shown to reduce acute rejection with minimal drug-related toxicity in kidney, liver, heart, and islet cell transplantation [21–24]. Unfortunately, these agents have not been as successful in leading to CNI avoidance or monotherapy maintenance immunosuppression compared with their depletional counterparts [25, 26].

Depletional induction therapy can be further subdivided into those that are polyclonal anti-T lymphocyte/thymocyte preparations (thymo-globulin (ATG-R), ATGAM, ATG-Fresenius) and monoclonal preparations specific for common lymphocyte antigens such as CD3 (muromonab), CD20 (rituximab), and CD52 (alemtuzumab). These agents typically lead to rapid lymphocyte depletion that can be prolonged [27]. Uncontrolled pilot studies report of the use of polyclonal antibody induction coupled with single drug maintenance therapy with comparable patient and graft survival

to standard therapy in selected patients [28, 29]. However, despite the theoretical benefits of reduced maintenance immunosuppression associated with these regimens, their results have not been adaptable to general clinical populations. Recently, the pairing of depletional induction with maintenance minimization has taken place with alemtuzumab. This chapter will provide an overview of the role of alemtuzumab in immunosuppression minimization regimens and summarize the current clinical evidence of its efficacy in achieving this goal.

History

Following the observation that lymphocytes were the primary mediators of organ transplant rejection [30], antilymphocyte agents were sought as potential drugs that might prolong allograft survival [31]. The important discovery of the technique for generating monoclonal antibodies allowed the rapid expansion of potential antilymphocyte-depleting antibodies [32]. After a series of studies, a set of antibodies was developed that could selectively deplete human lymphocytes through interactions with human complement. These antibodies were referred to as Cambridge Pathology or "Campath" antibodies. Alemtuzumab, a later humanized modification of a murine anti-human CD52 antibody, was originally developed by the laboratory of Waldmann in 1984. Alemtuzumab is a complement-fixing antibody specific for CD52, a glycoprotein expressed on most lymphocytes, natural killer cells, monocytes, and thymocytes [33, 34]. The initial preparations included both rat IgM (Campath-1M) and IgG (Campath-1G) isotypes. Early clinical trials with these rat-derived agents demonstrated their lymphocyte-depleting potential, but in combination with full dose maintenance or rescue regimens they were plagued by infectious complications [35, 36]. For perspective, these trials were performed prior to the currently available potent antiviral prophylactic agents. In addition, these agents were found to be potentially immunogenic, limiting their clinical utility [37]. Further work revealed human IgG1 as the best choice for complement lysis and antibody-dependent cellular cytotoxicity (ADCC), and advancements in bioengineering allowed the development of a humanized IgG1 CD52-specific monoclonal antibody, Campath-1H, which was developed for clinical use [38–40]. Initial clinical trials focused on treating lymphocyte neoplasms. Over time, Campath-1H was shown to be effective in cases of refractory vasculitis [41] and in late-stage progressive multiple sclerosis [42]. In 1999, the Food and Drug Administration approved Campath-1H as alemtuzumab for the treatment of lymphoid malignancies, and its role in transplantation has steadily grown, especially in concert with immunization minimization trials.

Mechanistic insights

CD52 is a 12-amino acid glycosylphosphatidylinositol (GPI)-anchored glycoprotein uniquely suited for use as a therapeutic target [43]. It is a high-density, nonmodulating molecule expressed on lymphocytes and monocytes that is absent on lymphoid progenitors. CD52's small size and proximity to the cell membrane facilitates efficient complement activation and membrane attack complex deposition upon alemtuzumab binding [44]. ADCC is also believed to account for its efficacy and is aided by the persistence of CD52 on the cell surface despite antibody binding (unlike CD3).

The presumed dominant mechanism by which alemtuzumab reduces the risk of allograft rejection is by lymphocyte death and a commensurate reduction in allospecific T cell precursor frequency. A single dose of alemtuzumab can lead to >99% peripheral blood lymphocyte depletion within 1 h of administration. There is also significant lymph node lymphocyte depletion within 2–4 days posttherapy [45]. While this is clearly mediated by complement-mediated lysis and ADCC, other mechanisms have been reported. Nuckel et al. reported that alemtuzumab may facilitate apoptosis of leukemic lymphocytes via the classical caspase-dependent cell death possibly secondary to activation of CD52-dependent signaling pathway associated with increased caspase 3 and 8 expression [46]. Alemtuzumab's pro-apoptotic effect was augmented in the presence of cross-linking anti-F_c

antibody which promoted cell clustering, suggesting a role of ADCC. Stanglmaier et al. have proposed that alemtuzumab may also lead to enhanced lymphocyte apoptosis via nonclassical caspase-independent cell death [47]. Recently, a human CD52 transgenic mouse model has been developed in order to assist in defining the mechanism of action and alemtuzumab's biological effects [48]. As anticipated, treatment with alemtuzumab led to depletion of peripheral blood lymphocytes with less profound changes in the secondary lymphoid tissues. Interestingly, initial results from this murine model suggest that the immunomodulatory impact of alemtuzumab appears to be independent of complement and may be mediated by innate immunity (neutrophils and natural killer cells), since the removal of these populations prior to alemtuzumab therapy strongly inhibited its activity. Clearly, ongoing future studies will provide additional insight into the mechanisms through which alemtuzumab impacts the immune response.

While depletion is profound in alemtuzumab-treated patients, the nuances of the drug's effect may have substantial influence on its efficacy. Pearl et al. have demonstrated that alemtuzumab leads to heterogeneous lymphocyte depletion showing specifically that antigen-experienced memory T cells are less susceptible to depletion than naive cells are, a trait also shared by polyclonal agents [49]. The mechanisms by which this effect occurs remain a matter of speculation, but may relate to survival pathways inherent to long-lived memory T cells, or differential distribution of antigen-experienced cells that sequester them from antibody exposure.

The inhomogeneous depletion seen in alemtuzumab-treated patients suggests that a recipient's pre-transplant heterologous allospecific immune memory dictates relative resistance or sensitivity to therapy, and this observation has been invoked as a potential mechanism of long-term efficacy. Trzonkowski et al. recently reported on their pilot study of alemtuzumab induction, reduced maintenance approach in 13 kidney allograft recipients [50]. The authors presented novel evidence demonstrating that the relative resistance of CD28-CD8+ T cells to depletion correlates with protection against acute rejection. These cells in an in vitro setting appear to compete with the recovery of CD4+ cells through either cell-to-cell contact or IL-10-dependent mechanisms and in doing so limit CD4 cell help for a de novo alloimmune response.

There is growing preliminary evidence suggesting that the residual post-alemtuzumab T cell population may be biased towards T cells with regulatory potential. Noris *et al.* recently reported on the results of a randomized, prospective trial with alemtuzumab induction and either sirolimus (SRL) or cyclosporine (CsA) with mycophenolate mofetil (MMF) maintenance therapy in kidney transplant recipients. The authors noted the emergence of T regulatory cells defined by CD4+CD25+FoxP3+ with in vitro regulatory function in setting of SRL but not CsA. Others report similar findings with alemtuzumab induction therapy in kidney transplant patients [27, 51]. Once again, alemtuzumab induction compared with Thymoglobulin or daclizumab led to an increased percentage of post-depletional T cells with a regulatory-like surface phenotype (CD4+CD25+) and more prominent FoxP3 mRNA expression. However, it should be noted that these observations of increased or disproportionate T regulatory cells have not been uniformly observed [49]. These discrepancies may be attributable to the influence of the maintenance immunosuppression on homeostatic repopulation and not be unique to alemtuzumab.

Pharmacologic properties

Alemtuzumab is a humanized monoclonal antibody of the IgG1 isotype that has been created by cloning the hypervariable regions of the murine parent Campath-1G into a framework provided by the human NEW and REI myeloma proteins [40]. The human IgG1 heavy chain was shown to have the best combination of FcR binding, ADCC, and complement activation. Similar to other clinical monoclonal antibody administration, selective patients are able to mount an anti-idiotypic response against the murine complement-determining regions (CDRs) after multiple exposures to this agent [52, 53]. The crystalline structure of the Campath antibody in complex with its antigens has been revealed, which has provided insight into

future generations of this agent with increased potency and less immunogenicity [54, 55].

Single-agent alemtuzumab is currently approved for the treatment of chronic lymphocytic leukemia as both initial therapy and to treat relapsing or refractory disease [56]. The approved dosage is a 30 mg infusion weekly for 12 weeks. There is a paucity of pharmacological reports in the field of organ transplantation to guide dosing in transplant patients. The most robust analysis of this topic was performed in studies involving lymphoproliferative and autoimmune disorders. Although alemtuzumab has been used in a variety of clinical settings, the specific pharmacological characteristics are not completely understood, partly because of the inherent difficulty with analyzing monoclonal antibodies.

The development of a reliable assay for alemtuzumab has been challenging given its xenogenic origin. Given its potency, the typical therapeutic concentration of 0.1–10 μg/mL proved to be difficult to discern from normal human immunoglobulin. An enzyme-linked immunosorbent assay (ELISA)-based assay has been shown to have a lower limit of quantification of 0.05 μg/mL [57]. In addition, a competitive immunofluorescence assay was developed which provided accurate and reproducible results from which future pharmacokinetic studies could be performed [58].

The pharmacokinetics of Campath were analyzed based on pooled data from various phase 1/2 or phase 2 noncomparative studies [59]. The most predictive pharmacokinetic model involved a two-compartment model with zero-order input and nonlinear Michaelis–Menten elimination. Not surprisingly, the critical covariate indentified was white blood cell (WBC) count, and thus the maximum rate of elimination was directly related to WBC count. The authors also found that there was tremendous interpatient variability that was felt to reflect patient diversity, disease status, and tumor burden. Rebello *et al.* were able to perform a pharmacokinetic study in bone marrow transplant patients who received intravenous administration of alemtuzumab and were also treated with cyclosporine and methotrexate [60]. Patients received a dose of 10 mg/day with two dosing schedules of 5 and 10 days. The mean peak concentrations at 5 days and 10 days were determined to be 6.1 µg/mL and 2.5 µg/mL respectively. Serum concentrations of alemtuzumab were detectable for 22–27 days after the 10th-day administration as compared with only being detectable between days 7 and 14 after the 5-day schedule. Peripheral lymphocytes were completely depleted by the second day after treatment and remained essentially undetectable for 1 month post-treatment. By day 180 post-treatment, there still remained over 50% depletion of peripheral lymphocytes. An industry-sponsored trial was performed in which the pharmacokinetics of intravenous once-weekly infusion for 12 weeks in an escalating-dose trial in patients with B-cell chronic lymphocytic leukemia (CLL) or non-Hodgkin's lymphoma was conducted [61]. Over a range of doses, the peak plasma concentration (C_{max}) and area under the plasma concentration-time curve (AUC) showed relative dose proportionality. The overall average plasma elimination half-life over the dosage interval was equivalent to 12 days [61]. A similar study involving intravenous dosages of alemtuzumab in patients with rheumatoid arthritis found the estimated half-life to be 9 days [62].

Most recently, the route of administration of alemtuzumab, either intravenous or subcutaneous, was evaluated [52]. Plasma alemtuzumab concentrations were monitored in 30 patients with relapsed CLL treated with intravenous alemtuzumab and were compared with 20 previously untreated patients who received similar doses subcutaneously. Higher blood concentrations did correlate with better clinical responses and minimal residual disease. Though the mean trough levels were similar in both groups, not unexpectedly, the subcutaneous arm required a high total cumulative dose (mean 90 µg vs 551 µg) to achieve the targeted level of 1 µg/mL. The authors concluded that subcutaneous alemtuzumab achieved similar concentrations to those of intravenous route. In addition, subcutaneous administration is more convenient and better tolerated. Consistent with these relationships, the clearance of alemtuzumab was more prolonged in those with a clinical

response than those with no response to treatment. Interestingly, this same report found two cases of antiglobulin response, both in the subcutaneous cohort. This response may have been due to the lack of prior immunosuppressive therapy in these patients. Yet the authors speculated that the subcutaneous route may allow for more effective antigen presentation, resulting in the higher antiglobulin response.

Ferrajoli *et al.* attempted a novel approach to rapidly achieve therapeutic drug concentrations in a limited cohort of 10 patients with refractory CLL by administration of alemtuzumab via continuous intravenous infusion of 30 mg/day for 7 days followed by subcutaneous doses of 30 mg three times a week for 11 weeks [63]. Plasma alemtuzumab concentrations were monitored after 24 h, 7 days, and 28 days after treatment in four patients. Alemtuzumab became detectable in three of four patients at the end of the continuous infusion and were at the minimum maintained with the subcutaneous doses. A larger cohort is necessary to determine if this regimen and the corresponding plasma alemtuzumab levels correlate with clinical outcome.

There have been numerous reports examining various factors which may impact exposure to alemtuzumab. First, soluble CD52 is present in the plasma of patients with CLL and, therefore, may lead to immune complexes with alemtuzumab, thereby reducing plasma concentrations of free agent [64]. The median plasma concentration of soluble CD52 in CLL patients was 709 nmol/L, compared with a median value of 73 nmol/L in normal individuals. Most importantly, patients who achieved a clinical response had significantly lower soluble CD52 levels, suggesting that those with higher soluble CD52 levels may require higher doses of alemtuzumab to saturate the soluble antigens and provide sufficient free agent to target CLL cells. Along the same line, Hale *et al.* demonstrated a negative relationship between initial lymphocyte count and peak concentration of alemtuzumab [52].

Factors that influence the clearance, metabolism, and elimination of alemtuzumab could potentially influence the pharmacokinetic and pharmacodynamic effects of this agent. Yet, there is minimal known information on the biological processes involved in the clearance of alemtuzumab from circulation and the extracellular space. To date, it is not known if hepatic function or macrophage activity could potentially affect the elimination and, therefore, the efficacy of alemtuzumab. Concurrent chemotherapy can change the exposure of alemtuzumab by directly altering the tumor burden. Patients who received both fludarabine and alemtuzumab achieved objective response compared with those who had been refractory to either single agent, suggesting a synergistic action of these agents [65].

CD52 is a glycoprotein expressed on approximately 95 % of peripheral blood lymphocytes, natural killer cells, monocytes, macrophages, and thymocytes. Therefore, near-complete mononuclear cell depletion occurs with treatment [34]. Though near-complete lymphocyte depletion occurs rapidly with single-dose therapy, there are differential rates of recovery of lymphocytic subpopulations [27]. Alemtuzumab therapy appears to cause minimal depletion of both memory T cells and plasma cells [45]. In addition, lymph node depletion is as complete as for peripheral blood lymphocytes, although delayed, in that it requires 3–5 days compared with less than 1 h seen in circulating lymphocytes [45]. Monocyte and B cell recovery is detectable at 3 months, while T cell recovery is frequently only at 50 % of baseline at 36 months [66, 67].

Clinical application of alemtuzumab in renal transplantation

Clinical trials have focused efforts on strategies minimizing exposure to either corticosteroids or CNIs. These efforts can be summarized by two general tactics: de novo minimization or progressive minimization in which one class of drug is either withdrawn or replaced by another agent.

Most of the clinical experience with alemtuzumab in the setting of solid organ transplantation has been in the field of renal transplantation. To date, however, most of the literature is based on single-center and/or

nonrandomized experiences. Nevertheless, most trials have been conceived with the vision of decreasing maintenance immunosuppression use. Calne and coworkers first reported on a series of patients who were treated with alemtuzumab induction and only low-dose CsA without azathioprine or steroids [68, 69]. The authors speculated that, in the absence of the initial pro-inflammatory state of the allograft, the healed graft could have a reduced capacity to immunize or activate the host T cell response and facilitate a state of "prope tolerance." A subsequent update of these 33 patients with 5-year follow-up reported equivalent patient and graft survival compared with a historical control group without induction using triple immunosuppression [70]. Although overall rejection rates were similar, the timing of rejections was markedly different: 14 % of alemtuzumab patients experienced acute rejection beyond 1 year post-transplant compared with 0 % of the control group. One possible explanation suggested by the authors was the lower targeted CsA levels in the alemtuzumab cohort were insufficient to suppress the allogeneic response of the recovering lymphocytes. Thus, alemtuzumab did not eliminate rejections, but rather shifted them to a later time point.

Building on Calne's early success combining alemtuzumab with truncated maintenance immunosuppression, numerous single centers have reported analyses involving alemtuzumab induction with lower immunosuppression (either CNI avoidance, steroid avoidance, or both) with comparisons with institutional standards of care [27, 71–75]. In general, these studies have consistently demonstrated that alemtuzumab regimens were well tolerated and equally efficacious in terms of short-term patient and graft survival, and rejection rates compared with the controls.

To date, there are only four published, randomized trials involving alemtuzumab induction therapy with nontraditional immunosuppression. At the University of Miami, 90 patients were randomized to receive induction with rATG, an anti-CD25 antibody, or alemtuzumab [27]. The alemtuzumab cohort received half-dose tacrolimus and rapid corticosteroid elimination, while the other arms received conventional maintenance regimens. After 15 months of follow-up, there was a reduced rate of rejection with no difference in infectious complications, but these promising early results gave way in a follow-up report to a higher incidence of chronic allograft nephropathy, higher mean creatinine, and a trend towards worse death-censored graft loss after 27 months follow-up [76].

Results from a multicenter, randomized control trial between three Asian transplant centers comparing alemtuzumab with low-dose CsA with triple immunosuppression with azathioprine, CsA, and corticosteroids have been reported [77]. Twenty patients received alemtuzumab and 10 were entered into the control arm. At 6 months, the limit of the study, there were no differences in rejection, but a higher rate of infectious complications in the alemtuzumab cohort occurred.

A prospective randomized trial was performed at the University of Wisconsin investigating the feasibility of CNI elimination in patients receiving alemtuzumab induction with standard triple immunosuppression [78]. Forty subjects with stable renal function were randomized between 2 and 16 months post-transplant to either continue or wean CNI. Twenty percent of the CNI-weaned cohort developed acute rejection within a median time of 4 months, while all of the controls remained stable. There was not a statistically significant difference between the rates of rejection in the two groups. The T regulatory cell population (CD4$^+$CD25$^+$FoxP3$^+$) in the control cohort underwent significant contraction, while the weaned patients maintained this population, although this observation was not related to outcome.

In the most recently reported study, Margreiter *et al.* performed a prospective randomized multicenter trial at four European centers with 131 deceased donor recipients comparing alemtuzumab induction and tacrolimus monotherapy with standard regimens [79]. Once again, the findings at 1 year post-transplant were similar to those in previous trials with alemtuzumab induction and tacrolimus monotherapy, showing sufficient efficacy and safety; longer term follow-up will be required to determine whether the admirable early results persist with time. Thus, CNIs remain an important element in the maintenance regimens

when alemtuzumab is used with the aim towards maintenance drug elimination. This may relate to the observations by Pearl *et al.* that alemtuzumab-resistant memory cells are sensitive to CNI but relatively resistant to other maintenance agents [49].

The importance of lymphocyte depletion in tolerance induction is a heavily debated issue in the transplant community. There is growing consensus that lymphocyte depletion may be beneficial by reducing the precursor frequency of allospecific lymphocytes and thus raise the threshold of clinical rejection allowing a window of opportunity for other maneuvers to influence the allospecific repertoire. However, it is clear that any "pro-tolerant" features of alemtuzumab are supportive and do not eliminate the need for maintenance immunosuppression. This has been most rigorously evaluated in a trial by Kirk *et al.* demonstrating that alemtuzumab's potent lymphocyte depletional effect alone with no maintenance immunosuppression was insufficient to induce tolerance in kidney transplant patients [45]. All of the patients developed reversible acute rejection with evidence of marked macrophage infiltration of the allograft. Knechtle *et al.* reported on the initial results of a similar pilot study involving alemtuzumab and sirolimus monotherapy. This trial demonstrated unacceptable high rates of acute humoral rejection (17%) in comparison with 10% in historical controls on traditional triple immunosuppression despite having equivalent patient and graft survival. The authors concluded that the combination of alemtuzumab and sirolimus monotherapy poorly protects against humoral immunity. The mechanism explaining the interaction between alemtuzumab and humoral immunity remains elusive, but may relate to occult sensitization. More likely, effects of alemtuzumab on B cell biology influence the higher risk of alloantibody, as has been recently published by Bloom *et al.* [80]. Specifically, patients treated with alemtuzumab have significantly higher B cell activating factor (BAFF) levels than control patients treated with basiliximab for at least 1 year after renal transplantation. Since BAFF may act to lower the B cell activation threshold, this may influence the likelihood of allo-B cell responses in treated transplant patients. However, it would also seem prudent to accurately screen patients for presensitization prior to transplantation in order to avoid promoting (by use of alemtuzumab) a pre-existing state of allo-B cell sensitization. Collectively, these studies imply that alemtuzumab induction in concert with reduced doses of maintenance immunosuppression can be safely performed, but require close follow-up late into the post-transplant course, and best include CNIs at least early post-transplant. The lessons learned must be translated into properly powered, randomized trials in order to fully understand the best late immunosuppressive strategy.

Interestingly, alemtuzumab's depletional effect has not been shown to increase the risk of post-transplant lymphoproliferative disease (PTLD). In a recent evaluation of the SRTR database, alemtuzumab was shown to have a significantly lower risk of PTLD compared with rATG and similar to that of patient receiving no induction [81]. This may relate to the B cell depletional effect of alemtuzumab, as B cells serve as the reservoir for Epstein–Barr virus and the source cell type for malignant transformation in PTLD.

Most recently, 3-year follow-up of a kidney transplant trial aimed at drug withdrawal and based on alemtuzumab induction, limited early tacrolimus use, and sirolimus maintenance showed that some (4 of 10) patients can successfully wean to minimal immunosuppression. Four of the study patients achieved stable graft function without clinical or biopsy evidence of rejection, and without alloantibody despite low-dose sirolimus therapy (1 mg daily with levels or 3–4 ng/mL) [82]. These patients have now been followed for over 4 years, again with stable allograft function. However, the pilot study also found a high incidence of alloantibody production in 5 of 10 patients, with clear antibody-mediated injury by biopsy in one patient. Other findings in the study included the emergence of increased naive B cells, increased gamma-delta T cells, and increased Vdelta1/Vdelta2 ratio of peripheral T cells [82]. These changes have also been noted in other tolerant transplant patient cohorts.

Liver, intestine, multivisceral transplantation

There is little evidence favoring a beneficial role for induction therapy in liver transplantation. Hence, published reports of the use of alemtuzumab in isolated liver transplantation are scarce. Tryphonopoulos et al. described the University of Miami's nonrandomized study of alemtuzumab induction in liver transplantation between 2001 and 2004. The authors compared 77 patients receiving alemtuzumab induction with low-dose tacrolimus monotherapy with historical controls [83]. There were no differences in patient or graft survival; yet, the incidence of rejection at 1 year was lower in the alemtuzumab-treated patients. A similar retrospective analysis of the University of Pittsburgh's experience with alemtuzumab induction with tacrolimus weaning/monotherapy compared with historical controls in liver transplantation has been reported [84]. One striking difference between the two studies is that the latter included hepatitis C recipients. Marcos et al. demonstrated that hepatitis C patients had poorer outcomes in both cohorts. The authors also showed that alemtuzumab-treated patients had significantly elevated levels of viral replication compared with the noninduction counterparts, which was interpreted as a result of viral-specific lymphocyte depletion. One of key conclusions was the recommendation against the use of alemtuzumab in hepatitis C seropositive patients.

Unlike the isolated liver transplant counterparts, there has been significant interest in the use of alemtuzumab in small-bowel and multivisceral transplantation, given the morbidity of acute rejection in this field. Reports have in general been retrospective or anecdotal [85]. Tzakis et al. recently reported on 21 intestinal or multivisceral transplant patients who received alemtuzumab and tacrolimus monotherapy. The authors reported that 13 patients remain with functioning grafts and tolerating enteral nutrition. There was a perceived reduction in incidence and severity of acute rejection with alemtuzumab induction therapy [85]. Nishidia et al. completed a subsequent updated report involving 76 adult intestinal transplants, 37 of whom received

alemtuzumab induction and tacrolimus monotherapy [86]. There was a significant reduction in
rejection rates compared with no induction and a
trend toward improved 1 year patient survival. In
addition, there was no graft-versus-host disease in
either cohort. In a recent report, Lauro *et al.*
compared alemtuzumab induction with daclizumab
(anti-IL-2 receptor) in 29 isolated bowel or
multivisceral recipients [87]. Alemtuzumab was
associated with a reduction in the incidence of acute
rejection within the first month post-transplant,
yet there were no differences in 3-year patient or
graft survival. Overall, the evidence suggests that
alemtuzumab induction with tacrolimus monotherapy provides sufficient immunosuppression in
most intestinal transplant settings.

Pancreas and islet cell transplantation

Similar to other solid organ transplants, the
published literature addressing alemtuzumab in
pancreas or islet transplantation is limited. Farney
et al. recently reported on their prospective,
randomized trial comparing alemtuzumab induction
with rATG in adult kidney and pancreas
transplantation. Of the 98 patients enrolled in the
study, 17 patients underwent simultaneous kidney–
pancreas (SPK) transplantation with four pancreas
after kidney transplantations [88]. There were no
differences in clinical outcomes between either
induction cohorts within 1 year follow-up. Although
this trial was randomized, its small number of
pancreas recipients limited its interpretation.

There have been several modest-sized retrospective analyses examining the role of alemtuzumab
in pancreas transplantation. Gruessner *et al.*
completed a nonrandomized cohort study to
compare 75 pancreas recipients of alemtuzumab
and MMF with historical controls (rATG and
tacrolimus monotherapy) [89]. Of note, these
patients received four doses of alemtuzumab within
the first 42 days post-transplant in addition to doses
of rATG to eliminate any CD52$^-$ cells. Total
lymphocyte counts were monitored and additional
alemtuzumab was administered for absolute

lymphocyte counts greater than 200 cells/mm^3.
There was no difference in patient or graft survival
at 6 months, although there was a trend toward
decreased isolated pancreas allograft survival
compared with controls. In addition, there was an
increased incidence of acute rejection in the
alemtuzumab cohort within the SPK transplant
cohort. Kaufman *et al.* performed a 3 year
retrospective analysis of alemtuzumab induction
($n = 50$) compared with rATG ($n = 38$) in SPK
recipients [90] with tacrolimus and sirolimus
maintenance. The only interesting difference was
the significantly lower incidence of viral infections
in the alemtuzumab cohort. The authors observed
no differences in 1 year actual or 3 year actuarial
patient or graft survival. Thai *et al.* recently published
on the University of Pittsburgh's experience with
alemtuzumab in pancreas transplantation [91].
Sixty patients (30 SPK, 20 pancreas after kidney,
and 10 pancreas alone) received alemtuzumab
induction with tacrolimus monotherapy. The
authors reported excellent patient and graft survival
with consistent infectious and acute rejection rates.
Most recently, Magliocca *et al.* have reported the
University of Wisconsin experience with SPK,
reporting similar graft and patient outcomes
between daclizumab and alemtuzumab induction
[92]. Initial results using two 30 mg doses were
associated with an increase in cytomegalovirus
(CMV) disease and prompted reduction to a single
30 mg induction dose. To date, there have only been
anecdotal reports addressing alemtuzumab in islet
cell transplantation [93, 94]. Results from ongoing
pilot studies are anticipated.

Pediatric transplantation

There has been a growing interest in the use of
alemtuzumab in children. The prospect of
maintenance immunosuppression reduction in
children is appealing given their lifelong exposure
to these agents. The initial description of its use in
pediatric population involved a small cohort of 11
high-risk intestinal recipients [85]. These patients
received alemtuzumab and low-dose tacrolimus
monotherapy with excellent short-term outcomes.

Kato *et al.* completed a retrospective review of 57 pediatric intestinal and multivisceral pediatric transplants performed between 1994 and 2004 comparing alemtuzumab and daclizumab induction. Both induction agents were well tolerated in children; however, patient survival was significantly worse in the alemtuzumab arm [95]. Kato *et al.* completed the University of Pittsburgh's review of the 10 pediatric liver transplants with alemtuzumab induction [96]. Tacrolimus monotherapy was used, except for two patients who were on steroids at the time of surgery. In comparison with historical controls, alemtuzumab induction recipients had significantly prolonged rejection-free survival. Shapiro *et al.* completed a retrospective review of the safety and efficacy of rATG or alemtuzumab induction in children in the setting of steroid avoidance and reduced CNI immunosuppression [97]. As anticipated, both regimens were tolerated and appeared to have equal efficacy. There were three cases of acute rejection in the alemtuzumab cohort that the authors attributed to noncompliance. Bartosh *et al.* reported the initial University of Wisconsin experience in pediatric renal transplantation with excellent outcomes and emphasized the importance of CNI maintenance in this patient group [98].

Thoracic organ transplantation

There is limited published literature on the use of alemtuzumab in thoracic organ transplantation. The first report of a series of lung transplant recipients receiving alemtuzumab was reported by McCurry *et al.* from the University of Pittsburgh [99]. The authors performed a retrospective analysis of 48 patients who both received rATG ($n=38$) or alemtuzumab induction ($n=10$) and were maintained on tacrolimus and corticosteroids, except for five alemtuzumab patients who were on tacrolimus monotherapy. The two cohorts were compared with historical controls, who received daclizumab induction and triple immunosuppression (prednisone, tacrolimus, and azathioprine). Alemtuzumab induction led to fewer and less severe acute rejection episodes compared with the other

two groups. There were no differences in patient or graft survival, pulmonary function, or infectious complications at 6 months. There was a trend for decreased CMV infection in the alemtuzumab cohort. The authors recently reported an updated report on these cohorts focused on the functional status of the recovered lymphocyte population in the alemtuzumab cohort [100]. In this study, global T cell function and CMV-specific T cell function were monitored longitudinally via intracellular ATP determination (ImmuKnow, Cylex, Columbia, MD). CMV-specific responses recovered as early as 2 weeks post-therapy in 80% of CMV-positive patients, while 72% of the subjects tested had a CMV memory response at 3 months post-transplant. These findings are consistent with previous reports of the preservation of memory T cell populations in the setting of lymphocyte depletion. In addition, these findings may account for the decreased CMV reactivation rates in these patients, as described in the earlier report. Yet longer follow-up is critical; particularly in the setting of immunosuppression minimization and tacrolimus monotherapy.

To date, there have been no published clinical trials involving alemtuzumab induction with immunosuppression minimization in thoracic transplantation. Das *et al.* describe a case of pediatric cardiac transplantation in which alemtuzumab induction was administered since the patient was sensitized and in an effort for steroid avoidance [101]. This patient received two standard doses of alemtuzumab and was maintained on MMF and tacrolimus therapy. At 1 year, the patient has maintained excellent allograft function with no episodes of acute rejection or infectious complications. The authors conclude that randomized prospective trials of alemtuzumab in pediatric organ transplant recipients is necessary in order to better define the risks and efficacy and that its use should be limited in children to special circumstances.

Safety and tolerability

The toxicity of alemtuzumab is predictable and typical of most immunoglobulin-based therapies. Adverse events include acute "first dose" administration-related reactions, infectious complications, and hematological toxicities. As prior, there is limited published literature in the field of solid organ transplantation.

Infusion-related events cover a wide variety of clinical signs and manifestations and include (but not limited to) rigor, fever, nausea, vomiting, skin rash, dyspnea, and hypotension [61]. The incidence of these events in the setting of hematologic malignancies was 90%, with 14% described at severe or life threatening. These "flu-like" symptoms typically manifest during the first alemtuzumab infusion and will decrease in severity with future doses. In the solid organ transplant setting, the single dose is frequently initiated while the patient is under general anesthesia. Therefore, the infusion-related symptoms may have been masked and, therefore, were imperceptible. These reactions can frequently be prevented by prophylactic anti-histamines, acetaminophen, or corticosteroids given 30 min prior to infusion [102,103]. Flu-like symptoms are reportedly reduced in the setting of subcutaneous injection; instead, these patients will experience injection-site skin reactions for 1–2 weeks post-treatment [104].

As anticipated, lymphopenia as a direct result of the mechanism of action of this agent is the most frequent hematologic change seen. This manifestation is self-limited and will resolve depending on the clinical indications for alemtuzumab therapy. Thrombocytopenia and neutropenia are also common and are also resolved over the ensuing few weeks [105]. Overall, hematological recovery can be achieved even without the assistance of growth factors. Recently, there was a case report of a patient who developed life-threatening alemtuzumab-induced coagulopathy in the setting of renal transplantation [106]. This patient demonstrated abnormal intrinsic and extrinsic coagulation pathway parameters, the need for multiple surgical procedures for hemorrhage, and unusual blood transfusion requirements. The coagulopathy resolved 2–3 days after infusion with little understanding of the exact etiology of this complication and it is not clear that it was due to alemtuzumab.

There are numerous reports in the oncology literature associating the lymphopenia from alemtuzumab with increased susceptibility to infectious complications [107]. Prophylactic antibiotics are routinely used during and after alemtuzumab therapy in transplant patients; specifically, for CMV and pneumocystis pneumonia. The most frequently seen opportunistic infection in this population is CMV and, fortunately, patients respond to intravenous ganciclovir [104, 105]. Once again, there are limited reports of infectious complications in solid organ transplant recipients secondary to alemtuzumab. Despite its profound immunosuppression, there does not appear to be any significant difference in the incidence or the morbidity of infectious complications with alemtuzumab therapy compared with conventional immunosuppression [108]. Perhaps this can be accounted for by the use of single-dose therapy in solid organ transplant in comparison with the multiple dosing regimens used in hematology. In a recent report, a group of 449 organ transplant recipients received alemtuzumab and were retrospectively followed for infectious complications [109]. The authors found that only 15 % of patients had bacteremia, but the pathogens were not those typically associated with lymphopenia (such as *Streptococcus pneumoniae* or *Mycobacterium avium* complex). A smaller study compared 50 renal transplant patients who received alemtuzumab induction therapy with historical controls. Those that received conventional immunosuppression had a higher incidence of infection (32 %) than with alemtuzumab (16 %) [109]. Finally, the use of alemtuzumab therapy in solid organ transplantation has thus far not been shown to have an increased incidence of post-transplant lymphoproliferative disorders (PTLD) [81].

Conclusions and future directions

Alemtuzumab reliably induces rapid and profound lymphocyte depletion. In doing so it reduces the risk of early acute rejection in unsensitized patients. It is well tolerated and facilitates (or perhaps requires, to avoid overimmunosuppression) reduction of some maintenance immunosuppressive drugs. There is growing evidence that CNI therapy is preferred following alemtuzumab, perhaps to thwart the activity of depletion-resistant memory T cells. Although it is clear that alemtuzumab reduces immunosuppressive drug requirements early after transplantation, there are limited pilot data from well-matched donor-recipient pairs [82] that the long-term maintenance requirements are substantially reduced. As such, the optimal dosing of alemtuzumab and its ideal combination with maintenance immunosuppression are yet to be determined. Alemtuzumab continues to be best considered an agent suitable for properly designed clinical trials until the long-term maintenance strategies are established. Future reports should focus on outcomes 3–5 years after transplantation.

References

1 Meier-Kriesche HU, Schold JD, Srinivas TR, Kaplan B. Lack of improvement in renal allograft survival despite a marked decrease in acute rejection rates over the most recent era. *Am J Transplant* 2004;4(3):378–383.

2 Meier-Kriesche HU, Li S, Gruessner RW *et al.* Immunosuppression: evolution in practice and trends, 1994–2004. *Am J Transplant* 2006;6(5 Pt 2):1111–1131.

3 Healthcare Systems Bureau, Division of Transplantation. 2007 Annual Report of the U.S. Organ Procurement and Transplantation Network and the Scientific Registry of Transplant Recipients: Transplant Data 1997–2006, Rockville, MD; 2007.

4 Danovitch GM. Immunosuppressive medications for renal transplantation: a multiple choice question. *Kidney Int* 2001;59(1):388–402.

5 Vincenti F. What's in the pipeline? New immunosuppressive drugs in transplantation. *Am J Transplant* 2002;2(10):898–903.

6 Gaber AO, First MR, Tesi RJ *et al.* Results of the double-blind, randomized, multicenter, Phase III clinical trial of Thymoglobulin versus Atgam in the treatment of acute graft rejection episodes after renal transplantation. *Transplantation* 1998;66(1):29–37.

7 Fishman JA. Infection in solid-organ transplant recipients. *N Engl J Med* 2007;357(25):2601–2614.

8 Fung J, Eghtesad B, Patel-Tom K *et al.* Liver transplantation in patients with HIV infection. *Liver Transpl* 2004;10(10 Suppl 2):S39–S53.

9 Schooley RT, Hirsch MS, Colvin RB *et al.* Association of herpesvirus infections with T-lymphocyte-subset

alterations, glomerulopathy, and opportunistic infections after renal transplantation. *N Engl J Med* 1983;308(6): 307–313.

10 Matas AJ, Humar A, Gillingham KJ *et al.* Five preventable causes of kidney graft loss in the 1990s: a single-center analysis. *Kidney Int* 2002;62(2): 704–714.

11 Miller LW. Cardiovascular toxicities of immunosuppressive agents. *Am J Transplant* 2002;2(9):807–818.

12 Brattstrom C, Wilczek H, Tyden G *et al.* Hyperlipidemia in renal transplant recipients treated with sirolimus (rapamycin). *Transplantation* 1998;65(9):1272–1274.

13 Singer DR, Jenkins GH. Hypertension in transplant recipients. *J Hum Hypertens* 1996;10(6):395–402.

14 Kobashigawa JA, Kasiske BL. Hyperlipidemia in solid organ transplantation. *Transplantation* 1997;63(3): 331–338.

15 Kirk AD. Induction immunosuppression. *Transplantation* 2006;82(5):593–602.

16 Szczech LA, Berlin JA, Feldman HI. The effect of antilymphocyte induction therapy on renal allograft survival. A meta-analysis of individual patient-level data. Anti-Lymphocyte Antibody Induction Therapy Study Group. *Ann Intern Med* 1998;128(10):817–826.

17 Szczech LA, Feldman HI. Effect of anti-lymphocyte antibody induction therapy on renal allograft survival. *Transplant Proc* 1999;31(3B Suppl):9S–11S.

18 Higgins R, Kirklin JK, Brown RN *et al.* To induce or not to induce: do patients at greatest risk for fatal rejection benefit from cytolytic induction therapy? *J Heart Lung Transplant* 2005;24(4):392–400.

19 Kaufman DB, Iii GW, Bruce DS *et al.* Prospective, randomized, multi-center trial of antibody induction therapy in simultaneous pancreas–kidney transplantation. *Am J Transplant* 2003;3(7):855–864.

20 Burke GW, 3rd, Kaufman DB, Millis JM *et al.* Prospective, randomized trial of the effect of antibody induction in simultaneous pancreas and kidney transplantation: three-year results. *Transplantation* 2004; 77(8):1269–1275.

21 Hershberger RE, Starling RC, Eisen HJ *et al.* Daclizumab to prevent rejection after cardiac transplantation. *N Engl J Med* 2005;352(26):2705–2713.

22 Vincenti F, Kirkman R, Light S *et al.* Interleukin-2-receptor blockade with daclizumab to prevent acute rejection in renal transplantation. Daclizumab Triple Therapy Study Group. *N Engl J Med* 1998;338(3): 161–165.

23 Neuhaus P, Clavien PA, Kittur D *et al.* Improved treatment response with basiliximab immunoprophylaxis after liver transplantation: results from a

double-blind randomized placebo-controlled trial. *Liver Transpl* 2002;8(2):132–142.

24 Shapiro AM, Lakey JR, Ryan EA *et al.* Islet transplantation in seven patients with type 1 diabetes mellitus using a glucocorticoid-free immunosuppressive regimen. *N Engl J Med* 2000;343(4):230–238.

25 Vincenti F, Ramos E, Brattstrom C *et al.* Multicenter trial exploring calcineurin inhibitors avoidance in renal transplantation. *Transplantation* 2001;71(9):1282–1287.

26 Parrott NR, Hammad AQ, Watson CJ *et al.* Multicenter, randomized study of the effectiveness of basiliximab in avoiding addition of steroids to cyclosporine a monotherapy in renal transplant recipients. *Transplantation* 2005;79(3):344–348.

27 Ciancio G, Burke GW, Gaynor JJ *et al.* The use of Campath-1H as induction therapy in renal transplantation: preliminary results. *Transplantation* 2004;78(3): 426–433.

28 Swanson SJ, Hale DA, Mannon RB *et al.* Kidney transplantation with rabbit antithymocyte globulin induction and sirolimus monotherapy. *Lancet* 2002;360(9346): 1662–1664.

29 Starzl TE, Murase N, Abu-Elmagd K *et al.* Tolerogenic immunosuppression for organ transplantation. *Lancet* 2003;361(9368):1502–1510.

30 Gowans JL, McGregor GD, Cowen DM, Ford CE. Initiation of immune responses by small lymphocytes. *Nature* 1962;196:651–655.

31 Lance EM, Medawar PB. Induction of tolerance with antilymphocytic serum. *Transplant Proc* 1969;1(1): 429–432.

32 Kohler G, Milstein C. Continuous cultures of fused cells secreting antibody of predefined specificity. *Nature* 1975;256(5517):495–497.

33 Waldmann H, Polliak A, Hale G *et al.* Elimination of graft-versus-host disease by in-vitro depletion of alloreactive lymphocytes with a monoclonal rat antihuman lymphocyte antibody (CAMPATH-1). *Lancet* 1984;2(8401):483–486.

34 Hale G, Xia MQ, Tighe HP *et al.* The CAMPATH-1 antigen (CDw52). *Tissue Antigens* 1990;35(3):118–127.

35 Friend PJ, Hale G, Waldmann H *et al.* Campath-1M – prophylactic use after kidney transplantation. A randomized controlled clinical trial. *Transplantation* 1989; 48(2):248–253.

36 Friend PJ, Waldmann H, Hale G *et al.* Reversal of allograft rejection using the monoclonal antibody, Campath-1G. *Transplant Proc* 1991;23(4):2253–2254.

37 Bruggemann M, Winter G, Waldmann H, Neuberger MS. The immunogenicity of chimeric antibodies. 1989;170(6):2153–2157.

38 Waldmann H, Hale G. CAMPATH: from concept to clinic. *Philos Trans R Soc London* 2005;360(1461): 1707–1711.

39 Bruggemann M, Williams GT, Bindon CI *et al.* Comparison of the effector functions of human immunoglobulins using a matched set of chimeric antibodies. *J Exp Med* 1987;166(5):1351–1361.

40 Riechmann L, Clark M, Waldmann H, Winter G. Reshaping human antibodies for therapy. *Nature* 1988;332(6162):323–327.

41 Mathieson PW, Cobbold SP, Hale G *et al.* Monoclonal-antibody therapy in systemic vasculitis. *N Engl J Med* 1990;323(4):250–254.

42 Coles AJ, Wing M, Smith S *et al.* Pulsed monoclonal antibody treatment and autoimmune thyroid disease in multiple sclerosis. *Lancet* 1999;354(9191): 1691–1695.

43 Xia MQ, Tone M, Packman L *et al.* Characterization of the CAMPATH-1 (CDw52) antigen: biochemical analysis and cDNA cloning reveal an unusually small peptide backbone. *Eur J Immunol* 1991;21(7):1677–1684.

44 Xia MQ, Hale G, Lifely MR *et al.* Structure of the CAMPATH-1 antigen, a glycosylphosphatidylinositol-anchored glycoprotein which is an exceptionally good target for complement lysis. *Biochem J* 1993;293(Pt 3): 633–640.

45 Kirk AD, Hale DA, Mannon RB *et al.* Results from a human renal allograft tolerance trial evaluating the humanized CD52-specific monoclonal antibody alemtuzumab (CAMPATH-1H). *Transplantation* 2003; 76(1):120–129.

46 Nuckel H, Frey UH, Roth A *et al.* Alemtuzumab induces enhanced apoptosis in vitro in B-cells from patients with chronic lymphocytic leukemia by antibody-dependent cellular cytotoxicity. *Eur J Pharmacol* 2005;514(2–3):217–224.

47 Stanglmaier M, Reis S, Hallek M. Rituximab and alemtuzumab induce a nonclassic, caspase-independent apoptotic pathway in B-lymphoid cell lines and in chronic lymphocytic leukemia cells. *Ann Hematol* 2004;83(10):634–645.

48 Hu Y, Turner MJ, Shields J *et al.* Investigation of the mechanism of action of alemtuzumab in a human CD52 transgenic mouse model. *Immunology* 2009; 128(2):260–270.

49 Pearl JP, Parris J, Hale DA *et al.* Immunocompetent T-cells with a memory-like phenotype are the dominant cell type following antibody-mediated T-cell depletion. *Am J Transplant* 2005;5(3):465–474.

50 Trzonkowski P, Zilvetti M, Chapman S *et al.* Homeostatic repopulation by CD28−CD8+ T cells in

alemtuzumab-depleted kidney transplant recipients treated with reduced immunosuppression. *Am J Transplant* 2008;8(2):338–347.

51 Bloom DD, Chang Z, Fechner JH *et al.* CD4+CD25+FOXP3+ regulatory T cells increase de novo in kidney transplant patients after immunodepletion with Campath-1H. *Am J Transplant* 2008;8(4):793–802.

52 Hale G, Rebello P, Brettman LR *et al.* Blood concentrations of alemtuzumab and antiglobulin responses in patients with chronic lymphocytic leukemia following intravenous or subcutaneous routes of administration. *Blood* 2004;104(4):948–955.

53 Isaacs JD. The antiglobulin response to therapeutic antibodies. *Semin Immunol* 1990;2(6):449–456.

54 Cheetham GM, Hale G, Waldmann H, Bloomer AC. Crystal structures of a rat anti-CD52 (CAMPATH-1) therapeutic antibody Fab fragment and its humanized counterpart. *J Mol Biol* 1998;284(1):85–99.

55 James LC, Hale G, Waldmann H, Bloomer AC. A structure of the therapeutic antibody CAMPATH-1H fab in complex with a synthetic peptide antigen. *J Mol Biol* 1999;289(2):293–301.

56 Demko S, Summers J, Keegan P, Pazdur R. FDA drug approval summary: alemtuzumab as single-agent treatment for B-cell chronic lymphocytic leukemia. *Oncologist* 2008;13(2):167–174.

57 Jilani I, Keating M, Giles FJ *et al.* Alemtuzumab: validation of a sensitive and simple enzyme-linked immunosorbent assay. *Leuk Res* 2004;28(12):1255–1262.

58 Rebello P, Hale G. Pharmacokinetics of CAMPATH-1H: assay development and validation. *J Immunol Methods* 2002;260(1–2):285–302.

59 Mould DR, Baumann A, Kuhlmann J *et al.* Population pharmacokinetics–pharmacodynamics of alemtuzumab (Campath) in patients with chronic lymphocytic leukaemia and its link to treatment response. *Br J Clin Pharmacol* 2007;64(3):278–291.

60 Rebello P, Cwynarski K, Varughese M *et al.* Pharmacokinetics of CAMPATH-1H in BMT patients. *Cytotherapy* 2001;3(4):261–267.

61 Pharmaceuticals G. Campath (alemtuzumab) package insert. Cambridge, MA; 2008.

62 Isaacs JD, Manna VK, Rapson N *et al.* CAMPATH-1H in rheumatoid arthritis – an intravenous dose-ranging study. *Br J Rheumatol* 1996;35(3):231–240.

63 Ferrajoli A, Wierda WG, LaPushin R *et al.* Pilot experience with continuous infusion alemtuzumab in patients with fludarabine-refractory chronic lymphocytic leukemia. *Eur J Haematol* 2008;80(4):296–298.

64 Albitar M, Do KA, Johnson MM *et al.* Free circulating soluble CD52 as a tumor marker in chronic lymphocytic leukemia and its implication in therapy with anti-CD52 antibodies. *Cancer* 2004;101(5):999–1008.

65 Elter T, Borchmann P, Schulz H *et al.* Fludarabine in combination with alemtuzumab is effective and feasible in patients with relapsed or refractory B-cell chronic lymphocytic leukemia: results of a phase II trial. *J Clin Oncol* 2005;23(28):7024–7031.

66 Bloom DD, Hu H, Fechner JH, Knechtle SJ. T-lymphocyte alloresponses of Campath-1H-treated kidney transplant patients. *Transplantation* 2006; 81(1):81–87.

67 Knechtle SJ, Pirsch JD, H. Fechner JJ *et al.* Campath-1H induction plus rapamycin monotherapy for renal transplantation: results of a pilot study. *Am J Transplant* 2003;3(6):722–730.

68 Calne R, Friend P, Moffatt S *et al.* Prope tolerance, perioperative Campath 1H, and low-dose cyclosporin monotherapy in renal allograft recipients. *Lancet* 1998;351(9117):1701–1702.

69 Calne R, Moffatt SD, Friend PJ *et al.* Campath IH allows low-dose cyclosporine monotherapy in 31 cadaveric renal allograft recipients. *Transplantation* 1999;68(10):1613–1616.

70 Watson CJ, Bradley JA, Friend PJ *et al.* Alemtuzumab (CAMPATH 1H) induction therapy in cadaveric kidney transplantation – efficacy and safety at five years. *Am J Transplant* 2005;5(6):1347–1353.

71 Knechtle SJ, Fernandez LA, Pirsch JD *et al.* Campath-1H in renal transplantation: The University of Wisconsin experience. *Surgery* 2004;136(4):754–760.

72 Shapiro R, Basu A, Tan H *et al.* Kidney transplantation under minimal immunosuppression after pretransplant lymphoid depletion with Thymoglobulin or Campath. *J Am Coll Surg* 2005;200(4):505–515; quiz A59–A61.

73 Kaufman DB, Leventhal JR, Axelrod D *et al.* Alemtuzumab induction and prednisone-free maintenance immunotherapy in kidney transplantation: comparison with basiliximab induction – long-term results. *Am J Transplant* 2005;5(10): 2539–2548.

74 Tan HP, Kaczorowski DJ, Basu A *et al.* Living donor renal transplantation using alemtuzumab induction and tacrolimus monotherapy. *Am J Transplant* 2006;6(10):2409–2417.

75 Ortiz J, Palma-Vargas J, Wright F *et al.* Campath induction for kidney transplantation: report of 297 cases. *Transplantation* 2008;85(11):1550–1556.

76 Ciancio G, Burke GW, Gaynor JJ *et al.* A randomized trial of thymoglobulin vs. alemtuzumab (with lower dose maintenance immunosuppression) vs. daclizumab in

renal transplantation at 24 months of follow-up. *Clin Transplant* 2008;22(2):200–210.

77 Vathsala A, Ona ET, Tan SY *et al.* Randomized trial of alemtuzumab for prevention of graft rejection and preservation of renal function after kidney transplantation. *Transplantation* 2005;80(6):765–774.

78 Pascual J, Bloom D, Torrealba J *et al.* Calcineurin inhibitor withdrawal after renal transplantation with alemtuzumab: clinical outcomes and effect on T-regulatory cells. *Am J Transplant* 2008;8(7):1529–1536.

79 Margreiter R, Klempnauer J, Neuhaus P *et al.* Alemtuzumab (Campath-1H) and tacrolimus monotherapy after renal transplantation: results of a prospective randomized trial. *Am J Transplant* 2008;8(7): 1480–1485.

80 Bloom D, Chang Z, Pauly K *et al.* BAFF is increased in renal transplant patients following treatment with alemtuzumab. *Am J Transplant* 2009;9(8):1835–1845.

81 Kirk AD, Cherikh WS, Ring M *et al.* Dissociation of depletional induction and posttransplant lymphoproliferative disease in kidney recipients treated with alemtuzumab. *Am J Transplant* 2007;7(11):2619–2625.

82 Knechtle SJ, Pascual J, Bloom DD *et al.* Early and limited use of tacrolimus to avoid rejection in an alemtuzumab and sirolimus regimen for kidney transplantation: clinical results and immune monitoring. *Am J Transplant* 2009;9(5):1087–1098.

83 Tryphonopoulos P, Madariaga JR, Kato T *et al.* The impact of Campath 1H induction in adult liver allotransplantation. *Transplant Proc* 2005;37(2):1203–1204.

84 Marcos A, Eghtesad B, Fung JJ *et al.* Use of alemtuzumab and tacrolimus monotherapy for cadaveric liver transplantation: with particular reference to hepatitis C virus. *Transplantation* 2004;78(7):966–971.

85 Tzakis AG, Kato T, Nishida S *et al.* Preliminary experience with campath 1H (C1H) in intestinal and liver transplantation. *Transplantation* 2003;75(8):1227–1231.

86 Nishida S, Levi DM, Moon JI *et al.* Intestinal transplantation with alemtuzumab (Campath-1H) induction for adult patients. *Transplant Proc* 2006;38(6):1747–1749.

87 Lauro A, Amaduzzi A, Dazzi A *et al.* Daclizumab and alemtuzumab as induction agents in adult intestinal and multivisceral transplantation: a comparison of two different regimens on 29 recipients during the early post-operative period. *Dig Liver Dis* 2007; 39(3):253–256.

88 Farney A, Sundberg A, Moore P *et al.* A randomized trial of alemtuzumab vs. anti-thymocyte globulin induction in renal and pancreas transplantation. *Clin Transplant* 2008;22(1):41–49.

89 Gruessner RW, Kandaswamy R, Humar A *et al.* Calcineurin inhibitor- and steroid-free immunosuppression in pancreas–kidney and solitary pancreas transplantation. *Transplantation* 2005;79(9):1184–1189.

90 Kaufman DB, Leventhal JR, Gallon LG, Parker MA. Alemtuzumab induction and prednisone-free maintenance immunotherapy in simultaneous pancreas–kidney transplantation comparison with rabbit antithymocyte globulin induction – long-term results. *Am J Transplant* 2006;6(2):331–339.

91 Thai NL, Khan A, Tom K *et al.* Alemtuzumab induction and tacrolimus monotherapy in pancreas transplantation: one- and two-year outcomes. *Transplantation* 2006;82(12):1621–1624.

92 Magliocca JF, Odorico JS, Pirsch JD *et al.* A comparison of alemtuzumab with basiliximab induction in simultaneous pancreas–kidney transplantation. *Am J Transplant* 2008;8(8):1702–1710.

93 Toso C, Edgar R, Pawlick R *et al.* Effect of different induction strategies on effector, regulatory and memory lymphocyte sub-populations in clinical islet transplantation. *Transpl Int* 2008;22(2):182–191.

94 Tan J, Yang S, Cai J *et al.* Simultaneous islet-kidney transplantation in 7 patients of type 1 diabetes with end-stage renal disease using a glucocorticoid-free immunosuppressive regimen with alemtuzumab induction. *Diabetes* 2008; 57(10): 2666–2671.

95 Kato T, Tzakis AG, Selvaggi G *et al.* Intestinal and multivisceral transplantation in children. *Ann Surg* 2006;243(6):756–764; discussion 764–766.

96 Kato T, Selvaggi G, Panagiotis T *et al.* Pediatric liver transplant with Campath 1H induction – preliminary report. *Transplant Proc* 2006;38(10):3609–3611.

97 Shapiro R, Ellis D, Tan HP *et al.* Antilymphoid antibody preconditioning and tacrolimus monotherapy for pediatric kidney transplantation. *J Pediatr* 2006; 148(6):813–818.

98 Bartosh SM, Knechtle SJ, Sollinger HW. Campath-1H use in pediatric renal transplantation. *Am J Transplant* 2005;5(6):1569–1573.

99 McCurry KR, Iacono A, Zeevi A *et al.* Early outcomes in human lung transplantation with Thymoglobulin or Campath-1H for recipient pretreatment followed by posttransplant tacrolimus near-monotherapy. *J Thorac Cardiovasc Surg* 2005;130(2):528–537.

100 Zeevi A, Husain S, Spichty KJ *et al.* Recovery of functional memory T cells in lung transplant recipients following induction therapy with alemtuzumab. *Am J Transplant* 2007;7(2):471–475.

101 Das B, Shoemaker L, Recto M *et al.* Alemtuzumab (Campath-1H) induction in a pediatric heart

transplant: successful outcome and rationale for its use. *J Heart Lung Transplant* 2008;27(2):242–244.

102 Kennedy B, Hillmen P. Immunological effects and safe administration of alemtuzumab (MabCampath) in advanced B-cLL. *Med Oncol* 2002;19(Suppl):S49–S55.

103 Pangalis GA, Dimopoulou MN, Angelopoulou MK *et al*. Campath-1H (anti-CD52) monoclonal antibody therapy in lymphoproliferative disorders. *Med Oncol* 2001;18(2):99–107.

104 Lundin J, Kimby E, Bjorkholm M *et al*. Phase II trial of subcutaneous anti-CD52 monoclonal antibody alemtuzumab (Campath-1H) as first-line treatment for patients with B-cell chronic lymphocytic leukemia (B-CLL). *Blood* 2002;100(3):768–773.

105 Keating MJ, Flinn I, Jain V *et al*. Therapeutic role of alemtuzumab (Campath-1H) in patients who have failed fludarabine: results of a large international study. *Blood* 2002;99(10):3554–3561.

106 Farid SG, Barwick J, Goldsmith PJ *et al*. Alemtuzumab (Campath-1H)-induced coagulopathy in renal transplantation. *Transplantation* 2009;87(11):1751–1752.

107 Dumont FJ. CAMPATH (alemtuzumab) for the treatment of chronic lymphocytic leukemia and beyond. *Expert Rev Anticancer Ther* 2002;2(1):23–35.

108 Morris PJ, Russell NK. Alemtuzumab (Campath-1H): a systematic review in organ transplantation. *Transplantation* 2006;81(10):1361–1367.

109 Silveira FP, Marcos A, Kwak EJ *et al*. Bloodstream infections in organ transplant recipients receiving alemtuzumab: no evidence of occurrence of organisms typically associated with profound T cell depletion. *J Infect* 2006;53(4):241–247.

CHAPTER 24

Rituximab, an Anti-CD20 Monoclonal Antibody

Mark D. Pescovitz
Indiana University Medical Center, Indianapolis, IN, USA

Introduction

While anti-T-cell targeted therapy has dramatically reduced the rate of acute rejection and enhanced 1-year graft survival, long-term graft survival has had only a marginal increase. As the transplant community addresses this issue and also focuses on circumventing the obstacle of transplanting across blood group ABO incompatibility and the sensitized recipient, attention is turning from purely attacking T-cell-mediated pathways and to a combined approach considering B cells and antibodies as major causative factors of allograft injury [1, 2]. Cai and Teraski annunciated three potential not mutually exclusive strategies to accomplish control of B cell/antibody-mediated rejection: (1) inhibition and depletion of antibody producing cells; (2) removal or blockage of antibodies; and (3) interference with the mechanism of tissue injury [3]. This chapter will focus on rituximab (Rituxan, Biogen-IDEC), an approved drug being used in protocols aimed at controlling B cell mediated immunity.

CD20

CD20 (human B-lymphocyte-restricted differentiation antigen, Bp35) is a hydrophobic transmembrane protein with a molecular weight of approximately 35 kDa located on pre-B and mature B lymphocytes [4]. It crosses the plasma membrane four times, resulting in a small and large extracellular loop [5]. The antigen is expressed on most B cell non-Hodgkin's lymphomas, but is not found on stem cells, pro B cells, normal plasma cells, or other normal tissues. Plasmablasts and stimulated plasma cells may express CD20 [6]. CD20 regulates an early step(s) in the activation process for cell cycle initiation and differentiation, and possibly functions as a calcium ion channel. Initially CD20 was considered to be stable on the cell surface and it does not internalize upon antibody binding [5]. In general, free CD20 antigen is not found in the circulation; thus, a drug that reacts with CD20, such as an antibody, would not be neutralized before binding to its target cell [7]. However, there is evidence in certain lymphomas that circulating CD20, perhaps as membrane fragments, can be detected in the blood [8] and that it can be "shaved" from the cell surface, both of which have been put forward as a possible explanation for cases of resistance to rituximab [9,10]. This dependence on the interaction of Fc portion of rituximab with Fcgamma receptors on macrophages was confirmed by Beum *et al.* [10]. The relevance to transplantation, where normal B cells are the target of rituximab, is not known.

Immunotherapy in Transplantation: Principles and Practice, First Edition. Edited by Bruce Kaplan, Gilbert J. Burckart and Fadi G. Lakkis.
© 2012 Blackwell Publishing Ltd. Published 2012 by Blackwell Publishing Ltd.

Rituximab: structure

Rituxan® (rituximab) is a chimeric murine/human monoclonal antibody that reacts with the CD20 antigen [11]. Rituximab is indicated for the treatment of patients with various types of CD20+ B cell lymphomas and, in combination with methotrexate, for treatment of moderately to severely active rheumatoid arthritis in adult patients who have failed tumor necrosis factor (TNF) antagonists [12]. It contains the antigen-binding regions from the original murine anti-human-CD20 antibody 2B8 in conjunction with human kappa and IgG1 heavy-chain constant region sequences [7]. As a typical IgG antibody, rituximab contains two heavy chains of 451 amino acids and two light chains of 213 amino acids with a total molecular weight of 145 kDa. Rituximab has a binding affinity for the CD20 antigen of approximately 8.0 nM, which is similar to the parent murine antibody, 2B8 [11]. Chinese hamster ovarian cells are used as the production source of the commercial immunoglobulin preparation [11]. Rituximab binds to the residues 163–187 of the larger extracellular loop of the CD20 antigen. Du *et al.* solved the crystal structure of the rituximab-Fab in complex using a synthesized peptide comprising the CD20 epitope at 2.6 Å resolution [13]. The bound peptide forms a cyclic conformation constrained by a disulfide bond and a proline residue (Pro172). The antigen–antibody interactions involve both hydrogen bonds and van der Waals contacts.

Mechanism of B cell depletion

The elimination of B cells by rituximab has been explained by induction of complement-dependent cytotoxicity (CDC) [11, 14], antibody-dependent cellular cytotoxicity (ADCC) [11], or stimulation of apoptosis [14]. In the apoptotic pathway for rituximab depletion, recent data indicate that caspase 9 (but not caspase 8) and mitochondria are critical [15]. Polymorphisms of Fc receptors gamma RIIIa (CD16) and gamma RIIa (CD32) have been associated with antilymphoma efficacy and efficacy in the treatment of lupus [16–18]. The relevance to

patients where rituximab is used for organ transplantation is not known. Studies using rituximab for transplant indications should consider including genomic analysis of the FcR until this issue is clarified. Recent data from a transgenic mouse strain that expresses the human CD20 antigen on B cells suggests that sensitivity of CD20-expressing cells to depletion by rituximab may depend on the microenvironment, integrin-regulated homeostasis, and circulatory dynamics of B cells [19]. For example, in these mice, marginal-zone B cells, thought to be involved in natural antibody responses [20] (and maybe the source of anti-ABO antibodies [21]), are not as completely depleted and their depletion is more dependent on complement than are B cells in other compartments. However, the marginal B cells are susceptible to elimination when they are mobilized by the addition of antibodies to α_L and α_4 integrin [22]. These differences in sensitivity may explain some of the variation in degree of depletion found in lymphoid tissue, as noted below.

Pharmacokinetics

The majority of pharmacokinetic and pharmacodynamic studies have been performed in patients with B cell lymphoma [7, 23]. In nine patients given 375 mg/m² as an intravenous (IV) infusion for four doses, the mean serum half-life was 59.8 h (range 11.1–104.6 h) after the first infusion and 174 h (range 26–442 h) after the fourth infusion. The serum concentration of rituximab was directly correlated with response and inversely correlated with tumor burden. The wide range of half-lives may, therefore, reflect the variable tumor burden among patients and the changes in CD20 positive (normal and malignant) B cell populations upon repeated administrations. In a study using rituximab in the treatment of rheumatoid arthritis, the half-life after the second dose was 20 days, which was similar to native IgG [24, 25]. This was significantly longer than that of a similar therapeutic chimeric antibody, basiliximab. In a single-dose study in subjects with renal failure, we found a half-life ranging from 10 to 14 days [26, 27]. In a study in patients with recent onset of type 1 diabetes [27], which included children down to the age of 8 years, there was a very strong effect of age, with a more rapid clearance of drug in the younger populations (unpublished results). The explanation for these differences is unknown.

The initial assays for rituximab concentration were based on idiotype-specific polyclonal anti-rituximab antibody. Blasco and coworkers [28, 29] developed an enzyme-linked immunosorbent assay (ELISA) for measurement of rituximab levels using a 20-mer peptide from the large extracellular loop sequence (residues 165–184). They compared this with a specific anti-rituximab anti-idiotype antibody MB2A4. While both methods were accurate and reproducible, the anti-idiotype was more sensitive. The results were discrepant when using patient samples, with the anti-idiotype producing higher levels consistently. They suggested that either circulating non-cell-bound CD20 or aggregated rituximab in the circulation as possible explanations for the differences. Thus, despite the association of rituximab levels to treatment efficacy for lymphoma, measurement of rituximab concentrations is not considered standard of care. Such detailed analyses are not available for rituximab use in transplantation, making the utility of pharmacokinetic measurement even weaker.

Pharmacodynamics

In all human disease states in which rituximab has been given, there has been a rapid elimination of circulating B cells. Among 166 lymphoma patients, circulating CD19+ B cells were depleted within the first three doses, with sustained depletion for up to 6–9 months post-treatment in 83 % of patients [30]. B cell recovery began at approximately 6 months following completion of treatment. Median B cell levels returned to normal by 12 months following completion of treatment. A similar rapid response was seen in the rheumatoid arthritis study [24], but recovery was prolonged, with some patients having depletion extending out 2 years. In patients receiving a renal transplant, a single dose of rituximab rapidly depletes circulating B cells [31, 32]. Even when the total B cell count returns to normal, as we

have shown [33], there appears to be a change in the phenotype, with the B cells present being relatively deficient in expression of CD27, a surface marker of memory B cells, findings that are confirmed by others [34]. This suggests that the B cells that do repopulate are primarily naive, at least as late as 2 years after a single dose.

The knowledge of the impact of rituximab on tissue B cells is limited by the invasive nature of the sampling methods (e.g., needle biopsy, lymph node excision, splenectomy). Cioc et al. in an autopsy study of lymphoma patients were able to demonstrate that after as few as three doses and as soon as 1 month after the last dose, rituximab depleted normal B cells in lymph node and spleen [35]. Repletion was not complete as long as 12 months after the last dose. These times and number of doses are outer limits, as earlier and later biopsies or from patients with fewer doses were not available. In another report, nephrectomy specimens 3.8 and 10.3 months after the last dose of rituximab (given for treatment of antibody-mediated rejection) CD20 cells could still be detected in tertiary lymphoid tissue [36]. These authors hypothesized that local BAFF (B cell Activation Factor of the TNF Family) production, confirmed by in situ staining, contributed to the long-term persistence in the face of near-complete elimination of circulating B cells. It is possible, however, that depletion was complete earlier after dosing and the cells present represent local clonal expansion as the concentration of rituximab fell. Steinmetz et al. [37] analyzed B cell clusters in patients with vascular renal rejection by immunohistochemistry. Nine of 16 (56 %) patients with vascular rejection displayed intrarenal B cell clusters that co-localized with expression of the B cell attractant chemokine BCA-1/CXCL13. Those patients who received rituximab had complete elimination of the intrarenal B cells ($P < 0.001$), whereas there was no effect on these intrarenal B cells in patients who did not get rituximab. Genberg et al. [38] used rituximab in 49 renal transplant recipients who were receiving an ABO-incompatible transplant or for treatment of rejection. A single dose of rituximab resulted in complete depletion of B cells in peripheral blood of 88 % of patients that was maintained for as long as 15 months. In kidney tissue, B cells were also completely eliminated. In contrast, the B cells were not eliminated in lymph nodes, although a reduction was observed. Lastly, even relatively low doses of rituximab are able to deplete CD20 cells in the spleen, as demonstrated in post-rituximab splenectomy samples [39]. Thus, while based on random sampling in a limited number of patients, it is clear that rituximab does eliminate tissue-based B cells.

Dosing

The appropriate dose of rituximab and the number of doses appears to be dependent on the clinical setting. For lymphoma, the approved dose is $375\,mg/m^2$, as an IV infusion, for four weekly doses; however, more doses have been studied with follicular lymphoma [40]. The dose used in adult patients with rheumatoid arthritis (and most autoimmune diseases) is 1 g every other week for two doses [25]. This is roughly equivalent to the standard four-dose regimen when applied to a $1.73\,m^2$ adult. Body surface area only contributed 19.7% to the variability in clearance and thus made an insignificant contribution to variability in drug exposure as measured by AUC. Therefore, for adult rheumatoid arthritis, it was determined that dosing by body surface area was not needed. Doses of 500 mg per dose give similar responses to the 1000 mg dose [41]. In our study in type 1 diabetes, the dose of $375\,mg/m^2$ for four doses was used and provided good long-term depletion and evidence of efficacy.

The appropriate dose to use in transplant recipients is even less well defined. In patients with renal failure, a single dose as low as $50\,mg/m^2$ resulted in the same degree and duration of peripheral B cell suppression and effect on antibody response as $375\,mg/m^2$ [26]. The dose of rituximab used for transplant patients is not fixed. Toki *et al.* treated single patients with a dose of rituximab at 10, 15, 35, 150, or $300\,mg/m^2$ at 3–13 days before ABO-incompatible transplantation [39]. Most informative was a splenectomy done at the time of transplant. This permitted a comparison of the impact of rituximab on both peripheral and tissue-based B cells.

While all five doses resulted in complete B cell depletion, the lowest dose resulted in early repopulation of the periphery and incomplete depletion of the splenic B cells. A dose of at least $35\,mg/m^2$ was required for complete depletion of the splenic B cells. In seven patients with early (less than 10 days post-transplant) and one with later (4 months post-transplant) antibody-mediated rejection (AMR) who failed plasmapheresis and intravenous immunoglobulin (IvIg), the addition of a single 500 mg dose of rituximab was effective in achieving long-term graft survival [42]. The authors claim that this is "low dose"; however, it is effectively the same as a dose of $375\,mg/m^2$ given as a single dose.

The ultimate resolution of dosing is important if for no other reason than cost. If using the body surface area dosing, for the average $1.73\,m^2$ person, a dose of 650 mg would be required which would translate to $3976 per infusion or $15904 for a four-dose course. If using the 1000 mg dose, it would be $5680 or $11360 for the two-dose course. The ultimate cost for a transplant patient would be based on the dose selected and the number of doses given. Depending on time of the dosing, it might be included within the initial global payment, thus competing with other costs.

A hindrance to the use of rituximab is the need for a slow infusion rate to decrease the severity of the side effects. Siano *et al.*, in a group of lymphoma patients who had received at least one prior infusion without major problems, were able to tolerate a second dose at the rate of 700 mg/h. This would translate into giving the complete dose in less than 1 h, thus facilitating infusions and decreasing patient inconvenience [39].

Implications for tissue typing

Rituximab is slowly eliminated from the circulation and thus can be detected in the serum for many months after the dose of drug [26]. This persistence of rituximab has implications for the tissue-typing laboratory. Since rituximab induces complement-dependent cytotoxicity, sera that contain rituximab produce a potentially false-positive B cell cytotoxic-positive cross-match. Furthermore, the human portion of the IgG1 reacts with the anti-human Ig fluorochromes used in flow cytometric cross-matches, potentially resulting in a false-positive B cell flow cross-match. We have demonstrated that either elimination of the cell surface CD20 by pronase treatment of the donor lymphocytes or removal of the circulating rituximab by immunomagnetic bead absorption through anti-mouse-IgG binding to the murine portion of the molecule eliminated the nonspecific reaction [43, 44]. We have recently improved this technique by using a synthesized CD20 peptide [13] attached to magnetic beads (Book *et al.*, unpublished results). This method allows for specific elimination of circulating rituximab. The beads are added to serum or plasma containing rituximab. The rituximab binds specifically to the bead-conjugated CD20 peptide. With removal of the beads with a magnet, the rituximab is specifically eliminated. This technique has no impact on the titer of anti-human leukocyte antigen (HLA) alloantibodies.

Toxicity

The toxicity of rituximab can be broken into two main types: immediate and late. The immediate variety, seen within the first 24 h, typically starts shortly after the first infusion begins. This is caused by cytokine release or necrosis of cells induced by rituximab binding to the cell surface. Agarwal *et al.* demonstrated that cytokine levels, particularly TNF, increase immediately after the first dose of rituximab and that this can be associated with a febrile response [45]. In a tumor population, side effects correlated with the number of circulating CD20 cells and consisted of fevers, chills, rigor, orthostatic hypotension, and bronchospasm. Fever is the most common side effect (43%) followed by bronchospasm (8%), and hypotension (10%) [7]. Other adverse events, including chills, headache, nausea, vomiting, rhinitis, and mild hypotension, occurred primarily during rituximab infusions and typically responded to an interruption of the infusion and resumption at a slower rate. Patients with preexisting cardiac conditions, including arrhythmia and angina, have had recurrences of

these cardiac events during rituximab infusions. In rare cases, severe and fatal cardiopulmonary events, including hypoxia, pulmonary infiltrates, acute respiratory distress syndrome, myocardial infarction, and cardiogenic shock, have occurred. Most fatal infusion-related events occurred in association with the first infusion. That these effects are not related to tumor lysis is clearly demonstrated in the similar pattern of adverse reactions seen when rituximab is used to treat autoimmune disease [27, 46, 47]. In a transplant setting in which corticosteroids might be given in conjunction with rituximab (e.g., treatment of rejection or at the time of transplant), the rate and severity of side effects might be decreased. In rheumatoid arthritis patients, a single 200 mg dose of methylprednisolone with the first dose of rituximab did reduce the frequency of side effects [48]. This is similar to the reduced side effects seen with steroids given at the time of OKT3 treatment [49]. Even in the absence of any corticosteroids, the side effects are generally minimal, can be ameliorated by slowing the infusion rate, and are substantially fewer with subsequent doses [27].

The late toxicity of rituximab is generally focused on increased rates of infection and long-term impact on immune parameters. Despite the profound B cell depletion, there were only mild to moderate reductions in IgM and IgG serum levels observed from 5 through 11 months following rituximab administration, with only 14% of patients having values below the normal range [30]. Longer courses of treatment [40] and some reports in renal transplant recipients [50] have been associated with increased rates of hypogammaglobulinemia; therefore, measuring of serum IgG levels should be considered along with appropriate treatment if levels fall below 300 mg/dL [51]. Neutropenia, particularly late onset, has been reported in patients receiving rituximab [52–54]. This has been associated with multiple doses of rituximab and chemotherapy and hypothesized to cause excess B cell generation induced by high levels of BAFF leading to neutropoesis competition in the bone marrow [54]. While the transplant population would not be getting cancer chemotherapy, they are typically receiving other agents associated with leukopenia, such as mycophenolic acid derivatives and ganciclovir. We did not see an increased rate of neutropenia in our series of patients with type 1 diabetes treated only with rituximab in the absence of other cytotoxic drugs [27].

The ultimate question for safety that is predominantly late in onset is the potential infectious risk. While there have been infections noted in patients treated with rituximab, these are generally anecdotal and no clear increase has been seen, including those of viral, bacterial, and fungal pathogens [24]. Grim *et al.* [55], when using rituximab as part of immunosuppressive protocols for ABO-incompatible and positive cross-match transplants, did a retrospective analysis of infections with the first 6 months of treatment. They note a rate of 48 % after rituximab compared with 11 % among historical controls who did not receive rituximab ($p=0.107$). In a separate review of 77 patients who received rituximab when compared with 902 patients who did not, there was a significantly higher rate of death from infection in those who received rituximab. This was particularly true in patients who also received T-cell-depleting drug [56].

While there has been a report of fatal reactivation of cytomegalovirus (CMV) in a transplant patient with post-transplant lymphoproliferative disease (PTLD) [57], others note that incidence of CMV infection and disease was not increased by a single low dose of rituximab given at the time of kidney transplant [58]. Furthermore, all of the patients who developed CMV infection and who were CMV seronegative at the time of transplant seroconverted, while those who were CMV at the time of transplant retained their anti-CMV titer. Vianna *et al.* added rituximab to thymoglobulin and tacrolimus for intestinal transplants and saw no cases of PTLD; i.e., a reduced incidence [59]. They suggest that this might be a useful combination leading to reduced PTLD in this troublesome population.

Reactivation of hepatitis has been noted, so that caution must be used with rituximab in patients with hepatitis B [60]. Concurrent use of lamivudine might mitigate this reactivation. Although not in transplant patients, Pei *et al.* reported that of 15 hepatitis B surface-antigen-positive lymphoma

patients, five who received lamivudine prophylaxis did not develop HBV-related hepatitis, whereas 8 of 10 who received lamivudine prophylaxis developed HBV-related hepatitis. Interestingly in this HBV endemic region, four (4.2 %) of 95 who were previously HBV-negative developed de novo HBV-related hepatitis and two died of fulminate hepatitis [61]. Thus, if a patient with hepatitis B requires rituximab therapy, it would probably be prudent to also provide antiviral therapy. This situation with hepatitis B should be contrasted with the situation with hepatitis C, where there does not appear to be an increase. On the contrary, rituximab has been used effectively to treat hepatitis C-associated cryoglobulinemia [62, 63]. Agarwal *et al.* reported their experience with the use of a single dose of rituximab in combination with Thymoglobulin, tacrolimus, and a short course of corticosteroids compared with a similar protocol without rituximab [64] in 118 patients. With hepatitis C as the cause of liver failure in about 45 %, there was no increase in recurrent hepatitis C in the 68 rituximab-treated subjects, with excellent graft and patient survival and low rates of rejection. This difference in response to rituximab between hepatitis B and C is probably related to the pathophysiology of the virus infection.

Over the past several years, the level of concern has increased dramatically for JC virus, a polyomavirus related to BK virus. As with BK virus, JC asymptomatically infects most healthy adults [65]. However, in the setting of a weakened immune response, JC virus can reactivate and cause progressive multifocal leukoencephalopathy (PML), a demyelinating disease of the central nervous system that frequently progresses to death. While an antibody response to JC is detectable in the blood, this does little to prevent progression to PML. The T cell arm of the immune response of both CD4 and CD8 cells is key to control of progression. Reactivity to a specific viral peptide, in HLA-A *0201 correlated with survival in 5/7 (71 %) versus none of six PML progressors ($P=0.02$) [66]. A handful of cases have been reported in patients who received rituximab, initially after chemotherapy, but more recently in patients getting rituximab for autoimmune diseases such as lupus [67]. This increased rate has resulted in a black-box warning. The rate of PML in transplant patients has been reported to be 14.4 cases/100 000 with a possible association to the use of mycophenolic acid [68]. However, no cases of post-transplant PML associated with rituximab have been reported. In a careful post-transplant monitoring program, Kamar *et al.* noted four cases of JC viremia out of 73 patients (5.5 %) [69]. All had also received T-cell-depleting drugs. None, however, developed PML.

Impact on in vivo immune responses

Despite the profound effect on B cells, studies analyzing its effect on the immune response lagged significantly behind those determining efficacy. Rituximab had little effect on circulating T cells or ex vivo T cell reactivity in humans [26, 45, 70]. There has been consistently reported preservation of protective antibody titers to such antigens as tetanus and measles. In one study, rituximab decreased antibody responses of lymphoma patients to recall antigens [71]. A similar report showed decreased primary and secondary antibody responses to keyhole limpet hemocyanin (KLH) in baboons [72]. Oren *et al.* [73], studying patients who had received rituximab for treatment of RA, found that the response to influenza virus vaccine was significantly lower among rituximab-treated patients, but that treatment with rituximab did not preclude administration of vaccination against influenza. We demonstrated profound inhibition in humans to the neoantigen phiX174 shortly after rituximab dosing with preservation, after B cell recovery to tetanus toxoid as a recall antigen [74]. We have recently completed a study immunizing type 1 diabetes patients after rituximab treatment versus control [27] (and Pescovitz *et al.* unpublished results). The patients were given four doses of rituximab and then immunized with a neoantigen (phiX174) when depleted and then again at 1 year after nearly complete B cell recovery. At the time of B cell recovery, the patients were also treated immunized with Td (tetanus/diphtheria) as recall antigens and with hepatitis A as another de novo immune response. As we found with the renal failure patients [74], antibody response to phiX174

was nearly completely suppressed at the time of B cell depletion. With recovery of B cells, responses to all immunizations had recovered, albeit not completely back to normal. This indicates that tolerance was not induced in this model and that memory B cells were completely deleted.

Animal models

Typically, an animal model is developed prior to the use of a drug in humans. The reverse is true with rituximab. Rituximab reacts only with human and cynomolgus macaque CD20 antigen. For example, Liu *et al.* [75] reported on a successful induction immunotherapy protocol consisting of rabbit antithymocyte globulin and rituximab in islet allograft survival in cynomolgus macaques combined with rapamycin monotherapy. Therefore, there were no major preclinical models. Furthermore, at the time that rituximab was initially developed, there were no anti-murine CD20 antibodies. These deficiencies have been remedied. Human-CD20 transgenic mouse strains were developed independently by Gong *et al.* [19] and Hu *et al.* [76]. When these animals are administered rituximab, the expressed human CD20 becomes an effective target and B cells are depleted in a manner analogous to humans treated with rituximab. Alternatively, potent anti-murine CD20 antibodies are able to deplete murine B cells [77]. Using these systems, Xiu *et al.* with anti-murine CD20 and Hu *et al.* with human CD20 transgenic treated with rituximab [76] have been able to prevent and treat diabetes in the non-obese diabetic mouse model.

Off-label rituximab use in transplant patients

As noted above, rituximab is only indicated for treatment of B cell lymphomas and rheumatoid arthritis. Despite this limited indication, rituximab has seen widespread use in organ transplant patients in several settings: (1) treatment of PTLD; (2) prevention of rejection; (3) ABO-incompatible transplantation; (4) treatment of rejection; (5)

Table 24.1 Reference review of proposed off-label uses of rituximab in solid organ transplantation.

Proposed therapy	Reference
Post-transplant lymphoma	[51, 78–96]
ABO-incompatible transplant	[32, 97–103]
Rejection prevention/treatment	[104–110]
Desensitization	[26, 48, 111, 112]
Post-transplant nephrotic syndrome	[113]

desensitization in HLA-sensitized patients; (6) treatment of nephrotic syndrome, such as focal segmental glomerulosclerosis (FSGS). A partial summary of the literature, including published abstracts, related to each of these uses is summarized in Table 24.1. The primary focus of this chapter is the use of rituximab in solid organ transplantation. However, its use in the treatment of both acute and chronic graft-versus-host disease is expanding with case reports and small series of successful outcomes [114]. As with the use in organ transplants, there is a scarcity of prospective randomized trials.

Treatment of PTLD has probably seen the greatest use of rituximab with great success, but there is no formal indication for this use [78, 79, 115]. Simple reduction in immunosuppression at the time of PTLD treatment is probably inadequate [116]. In nontransplant patients with lymphoma, rituximab is typically combined with other chemotherapeutic agents with somewhat worse results [117]. While there is fairly uniform acceptance of rituximab in the treatment of PTLD, some report less than stellar results. Choquet and coworkers using single-agent rituximab in 60 patients reported that, at 12 months after treatment, 34 of 60 patients (57%) had disease progressive with a median progression-free survival of 6.0 [118, 119]. Depending on a PTLD-specific prognostic index separated by low, intermediate, and high risk, 2-year overall survival rates were 88%, 50%, and 0% respectively.

A recent brief report of a randomized induction trial with rituximab after kidney transplantation indicated that those patients getting rituximab had an increased rate of rejection that led to early termination of the study [120]. This is in contrast to a randomized study by Tyden *et al.* where rituximab was safe and resulted in a trend to a reduced frequency of rejections [31]. Regardless, the data for induction with rituximab are not clear, and more and larger studies are warranted.

Tyden's group has a very large experience with rituximab in ABO-incompatible kidney transplantation including as part of a randomized trial [31]. Fifteen ABO-incompatible kidney recipients had the same patient and graft survival as 27 compatible patients [121].

Although not a randomized trial, Kaposztas *et al.* reported a large group of patients treated with rituximab for AMR over a 5 year period [122]. This study included 26 patients who received plasmapheresis with rituximab and 28 patients who had plasmapheresis alone. The 2-year graft survival for patients receiving the combined treatment was 90%, significantly better than only getting pheresis (60%) ($p=0.005$). With multivariate analysis rituximab use was the most significant factor ($p=0.009$) for improved graft survival. Mulley *et al.* also reported success with a single 500 mg dose of rituximab [42]. While most of the use of rituximab has been for acute antibody rejection, Fehr *et al.* reported four cases with chronic rejection successfully treated with a combination of IvIg and rituximab [123].

The initial use of rituximab as an agent to reduce alloantibody was as a single agent in a small dose-escalation trial [26]. At the time this study was designed and conducted, there was only limited information on the safety of rituximab, so that it primarily focused on pharmacokinetics, pharmacodynamics, and safety as part of a Phase 1 dose-escalation study. Despite this, there was some noticeable impact on alloantibody, with one patient successfully receiving a transplant. Subsequent studies were of limited success, indicating that rituximab immunotherapy has limited value in reduction in alloantibody, perhaps from the lack of impact on long-lived plasma cells [124]. Combination treatment, however, appears to be substantially more effective. Vo *et al.* combined IvIg with rituximab in 20 sensitized renal transplant candidates. They were able to transplant 18 of these [125]. The combined effect may result from the elimination of plasma cells by the IvIg through Fc receptor cross-linking [126]. The rituximab contributes by preventing further recruitment of allospecific B cells.

The efficacy of rituximab in the treatment of FSGS has been variable. We initially reported success in the treatment of post-transplant recurrence [127]. Dello Strologo *et al.* reported success in six cases out of seven [128]. Hickson *et al.* noted that those patients treated with the combination of rituximab and plasmapheresis was the only group with long-term response [129]. Others, such as Yabu *et al.* [130] and Rodríguez-Ferrero *et al.* [131], each with four cases, reported that rituximab was not beneficial. Until the complete pathophysiology of FSGS is elucidated it will be difficult to predict responders.

Mode of action in clinical use

Rituximab clearly depletes B cells, and while this is the mode of action in lymphoma, where the target lymphoma cells are eliminated by rituximab, it is unclear how it works in these various off-label uses. If one allows that the positive results were seen because of rituximab and not in spite of it, then the mechanism must be established. There are three potential, and not necessarily mutually exclusive, mechanisms.

First, rituximab may be acting as a nonspecific IvIg [132]. While the clinically used dose might seem too low to see an effect, IvIg and a humanized monoclonal antibody inhibit anaphylatoxin-C3a and -C5a respectively. IvIg blocked induced calcium responses in vitro and blocked cellular migration and lethal C5a-mediated circulatory effects in vivo

in mice and pigs [133] at a concentration of 10 mg/mL, a concentration that is easily surpassed at the peak of a rituximab infusion [26]. Ecalizumab, however, directly inhibits ongoing rejection [134].

Second, rituximab may deplete specific antidonor antibody. In our own study of nine sensitized dialysis patients treated with single doses of rituximab, there was some change in panel reactive antibody 7/9 (78%) [26]. In a more detailed analysis using single antigen beads, we found that specificities with lower titers were more likely to fall after rituximab treatment [111]. Such an effect, however, is not likely as an explanation of the reported efficacy in treatment of rejection, because of the relatively rapid response noted in those patients treated with rituximab. With a half-life of 21 days, to eliminate 99% of circulating specific antibody would require at least 4 months, and this only if antibody production completely and immediately ceased with rituximab. Since antibodies are made primarily by plasma cells that have minimal expression of CD20 and, therefore, are not eliminated by rituximab, such a mechanism is further questioned. As noted above, this may explain the success with the combination of IvIg and rituximab.

Third, rituximab may be acting by eliminating B cells. B cells are very efficient antigen-presenting cells, particularly after they have been activated [135, 136]. Such activation could occur at the time of rejection. The rapidity with which rituximab eliminates circulating and presumably tissue CD20$^+$ B cells is consistent with this mechanism of its action. The control of the rejection would occur because of loss of antigen presentation, resulting in less stimulation of T cells. However, it could include elimination of B-cell-produced cytokines that are either directly damaging to the organ or that stimulate or recruit other cells that are damaging. Supporting the direct role of B cells in rejection is the report of Sarwal *et al.* showing that CD20 gene expression was associated with worse prognosis [137]. Hippen *et al.* showed that subjects with CD20 positive rejection had worse long-term renal graft survival [138]. Of 27 patients with biopsy-proven Banff 1-A or Banff 1-B rejection in the first year after transplantation, six had CD20-positive B cell clusters in the interstitium and 21 did not. The

CD20-positive group had reduced graft survival compared with CD20-negative controls. Treatment with rituximab of a patient with such CD20 cells in the biopsy and rejection resistant to steroids and antithymocyte globulin was successful [104].

Conclusions and future directions

This renewed interest in B cells and antibodies in transplantation, and autoimmune disease, has stimulated the search for new drugs. Already, improved versions of "rituximab" [139] that might improve efficacy have been developed and are being studied. One of these, veltuzumab, has a single amino acid change in the CDR3 of the variable heavy chain (V(H)), having aspartic acid (Asp) instead of asparagine (Asn). This change leads to increased efficacy in preclinical models and clinical lymphoma cases [140, 141]. Veltuzumab is humanized, as is another anti-CD20 monoclonal antibody in clinical development for treatment of rheumatoid arthritis. This modification decreases the likelihood of development of neutralizing human antibodies against the chimeric murine portion of the molecule (HACA) and facilitates chronic dosing. Further modifications, such as increasing valency of the antigen-combining region, are being explored [142]. The lack of effect of anti-CD20 treatment on plasma cells is directing research toward other B-cell-surface proteins, such as APRIL (A PRoliferation-Inducing Ligand), transmembrane activator and CAML interactor (TACI), and BAFF that might eliminate plasma cells [19, 143, 144]. TACI-Ig has been shown to have some efficacy in a preclinical monkey model and has efficacy in the treatment of lupus [145]. This intense interest in B cells and antibody in transplant is an area that is ripe for application of carefully designed clinical trials.

References

1 Inoue K, Niesen N, Milgrom F, Albini B. Humoral transplantation antibodies play a role in protracted rejection of murine renal allografts. *Int Arch Allergy Appl Immunol* 1991;96:253–258.

2 Milgrom F. Humoral transplantation antibodies. *Transplant Proc* 1999;31:30–33.

3 Cai J, Terasaki PI. Humoral theory of transplantation: mechanism, prevention, and treatment. *Hum Immunol* 2005;66(4):334–342.

4 Nadler LM, Ritz J, Hardy R et al. A unique cell surface antigen identifying lymphoid malignancies of B cell origin. *J Clin Invest* 1981;67:134–140.

5 Einfeld DA, Brown JP, Valentine MA et al. Molecular cloning of the human B cell CD20 receptor predicts a hydrophobic protein with multiple transmembrane domains. *EMBO J* 1988;7(3):711–717.

6 Treon SP, Shima Y, Raje N et al. Interferon-γ induces CD20 expression on multiple myeloma cells via induction of Pu.1 and augments rituximab binding to myeloma cells. *Blood* 2000; 94(Suppl 1):119a.

7 Maloney DG, Liles TM, Czerwinski DK et al. Phase I clinical trial using escalating single-dose infusion of chimeric anti-CD20 monoclonal antibody (IDEC-C2B8) in patients with recurrent B-cell lymphoma. *Blood* 1994;84:2457–2466.

8 Giles FJ, Vose JM, Do KA et al. Circulating CD20 and CD52 in patients with non-Hodgkin's lymphoma or Hodgkin's disease. *Br J Haematol* 2003;123(5):850–857.

9 Li Y, Williams ME, Cousar JB et al. Rituximab-CD20 complexes are shaved from Z138 mantle cell lymphoma cells in intravenous and subcutaneous SCID mouse models. *J Immunol* 2007;179(6):4263–4271.

10 Beum PV, Kennedy AD, Williams ME et al. The shaving reaction: rituximab/CD20 complexes are removed from mantle cell lymphoma and chronic lymphocytic leukemia cells by THP-1 monocytes. *J Immunol* 2006;176(4):2600–2609.

11 Reff ME, Carner K, Chambers KS et al. Depletion of B cells in vivo by a chimeric mouse human monoclonal antibody to CD20. *Blood* 1994;83:435–445.

12 Edwards JC, Szczepanski L, Szechinski J et al. Efficacy of B-cell-targeted therapy with rituximab in patients with rheumatoid arthritis. *N Engl J Med* 2004; 350(25):2572–2581.

13 Du J, Wang H, Zhong C et al. Structural basis for recognition of CD20 by therapeutic antibody Rituximab. *J Biol Chem* 2007;282(20):15073–15080.

14 Maloney DG, Smith B, Appelbaum FR. The anti-tumor effect of monoclonal anti-CD20 antibody (mAb) therapy includes direct anti-proliferative activity and induction of apoptosis in CD20 positive non-Hodgkin's lymphoma (NHL) cell lines. *Blood* 1996;88(Suppl 1):637.

15 Eeva J, Nuutinen U, Ropponen A et al. The involvement of mitochondria and the caspase-9 activation

pathway in rituximab-induced apoptosis in FL cells. *Apoptosis* 2009;14(5):687–698.

16 Anolik JH, Campbell D, Felgar RE *et al.* The relationship of FcgammaRIIIa genotype to degree of B cell depletion by rituximab in the treatment of systemic lupus erythematosus. *Arthritis Rheum* 2003;48(2):455–459.

17 Weng WK, Levy R. Two immunoglobulin G fragment C receptor polymorphisms independently predict response to rituximab in patients with follicular lymphoma. *J Clin Oncol* 2003;21:3940–3947.

18 Paiva M, Marques H, Martins A, Ferreira P, Catarino R, Medeiros R. FcgammaRIIa polymorphism and clinical response to rituximab in non-Hodgkin lymphoma patients. *Cancer Genet Cytogenet* 2008;183(1):35–40.

19 Gong Q, Ou Q, Ye S *et al.* Importance of cellular microenvironment and circulatory dynamics in B cell immunotherapy. *J Immunol* 2005;174(2):817–826.

20 Pillai S, Cariappa A, Moran ST. Marginal zone B cells. *Annu Rev Immunol* 2005;23:161–196.

21 Goodyear CS, Silverman GJ. B cell superantigens: a microbe's answer to innate-like B cells and natural antibodies. *Springer Semin Immunopathol* 2005;26(4):463–484.

22 Qian J-H, Hashimoto T, Fujiwara H, Hamaoka T. Studies on the induction of tolerance to alloantigens I. The abrogation of potentials for delayed-type-hypersensitivity responses to alloantigens by portal venous inoculation with allogeneic cells. *J Immunol* 1985;134(6):3656–3661.

23 Tobinai K, Kobahashi Y, Narabayashi M *et al.* Feasibility and pharmacokinetic study of a chimeric anti-CD20 monoclonal antibody (IDEC-C2B8, rituximab) in relapsed B-cell lymphoma. *Ann Oncol* 1998;9:527–534.

24 Edwards JC, Leandro MJ, Cambridge G. B lymphocyte depletion therapy with rituximab in rheumatoid arthritis. *Rheum Dis Clin North Am* 2004;30(2):393–403, viii.

25 Ng CM, Bruno R, Combs D, Davies B. Population pharmacokinetics of rituximab (anti-CD20 monoclonal antibody) in rheumatoid arthritis patients during a Phase II clinical trial. *J Clin Pharmacol* 2005;45(7):792–801.

26 Vieira CA, Agarwal A, Book BK *et al.* Rituximab for reduction of anti-HLA antibodies in patients awaiting renal transplantation: 1. Safety, pharmacodynamics, and pharmacokinetics. *Transplantation* 2004;77(4):542–548.

27 Pescovitz MD, Greenbaum CJ, Krause-Steinrauf H *et al.* Rituximab, B-lymphocyte depletion and preservation of beta-cell function. *N Engl J Med* 2009;361(22):2143–2152.

28 Blasco H, Lalmanach G, Godat E *et al.* Evaluation of a peptide ELISA for the detection of rituximab in serum. *J Immunol Methods* 2007;325(1–2):127–139.

29 Cartron G, Blasco H, Paintaud G *et al.* Pharmacokinetics of rituximab and its clinical use: thought for the best use? *Crit Rev Oncol Hematol* 2007;62(1):43–52.

30 McLaughlin P, Grillo-Lopez A, Link BK *et al.* Rituximab chimeric anti-CD20 monoclonal antibody therapy for relapsed indolent lymphoma: half of patients respond to a four-dose treatment program. *J Clin Oncol* 1998;16:2825–2833.

31 Tyden G, Genberg H, Tollemar J *et al.* A randomized, doubleblind, placebo-controlled, study of single-dose rituximab as induction in renal transplantation. *Transplantation* 2009;87(9):1325–1329.

32 Tyden G, Kumlien G, Genberg H *et al.* ABO incompatible kidney transplantations without splenectomy, using antigen-specific immunoadsorption and rituximab. *Am J Transplant* 2005;5(1):145–148.

33 Sidner RA, Book BK, Agarwal A *et al.* In vivo human B-cell subset recovery after in vivo depletion with rituximab, anti-human CD20 monoclonal antibody. *Hum Antibodies* 2004;13(3):55–62.

34 Roll P, Palanichamy A, Kneitz C *et al.* Regeneration of B cell subsets after transient B cell depletion using anti-CD20 antibodies in rheumatoid arthritis. *Arthritis Rheum* 2006;54(8):2377–2386.

35 Cioc AM, Vanderwerf SM, Peterson BA *et al.* Rituximab-induced changes in hematolymphoid tissues found at autopsy. *Am J Clin Pathol* 2008;130(4):604–612.

36 Thaunat O, Patey N, Gautreau C *et al.* B cell survival in intragraft tertiary lymphoid organs after rituximab therapy. *Transplantation* 2008;85(11):1648–1653.

37 Steinmetz OM, Lange-Husken F, Turner JE *et al.* Rituximab removes intrarenal B cell clusters in patients with renal vascular allograft rejection. *Transplantation* 2007;84(7):842–850.

38 Genberg H, Hansson A, Wernerson A *et al.* Pharmacodynamics of rituximab in kidney allotransplantation. *Am J Transplant* 2006;6(10):2418–2428.

39 Toki D, Ishida H, Horita S *et al.* Impact of low-dose rituximab on splenic B cells in ABO-incompatible renal transplant recipients. *Transpl Int* 2009;22(4):447–454.

40 Ghielmini M, Rufibach K, Salles G *et al.* Single agent rituximab in patients with follicular or mantle cell lymphoma: clinical and biological factors that are predictive of response and event-free survival as well as the effect of rituximab on the immune system: a study of the Swiss Group for Clinical Cancer Research (SAKK). *Ann Oncol* 2005;16:1675–1682.

41 Emery P, Filipowicz-Sosnowska A, Szczepanski L *et al.* Primary analysis of a double-blind, placebo-controlled,

dose-ranging trial of rituximab, an anti-CD20 monoclonal antibody, in patients with rheumatoid arthritis receiving methotrexate (DANCER trial). *Ann Rheum Dis* 2005;64(Suppl III):434.

42 Mulley WR, Hudson FJ, Tait BD *et al*. A single low-fixed dose of rituximab to salvage renal transplants from refractory antibody-mediated rejection. *Transplantation* 2009;87(2):286–289.

43 Book BK, Agarwal A, Milgrom AB *et al*. New cross-match technique eliminates interference by humanized and chimeric monoclonal antibodies. *Transplant Proc* 2005;37(2):640–642.

44 Bearden CM, Book BK, Sidner RA, Pescovitz MD. Removal of therapeutic anti-lymphocyte antibodies from human sera prior to anti-human leukocyte antibody testing. *J Immunol Methods* 2005;300(1–2):192–199.

45 Agarwal A, Vieira CA, Book BK, Sidner RA, Fineberg NS, Pescovitz MD. Rituximab, anti-CD20, induces in vivo cytokine release but does not impair ex vivo T-cell responses. *Am J Transplant* 2004;4(8):1357–1360.

46 Edwards JC, Cambridge G. Sustained improvement in rheumatoid arthritis following a protocol designed to deplete B-lymphocytes. *Rheumatology* 2001;40:205–211.

47 Leandro MJ, Edwards JC, Cambridge G. Clinical outcome in 22 patients with rheumatoid arthritis treated with B lymphocyte depletion. *Ann Rheum Dis* 2002; 61:883–888.

48 Balfour IC, Fiore A, Graff RJ, Knutsen AP. Use of rituximab to decrease panel-reactive antibodies. *J Heart Lung Transplant* 2005;24(5):628–630.

49 Pescovitz MD, Breen N, Book BK *et al*. OKT3 treatment of acute renal allograft rejection in children. *Clin Transplant* 1992;6:184–190.

50 Genberg H, Hansson A, Wernerson A, Tyden G. Effective B-cell depletion in peripheral blood and tissue by single-dose rituximab in kidney transplant recipients: a pilot study. *Am J Transplant* 2005;5(Suppl 11):397.

51 Verschuuren EA, Stevens SJ, van Imhoff GW *et al*. Treatment of posttransplant lymphoproliferative disease with rituximab: the remission, the relapse, and the complication. *Transplantation* 2002;73:100–104.

52 Marotte H, Paintaud G, Watier H, Miossec P. Rituximab-related late-onset neutropenia in a patient with severe rheumatoid arthritis. *Ann Rheum Dis* 2008;67(6):893–894.

53 Cattaneo C, Spedini P, Casari S *et al*. Delayed-onset peripheral blood cytopenia after rituximab: frequency and risk factor assessment in a consecutive series of 77 treatments. *Leuk Lymphoma* 2006;47(6):1013–1017.

54 Terrier B, Ittah M, Tourneur L *et al*. Late-onset neutropenia following rituximab results from a hematopoietic

lineage competition due to anexcessive BAFF-induced B-cell recovery. *Haematologica* 2007;92:ECR10.

55 Grim SA, Pham T, Thielke J *et al*. Infectious complications associated with the use of rituximab for ABO-incompatible and positive cross-match renal transplant recipients. *Clin Transplant* 2007;21(5):628–632.

56 Kamar N, Milioto O, Puissant-Lubrano B *et al*. Incidence and predictive factors for infectious disease after rituximab therapy in kidney-transplant patients. *Am J Transplant* 2010;10(1):89–98.

57 Suzan F, Ammor M, Ribrag V. Fatal reactivation of cytomegalovirus infection after use of rituximab for a post-transplantation lymphoproliferative disorder. *N Engl J Med* 2001;345(13):1000.

58 Nishida H, Ishida H, Tanaka T *et al*. Cytomegalovirus infection following renal transplantation in patients administered low-dose rituximab induction therapy. *Transpl Int* 2009;22(10):961–969.

59 Vianna RM, Mangus RS, Fridell JA *et al*. Induction immunosuppression with thymoglobulin and rituximab in intestinal and multivisceral transplantation. *Transplantation* 2008;85(9):1290–1293.

60 Tsutsumi Y, Kanamori H, Mori A *et al*. Reactivation of hepatitis B virus with rituximab. *Expert Opin Drug Saf* 2005;4(3):599–608.

61 Pei SN, Chen CH, Lee CM *et al*. Reactivation of hepatitis B virus following rituximab-based regimens: a serious complication in both HBsAg-positive and HBsAg-negative patients. *Ann Hematol* 2010;89(3):255–262.

62 Roccatello D, Baldovino S, Rossi D *et al*. Long-term effects of anti-CD20 monoclonal antibody treatment of cryoglobulinaemic glomerulonephritis. *Nephrol Dial Transplant* 2004;19(12):3054–3061.

63 Da Silva Fucuta Pereira P, Lemos LB, de Oliveira Uehara SN *et al*. Long-term efficacy of rituximab in hepatitis C virus-associated cryoglobulinemia. *Rheumatol Int* 2010;30(11):1515–1518.

64 Agarwal A, Sidner RA, Fridell JA *et al*. Immunomodulatory impact of rituximab and thymoglobuin therapy in liver transplantation. *Am J Transplant* 2005;5(Suppl 11):1239.

65 Garcia-Suarez J, de Miguel D, Krsnik I *et al*. Changes in the natural history of progressive multifocal leukoencephalopathy in HIV-negative lymphoproliferative disorders: impact of novel therapies. *Am J Hematol* 2005; 80(4):271–281.

66 Koralnik IJ. Overview of the cellular immunity against JC virus in progressive multifocal leukoencephalopathy. *J Neurovirol* 2002;8(Suppl 2):59–65.

67 Harris HE. Progressive multifocal leucoencephalopathy in a patient with systemic lupus erythematosus treated

with rituximab. *Rheumatology (Oxford)* 2008;47(2):224–225.

68 Neff RT, Hurst FP, Falta EM *et al*. Progressive multifocal leukoencephalopathy and use of mycophenolate mofetil after kidney transplantation. *Transplantation* 2008;86(10):1474–1478.

69 Kamar N, Mengelle C, Rostaing L. Incidence of JC-virus replication after rituximab therapy in solid-organ transplant patients. *Am J Transplant* 2009;9(1):244–245.

70 Saville MW, Benyunes MC, Multani PS. No clinical evidence for CD4+ cell depletion caused by rituximab. *Blood* 2003;102(1):408; author reply 408–409.

71 Van der Kolk LE, Baars JW, Prins MH, van Oers MHJ. Rituximab treatment results in impaired secondary humoral immune responsiveness. *Blood* 2002;100(6):2257–2259.

72 Gonzalez-Stawinski GV, Yu PB, Love SD *et al*. Hapten-induced primary and memory humoral responses are inhibited by the infusion of anti-CD20 monoclonal antibody (IDEC-C2B8, rituximab). *Clin Immunol* 2001;98(2):175–179.

73 Oren S, Mandelboim M, Braun-Moscovici Y *et al*. Vaccination against influenza in patients with rheumatoid arthritis: the effect of rituximab on the humoral response. *Ann Rheum Dis* 2008;67(7):937–941.

74 Bearden CM, Agarwal A, Book BK *et al*. Rituximab inhibits the in vivo primary and secondary antibody response to a neoantigen, bacteriophage phiX174. *Am J Transplant* 2005;5(1):50–57.

75 Liu C, Noorchashm H, Sutter JA *et al*. B lymphocyte-directed immunotherapy promotes long-term islet allograft survival in nonhuman primates. *Nat Med* 2007;13(11):1295–1298.

76 Hu CY, Rodriguez-Pinto D, Du W *et al*. Treatment with CD20-specific antibody prevents and reverses autoimmune diabetes in mice. *J Clin Invest* 2007;117(12):3857–3867.

77 Xiu Y, Wong CP, Bouaziz JD *et al*. B lymphocyte depletion by CD20 monoclonal antibody prevents diabetes in nonobese diabetic mice despite isotype-specific differences in Fc gamma R effector functions. *J Immunol* 2008;180(5):2863–2875.

78 Shimabukuro-Vornhagen A, Hallek MJ, Storb RF, von Bergwelt-Baildon MS. The role of B cells in the pathogenesis of graft-versus-host disease. *Blood* 2009;114(24):4919–4927.

79 Norin S, Kimby E, Ericzon BG *et al*. Posttransplant lymphoma – a single-center experience of 500 liver transplantations. *Med Oncol* 2004;21(3):273–284.

80 Caillard S, Pessione F, Moulin B, French PTLD Working Group. Post-transplant lymphoproliferative disorders (PTLD) in kidney transplantation: report of 220 cases of a French registry. *Am J Transplant* 2005;5(Suppl 11):360.

81 Blaes AH, Peterson BA, Bartlett N *et al*. Rituximab therapy is effective for posttransplant lymphoproliferative disorders after solid organ transplantation: results of a phase II trial. *Cancer* 2005;104(8):1661–1667.

82 Swinnen LJ, LeBlanc M, Grogan TM *et al*. Prospective study of sequential reduction in immunosuppression, interferon alpha-2B, and chemotherapy for posttransplantation lymphoproliferative disorder. *Transplantation* 2008;86(2):215–222.

83 Tobinai K. Rituximab and other emerging monoclonal antibody therapies for lymphoma. *Expert Opin Emerg Drugs* 2002;7(2):289–302.

84 Choquet S, Leblond V, Herbrecht R *et al*. Efficacy and safety of rituximab in B-cell post-transplantation lymphoproliferative disorders: results of a prospective multicenter Phase 2 study. *Blood* 2006;107(8):3053–3057.

85 Choquet S, Oertel S, LeBlond V *et al*. Rituximab in the management of post-transplantation lymphoproliferative disorder after solid organ transplantation: proceed with caution. *Ann Hematol* 2007;86(8):599–607.

86 Clatworthy MR, Watson CJ, Plotnek G *et al*. B-cell-depleting induction therapy and acute cellular rejection. *N Engl J Med* 2009;360(25):2683–2685.

87 Tyden G, Donauer J, Wadstrom J *et al*. Implementation of a protocol for ABO-incompatible kidney transplantation – a three-center experience with 60 consecutive transplantations. *Transplantation* 2007;83(9):1153–1155.

88 Kaposztas Z, Podder H, Mauiyyedi S *et al*. Impact of rituximab therapy for treatment of acute humoral rejection. *Clin Transplant* 2009;23(1):63–73.

89 Fehr T, Rusi B, Fischer A *et al*. Rituximab and intravenous immunoglobulin treatment of chronic antibody-mediated kidney allograft rejection. *Transplantation* 2009;87(12):1837–1841.

90 Slifka MK, Ahmed R. Long-lived plasma cells: a mechanism for maintaining persistent antibody production. *Curr Opin Immunol* 1998;10:252–258.

91 Vo AA, Lukovsky M, Toyoda M *et al*. Rituximab and intravenous immune globulin for desensitization during renal transplantation. *N Engl J Med* 2008;359(3):242–251.

92 Xiang Z, Cutler AJ, Brownlie RJ *et al*. FcγRIIb controls bone marrow plasma cell persistence and apoptosis. *Nat Immunol* 2007;8(4):419–429.

93 Pescovitz MD, Book BK, Sidner RA. Resolution of recurrent focal segmental glomerulosclerosis proteinuria after rituximab treatment. *N Engl J Med* 2006;354(18):1961–1963.

94 Dello Strologo L, Guzzo I, Laurenzi C *et al*. Use of rituximab in focal glomerulosclerosis relapses after renal transplantation. *Transplantation* 2009;88(3): 417–420.

95 Hickson LJ, Gera M, Amer H *et al*. Kidney transplantation for primary focal segmental glomerulosclerosis: outcomes and response to therapy for recurrence. *Transplantation* 2009;87(8):1232–1239.

96 Yabu JM, Ho B, Scandling JD, Vincenti F. Rituximab failed to improve nephrotic syndrome in renal transplant patients with recurrent focal segmental glomerulosclerosis. *Am J Transplant* 2008;8(1):222–227.

97 Rodriguez-Ferrero M, Ampuero J, Anaya F. Rituximab and chronic plasmapheresis therapy of nephrotic syndrome in renal transplantation patients with recurrent focal segmental glomerulosclerosis. *Transplant Proc* 2009;41(6):2406–2408.

98 Luke PP, Scantlebury VP, Jordan ML *et al*. Reversal of steroid- and anti-lymphocyte antibody-resistant rejection using intravenous immunoglobulin (IVIG) in renal transplant recipients. *Transplantation* 2001; 72:419–422.

99 Basta M, van Goor F, Luccioli S *et al*. F(ab)′₂-mediated neutralization of C3a and C5a anaphylatoxins: a novel effector function of immunoglobulins. *Nat Med* 2003;9:431–438.

100 Locke JE, Magro CM, Singer AL *et al*. The use of antibody to complement protein C5 for salvage treatment of severe antibody-mediated rejection. *Am J Transplant* 2009;9(1):231–235.

101 Pescovitz MD, Book BK, Rahman A *et al*. Measurement of HLA antibody specificity by single antigen beads and MESF quatitation demonstrates efficacy of rituximab desensitization. *Am J Transplant* 2005;5(Suppl 11):324.

102 Lapointe R, Bellemare-Pelletier A, Housseau F *et al*. CD40-stimulated B lymphocytes pulsed with tumor antigens are effective antigen-presenting cells that can generate specific T cells. *Cancer Res* 2003;63:2836–2843.

103 Rivera A, Chen CC, Ron N *et al*. Role of B cells as antigen-presenting cells in vivo revisited: antigen-specific B cells are essential for T cell expansion in lymph nodes and for systemic T cell responses to low antigen concentrations. *Int Immunol* 2001;13: 1583–1593.

104 Sarwal M, Chua MS, Kambham N *et al*. Molecular heterogeneity in acute renal allograft rejection identified by DNA microarray profiling. *N Engl J Med* 2003;349:125–138.

105 Hippen BE, DeMattos A, Cook WJ *et al*. Association of CD20⁺ infiltrates with poorer clinical outcomes in acute cellular rejection of renal allografts. *Am J Transplant* 2005;5(9):2248–2252.

106 Alausa M, Almagro U, Siddiqi N *et al*. Refractory acute kidney transplant rejection with CD20 graft infiltrates and successful therapy with rituximab. *Clin Transplant* 2005;19(1):137–140.

107 Vugmeyster Y, Beyer J, Howell K *et al*. Depletion of B cells by a humanized anti-CD20 antibody PRO70769 in *Macaca fascicularis*. *J Immunother* 2005;28(3):212–219.

108 Goldenberg DM, Rossi EA, Stein R *et al*. Properties and structure-function relationships of veltuzumab (hA20), a humanized anti-CD20 monoclonal antibody. *Blood* 2009;113(5):1062–1070.

Morschhauser F, Leonard JP, Fayad L *et al*. Humanized anti-CD20 antibody, veltuzumab, in refractory/recurrent non-Hodgkin's lymphoma: Phase I/II results. *J Clin Oncol* 2009;27(20):3346–3353.

109 Rossi EA, Goldenberg DM, Cardillo TM *et al*. Novel designs of multivalent anti-CD20 humanized antibodies as improved lymphoma therapeutics. *Cancer Res* 2008;68(20):8384–8392.

110 Schneider P. The role of APRIL and BAFF in lymphocyte activation. *Curr Opin Immunol* 2005;17(3):282–289.

111 Peter HH, Warnatz K. Molecules involved in T–B co-stimulation and B cell homeostasis: possible targets for an immunological intervention in autoimmunity. *Expert Opin Biol Ther* 2005;5(Suppl 1):S61–S71.

112 Pena-Rossi C, Nasonov E, Stanislav M *et al*. An exploratory dose-escalating study investigating the safety, tolerability, pharmacokinetics and pharmacodynamics of intravenous atacicept in patients with systemic lupus erythematosus. *Lupus* 2009;18(6):547–555.

113 Milpied N, Vasseur B, Parquet N *et al*. Humanized anti-CD20 monoclonal antibody (rituximab) in post transplant B-lymphoproliferative disorder: a retrospective analysis on 32 patients. *Ann Oncol* 2000; 11(Suppl 1):113–116.

114 Culic S, Culic VV, Armanda V *et al*. Anti-CD20 monoclonal antibody (rituximab) for therapy of mediastinal CD20-positive large B-cell non-Hodgkin lymphoma with a local tumor extension into the lung of a 10-year-old girl. *Pediatr Hematol Oncol* 2003;20:339–344.

115 Bueno J, Ramil C, Somoza I *et al*. Treatment of monomorphic B-cell lymphoma with rituximab after liver transplantation in a child. *Pediatr Transplant* 2003;7:153–156.

116 Herman J, Vandenberghe P, van den Heuvel I *et al*. Successful treatment with rituximab of lymphoproliferative disorder in a child after cardiac transplantation. *J Heart Lung Transplant* 2002;21:1304–1309.

117 Berney T, Delis S, Kato T *et al*. Successful treatment of posttransplant lymphoproliferative disease with prolonged rituximab treatment in intestinal transplant recipients. *Transplantation* 2002;74:1000–1006.

118 Serinet MO, Jacquemin E, Habes D *et al*. Anti-CD20 monoclonal antibody (rituximab) treatment for Epstein–Barr virus-associated, B-cell lymphoproliferative disease in pediatric liver transplant recipients. *J Pediatr Gastroenterol Nutr* 2002;34:389–393.

119 Webber SA, Fine RN, McGhee W *et al*. Anti-CD20 monoclonal antibody (rituximab) for pediatric post-transplant lymphoproliferative disorders: a preliminary multicenter experience. *Am J Transplant* 2001; 1(Suppl 1):469.

120 Chen LJ, Nepomuceno RR, Beatty PR *et al*. CD20 ligation using rituximab (anti-CD20 monoclonal antibody) inhibits growth of EBV infected B cells from a patient with PTLD. *Transplantation* 2000;69(Suppl):S331.

121 Roithmann S, Bonamigo-Filho JL, Neumann J *et al*. Anti-CD20 monoclonal antibody (rituximab) for post-transplant lymphoproliferative disease treatment (PTLD). *Blood* 2000;96:246b.

122 Zilz ND, Olson LJ, McGregor CG. Treatment of posttransplant lymphoproliferative disorder with monoclonal CD20 antibody (rituximab) after heart transplantation. *J Heart Lung Transplant* 2001;20: 770–772.

123 Dotti G, Rambaldi A, Frocchi R *et al*. Anti-CD20 antibody rituximab administration in patients with late-occurring lymphomas after solid organ transplant. *Haematologica* 2001;86:618–623.

124 Horwitz SM, Tsai D, Twist C *et al*. Rituximab is effective therapy for post-transplant lymphoproliferative disorder (PTLD) not responding to reduction in immunosuppression: a prospective trial in adults and children. *Proc Am Soc Clin Oncol* 2001;20:284a.

125 Ganjoo J, Green M, Sindhi R *et al*. Lymphocyte subsets may discern treatment effects in children with post-transplant lymphoproliferative disorder (PTLD). *Am J Transplant* 2001;1(Suppl 1):287.

126 Mazariegos GV, McGhee W, Sindhi R, Reyes J. Thymoglobulin (T) in the management of steroid resistant acute cellular rejection (SRACR) in children. *Am J Transplant* 2001;1(Suppl 1):311.

127 Pescovitz MD. The use of rituximab, anti-CD20 monoclonal antibody, in pediatric transplantation. *Pediatr Transplant* 2004;8(1):9–21.

128 Oertel SH, Verschuuren E, Reinke P *et al*. Effect of anti-CD 20 antibody rituximab in patients with post-transplant lymphoproliferative disorder (PTLD). *Am J Transplant* 2005;5(12):2901–2906.

129 Choquet S, Leblond V, Herbrecht R *et al*. Efficacy and safety of rituximab in B-cell post-transplant lymphoproliferative disorders: results of a prospective multicentre Phase II study. *Blood* 2006;107(8):3053–3057.

130 Kawagishi N, Satoh K, Enomoto Y *et al*. New strategy for ABO-incompatible living donor liver transplantation with anti-CD20 antibody (rituximab) and plasma exchange. *Transplant Proc* 2005;37(2):1205–1206.

131 Sonnenday CJ, Warren DS, Cooper M *et al*. Plasmapheresis, CMV hyperimmune globulin, and anti-CD20 allow ABO-incompatible renal transplantation without splenectomy. *Am J Transplant* 2004; 4(8):1315–1322.

132 Sawada T, Fuchinoue S, Kawase T *et al*. Preconditioning regimen consisting of anti-CD20 monoclonal antibody infusions, splenectomy and DFPP-enabled non-responders to undergo ABO-incompatible kidney transplantation. *Clin Transplant* 2004;18(3):254–260.

133 Usuda M, Fujimori K, Koyamada N *et al*. Successful use of anti-CD20 monoclonal antibody (rituximab) for ABO-incompatible living-related liver transplantation. *Transplantation* 2005;79(1):12–16.

134 Segev DL, Simpkins CE, Warren DS *et al*. ABO Incompatible high-titer renal transplantation without splenectomy or anti-CD20 treatment. *Am J Transplant* 2005;5(10):2570–2575.

135 Koyama I, Fuchinoue S, Kai K *et al*. Successful ABO-incompatible kidney transplantation for non-responders with the use of anti-CD20 monoclonal antibody and plasmapheresis. *Am J Transplant* 2005;5 (Suppl 11):183.

136 Diaz A, Thielke J, Pham T *et al*. Successful kidney transplant in ABO incompatible patients after plasmapheresis and thymoglobulin under a steroid avoidance protocol. *Am J Transplant* 2005; 5(Suppl 11):324–325.

137 Gloor J, Moore S, Pineda AA *et al*. Living donor kidney transplantation in positive crossmatch patients. *Am J Transplant* 2003;3(Suppl 5):200.

138 Samaniego M, Zachary A, Lucas D *et al*. Early allograft outcomes in patients with antibody mediated rejection treated with rituximab. *Am J Transplant* 2002;2(Suppl 3):259.

139 Garrett HE, Jr, Groshart K, Duvall-Seaman D *et al*. Treatment of humoral rejection with rituximab. *Ann Thorac Surg* 2002;74:1240–1242.

140 Aranda JM, Jr, Scornik JC, Normann SJ *et al*. Anti-CD20 monoclonal antibody (rituximab) therapy for acute cardiac humoral rejection: a case report. *Transplantation* 2002;73:907–910.

141 Goldstein MJ, Lee S, Guarrera JV *et al*. Rituximab rescue for refractory antibody mediated rejection after kidney transplantation. *Am J Transplant* 2005; 5(Suppl 11):397–398.

142 Becker YT, Becker BN, Pirsch JD, Sollinger HW. Rituximab as treatment for refractory kidney transplant rejection. *Am J Transplant* 2004;4(6):996–1001.

143 Stegall MD, Moore SB, Gloor JM, von Liebig WJ. Achieving desensitization and preventing humoral rejection in positive crossmatch living donor kidney transplantation. *Am J Transplant* 2005;5(Suppl 11): 292–293.

144 Nozu K, Iijima K, Fujisawa M *et al*. Rituximab treatment for posttransplant lymphoproliferative disorder (PTLD) induces complete remission of recurrent nephrotic syndrome. *Pediatr Nephrol* 2005;20(11): 1660–1663.

CHAPTER 25

The Anti-Interleukin 2 Receptor Antibodies

Muna Alnimri and Flavio Vincenti

University of California, San Francisco, Transplant Service, San Francisco, CA, USA

Introduction

The discovery of interleukin 2 (IL-2) and its multiple receptor complex led to the development of monoclonal antibodies (mAbs) to the α chain (also referred to as CD25) component of the IL-2 receptor (IL-2R) [1]. The IL-2R can be expressed in two forms: the constitutively expressed β and the common γ chain represent the low-affinity IL-2R, while the addition of the upregulated α chain leads to the formation of the high-affinity ILR2R [1]. In preclinical development mAbs were developed to each of the ILR2R chains; however, antibodies to the α chain were eventually targeted for clinical development because of the selectivity of the α chain, which is upregulated primarily on activated T cells (obviously, CD25 expression on regulatory T cells was yet to be discovered) [2, 3]. Two anti-CD25 mAbs were selected for clinical development: basiliximab, a chimeric mAb, and daclizumab, a humanized mAb [4, 5]. While both antibodies were tested in rigorous double-blind randomized trials as induction agents, no trial was ever designed to test the relative efficacy and safety of these two mAbs head to head [6–9]. This issue, however, is not going to be relevant, since in 2010 daclizumab was withdrawn from the market.

Outcome of clinical trials

Basiliximab and daclizumab were each tested as induction agents in two parallel Phase III trials [6–9]. Both antibodies were tested in regimens that lacked mycophenolate mofetil (MMF), as it was not approved for use in transplantation at the time of the Phase III trials. When the clinical trials with anti-CD25 mAbs were initiated, acute rejection rates were in the range 40–50%. Immunosuppression regimens in these trials consisted of cyclosporine plus/minus azathioprine and steroids. While the design of the Phase III trials of the two anti-CD25 antibodies differed, they had similar endpoints: acute rejection at 6 months, patient and graft survival at 1 year. Basiliximab was administered in two doses of 20 mg IV at day 0 (day of transplant surgery) and day 4 after transplantation [8, 19]. The maintenance immunosuppression regimen consisted of cyclosporine and azathioprine. The regimen and dose of basiliximab that was selected in the Phase III trials was based on the results of the Phase II dose-finding study reported by Amlot *et al.* [5]. In the Phase II dose-finding trial, post-transplant lymphoproliferative disease (PTLD) developed in patients treated with doses of basiliximab higher than 40 mg or regimens that included azathioprine. Thus, for safety reasons, the Phase III

Immunotherapy in Transplantation: Principles and Practice, First Edition. Edited by Bruce Kaplan, Gilbert J. Burckart and Fadi G. Lakkis.

trials with basiliximab used a cumulative dose of 40 mg (20 mg dose × 2) and maintenance immunosuppression consisting of cyclosporine and prednisone. Subsequent trials using triple immunosuppression therapy with the addition of either azathioprine or MMF did not show an increase in the risk of PTLD or opportunistic infections [4, 10–12].

In Phase III trials, daclizumab was administered IV at a dose of 1 mg/kg preoperatively and every 2 weeks for a total of five doses [6, 7]. In a Phase I/II trial of daclizumab, this regimen was found to be both safe and effective and provided saturation of the CD25 receptor on circulating lymphocytes for up to 120 days [13]. Two Phase III trials with daclizumab were performed [6, 7]. In one trial the maintenance immunosuppression regimen consisted of cyclosporine, azathioprine, and steroids; in the second trial, patients were maintained on double therapy consisting of cyclosporine and prednisone. The outcome of the Phase III trials with basiliximab and daclizumab were similar: acute rejection rates in patients treated with the anti-CD25 mAbs were reduced by 30–40 % compared with placebo, with comparable patient and graft survival and no increase in opportunistic infection or PTLD. Daclizumab was approved by the Food and Drug Administration in 1997 and a year later basiliximab gained approval. The addition of MMF to maintenance immunosuppression regimens and the observation that the combination of cyclosporine–MMF and steroids or tacrolimus–MMF and steroids reduced acute rejection rates to 20 % or less in clinical trials raised the question of whether induction with the anti-CD25 antibodies was relevant in the era of more potent immunosuppression drugs. Two nonpowered trials were performed to evaluate the outcome of basiliximab and daclizumab with regimens that included a calcineurin inhibitor, MMF, and steroids [12, 14]. In both studies, the addition of the anti-CD25 mAbs resulted in numerically lower rates of acute rejection; although statistical significance could not be demonstrated, these trials were not adequately powered. While the percentage of patients receiving induction therapy in the USA has increased over the past 5 years (approximately 80 % in de novo transplant patients), the proportion receiving anti-CD25 mAbs (approximately 40 %) has decreased owing to the increasing popularity of Thymoglobulin and alemtuzumab, especially in patients with high immunologic risk profiles. Recent trials comparing Thymoglobulin with basiliximab in patients with higher immunologic risk profiles showed that Thymoglobulin was superior to basiliximab in reducing acute rejection [15, 16]. No such advantage, however, is observed in low-risk patients, who benefit from the lower risk associated with the anti-IL-2 mAbs [17–19]. Furthermore, anti-IL-2 mAb induction has also been effective in low immunologic risk patients undergoing rapid steroid withdrawal [4]. While both anti-CD25mAbs have been extensively used in clinical trials, basiliximab has emerged as the preferred antibody in clinical practice owing to ease of administration, and it is the only anti-CD25 mAb currently available for use in transplantation.

Chemistry and structure

Both daclizumab and basiliximab are identical in their specificity, although they have different structures. Basiliximab is an IgG1 chimeric mAb, 75 % human and 25 % retaining the entire murine variable region. Daclizumab is a humanized mAb, 90 % human, retaining only the murine complementarity-determining regions that bind to CD25.

Mechanism of action

The main mechanism of action of the anti-IL-2 mAbs is interference with binding of IL-2 to its receptor. The anti-IL-2R mAbs do not fix complement and do not induce measurable depletion of effector T cells [5, 20]. Basiliximab and daclizumab bind to the same epitope (the motif ERI Y HFV) compromising amino acid positions 116 to 122 within the extracellular domain of the α chain and overlap the interaction site between IL-2 and CD25

[21]. The effect of daclizumab on circulating T cells and the expression of CD25 have been analyzed in a Phase III trial [6]. Lymphocytes from 20 patients (10 in the placebo group, 10 in the daclizumab group) were compared in a blinded fashion pre-transplant and after transplantation. No significant difference in absolute lymphocyte number was found between placebo and daclizumab-treated patients at day 14 (0.9 ± 0.4 versus $1.0 \pm 0.8 \times 10^3$ mm^3) or at day 56 (1.1 ± 0.7 versus $0.9 \pm 0.5 \times 10^3$ mm^3) after transplantation. CD3 levels and T cell subsets were not affected by daclizumab therapy. The percentage of circulating lymphocytes from daclizumab-treated patients showed a significant decrease in staining with exogenous fluorescein-conjugated 2A3, an antibody that binds to the same epitope on the IL-2Rα as daclizumab, when compared with control patients. The total IL-2Rα expression was measured by staining cells with the fluorescein-conjugated antibody 7g7, which binds to an IL-2Rα epitope distinct from the epitope recognized by daclizumab. Staining for the 7g7 epitope was present but also significantly reduced in daclizumab patients compared with control patients at day 14 ($13 \pm 6\%$ versus $24 \pm 12\%$, $P=0.04$), day 56 ($9 \pm 5\%$ versus $18 \pm 10\%$, $P=0.04$), and at 4 months ($5 \pm 3\%$ versus $22 \pm 10\%$, $P=0.03$).

These findings are consistent with the proposed mechanism of action of the anti-IL-2R mAbs, having a predominantly immunomodulatory rather than depleting effect on T cells. The decrease in total IL-2R expression is likely due to antibody-bound IL-2R being internalized or shed in circulation. Similar results were reported by Amlot *et al.* in a Phase II trial with basiliximab [5]. However, marginal depletion of CDD25-positive T cells through antibody-dependent cell-mediated cytotoxicity cannot be ruled out. In fact, transient depletion of CD25$^+$ cells which express FoxP3 (the forkhead transcription factor that is a marker of T regulatory cells) has been demonstrated following therapy with basiliximab [22]. The clinical relevance of the effect of basiliximab on regulating T cells remains unclear. However, since effector CD25$^+$ cells are affected to a greater extent than regulatory cells by anti-CD25 therapy, the net balance is tilted towards immunosuppression.

Pharmacokinetics and pharmacodynamics of the anti-CD25 mAbs

Basiliximab

The pharmacokinetics of basiliximab were analyzed extensively in the Phase II and III trials [23–25]. After the first administration of basiliximab 20 mg the C_{max} range was 5.2–8.2 µg/mL and after the second dose at day 4, it was 6.9–13.1 µg/mL [23, 24]. The AUC was 104 µg/(day mL). Serum concentration of basiliximab above 0.2 µg/mL, which had been shown to result in full saturation of the IL-2R, was maintained for 36 ± 14 days (range 12–91 days) [5]. Basiliximab clearance was 36 ± 15.2 mL/h; the distribution volume was 8.0 ± 2.4 L, and the half-life was 7.4 ± 3.0 days. Gender, ethnic group, and the presence of proteinuria had no clinical relevance to basiliximab disposition. There was no apparent relationship between the incidence or day of appearance of acute rejection during CD25 saturation and basiliximab concentration (range 0.2–5.0 µg/mL) [24]. In patients who experienced a rejection episode after basiliximab was eliminated from serum, basiliximab had not been cleared faster than in their rejection-free peers ($p=0.322$) nor had CD25 been saturated for a shorter period of time (33 ± 13 days versus 37 ± 14 days for rejection-free patients, $p=0.162$) [25].

The pharmacokinetics of basiliximab were analyzed in a single-center trial in liver transplantation [26]. Patients received a 40 mg dose of basiliximab either with a regimen of 20 mg × 2 at days 0 and 4 or 10 mg × 4 at days 0, 2, 4, and 6. The higher regimen had higher C_{max} than the lower dose, and clearance was faster with the multiple-dose regimen. In pediatric renal transplant recipients the pharmacokinetics of basiliximab were similar to adults in patients aged 12–16 years. However, the dose and clearance of basiliximab were reduced by 50% in pediatric patients aged 1–11 years; thus, this age group required 50% of the adult dose [27]. A second pediatric study confirmed the decreased clearance of basiliximab in children (weight below 35 kg) treated with two doses of 10 mg of basiliximab [28]. Furthermore, concomitant therapy with

MMF reduced clearance of basiliximab and increased saturation of CD25 on circulating T cells from 5 to 10 weeks.

Daclizumab

The pharmacokinetic analysis of daclizumab was performed in the Phase III trials in patients treated with five doses of 1 mg/kg of daclizumab administered at day 0 and every 2 weeks thereafter [6, 21]. Peak and trough levels of daclizumab were obtained with the first and fifth (last) doses of daclizumab, as well as at 14 and 58 days after administration of the last dose. The population pharmacokinetic analysis indicated the half-life of daclizumab to be approximately 480 h (20 days). The volume distribution was 3 L. The five-dose regimen of daclizumab provided saturation of the circulating IL-2R for up to 120 days. Because the five-dose regimen of daclizumab was not convenient, we performed a study to evaluate the pharmacokinetics of daclizumab in a limited dosing regimen [29]. Twenty patients undergoing primary deceased donor or living donor transplantation were randomized to receive a regimen of one dose 2 mg/kg or two doses (2 mg/kg at day 0 and 1 mg/kg at day 4) of daclizumab [29]. In patients treated with one dose of daclizumab, the blood concentration declined to 1 µg/mL at 43 ± 7 days after transplantation; and following two doses of daclizumab, the blood concentration declined to 1 µg/mL at 59 ± 13 days after transplantation. In vivo daclizumab levels of 1 µg/mL or greater are associated with saturation of the IL-2Rα on circulating lymphocytes (Figure 25.1). Thus, one or two doses of daclizumab were comparable to the regimen of basiliximab in the saturation of the IL-2R. We further explored the differential effect of the anti-IL-2R mAbs on saturation of the IL-2R versus inhibition of the biological effects of anti-IL-2 mAbs. Lymphocytes obtained in the 4 day mixed-lymphocyte reaction were incubated with increasing concentrations of daclizumab. In vitro saturation of the ILR on lymphocytes was demonstrated at a daclizumab concentration of 0.1 µg/mL (Figure 25.2a). However, suppression of the mixed-lymphocyte reaction required a daclizumab concentration of 1 µg/ml (Figure 25.2b). This in vitro analysis suggests that a higher concentration of anti-CD25 mAbs may be required to block biological

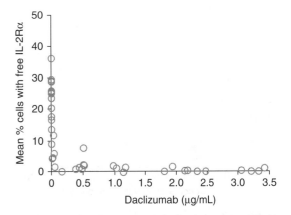

Figure 25.1 Percentage of lymphocytes with free CD25 (II-2Ra) receptors in patients treated with daclizumab.

response than simply saturating the ILR, likely related to the much higher affinity of IL-2 to the receptor compared with the anti-IL-2 mAbs. At higher levels of IL-2, increasing concentrations of daclizumab cannot displace IL-2 from binding to IL-2 and inhibit proliferation of the Kit 225 human T cells that express CD25 receptors (Figure 25.3).

Drug interactions

Since basiliximab was used in combination with double therapy (cyclosporine and prednisone), the effect of adding azathioprine or MMF on the clearance of basiliximab and duration of saturation of the IL-2R was analyzed in a study by Kovarik *et al.* [30]. Blood samples were collected over 12 weeks post-transplant from 31 patients treated with triple therapy with azathioprine and 66 patients treated with triple therapy with MMF. Empirical Bayes estimates of each patient's basiliximab disposition parameters were derived, and the duration of CD25 saturation on circulating lymphocytes was estimated as the time over which serum concentrations exceeded 0.2 µg/mL as confirmed by flow-cytometry measurements. Basiliximab clearance was 29 ± 14 mL/h when co-administered with azathioprine and 18 ± 8 mL/h with MMF. Both were significantly lower, compared with the clearance of 37 ± 15 mL/h from a previous study of basiliximab with dual therapy with cyclosporine and prednisone

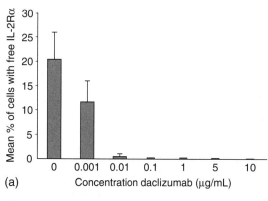 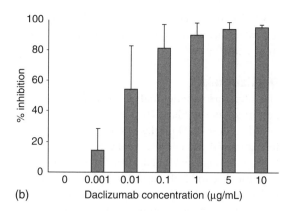

Figure 25.2 (a) Percentage of lymphocytes with free CD25 (IL-2Ra) in 4-day mixed-lymphocyte reaction in the presence of daclizumab. (b) The inhibitory effect of daclizumab on mixed-lymphocyte reaction.

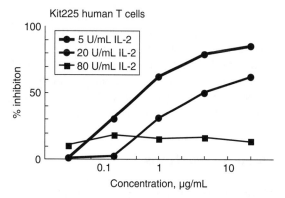

Figure 25.3 Inhibition of IL-2-dependent proliferation in vitro is dependent on IL-2 concentrations. Figure courtesy of John Hakimi.

($p < 0.001$). As a consequence of the lower clearance of basiliximab, the durations of CD25 saturation were prolonged in the presence of azathioprine (50 ± 20 days; range, 13–84 days) and MMF (59 ± 17 days; range, 28–94 days) compared with dual therapy (36 ± 14 days; range, 12–91 days). The average duration of CD25 saturation was prolonged by 39% and 64% in the presence of azathioprine and MMF respectively. Similar results were noted in pediatric patients when basiliximab was combined with MMF [29]. Whether a blunted humoral response to basiliximab (i.e., neutralizing anti-idiopathic antibodies) with azathioprine or MMF accounts for the reduced clearance of basiliximab or a direct drug–drug interaction is unclear.

Conclusion

The anti-IL-2R mAbs provide moderate but safe immunosuppression as induction agents in all patients except patients at high immunologic risk. Acute rejection episodes during anti-CD25 mAb therapy are not associated with failure of saturation of the α chain on circulating T cells. The anti-CD25 mAbs are the only class of immunosuppressive agents that is not associated with increase in PTLD or opportunistic infections.

References

1 Waldmann TA. The IL-2/IL2 receptor system: a target for rational immune intervention. *Immunol Today* 1993; 14:264–270.
2 Kirkman RL, Barrett LV, Gaulton GN *et al.* Administration of an anti-interleukin 2 receptor monoclonal antibody prolongs allograft survival in mice. *J Exp Med* 1985;162:358–362.
3 Reed MH, Shapiro ME, Strom TB *et al.* Prolongation of primate renal allograft survival by anti-Tac, an anti-human IL-2 receptor monoclonal antibody. *Transplantation* 1989;47:55–59.

4 Vincenti F, de Andres A, Becker T *et al*. Interleukin-2 receptor antagonist induction in modern immunosuppression regimens for renal transplant recipients. *Transpl Int* 2006;19:446–457.

5 Amlot PL, Rawlings E, Fernando ON *et al*. Prolonged action of a chimeric interleukin-2 receptor (CD25) monoclonal antibody used in cadaveric renal transplantation. *Transplantation* 1995;60:748–756.

6 Vincenti F, Kirkman R, Light S *et al*. Interleukin-2-receptor blockade with daclizumab to prevent acute rejection in renal transplantation. Daclizumab Triple Therapy Study Group. *N Engl J Med* 1998;338:161–165.

7 Nashan B, Light S, Hardie IR *et al*. Reduction of acute renal allograft rejection by daclizumab. Daclizumab Double Therapy Study Group. *Transplantation* 1999; 67:110–115.

8 Nashan B, Moore R, Amlot P *et al*. Randomised trial of basiliximab versus placebo for control of acute cellular rejection in renal allograft recipients. CHIB 201 International Study Group. *Lancet* 1997;350:1193–1198.

9 Kahan BD, Rajagopalan PR, Hall M. Reduction of the occurrence of acute cellular rejection among renal allograft recipients treated with basiliximab, a chimeric anti-interleukin-2-receptor monoclonal antibody. United States Simulect Renal Study Group. *Transplantation* 1999;67:267–284.

10 Webster AC, Playford EG, Higgins G *et al*. Interleukin 2 receptor antagonists for renal transplant recipients: a meta-analysis of randomized trials. *Transplantation* 2004;77:166–176.

11 Ponticelli C, Yussim A, Cambi V *et al*. A randomized, double-blind trial of basiliximab immunoprophylaxis plus triple therapy in kidney transplant recipients. *Transplantation* 2001;72:1261–1267.

12 Lawen JG, Davies EA, Mourad G *et al*. Randomized double-blind study of immunoprophylaxis with basiliximab, a chimeric anti-interleukin-2 receptor monoclonal antibody, in combination with mycophenolate mofetil-containing triple therapy in renal transplantation. *Transplantation* 2003;75:37–43.

13 Vincenti F, Lantz M, Birnbaum J *et al*. A Phase I trial of humanized anti-interleukin 2 receptor antibody in renal transplantation. *Transplantation* 1997;63:33–38.

14 Pescovitz MD, Bumgardner GL, Gaston RS *et al*. Pharmacokinetics of daclizumab and mycophenolate mofetil with cyclosporine and steroids in renal transplantation. *Clin Transplant* 2003;17:511–517.

15 Brennan DC, Daller JA, Lake KD *et al*. Rabbit antithymocyte globulin versus basiliximab in renal transplantation. *N Engl J Med* 2006;355:1967–1977.

16 Noël C, Abramowicz D, Durand D *et al*. Daclizumab versus antilymphocyte globulin in high-immunological risk renal transplant recipients. *J Am Soc Nephrol* 2009;20:1385–1392.

17 Lebranchu Y, Bridoux F, Buchler M *et al*. Immunoprophylaxis with basiliximab compared with antithymocyte globulin in renal transplant patients receiving MMF-containing triple therapy. *Am J Transplant* 2002;2:48–56.

18 Sollinger H, Kaplan B, Pescovitz MD *et al*. Basiliximab versus antilymphocyte globulin for prevention of acute renal allograft rejection. *Transplantation* 2001;72:1915–1919.

19 Mourad G, Rostaing L, Legendre C *et al*. Sequential protocols using basiliximab versus antithymocyte globulins in renal-transplant patients receiving mycophenolate mofetil and steroids. *Transplantation* 2004;78:584–590.

20 Vincenti F, Nashan B, Light S. Daclizumab: outcome of Phase III trials and mechanism of action. Double Therapy and the Triple Therapy Study Groups. *Transplant Proc* 1998;30:2155–2158.

21 Binder M, Vogtle FN, Michelfelder S *et al*. Identification of their epitope reveals the structural basis for the mechanism of action of the immunosuppressive antibodies basiliximab and daclizumab. *Cancer Res* 2007;67:3518–3523.

22 Bluestone JA, Liu W, Yabu JM *et al*. The effect of costimulatory and interleukin-2 receptor blockade on regulatory T cells in renal transplantation. *Am J Transplant* 2008;8:2086–2096.

23 Chapman TM, Keating GM. Basiliximab: a review of its use as induction therapy in renal transplantation. *Drugs* 2003;63:2803–2835.

24 Kovarik J, Wolf P, Cisterne JM *et al*. Disposition of basiliximab, an interleukin-2 receptor monoclonal antibody, in recipients of mismatched cadaver renal allografts. *Transplantation* 1997;64:1701–1705.

25 Kovarik JM, Kahan BD, Rajagopalan PR *et al*. Population pharmacokinetics and exposure–response relationships for basiliximab in kidney transplantation. *Transplantation* 1999;68:1288–1294.

26 Koch M, Niemeyer G, Patel I *et al*. Pharmacokinetics, pharmacodynamics, and immunodynamics of daclizumab in a two-dose regimen in liver transplantation. *Transplantation* 2002;73:1640–1646.

27 Strelau J, Pape L, Offner G *et al*. Interleukin-2 receptor antibody-induced alterations of ciclosporin dose requirements in paediatric transplant recipients. *Lancet* 2000;356:1327–1328.

28 Vincenti F, Pace D, Birnbaum J, Lantz M. Pharma-cokinetic and pharmacodynamic studies of one or two doses of daclizumab in renal transplantation. *Am J Transplant* 2003;3:50–52.

29 Hocker B, Kovarik JM, Daniel V *et al.* Pharmacokinetics and immunodynamics of basiliximab in pediatric renal transplant recipients on mycophenolate mofetil comedication. *Transplantation* 2008;86:1234–1233.

30 Kovarik JM, Pescovitz MD, Sollinger HW *et al.* Differential influence of azathioprine and mycophe-nolate mofetil on the disposition of basiliximab in renal transplant patients. *Clin Transplant* 2001;15: 123–130.

CHAPTER 26
Infliximab/Anti-TNF

Marina Vardanyan, Edward C. Parkin, and Horacio L. Rodriguez Rilo
Department of Surgery, College of Medicine, University of Arizona, Tucson, AZ, USA

History

The biologic activity of tumor necrosis factor-alpha (TNF-α) was first observed more than a century ago by Coley, who used extracts from Gram-positive and Gram-negative bacteria to show tumor regression in patients with inoperable tumors [1]. In 1944, Shear demonstrated that lipopolysaccharide (LPS), isolated from bacterial extracts, was responsible for tumor regression. Subsequently, in 1963, O'Malley found that the effects of LPS on tumor regression were mediated through induction of serum tumor necrotizing factor [2], later renamed tumor necrosis factor [3].

TNF-α

TNF-α, also known as cachectin and TNFSF1A, is the prototypic ligand in the TNF superfamily, acting as a pleiotropic molecule that orchestrates initiation of the inflammatory response, induction of apoptosis, and development of immune system components. TNF-α has been called the "body's fire alarm" [4], since it initiates defense mechanisms to local tissue injury. Many immune cell types produce TNF-α, including macrophages, T and B lymphocytes, granulocytes, mast cells, and natural killer cells; so do nonimmune smooth muscle and epithelial cell types. Human TNF-α consists of a 35-amino-acid (aa) cytoplasmic domain, a single-pass 21-aa transmembrane domain, and a 177-aa extracellular domain. Membrane-bound TNF-α is released into the circulation as a 17 kDa protein subunit after cleavage by proteolytic enzyme TACE (TNF-α-converting enzyme), which, in turn, self-associates into the trimeric 51 kDa soluble cytokine.

Receptors

TNF-α is biologically active in the membrane-bound and the soluble form. Both forms serve as extracellular ligands to two receptor isoforms: TNFR1 (p55, CD120a) and TNFR2 (p75, CD120b). TNFR1 is the constitutively expressed isoform found in virtually all nucleated cell types. TNFR2 is inducible, with more restricted expression of endothelial, hematopoietic, and lymphoid cell types. Soluble TNF-α binds to both receptors on human cells, with a higher affinity to TNFR1 ($K_d \approx$ 20 pM) than to TNFR2 ($K_d \approx 400$ pM) [5]. In contrast, in vitro studies have shown that membrane-bound TNF-α preferentially binds to TNFR2 [6]. TNF-α signaling initiated via TNFR1 and TNFR2 is mediated by adapter proteins that bind to the cytoplasmic domains of the receptors upon ligand binding. The cytoplasmic region of TNFR1 contains

Immunotherapy in Transplantation: Principles and Practice, First Edition. Edited by Bruce Kaplan, Gilbert J. Burckart and Fadi G. Lakkis.
© 2012 Blackwell Publishing Ltd. Published 2012 by Blackwell Publishing Ltd.

a death domain (DD) that couples TNFR1 to signaling pathways via binding of the adapter protein TNFR-associated death domain (TRADD). The primary pathway leads to caspase-8- and caspase-3-dependent apoptosis (Plate 26.1). Additionally, ligand binding to TNFR1 activates nuclear factor kappa-B (NF-κB), a family of transcription factors that controls a large number of inflammatory genes (Plate 26.2). The majority of functions of TNF require TNFR1 signaling; however, TNFR2 has signaling capabilities on its own, including induction of T cells and thymocytes [9]. Several studies have indicated that TNFR2 is a weak activator of the NF-κB signaling pathway [10,11]. The major difference between TNFR1 and TNFR2 is in the mode of signal transduction: unlike TNFR1, TNFR2 belongs to a non-DD group of receptors that signal by directly binding members of the TNF receptor-associated factor (TRAF) family.

Biologic roles of TNF-α

The good
Anticancer potential
Although originally considered an antitumor agent, thanks to work extended from Coley's initial observation, TNF-α does not induce apoptosis in the majority of evaluated cell lines [12]. Studies of tumor models and patients undergoing treatment with TNF-α have shown limited activity in suppressing cancer, primarily owing to its systemic toxicity, including hypertension, hyperkalemia, and multiple organ failure [13, 14]. This toxicity restricts the use of TNF-α to locally advanced limb sarcomas, with administration by isolated perfusion of the limb. When used in this way, TNF-α eliminates the need for amputation [15, 16]. In a multicenter European trial, the response rate to isolated limb perfusion with TNF-α plus melphalan was 76%, and the limb was saved in 71% of patients. The trial demonstrated the efficacy of isolated limb perfusion of TNF-α in patients with drug-resistant skin cancers and bone sarcomas; in addition, it showed that adding TNF-α to the perfusate results in a three- to six-fold increase in uptake of chemotherapeutic agents by tumors [15].

Regulation of the immune system
TNF superfamily members coordinate the interplay between the cells in the immune system by providing important signals for the function of cytotoxic T lymphocytes. TNF–TNFR interactions regulate T cell immune function by influencing inflammation and innate immunity [17], lymphoid organization [18, 19], and activation of antigen-presenting cells (APCs) [20, 21], as well as by providing direct signals to T cells [22].

TNF superfamily members play a crucial role in secondary lymphoid organ development and function. Several strains of TNF-α-deficient mice have been generated [23–25] that are viable and fertile, with no gross structural defects; however, they exhibit morphologic alterations in lymph nodes. Specifically, they lack both B cell follicles and germinal centers in the spleen, with severely reduced responses to T-cell-dependent antigens. In particular, mice lacking either TNF superfamily member lymphotoxin B or its receptor fail to develop lymph nodes or Peyer patches [26–28]. Genomic deletion of another TNF superfamily member, RANKL (receptor activator of the NF-κB ligand), results in the absence of all peripheral lymph nodes, but Peyer patches remain intact [29–31].

Protection against microbial infection
TNF-α knockout mice are resistant to LPS challenge, when compared with wild-type littermates. However, they are more susceptible to developing infections, from *Listeria monocytogenes*, *Candida albicans*, and *Cryptosporidium parvum*. A similar increase in susceptibility to *Mycobacterium tuberculosis* has been reported in mice treated with anti-TNF monoclonal antibody [32], thus suggesting that anti-TNF therapies considerably increase a patient's risk of developing certain infectious diseases (in particular, tuberculosis).

The bad
Side effects and efficacy
Infusion of TNF-α into rats causes hypotension, metabolic acidosis and hyperkalemia, hyperglycemia, and finally death (as a result of respiratory depression) [33]. Although treatment with TNF-neutralizing antibodies has been shown to play a

protective role in several animal models, including nonhuman primates [34,35], clinical trials with anti-TNF monoclonal antibodies in human patients with septic conditions have been disappointing [36].

Cancer

Intensive research in the cytokine area has revealed that TNF-α, despite its name, can act as a tumorigenic factor by mediating the proliferation, invasion, and metastasis of cancer cells [37, 38]. TNF-α induces the expression of several tumor metastasis and invasion genes through the activation of NF-κB, such as matrix metalloproteinase 9 (MMP-9), cyclooxygenase 2 (COX2), and vascular endothelial growth factor (VEGF). Moore *et al.* found that TNF-α-deficient mice are resistant to the development of benign and malignant skin tumors, indicating that TNF-α is highly carcinogenic [39].

Autoimmunity

TNF-α has been shown to play a central role in the pathogenesis of several autoimmune disorders, such as rheumatoid arthritis (RA), Crohn's disease (CD), psoriasis, and type 2 diabetes.

Increased levels of TNF-α mRNA and protein have been detected in synovial fluid from joints of RA patients [40, 41], suggesting that TNF-α may be at the top of the cascade that leads to sequential upregulation of other proinflammatory cytokines, such as interleukin-1 (IL-1), interleukin-6 (IL-6), interleukin-8 (IL-8), and granulocyte-macrophage colony-stimulating factor (GM-CSF) [42–44]. Explanted cartilage treated with recombinant human TNF-α showed evidence of tissue destruction via reduction of proteoglycan mass [45]. Mice that constitutively express human TNF-α developed clinical and histologic changes characteristic of RA, whose progression significantly decreased with anti-TNF antibody treatment [46]. Those observations were further confirmed by studies showing that anti-TNF antibodies could reduce disease activity in a collagen-induced arthritis model [47–49] and that pre- or post-treatment with anti-TNF antibodies was effective even when considerable disease was present [49].

Elevated concentrations of TNF-α mRNA and protein in both the intestinal mucosa and stools of CD patients suggest an association between TNF-α and inflammation of the bowel [50, 51]. Cottontop tamarin monkeys spontaneously develop colitis with attributes that are similar to symptoms of ulcerative colitis in humans [52]. When treated with anti-TNF antibodies, the tamarin monkeys showed a significant improvement in body weight, fecal matter consistency, and, per biopsy results, rectal pathology [53, 54]. In addition, several mouse models mimicking human colitis have been developed [55]. A recently described mouse strain developed chronic ileitis, similar to CD, with perianal fistulas; administering a single injection of anti-TNF antibody diminished the degree of intestinal inflammation and epithelial cell damage, compared with control mice [56]. These data suggest that TNF-α plays a key role in maintaining CD's chronic inflammation characteristics.

A recent animal model showed that skin lesions spontaneously developed when prepsoriatic human skin was engrafted onto mice deficient in type I and type II interferon receptors and deficient in the recombination-activating gene 2 (rag2) [57]. Clinical and histologic features of psoriasis appeared within 6–8 weeks after engraftment, together with enhanced expression of Ki-67, TNF, IL-12, and ICAM-1. TNF-neutralizing antibody treatment resulted in a marked reduction of papillomatosis and acanthosis, along with a decrease in the number of T lymphocytes in the graft. These findings highlight the role of resident T lymphocytes in TNF-α production during development of a psoriatic lesion.

Finally, TNF-α has been shown to be a key mediator of insulin resistance in type 2 diabetes [58]. TNF-α blocks insulin signaling by disrupting the autophosphorylation of the insulin receptor and inhibiting phosphorylation of the insulin receptor substrate 1 [58]. Deletion of the TNF-α or TNFR gene results in a significant improvement in insulin sensitivity in mice with diet-induced obesity and in the ob/ob mouse model of obesity, indicating a role for TNF-α in insulin resistance in obesity [59].

Infliximab structure and properties

Infliximab is a high-molecular-weight (~149 kDa) chimeric monoclonal antibody against TNF-α. The molecule comprises two components: a murine variable region (25%) and a human constant region (75%) [60]. In contrast to murine monoclonal antibodies, infliximab has a higher efficacy because of its decreased immunogenicity and longer half-life [60]. The strategy used to produce infliximab (previously cA2) was creation of a chimeric molecule where the murine constant domains were replaced by human constant domains. That strategy generated a chimeric antibody combining the binding characteristics of a murine antibody with the functional properties of the human IgG1 Fc region [61].

In contrast, adalimumab is a humanized monoclonal antibody with both human IgG1 constant and variable regions, and the etanercept molecule consists of two extracellular domains of the human TNFR2 fused to the constant fragment of human IgG1 (Plate 26.3).

Infliximab binds human TNF-α with high affinity and specificity; it inhibits the biologic activity of both soluble and membrane-bound TNF-α [62, 63] and inhibits binding of the cytokine to its receptors by the formation of infliximab–TNF-α trimer complexes, thereby neutralizing its biologic activity. Infliximab is also associated with complement- and antibody-dependent lysis of TNF-producing cells; moreover, it may cause apoptosis of T lymphocytes and monocytes [61, 64].

In several studies, infliximab reduced the production of cytokines in biopsy samples and the cytokine levels in blood – findings that correlate with a positive clinical response [65–67]. Infliximab also decreased the migration of inflammatory cells to the site of inflammation by reducing levels of chemokines (e.g., monocyte chemotactic protein-1) and of endothelial adhesion molecules [65–67]. Although transitory changes in the numbers of peripheral blood leukocytes occur with infliximab therapy, generalized suppression of cellular immune function has not been observed [68]. Infliximab decreases the plasma levels of phospholipase A2, serum MMP-1 and MMP-3, VEGF, and acute-phase proteins [65]; it increases NF-κB inhibitor levels in intestinal mucosa [69].

Pharmacokinetics of infliximab

Infliximab is administered intravenously under various dosing regimens specific to each patient population. The volume of distribution of infliximab, which ranges from 3.1 to 5.6 L, has been shown to be independent of dose, indicating that it is distributed primarily within the vascular compartment [70]. For intravenous infliximab, the relationship between the administered dose and the maximum serum concentration is linear within the dose range of 3–20 mg/kg [71]. High serum levels of infliximab are achieved within 1 h after infusion, with a median concentration of 68.6 μg/mL after a dose of 3 mg/kg and 219.1 μg/mL after a dose of 10 mg/kg [72]. These high serum levels of infliximab effectively neutralize local levels of TNF-α in the skin, gut mucosa, and synovium. After multiple-dose infliximab administration, the median serum concentration 1 h after infusion was 110.5 μg/mL in CD patients receiving 5 mg/kg (five doses) and 69.7 μg/mL in RA patients receiving 3 mg/kg (four doses) with concomitant methotrexate [72]. Serum infliximab concentrations were still detectable in patients 10 to 12 weeks after the last dose [70, 73]; however, no clinically relevant reports have focused on systemic accumulation after repeated treatment with infliximab at either 3 or 10 mg/kg [74].

Limited data are available on the metabolism and excretion of infliximab; no metabolite of infliximab has been detected in urine. Infliximab is probably degraded by nonspecific proteases [75], but studies have not been conducted to characterize the pathways of infliximab elimination [71]. Its median half-life ranges from 7.7 to 9.5 days [76]; clearance is known to be nonlinear and reduced in the presence of methotrexate [66, 77]. In patients who develop antibodies to infliximab, its clearance increases and serum concentrations decrease [78]. One study found no major differences in clearance or in volume of distribution in patient subpopulations defined by age, weight, or gender [71]. To date, whether or not marked hepatic or renal impairment affects infliximab clearance or volume of distribution remains unknown, and no formal drug–drug interaction studies have been performed [77, 79].

Pharmacodynamics of infliximab

The mechanism of action of infliximab has been extensively studied. It binds to and inhibits both the soluble and membrane-bound forms of TNF-α and does not neutralize TNF-β [61, 63, 80].

Markers of apoptosis

A decreased rate of apoptosis, or defective apoptosis, may cause chronic inflammation in diseases such as CD and RA [81, 82]. Several studies have addressed the question of whether or not TNF-α antagonists induce apoptosis in vivo by measuring the number of apoptotic cells in peripheral blood and biopsy samples of patients with CD, RA, and psoriasis post-treatment. Using the terminal deoxynucleotidyl transferase dUTP nick end labeling (TUNEL) assay, researchers showed that infliximab induced apoptosis of lamina propria T lymphocytes 24h after treatment [83], as well as 4 weeks after the last of three infliximab infusions [84–86]. Furthermore, a significant increase in the annexin V-positive cells was observed in CD patients after infliximab infusion [87].

In a study of RA patients, the number of TUNEL-positive cells in synovial biopsies was determined before, 48h after, and 28days after the first infliximab infusion [88]. In that study, infliximab significantly reduced the number of inflammatory cells in the synovial fluid, but did not increase the number of TUNEL-positive cells. However, another study looking at synovial biopsies in RA patients treated with infliximab detected a two- to five-fold increase in the percentage of TUNEL-positive or active caspase-3-positive cells [89].

Infliximab-induced apoptosis has also been studied in patients with psoriasis. No increase in the number of apoptotic cells, either in the skin or in synovial biopsy samples, could be detected [90].

Markers of inflammation

Many of the hallmarks of chronic inflammation are reduced by TNF-α antagonist therapy. Infliximab therapy leads to a reduction in synovial tissue expression of IL-6 in RA patients [91] and in CD patients [92, 93]. In addition, infliximab reduces the levels of IL-1 and IL-1β in the synovium of RA patients [94, 95] and decreases the serum concentration of IL-18 [52, 90]. Additionally in RA patients, infliximab reduces the levels of acute-phase proteins such as amyloid A, fibrinogen, and C-reactive protein (CRP) [96]. CRP levels are also reduced in patients with psoriasis [91, 97] and CD [98, 99] after infliximab treatment.

Infliximab decreases the expression of vascular adhesion molecules, VCAM-1, ICAM-1, and E-selectin [100], in both the synovial tissue and the serum of RA patients. ICAM-1 expression is markedly reduced in the skin biopsies of patients with psoriasis [101, 102] and in the intestine of CD patients [52]. In addition, infliximab treatment reduces the number of the chemokines MCP-1 (monocyte chemotactic protein-1) and RANTES (regulated on activation, normal T cells expressed and secreted) detected in the bowel mucosa of CD patients [103].

Angiogenesis is a predominant feature in RA, psoriasis, and other chronic inflammatory conditions; elevations of VEGF are seen in RA synovial tissue [104] and in psoriatic skin [105, 106]. In RA patients, infliximab treatment suppresses VEGF expression [107, 108].

Markers of bone and cartilage destruction

Chronic inflammatory diseases such as RA are characterized by bone loss within the affected joints that is caused by an increase in bone resorption by osteoclasts. Bone resorption is mediated by excessive production of proinflammatory cytokines, including TNF-α. In vivo and in vitro studies have shown that TNF-α promotes bone degradation both directly (by promoting formation, activation, and survival of osteoclasts) and indirectly (by sustaining inflammation within the synovial cavity) [46, 109]. Studies of transgenic mice overexpressing TNF-α have shown that these mice develop erosive arthritis similar to that in humans [110].

Cartilage erosion in RA is mediated by the upregulation of MMPs, downstream of several cytokines, including TNF-α. TNF-α synergy with IL-17 activates MMP-1, MMP-3, and MMP-9, leading to the degradation of type II collagen [111–113]. In RA patients, infliximab treatment significantly reduces levels of MMP-1, MMP-3, and MMP-9 [114] and increases bone mineral density [115, 116].

Reduced bone mineral density often accompanies CD [117]. The bone loss observed in CD appears to be related to increased bone resorption, rather than to decreased bone production [118, 119]. Recent studies have shown that infliximab treatment of CD patients also increases their bone mineral density, thereby reducing the risk of fractures [120, 121].

Pharmacogenetics of infliximab

Despite the clinical efficacies of all three TNF-α antagonists, only about 70% of patients show improvement in symptoms. The 30% who do not show improvement in symptoms can be arbitrarily divided into *primary nonresponders* (those in whom anti-TNF treatment lacks efficacy from the first dose) and *secondary nonresponders* (those who benefit initially, but in whom, over time, anti-TNF treatment exhibits diminished efficacy) [74, 122]. Lack of efficacy has led to the search for markers that can predict treatment outcome. Anti-TNF pharmacogenetics is an area of research focusing on genetic variations that can be used to predict treatment outcome.

Both the TNFA, the gene that codes for TNF-α, and the genes encoding TNF-α receptors have been investigated for any association with anti-TNF treatment outcome. The effect of polymorphisms in TNFA has been examined in relation to the response to infliximab. Mugnier *et al.* published the first study investigating the relationship between the response to infliximab and the −308G>A SNP in the TNFA promoter in 59 RA patients [123]. Patients with the GC genotype were twice as likely to respond to infliximab, compared with patients with the AG or AA genotype ($P = 0.0086$). A different study demonstrated that patients with the GG genotype had a better response to infliximab

than patients with the AG genotype [124]. Still another study demonstrated that patients with the GG genotype had a better response to any of the three anti-TNF treatments, compared with patients with the AG or AA genotype [125].

In contrast, a study of the −308G>A promoter polymorphism of TNFA, the −238G>A promoter polymorphism, and polymorphisms in the IL1B and IL1RN genes found no significant association between the response to infliximab and polymorphisms [126]. Fabris *et al.* showed that the presence of a G-allele at position +676 in TNFR2 predisposed patients to be unresponsive to infliximab [127].

Infliximab side effects

Several studies have evaluated the safety of infliximab in healthy volunteers and in patients with RA, CD, and ulcerative colitis [128].

Death

In clinical trials of infliximab, no patients died. But nine deaths have been reported during the 3-year long-term follow-up period. Of those nine patients, two had CD and seven had RA. The causes of death included cardiovascular disease, malignancy or its treatment, or infection [129, 130].

Tolerability

For up to 102 weeks, infliximab (3–10 mg/kg) was generally well tolerated in patients with CD or RA in clinical trials [131]. The most commonly reported adverse events were upper respiratory tract infection, nausea, headache, sinusitis, diarrhea, cough, pharyngitis, abdominal pain, dyspepsia, bronchitis, and skin rash [71]. The incidence of adverse events was higher in RA patients receiving infliximab at a dose of 10 mg/kg, compared with 3 mg/kg; however, in CD patients, the incidence was similar at doses of 5 and 10 mg/kg [71].

Infusion reactions

An infusion reaction was defined as any adverse reaction reported during an infusion or within 2 h after the infusion. Infusion reactions occurred in about 20% of infliximab recipients and in 10% of placebo recipients [71]. The most commonly reported infusion reactions were headache, nausea, dizziness, flushing, pruritus, urticaria, and chest pain. Infusion reactions resulted in immediate discontinuation of the drug in about 3 % of patients.

In fewer than 1 % of infliximab recipients, infusion reactions were considered serious (e.g., anaphylaxis). However, no sequelae have been reported, and symptoms were controlled with antihistamine treatment and discontinuation of the infliximab infusion [78, 129, 132, 133]. The risk of experiencing an infusion reaction increased by two- to three-fold in patients who developed antibodies to infliximab, whereas concomitant use of methotrexate was associated with a decrease in the incidence [78].

Serum sickness-type reactions have also been reported, generally after one to five infusions, in 2 % of placebo recipients and 3 % of infliximab recipients [134–136].

Oncogenic potential

Malignancies have been reported in infliximab recipients, including metastatic breast cancer, malignant melanoma, and papillary thyroid cancer in patients with a nodular thyroid gland. The medical histories in all patients with solid tumors suggested that malignancy was present at the time of infliximab infusion. Further studies have demonstrated that, with the exception of lymphomas, the incidence of malignancies in infliximab recipients was similar to what would be expected in an equivalent population not receiving the drug [71]. The incidence of lymphomas in infliximab recipients (0.08–0.12 %) represented an increase of three- to five-fold, compared with the general population [71].

B cell malignancies occurred in patients with a long duration of RA or CD who had previous exposure to immunosuppressive therapy, such as methotrexate and azathioprine, which are known to increase the risk of lymphoproliferative disorders [137].

Serious infections

Because TNF-α is a mediator of inflammation and modulates cellular immune response, it is an important component in the defense against some intracellular pathogens.

Infliximab treatment is associated with tuberculosis [138, 139], and when compared with etanercept, infliximab is associated with an increase of two- to seven-fold in the risk of developing tuberculosis, coccidioidomycosis, and histoplasmosis. Infliximab has also been associated with an earlier onset of tuberculosis [137]: in one study, the median time from initiation of infliximab treatment to detection of tuberculosis was 12 weeks (range: 1–52 weeks) [140]. Although some tuberculosis infections have been reported in patients with no known history of the disease, most have occurred in patients with a previous history of tuberculosis, suggesting a reactivation of the latent disease [141]. Moreover, the rate of reactivation of latent tuberculosis infection by infliximab has been reported to be more than 20 % per month, a 12.1-fold increase compared with etanercept [78, 129, 130, 142].

Cryptococcal meningitis is a rare but potentially lethal complication of infliximab treatment [143, 144].

Autoantibodies

Infliximab treatment has been associated with the production of antinuclear antibodies (ANAs) and antibodies to infliximab. In patients receiving maintenance infliximab treatment, ANAs and antibodies against double-stranded DNA (dsDNA) developed in a higher proportion of infliximab recipients, compared with placebo recipients [145, 146]. Such autoantibodies are generally of the IgM or IgA class and rarely of the IgG subclass. Greater frequencies and concentrations of them have been reported with infliximab, compared with etanercept or adalimumab [78, 129, 147]. Although anti-TNF-α treatment with infliximab has been associated with development of anti-dsDNA antibodies, clinical manifestations (such as lupus and lupus-like reactions) in patients with such antibodies have been rare [132].

In one study, an antibody titer of $\geq 8 \mu g/mL$ before infusion was associated with a reduced duration of response, compared with a titer of $< 8 \mu g/mL$ [132]. The risk of the antibody titer being $\geq 8 \mu g/mL$ was lower by at least twofold in patients receiving concomitant immunosuppressants, compared with those not receiving immunosuppressants [148].

Indeed, of the patients receiving infliximab alone, 53% (1 mg/kg), 21% (3 mg/kg), and 7% (10 mg/kg) developed anti-dsDNA antibodies; in contrast, of the patients receiving infliximab in combination with methotrexate, 15% (1 mg/kg), 7% (3 mg/kg), and 0% (10 mg/kg) developed anti-dsDNA antibodies [130, 145, 148].

The mechanism of autoantibody induction by infliximab is not completely understood, but can perhaps be attributed to a release of autoimmunogenic nucleosomes from apoptotic cells or to inhibition of the cytotoxic T lymphocyte response [149].

Other adverse events

The use of infliximab is associated with heart failure [150], hepatic complications – ranging from mild to severe increases in alanine transaminase (ALT) and aspartate transaminase (AST) levels to severe reactions requiring liver transplantation (http://www.fda.gov/medwatch) – and, albeit rarely, with neurologic complications, including optic neuritis, seizures, and new onset or exacerbation of clinical symptoms of demyelinating disorders [150]. Within addition, infliximab has been associated with the development of psoriasiform lesions in patients with chronic arthritic diseases [151], including juvenile idiopathic arthritis [152].

Emerging directions of anti-TNF therapy

Given the important role of TNF-α in regulating the immune system, it represents an attractive target of new treatment strategies for organ transplant recipients. Yet very few studies have evaluated the efficacy of anticytokine monoclonal antibodies as novel immunosuppressants. Infliximab has been used in clinical trials as an alternative to conventional immunosuppressants in several areas of transplantation. It has been successfully applied as rescue treatment for intestinal transplant recipients with acute graft rejection [121], as well as for skin transplant recipients with graft-versus-host disease. Pech *et al.* recently demonstrated that preoperative infliximab administration was a viable option for overcoming graft dysfunction after a small-bowel transplant [153]. However, the efficacy of infliximab in solid-organ transplantation requires further investigation [121]. Infliximab was used in two heart transplant recipients, but larger studies are needed [154].

Infliximab was administered in an attempt to improve engraftment of allogeneic islets, but no clinical benefit of the TNF-α blockade was demonstrated [155]. No dose–response or long-term studies of infliximab have been done, but blockade of a single molecule will likely not be sufficient to surmount the immune response in allogeneic islet transplant recipients. A case report by Leroy *et al.* [156] demonstrated success with infliximab in preventing the post-transplant recurrence of focal segmental glomerulosclerosis in a pediatric patient. But further studies are necessary to investigate the clinical utility of anti-TNF treatment in preventing and treating acute graft rejection.

References

1 Coley WB, II. Contribution to the knowledge of sarcoma. *Ann Surg* 1891;14(3):199–220.

2 O'Malley WE, Achinstein B, Shear MJ. Action of bacterial polysaccharide on tumors. III. Repeated response of sarcoma 37, in tolerant mice, to *Serratia marcescens endotoxin*. *Cancer Res* 1963;23:890–895.

3 Carswell EA, Old LJ, Kassel RL *et al.* An endotoxin-induced serum factor that causes necrosis of tumors. *Proc Natl Acad Sci U S A* 1975;72(9):3666–3670.

4 Feldmann M. Development of anti-TNF therapy for rheumatoid arthritis. *Nat Rev Immunol* 2002;2(5):364–371.

5 Grell M, Wajant H, Zimmermann G *et al.* The type 1 receptor (CD120a) is the high-affinity receptor for soluble tumor necrosis factor. *Proc Natl Acad Sci U S A* 1998;95(2):570–575.

6 Grell M, Douni E, Wajant H *et al.* The transmembrane form of tumor necrosis factor is the prime activating ligand of the 80 kDa tumor necrosis factor receptor. *Cell* 1995;83(5):793–802.

7 Tracey D, Klareskog L, Sasso EH *et al.* Tumor necrosis factor antagonist mechanisms of action: a comprehensive review. *Pharmacol Therapeut* 2008;117:244–279.

8 Aggarwal BB. Signalling pathways of the TNF superfamily: a double-edged sword. *Nat Rev* 2003;3:745–756.

9 Tartaglia LA, Weber RF, Figari IS *et al.* The two different receptors for tumor necrosis factor mediate distinct cellular responses. *Proc Natl Acad Sci U S A* 1991;88(20):9292–9296.

10 Chainy GB, Singh S, Raju U *et al.* Differential activation of the nuclear factor-kappa B by TNF muteins specific for the p60 and p80 TNF receptors. *J Immunol* 1996;157(6):2410–2417.

11 Laegreid A, Medvedev A, Nonstad U *et al.* Tumor necrosis factor receptor p75 mediates cell-specific activation of nuclear factor kappa B and induction of human cytomegalovirus enhancer. *J Biol Chem* 1994;269(10):7785–7791.

12 Sugarman BJ, Aggarwal BB, Hass PE *et al.* Recombinant human tumor necrosis factor-alpha: effects on proliferation of normal and transformed cells in vitro. *Science* 1985;230(4728):943–945.

13 Feinberg B, Kurzrock R, Talpaz M *et al.* A Phase I trial of intravenously-administered recombinant tumor necrosis factor-alpha in cancer patients. *J Clin Oncol* 1988;6(8):1328–1334.

14 Burke F. Cytokines (IFNs, TNF-alpha, IL-2 and IL-12) and animal models of cancer. *Cytokines Cell Mol Ther* 1999;5(1):51–61.

15 Eggermont AM, de Wilt JH, ten Hagen TL. Current uses of isolated limb perfusion in the clinic and a model system for new strategies. *Lancet Oncol* 2003;4(7):429–437.

16 Lejeune FJ, Liénard D, Matter M, Rüegg C. Efficiency of recombinant human TNF in human cancer therapy. *Cancer Immun* 2006;6:6.

17 Kollias G, Kontoyiannis D. Role of TNF/TNFR in autoimmunity: specific TNF receptor blockade may be advantageous to anti-TNF treatments. *Cytokine Growth Factor Rev* 2002;13(4–5):315–321.

18 Gommerman JL, Browning JL. Lymphotoxin/light, lymphoid microenvironments and autoimmune disease. *Nat Rev Immunol* 2003;3(8):642–655.

19 Pfeffer K. Biological functions of tumor necrosis factor cytokines and their receptors. *Cytokine Growth Factor Rev* 2003;14(3–4):185–191.

20 Bachmann MF, Wong BR, Josien R *et al.* TRANCE, a tumor necrosis factor family member critical for CD40 ligand-independent T helper cell activation. *J Exp Med* 1999;189(7):1025–1031.

21 Josien R, Li HL, Ingulli E *et al.* TRANCE, a tumor necrosis factor family member, enhances the longevity and adjuvant properties of dendritic cells in vivo. *J Exp Med* 2000;191(3):495–502.

22 Croft M. Co-stimulatory members of the TNFR family: keys to effective T-cell immunity? *Nat Rev Immunol* 2003;3(8):609–620.

23 Korner H, Cook M, Riminton DS *et al.* Distinct roles for lymphotoxin-alpha and tumor necrosis factor in organogenesis and spatial organization of lymphoid tissue. *Eur J Immunol* 1997;27(10):2600–2609.

24 Marino MW, Dunn A, Grail D *et al.* Characterization of tumor necrosis factor-deficient mice. *Proc Natl Acad Sci U S A* 1997;94(15):8093–8098.

25 Pasparakis M, Alexopoulou L, Episkopou V *et al.* Immune and inflammatory responses in TNF alpha-deficient mice: a critical requirement for TNF alpha in the formation of primary B cell follicles, follicular dendritic cell networks and germinal centers, and in the maturation of the humoral immune response. *J Exp Med* 1996;184(4):1397–1411.

26 Banks TA, Rouse BT, Kerley MK *et al.* Lymphotoxin-alpha-deficient mice. Effects on secondary lymphoid organ development and humoral immune responsiveness. *J Immunol* 1995;155(4):1685–1693.

27 De Togni P, Goellner J, Ruddle NH *et al.* Abnormal development of peripheral lymphoid organs in mice deficient in lymphotoxin. *Science* 1994;264(5159):703–707.

28 Koni PA, Sacca R, Lawton P *et al.* Distinct roles in lymphoid organogenesis for lymphotoxins alpha and beta revealed in lymphotoxin beta-deficient mice. *Immunity* 1997;6(4):491–500.

29 Dougall WC, Glaccum M, Charrier K *et al.* RANK is essential for osteoclast and lymph node development. *Genes Dev* 1999;13(18):2412–2424.

30 Kim D, Mebius RE, MacMicking JD *et al.* Regulation of peripheral lymph node genesis by the tumor necrosis factor family member TRANCE. *J Exp Med* 2000;192(10):1467–1478.

31 Kong YY, Feige U, Sarosi I *et al.* Activated T cells regulate bone loss and joint destruction in adjuvant arthritis through osteoprotegerin ligand. *Nature* 1999;402(6759):304–309.

32 Flynn JL, Goldstein MM, Chan J *et al.* Tumor necrosis factor-alpha is required in the protective immune response against *Mycobacterium tuberculosis* in mice. *Immunity* 1995;2(6):561–572.

33 Tracey KJ, Beutler B, Lowry SF *et al.* Shock and tissue injury induced by recombinant human cachectin. *Science* 1986;234(4775):470–474.

34 Beutler B, Greenwald D, Hulmes JD *et al.* Identity of tumour necrosis factor and the macrophage-secreted factor cachectin. *Nature* 1985;316(6028):552–554.

35 Bodmer M, Fournel MA, Hinshaw LB. Preclinical review of anti-tumor necrosis factor monoclonal antibodies. *Crit Care Med* 1993;21(10 Suppl):S441–S446.

36 Freeman BD, Natanson C. Anti-inflammatory therapies in sepsis and septic shock. *Expert Opin Investig Drugs* 2000;9(7):1651–1663.

37 Karin M, Greten FR. NF-kappaB: linking inflammation and immunity to cancer development and progression. *Nat Rev Immunol* 2005;5(10):749–759.

38 Szlosarek P, Charles KA, Balkwill FR. Tumour necrosis factor-alpha as a tumour promoter. *Eur J Cancer* 2006;42(6):745–750.

39 Moore RJ, Owens DM, Stamp G *et al.* Mice deficient in tumor necrosis factor-alpha are resistant to skin carcinogenesis. *Nat Med* 1999;5(7):828–831.

40 Feldmann M, Brennan FM, Maini RN. Role of cytokines in rheumatoid arthritis. *Annu Rev Immunol* 1996;14:397–440.

41 Feldmann M, Elliott MJ, Woody JN *et al.* Anti-tumor necrosis factor-alpha therapy of rheumatoid arthritis. *Adv Immunol* 1997;64:283–350.

42 Brennan FM, Chantry D, Jackson A *et al.* Inhibitory effect of TNF alpha antibodies on synovial cell interleukin-1 production in rheumatoid arthritis. *Lancet* 1989;2(8657):244–247.

43 Butler DM, Maini RN, Feldmann M *et al.* Modulation of proinflammatory cytokine release in rheumatoid synovial membrane cell cultures. Comparison of monoclonal anti TNF-alpha antibody with the interleukin-1 receptor antagonist. *Eur Cytokine Netw* 1995;6(4):225–230.

44 Haworth C, Brennan FM, Chantry D *et al.* Expression of granulocyte-macrophage colony-stimulating factor in rheumatoid arthritis: regulation by tumor necrosis factor-alpha. *Eur J Immunol* 1991;21(10):2575–2579.

45 Saklatvala J. Tumour necrosis factor alpha stimulates resorption and inhibits synthesis of proteoglycan in cartilage. *Nature* 1986;322(6079):547–549.

46 Keffer J, Probert L, Cazlaris H *et al.* Transgenic mice expressing human tumour necrosis factor: a predictive genetic model of arthritis. *EMBO J* 1991;10(13):4025–4031.

47 Piguet PF, Grau GE, Vesin C *et al.* Evolution of collagen arthritis in mice is arrested by treatment with anti-tumour necrosis factor (TNF) antibody or a recombinant soluble TNF receptor. *Immunology*,1992;77(4):510–514.

48 Thorbecke GJ, Shah R, Leu CH *et al.* Involvement of endogenous tumor necrosis factor alpha and transforming growth factor beta during induction of collagen type II arthritis in mice. *Proc Natl Acad Sci U S A* 1992;89(16):7375–7379.

49 Williams RO, Feldmann M, Maini RN. Anti-tumor necrosis factor ameliorates joint disease in murine collagen-induced arthritis. *Proc Natl Acad Sci U S A* 1992;89(20):9784–9788.

50 Braegger CP, Nicholls S, Murch SH *et al.* Tumour necrosis factor alpha in stool as a marker of intestinal inflammation. *Lancet* 1992;339(8785):89–91.

51 Breese EJ, Michie CA, Nicholls SW *et al.* Tumor necrosis factor alpha-producing cells in the intestinal mucosa of children with inflammatory bowel disease. *Gastroenterology* 1994;106(6):1455–1466.

52 Van Deventer SJ. Tumour necrosis factor and Crohn's disease. *Gut* 1997;40(4):443–448.

53 Watkins PE, Warren BF, Stephens S *et al.* Treatment of ulcerative colitis in the cottontop tamarin using antibody to tumour necrosis factor alpha. *Gut* 1997;40(5):628–633.

54 Neurath MF, Fuss I, Pasparakis M *et al.* Predominant pathogenic role of tumor necrosis factor in experimental colitis in mice. *Eur J Immunol* 1997;27(7):1743–1750.

55 Pizarro TT, Arseneau KO, Bamias G *et al.* Mouse models for the study of Crohn's disease. *Trends Mol Med* 2003;9(5):218–222.

56 Marini M, Bamias G, Rivera-Nieves J *et al.* TNF-alpha neutralization ameliorates the severity of murine Crohn's-like ileitis by abrogation of intestinal epithelial cell apoptosis. *Proc Natl Acad Sci U S A* 2003; 100(14):8366–8371.

57 Boyman O, Hefti HP, Conrad C *et al.* Spontaneous development of psoriasis in a new animal model shows an essential role for resident T cells and tumor necrosis factor-alpha. *J Exp Med* 2004;199(5):731–736.

58 Hotamisligil GS, Murray DL, Choy LN *et al.* Tumor necrosis factor alpha inhibits signaling from the insulin receptor. *Proc Natl Acad Sci U S A* 1994;91(11):4854–4858.

59 Uysal KT, Wiesbrock SM, Marino MW *et al.* Protection from obesity-induced insulin resistance in mice lacking TNF-alpha function. *Nature* 1997;389(6651):610–614.

60 Bell SJ, Kamm MA. Review article: the clinical role of anti-TNFalpha antibody treatment in Crohn's disease. *Aliment Pharmacol Ther* 2000;14(5):501–514.

61 Scallon BJ, Moore MA, Trinh H *et al.* Chimeric anti-TNF-alpha monoclonal antibody cA2 binds recombinant transmembrane TNF-alpha and activates immune effector functions. *Cytokine* 1995;7(3):251–259.

62 Scallon B, Cai A, Solowski N *et al.* Binding and functional comparisons of two types of tumor necrosis factor antagonists. *J Pharmacol Exp Ther* 2002;301(2):418–426.

63 Knight DM, Trinh H, Le J *et al.* Construction and initial characterization of a mouse-human chimeric anti-TNF antibody. *Mol Immunol* 1993;30(16):1443–1453.

64 Van den Brande J, Hommes DW, Peppelenbosch MP. Infliximab induced T lymphocyte apoptosis in Crohn's disease. *J Rheumatol Suppl* 2005;74:26–30.

65 Keating GM, Perry CM. Infliximab: an updated review of its use in Crohn's disease and rheumatoid arthritis. *BioDrugs* 2002;16(2):111–148.

66 Markham A, Lamb HM. Infliximab: a review of its use in the management of rheumatoid arthritis. *Drugs* 2000;59(6):1341–1359.

67 Onrust SV, Lamb HM. Infliximab: a review of its use in Crohn's disease and rheumatoid arthritis. *BioDrugs* 1998;10(5):397–422.

68 Cornillie F, Shealy D, D'Haens G *et al.* Infliximab induces potent anti-inflammatory and local immunomodulatory activity but no systemic immune suppression in patients with Crohn's disease. *Aliment Pharmacol Ther* 2001;15(4):463–473.

69 Guidi L, Costanzo M, Ciarniello M *et al.* Increased levels of NF-kappaB inhibitors (IkappaBalpha and IkappaBgamma) in the intestinal mucosa of Crohn's disease patients during infliximab treatment. *Int J Immunopathol Pharmacol* 2005;18(1):155–164.

70 Kavanaugh A, St Clair EW, McCune WJ *et al.* Chimeric anti-tumor necrosis factor-alpha monoclonal antibody treatment of patients with rheumatoid arthritis receiving methotrexate therapy. *J Rheumatol* 2000;27(4): 841–850.

71 Centocor Inc.Product Information (US), 2009; available from: http://www.remicade.com.

72 St Clair EW, Wagner CL, Fasanmade AA *et al.* The relationship of serum infliximab concentrations to clinical improvement in rheumatoid arthritis: results from ATTRACT, a multicenter, randomized, double-blind, placebo-controlled trial. *Arthritis Rheum* 2002;46(6):1451–1459.

73 Rutgeerts P, D'Haens G, Targan S *et al.* Efficacy and safety of retreatment with anti-tumor necrosis factor antibody (infliximab) to maintain remission in Crohn's disease. *Gastroenterology* 1999;117(4):761–769.

74 Maini RN, Breedveld FC, Kalden JR *et al.* Sustained improvement over two years in physical function, structural damage, and signs and symptoms among patients with rheumatoid arthritis treated with infliximab and methotrexate. *Arthritis Rheum* 2004;50(4):1051–1065.

75 Klotz U, Teml A, Schwab M. Clinical pharmacokinetics and use of infliximab. *Clin Pharmacokinet* 2007;46(8): 645–660.

76 Scheinfeld N. Off-label uses and side effects of infliximab. *J Drugs Dermatol* 2004;3(3):273–284.

77 Schwab M, Klotz U. Pharmacokinetic considerations in the treatment of inflammatory bowel disease. *Clin Pharmacokinet* 2001;40(10):723–751.

78 Hanauer SB, Feagan BG, Lichtenstein GR *et al.* Maintenance infliximab for Crohn's disease: the ACCENT I randomised trial. *Lancet* 2002;359(9317): 1541–1549.

79 Siddiqui MA, Scott LJ. Infliximab: a review of its use in Crohn's disease and rheumatoid arthritis. *Drugs* 2005;65(15):2179–2208.

80 Siegel SA, Shealy DJ, Nakada MT *et al.* The mouse/human chimeric monoclonal antibody cA2 neutralizes TNF in vitro and protects transgenic mice from cachexia and TNF lethality in vivo. *Cytokine* 1995;7(1):15–25.

81 Sands BE. Why do anti-tumor necrosis factor antibodies work in Crohn's disease? *Rev Gastroenterol Disord* 2004;4(Suppl 3):S10–S17.

82 Tak PP. Effects of infliximab treatment on rheumatoid synovial tissue. *J Rheumatol Suppl* 2005;74:31–34.

83 Ten Hove T, van Montfrans C, Peppelenbosch MP *et al.* Infliximab treatment induces apoptosis of lamina propria T lymphocytes in Crohn's disease. *Gut* 2002;50(2):206–211.

84 Di Sabatino A, Ciccocioppo R, Cinque B *et al.* Defective mucosal T cell death is sustainably reverted by infliximab in a caspase dependent pathway in Crohn's disease. *Gut* 2004;53(1):70–77.

85 Lugering A, Schmidt M, Lugering N *et al.* Infliximab induces apoptosis in monocytes from patients with chronic active Crohn's disease by using a caspase-dependent pathway. *Gastroenterology* 2001;121(5):1145–1157.

86 Van den Brande JM, Koehler TC, Zelinkova Z *et al.* Prediction of antitumour necrosis factor clinical efficacy by real-time visualisation of apoptosis in patients with Crohn's disease. *Gut* 2007;56(4):509–517.

87 Smeets TJ, Kraan MC, van Loon ME *et al.* Tumor necrosis factor alpha blockade reduces the synovial cell infiltrate early after initiation of treatment, but apparently not by induction of apoptosis in synovial tissue. *Arthritis Rheum* 2003;48(8):2155–2162.

88 Catrina AI, Trollmo C, af Klint E *et al.* Evidence that anti-tumor necrosis factor therapy with both etanercept and infliximab induces apoptosis in macrophages, but not lymphocytes, in rheumatoid arthritis joints: extended report. *Arthritis Rheum* 2005;52(1):61–72.

89 Goedkoop AY, Kraan MC, Picavet DI *et al.* Deactivation of endothelium and reduction in angiogenesis in psoriatic skin and synovium by low dose infliximab therapy in combination with stable methotrexate therapy: a prospective single-centre study. *Arthritis Res Ther* 2004;6(4):R326–R334.

90 Charles P, Elliott MJ, Davis D *et al.* Regulation of cytokines, cytokine inhibitors, and acute-phase proteins following anti-TNF-alpha therapy in rheumatoid arthritis. *J Immunol* 1999;163(3):1521–1528.

91 Van Dullemen HM, van Deventer SJ, Hommes DW *et al.* Treatment of Crohn's disease with anti-tumor necrosis factor chimeric monoclonal antibody (cA2). *Gastroenterology* 1995;109(1):129–135.

92 Ulfgren AK, Andersson U, Engstrom M *et al.* Systemic anti-tumor necrosis factor alpha therapy in rheumatoid arthritis down-regulates synovial tumor necrosis factor alpha synthesis. *Arthritis Rheum* 2000;43(11):2391–2396.

93 Barrera P, Joosten LA, den Broeder AA *et al.* Effects of treatment with a fully human anti-tumour necrosis factor alpha monoclonal antibody on the local and systemic homeostasis of interleukin 1 and TNFalpha in patients with rheumatoid arthritis. *Ann Rheum Dis* 2001;60(7):660–669.

94 Pittoni V, Bombardieri M, Spinelli FR *et al.* Anti-tumour necrosis factor (TNF) alpha treatment of rheumatoid arthritis (infliximab) selectively down regulates the production of interleukin (IL) 18 but not of IL12 and IL13. *Ann Rheum Dis* 2002; 61(8):723–725.

95 Van Oosterhout M, Levarht EW, Sont JK *et al.* Clinical efficacy of infliximab plus methotrexate in DMARD naive and DMARD refractory rheumatoid arthritis is associated with decreased synovial expression of TNF alpha and IL18 but not CXCL12. *Ann Rheum Dis* 2005;64(4):537–543.

96 Feletar M, Brockbank JE, Schentag CT *et al.* Treatment of refractory psoriatic arthritis with infliximab: a 12 month observational study of 16 patients. *Ann Rheum Dis* 2004;63(2):156–161.

97 Baldassano R, Braegger CP, Escher JC *et al.* Infliximab (REMICADE) therapy in the treatment of pediatric Crohn's disease. *Am J Gastroenterol* 2003;98(4):833–838.

98 Goedkoop AY, Kraan MC, Teunissen MB *et al.* Early effects of tumour necrosis factor alpha blockade on skin and synovial tissue in patients with active psoriasis and psoriatic arthritis. *Ann Rheum Dis* 2004; 63(7):769–773.

99 Paleolog EM, Hunt M, Elliott MJ *et al.* Deactivation of vascular endothelium by monoclonal anti-tumor necrosis factor alpha antibody in rheumatoid arthritis. *Arthritis Rheum* 1996;39(7):1082–1091.

100 Gottlieb AB, Masud S, Ramamurthi R *et al.* Pharmacodynamic and pharmacokinetic response to anti-tumor necrosis factor-alpha monoclonal antibody (infliximab) treatment of moderate to severe psoriasis vulgaris. *J Am Acad Dermatol* 2003;48(1):68–75.

101 Baert FJ, D'Haens GR, Peeters M *et al.* Tumor necrosis factor alpha antibody (infliximab) therapy profoundly down-regulates the inflammation in Crohn's ileocolitis. *Gastroenterology* 1999;116(1):22–28.

102 Geboes K, Dalle I. Influence of treatment on morphological features of mucosal inflammation. *Gut* 2002;50(Suppl 3):iii37–iii42.

103 Fraser A, Fearon U, Reece R *et al.* Matrix metalloproteinase 9, apoptosis, and vascular morphology in early arthritis. *Arthritis Rheum* 2001;44(9): 2024–2028.

104 Dvorak HF, Brown LF, Detmar M *et al.* Vascular permeability factor/vascular endothelial growth factor, microvascular hyperpermeability, and angiogenesis. *Am J Pathol* 1995;146(5):1029–1039.

105 Maini RN, Taylor PC, Paleolog E *et al.* Anti-tumour necrosis factor specific antibody (infliximab) treatment provides insights into the pathophysiology of rheumatoid arthritis. *Ann Rheum Dis* 1999;58 (Suppl 1):I56–I60.

106 Strunk J, Bundke E, Lange U. Anti-TNF-alpha antibody Infliximab and glucocorticoids reduce serum vascular endothelial growth factor levels in patients with rheumatoid arthritis: a pilot study. *Rheumatol Int* 2006;26(3):252–256.

107 Boyce BF, Li P, Yao Z *et al.* TNF-alpha and pathologic bone resorption. *Keio J Med* 2005;54(3):127–131.

108 Schett G, Hayer S, Zwerina J *et al.* Mechanisms of disease: the link between RANKL and arthritic bone disease. *Nat Clin Pract Rheumatol* 2005;1(1):47–54.

109 Li P, Schwarz EM, O'Keefe RJ *et al.* RANK signaling is not required for TNFalpha-mediated increase in CD11(hi) osteoclast precursors but is essential for mature osteoclast formation in TNFalpha-mediated inflammatory arthritis. *J Bone Miner Res* 2004;19(2): 207–213.

110 Koshy PJ, Henderson N, Logan C *et al.* Interleukin 17 induces cartilage collagen breakdown: novel synergistic effects in combination with proinflammatory cytokines. *Ann Rheum Dis* 2002;61(8):704–713.

111 Brennan FM, Browne KA, Green PA *et al.* Reduction of serum matrix metalloproteinase 1 and matrix metalloproteinase 3 in rheumatoid arthritis patients following anti-tumour necrosis factor-alpha (cA2) therapy. *Br J Rheumatol* 1997;36(6):643–650.

112 Catrina AI, Lampa J, Ernestam S *et al.* Anti-tumour necrosis factor (TNF)-alpha therapy (etanercept) down-regulates serum matrix metalloproteinase (MMP)-3 and MMP-1 in rheumatoid arthritis. *Rheumatology (Oxford)* 2002;41(5):484–489.

113 Klimiuk PA, Sierakowski S, Domyslawska I *et al.* Effect of repeated infliximab therapy on serum matrix metalloproteinases and tissue inhibitors of metalloproteinases in patients with rheumatoid arthritis. *J Rheumatol* 2004;31(2):238–242.

114 Vis M, Havaardsholm EA, Haugeberg G *et al.* Evaluation of bone mineral density, bone metabolism, osteoprotegerin and receptor activator of the NFkappaB ligand serum levels during treatment with infliximab in patients with rheumatoid arthritis. *Ann Rheum Dis* 2006;65(11):1495–1499.

115 Adachi JD, Rostom A. Metabolic bone disease in adults with inflammatory bowel disease. *Inflamm Bowel Dis* 1999;5(3):200–211.

116 Lichtenstein GR. Evaluation of bone mineral density in inflammatory bowel disease: current safety focus. *Am J Gastroenterol* 2003;98(12 Suppl):S24–S30.

117 Bjarnason I. Metabolic bone disease in patients with inflammatory bowel disease. *Rheumatology (Oxford)* 1999;38(9):801–804.

118 Bernstein M, Irwin S, Greenberg GR. Maintenance infliximab treatment is associated with improved bone mineral density in Crohn's disease. *Am J Gastroenterol* 2005;100(9):2031–2035.

119 Franchimont N, Putzeys V, Collette J *et al.* Rapid improvement of bone metabolism after infliximab treatment in Crohn's disease. *Aliment Pharmacol Ther* 2004;20(6):607–614.

120 Pascher A, Radke C, Dignass A *et al.* Successful infliximab treatment of steroid and OKT3 refractory acute cellular rejection in two patients after intestinal transplantation. *Transplantation* 2003;76(3):615–618.

121 Couriel DR, Hicks K, Giralt S *et al.* Role of tumor necrosis factor-alpha inhibition with inflixiMAB in cancer therapy and hematopoietic stem cell transplantation. *Curr Opin Oncol* 2000;12(6):582–587.

122 Sidiropoulos P, Bertsias G, Kritikos HD *et al.* Infliximab treatment for rheumatoid arthritis, with dose titration based on the Disease Activity Score: dose adjustments are common but not always sufficient to assure sustained benefit. *Ann Rheum Dis* 2004; 63(2):144–148.

123 Mugnier B, Balandraud N, Darque A *et al.* Polymorphism at position −308 of the tumor necrosis factor alpha gene influences outcome of infliximab therapy in rheumatoid arthritis. *Arthritis Rheum* 2003;48(7):1849–1852.

124 Fonseca JE, Carvalho T, Cruz M *et al.* Polymorphism at position −308 of the tumour necrosis factor alpha gene and rheumatoid arthritis pharmacogenetics. *Ann Rheum Dis* 2005;64(5):793–794.

125 Seitz M, Wirthmuller U, Moller B *et al.* The −308 tumour necrosis factor-alpha gene polymorphism predicts therapeutic response to TNFalpha-blockers in rheumatoid arthritis and spondyloarthritis patients. *Rheumatology (Oxford)* 2007;46(1):93–96.

126 Marotte H, Pallot-Prades B, Grange L *et al.* The shared epitope is a marker of severity associated with selection for, but not with response to, infliximab in a large rheumatoid arthritis population. *Ann Rheum Dis* 2006;65(3):342–347.

127 Fabris M, Tolusso B, Di Poi E *et al.* Tumor necrosis factor-alpha receptor II polymorphism in patients from southern Europe with mild–moderate and severe rheumatoid arthritis. *J Rheumatol* 2002;29(9): 1847–1850.

128 Wolfe F, Mitchell DM, Sibley JT *et al.* The mortality of rheumatoid arthritis. *Arthritis Rheum* 1994;37(4): 481–494.

129 Sands BE, Anderson FH, Bernstein CN *et al.* Infliximab maintenance therapy for fistulizing Crohn's disease. *N Engl J Med* 2004;350(9):876–885.

130 St Clair EW, van der Heijde DM, Smolen JS *et al.* Combination of infliximab and methotrexate therapy for early rheumatoid arthritis: a randomized, controlled trial. *Arthritis Rheum* 2004;50(11): 3432–3443.

131 Cheifetz A, Smedley M, Martin S *et al.* The incidence and management of infusion reactions to infliximab: a large center experience. *Am J Gastroenterol* 2003; 98(6):1315–1324.

132 Baert F, Noman M, Vermeire S *et al.* Influence of immunogenicity on the long-term efficacy of infliximab in Crohn's disease. *N Engl J Med* 2003;348(7): 601–608.

133 Farrell RJ, Alsahli M, Jeen YT *et al.* Intravenous hydrocortisone premedication reduces antibodies to infliximab in Crohn's disease: a randomized controlled trial. *Gastroenterology* 2003;124(4):917–924.

134 Jones M, Symmons D, Finn J *et al.* Does exposure to immunosuppressive therapy increase the 10 year malignancy and mortality risks in rheumatoid arthritis? A matched cohort study. *Br J Rheumatol* 1996;35(8):738–745.

135 Prior P. Cancer and rheumatoid arthritis: epidemiologic considerations. *Am J Med* 1985;78(1A):15–21.

136 Williams CA, Bloch DA, Sibley J *et al.* Lymphoma and luekemia in rheumatoid arthritis: are they associated with azathioprine, cyclophosphamide, or methotrexate? *J Clin Rheumatol* 1996;2(2):64–72.

137 Keane J, Gershon S, Wise RP *et al.* Tuberculosis associated with infliximab, a tumor necrosis factor alpha-neutralizing agent. *N Engl J Med* 2001;345(15): 1098–1104.

138 Wallis RS, Broder M, Wong J *et al.* Granulomatous infections due to tumor necrosis factor blockade: correction. *Clin Infect Dis* 2004;39(8):1254–1255.

139 Wallis RS, Broder MS, Wong JY *et al*. Granulomatous infectious diseases associated with tumor necrosis factor antagonists. *Clin Infect Dis* 2004;38(9):1261–1265.

140 Scheinfeld N. A comprehensive review and evaluation of the side effects of the tumor necrosis factor alpha blockers etanercept, infliximab and adalimumab. *J Dermatolog Treat* 2004;15(5):280–294.

141 Wallis RS. Mathematical modeling of the cause of tuberculosis during tumor necrosis factor blockade. *Arthritis Rheum* 2008;58(4):947–952.

142 Lipsky PE, van der Heijde DM, St Clair EW *et al*. Infliximab and methotrexate in the treatment of rheumatoid arthritis. Anti-Tumor Necrosis Factor Trial in Rheumatoid Arthritis with Concomitant Therapy Study Group. *N Engl J Med* 2000;343(22): 1594–1602.

143 Kluger N, Poirier P, Guilpain P *et al*. Cryptococcal meningitis in a patient treated with infliximab and mycophenolate mofetil for Behcet's disease. *Int J Infect Dis* 2009;13(5):e325.

144 Munoz P, Giannella M, Valerio M *et al*. Cryptococcal meningitis in a patient treated with infliximab. *Diagn Microbiol Infect Dis* 2007;57(4):443–446.

145 Atzeni F, Turiel M, Capsoni F *et al*. Autoimmunity and anti-TNF-alpha agents. *Ann N Y Acad Sci* 2005; 1051:559–569.

146 De Rycke L, Baeten D, Kruithof E *et al*. Infliximab, but not etanercept, induces IgM anti-double-stranded DNA autoantibodies as main antinuclear reactivity: biologic and clinical implications in autoimmune arthritis. *Arthritis Rheum* 2005;52(7):2192–2201.

147 Colombel JF, Loftus EV, Jr, Tremaine WJ *et al*. The safety profile of infliximab in patients with Crohn's disease: the Mayo Clinic experience in 500 patients. *Gastroenterology* 2004;126(1):19–31.

148 Maini RN, Breedveld FC, Kalden JR *et al*. Therapeutic efficacy of multiple intravenous infusions of anti-tumor necrosis factor alpha monoclonal antibody combined with low-dose weekly methotrexate in rheumatoid arthritis. *Arthritis Rheum* 1998;41(9):1552–1563.

149 Kwon HJ, Cote TR, Cuffe MS *et al*. Case reports of heart failure after therapy with a tumor necrosis factor antagonist. *Ann Intern Med* 2003;138(10):807–811.

150 Mohan N, Edwards ET, Cupps TR *et al*. Demyelination occurring during anti-tumor necrosis factor alpha therapy for inflammatory arthritides. *Arthritis Rheum* 2001;44(12):2862–2869.

151 Pontikaki I, Shahi E, Frasin LA *et al*. Skin manifestations induced by TNF-alpha inhibitors in juvenile idiopathic arthritis. *Clin Rev Allergy Immunol*. 2011; in press.

152 Sfikakis PP, Iliopoulos A, Elezoglou A *et al*. Psoriasis induced by anti-tumor necrosis factor therapy: a paradoxical adverse reaction. *Arthritis Rheum* 2005;52(8): 2513–2518.

153 Pech T, Finger T, Fujishiro J *et al*. Perioperative infliximab application ameliorates acute rejection associated inflammation after intestinal transplantation. *Am J Transplant* 2010;10(11):2431–2441.

154 Metyas S, La D, Arkfeld DG. The use of the tumour necrosis factor antagonist infliximab in heart transplant recipients: two case reports. *Ann Rheum Dis* 2007;66(11):1544–1545.

155 Froud T, Ricordi C, Baidal DA *et al*. Islet transplantation in type 1 diabetes mellitus using cultured islets and steroid-free immunosuppression: Miami experience. *Am J Transplant* 2005;5(8):2037–2046.

156 Leroy S, Guigonis V, Bruckner D *et al*. Successful anti-TNFalpha treatment in a child with posttransplant recurrent focal segmental glomerulosclerosis. *Am J Transplant* 2009;9(4):858–861.

CHAPTER 27
CTLA4-Ig

Sarah E. Yost and Bruce Kaplan
University of Arizona Medical Center, Tucson, AZ, USA

History

The most commonly used immunosuppressive strategies are mainly based on induction with monoclonal or polyclonal antibodies, and a triple-based maintenance regimen including calcineurin inhibitors, antiproliferatives, and steroids. There is a trend for novel drugs and biologic agents for new immunosuppressive therapies that are based on steroid avoidance or calcineurin inhibitor avoidance or withdrawal.

During the alloimmune response, both naive and memory alloreactive T cells are engaged by dendritic cells of both the donor and the recipient. T lymphocyte activation requires three signals. Signal 1 involves T cell receptor triggered by donor antigen on the surface of dentritic cells or other antigen presenting cells (APCs). Signal 2, or the "costimulation signal," is not antigen specific and many pairs of molecules on the surface of T lymphocytes and APCs can contribute as well to the costimulation. The B7/CD28 and CD40/CD40L pathways are very important in T cell activation. The costimulation signal is delivered when B7-1/CD28 and B7-2/CD86 on the surface of dentritic cells engage CD28 on T cells. This costimulation from signals 1 and 2 activates the transduction pathways that result in the production of interleukin-2 (IL-2) and the α-chain of its receptor CD25 and CD40 ligand. The CD40 is expressed on all APCs and its ligand is on activated CD4 T cells and on a subset of CD8 T cells and natural killer cells. CD40 stimulation triggers important signals for antibody production by B cells and strongly induces B7 and major histocompatibility complex (MHC) expression on APCs [1–4].

The B7/CD28/CTLA-4 pathway is characterized by the dual specificity of two B7 family members, B7-1 and B7-2, for both the stimulatory receptor CD28 and the inhibitory receptor CTLA-4 (cytotoxic T-lymphoctye-associated antigen 4/CD152). CD 28 provides a T cell activation signal and CTLA-4 inhibits T cell responses. CD28 is constitutively expressed on T cells, whereas CTLA-4 expression is rapidly upregulated following T cell activation. CTLA-4 has a higher receptor affinity for both B7-1 and B7-2 than CD28 [1, 2, 5].

The CTLA4-Ig molecule was used to target the B7/CD28 pathway, a fusion protein consisting of the extracellular domain of CTLA-4 and the Fc domain of IgG. CTLA4-Ig may act by directly disrupting B7/CD28 cross-talk and or by activating the immunosuppressive pathway of tryptophan catabolism on dendritic cells [2]. In nonhuman primates (NHPs), kidney graft survival increases from 8 to 30 days using CTLA4-Ig alone and up to 6 months if CTLA4-Ig plus humanized danti-CD40L antibody are used [2,6]. Survival was similar with the humanized anti-CD40L antibody alone, suggesting that CD40/CD40L pathway is significant [2, 6].

The humanized anti-CD40L antibody (huC58) was the first agent used to block costimulation in human trials. This agent was tolerated in NHPs but was discontinued for human use after seven

Immunotherapy in Transplantation: Principles and Practice, First Edition. Edited by Bruce Kaplan, Gilbert J. Burckart and Fadi G. Lakkis.
© 2012 Blackwell Publishing Ltd. Published 2012 by Blackwell Publishing Ltd.

patients suffered thromboembolic events. The CD40L has been detected on the surface of activated platelets and has been shown to activate endothelium [7].

The production of a soluble fusion protein comprising of the extracellular domain of CTLA4 and a human IgG1 Fc domain that binds to the CD28 ligands, CD80, and CD86 with a higher affinity than CD28 was made [1]. Abatacept (Orencia®) was developed as a CTLA4-Ig molecule with a mutated Fc domain for treatment of rheumatoid arthritis [2]. The affinity of CTLA4-Ig for CD80 is 200 times higher than that for CD86 and is 100 times more potent for the blockade of CD80-dependent costimulation than that of CD86 costimulation [21]. Belatacept (LEA29Y) was developed as a second-generation compound with more immunosuppressive effects than abatacept by creating a derivative with slower dissociation rates from CD80 and CD86 [8–10].

A review of the clinical trials

A large Phase II study was conducted to evaluate the safety and efficacy of belatacept versus a cyclosporine based regimen in kidney transplant recipients [11]. This multicenter study included 218 patients randomly assigned to receive one of three regimens for primary immunosuppression; intensive regimen of belatacept, less intensive regimen of belatacept, or cyclosporine. The belatacept regimens included an early phase of 10 mg/kg and a late phase of 5 mg/kg at 4 or 8 week intervals and was administered as a 30 min intravenous infusion. All patients received induction therapy with basiliximab (20 mg on day 0 and day 4), mycophenolate mofetil, and a corticosteroid taper regimen. The incidence of acute rejection at 6 months was similar among the groups with 7% in the intensive belatacept group, 6% in less intensive group, and 8% in the cyclosporine group. The glomerular filtration rate (GFR) was calculated by the modification of diet in renal disease (MDRD) and at 12 months the GFR was significantly higher among the intensive and less-intensive belatacept groups (66.3 mL/min per 1.73 m^2, 62.1 mL/min per 1.73 m^2) than the cyclosporine group (53.5 mL/min per 1.73 m^2; $p=0.01$). In patients who underwent a 12 month biopsy the incidence of chronic allograft nephropathy was lower in the intensive and less-intensive belatacept groups (29%, 20%) than the cyclosporine group (44%) [11].

The Phase II study results suggested belatacept may provide adequate maintenance immunosuppression and possibly have renal sparing effects. Two Phase III studies were conducted to assess whether a belatacept-based regimen would achieve adequate renal function and patient and graft survival compared with cyclosporine in standard and extended-criteria donor kidneys [12, 13]. The BENEFIT (Belatacept Evaluation of Nephroprotection and Efficacy as First-line Immunosuppression Trial) is a multicenter 3 year randomized trial with primary outcomes assessed at 12 months [12]. This study included 686 patients randomly assigned to receive one of three regimens: intensive regimen of belatacept, less intensive regimen of belatacept, or cyclosporine. Patients received basiliximab induction therapy (20 mg at days 0 and 4), mycophenolate mofetil, and corticosteroid taper. At 12 months there was no difference between the belatacept regimens and cyclosporine groups in patient and graft survival. Renal function was found to be higher in the belatacept arms of the study than in the cyclosporine arm. The measured mean GFR was 13–15 mL/min higher in the belatacept groups than with cyclosporine. The prevalence of biopsy-proven chronic allograft nephropathy was 18% in the intensive regimen, 24% in the less intensive regimen, and 32% in the cyclosporine group (in the subset of patients who underwent a protocol 12 month renal biopsy). However, the incidence of acute rejection at 12 months was higher in the belatacept groups than in the cyclosporine group: 22% intensive regimen, 17% less intensive regimen, and 7% in the cyclosporine group [12].

The 2 year BENEFIT data were published and continued to show patient and graft survival was similar across all three treatment groups (94% intensive group, 95% less intensive, 91% cyclosporine) [14]. The mean GFR was higher in the belatacept groups than in the cyclosporine group. There were eight additional patients with an acute rejection episode between the first and second years ($n=4$ intensive, $n=4$ cyclosporine). The incidence rate of malignancies and infections was the same across all groups with the addition of two cases of post-transplant lymphoproliferative disorder (PTLD) between the first and second years. Currently, at 24 months, the belatacept regimens provide similar efficacy and superior renal function compared with cyclosporine [14]. BENEFIT-EXT (Belatacept Evaluation of Nephroprotection and Efficacy as First-line Immunosuppression Trial-EXTended criteria donors) is a multicenter 3 year randomized trial that includes 578 patients that received an extended-criteria donor kidney who were randomly assigned to receive one of three regimens: intensive regimen of belatacept, less-intensive regimen of belatacept, or cyclosporine [15]. This study evaluated the same primary outcomes at 12 months as the BENEFIT study and received the same immunosuppression. The belatacept arms showed noninferiority to cyclosporine for patient and graft survival at 1 year and the proportion of patients surviving with a functioning graft was similar among all groups. The incidence of acute rejection at 12 months was similar among the groups, with 17.9% in the intensive group, 17.7% in the less-intensive group, and 14.1% in the cyclosporine group. The GFR was 6–8 mL/min higher from the beginning of the study to 12 months in the belatacept arms compared with cyclosporine despite a similar number of patients with delayed graft function among the treatment groups. The incidence of chronic allograft nephropathy was similar among all three treatment groups in the subset of patients who received a biopsy [13].

The 2 year BENEFIT-EXT data show similar graft and patient survival amongst the three treatment groups (83% intensive regimen, 84% less intensive, and 83% cyclosporine). The GFR was 8–10 mL/min higher in the belatacept groups than with cyclosporine. There were three additional episodes of acute rejection after the first year ($n = 1$ less-intensive group, $n = 1$ cyclosporine). The incidence of malignancies and serious infections was similar among the treatment groups with the same number of PTLD cases equaling five patients. Currently, the benefits of belatacept are similar to the BENEFIT study but in patients with extended-criteria donors [15].

Chemistry and structure

Abatacept (CTLA4-Ig) is the first recombinant immunoglobulin fusion protein that contains an extracellular portion of CTLA4 and the Fc domain of IgG. Belatacept is a fusion protein composed of the Fc fragment of a human IgG1 immunoglobulin linked to the extracellular domain of CTLA4 and differs from abatacept only by two amino acids (L104E and A29Y). This small difference confers greater binding affinity to CD80 and CD86 (twofold and fourfold respectively). CTLA4-Ig binds to both CD80 and CD86 rather than CD28; however, it is 100-fold less potent at inhibiting CD86-dependent costimulation than CD80 [8, 16].

Mechanism of action

Abatacept is a biological response modifier that demonstrates anti-inflammatory affects by downregulating T cell activation. Abatacept is a cytotoxic T lymphocyte antigen immunoglobulin (CTLA4-Ig), a novel fusion protein, which consist of CTLA linked to the modified heavy-chain constant region of human IgG1. One mechanism for the initiation of the inflammatory process is the activation of the T cell. Costimulation is one of two pathways necessary for optimal T cell activation. Costimulation consists of two sites on the APC binding to the two sites on the T cell. The two sites on the APC are the MHC and the CD80/86. The two sites on the T cell are T cell receptor and the CD28. The initial event is the MHC binding to the T cell receptor and the costimulatory event is the CD80 or CD86 binding to the CD28. Abatacept blocks the costimulation pathway by binding to CD80 and CD86 on APC, thus preventing them from binding to CD28 on the T cells [17–20]. Abatacept provided selective costimulation blockade of T cell activation and binds CD80 and CD86 [21]. This agent is currently Food and Drug Administration (FDA) approved for the treatment of rheumatoid arthritis and with the trade name of Orencia®. CTLA4-Ig was studied in rodents and showed prolonged transplanted organ survival which led to studies in NHP transplant models. These studies showed

CTLA4-Ig did not completely inhibit B7-mediated responses and did not completely inhibit T cell activation and thus was felt not to allow adequate immunosuppression without the use of a calcineurin inhibitor [9]. A new molecule was developed, belatacept, to have a higher affinity for B7 ligands, specifically CD86; this molecule, first termed LEA29Y, was found to have increased affinity for CD86 and CD80 on lymphocytes [9, 22, 23]. Belatacept is a human fusion protein which prevents CD28 signaling and inhibits T cell activation.

Pharmacokinetics and pharmacodynamics

The pharmacokinetics of belatacept is characterized by a linear and time-invariant model with a clearance of 0.86 L/day, volume of distribution of 10.3 L, and terminal half-life of 11 days. Belatacept's concentrations for any given dose were lower with an increase in body weight (either increased clearance or increased volume of distribution leading to a shorted terminal half-life), thus supporting weight-based dosing. However, clearance is not affected by age, gender, renal or hepatic function, diabetes, or dialysis [24]. The peak concentration was 295 mcg/mL and the C_{max} of abatacept after multiple intravenous doses of 10 mg/kg was 295 mcg/mL (171–398 mcg/mL) in 14 rheumatoid arthritis patients. Proportional increases in C_{max} was demonstrated over the dose range 2–10 mg/kg. No systemic accumulation of abatacept occurred upon continued repeated treatment with 10 mg/kg at monthly intervals in rheumatoid patients. The C_{max} of abatacept after the fourth dose was 17±4.6 mcg/mL for the 0.5 mg/kg dose ($n=4$) and 2201±578 mcg/mL for the 50 mg/kg dose ($n=5$) in a Phase I dose-escalation study. Abatacept was administered on days 1, 3, 16, and 29 [18, 25]. Proportional increases in the area under the curve were demonstrated over the dose range 2–10 mg/kg [18].

Adverse effects

The investigators of belatacept have pooled safety from the Phase II and Phase III studies, which includes 1425 intent-to-treat patients with a median follow up of 2.4 years with some of the patients being followed 7 years. The belatacept-based regimens was found to be generally safe (Table 27.1), with the incidence of PTLD higher in the belatacept groups, especially in Epstein–Barr virus serologically negative patients and the intensive regimen. There were no cases of PTLD after 18 months in the belatacept groups. The incidence of deaths and serious infections was lowest in the belatacept less-intensive regimen. Tuberculosis occurred in 10 patients, mostly in endemic areas. There were no reports of anaphylaxis or hypersensitivity reactions to belatacept [26].

Recently, the 5 year safety and efficacy data were published; this included 78 (out of 102) belatacept patients and 16 (out of 26) patients in the

Table 27.1 Summary of safety profile of belatacept [26].

	Belatacept MI ($n=477$)	Belatacept LI ($n=472$)	Cyclosporine ($n=476$)
Incidence of death (%)	7	5	7
Serious adverse events (%)	71	68	69
Overall malignancy (%)	10	6	7
Overall PTLD (n)	8	5	2
PTLD, CNS involvement	6	2	0
Serious infections (%)	37	32	36
Polyoma (%)	7	3	6
Fungal infections (%)	22	17	21
PML (n)	1	0	0
Tuberculosis (n)	5	4	1

Table 27.2 Cardiovascular risk factors in the 5 year follow-up study [27].

Parameter	24 months	36 months	48 months	60 months
Systolic BP				
Belatacept (mmHg; mean [SD])	129 [15.3]	129 [13.4]	126 [15.6]	125 [13.9]
Cyclosporine (mmHg; mean [SD])	132 [20.2]	129 [8.9]	140 [21.0]	138 [18.9]
Diastolic BP				
Belatacept (mmHg; mean [SD])	76 [10.5]	76 [9.5]	76 [9.9]	76 [10.1]
Cyclosporine (mmHg; mean [SD])	78 [9.3]	76 [7.5]	77 [11.9]	83 [8.9]
Non-HDL cholesterol				
Belatacept (mg/dL; mean [SD])	150 [35.7]	144 [37.5]	138 [38.8]	128 [37.3]
Cyclosporine (mg/dL; mean [SD])	140 [44.9]	130 [31.7]	131 [38.6]	119 [29.5]
New-onset diabetes after transplant				
Belatacept	7 [7]	8 [9]	8 [9]	9 [10]
Cyclosporine	2 [9]	2 [9]	2 [9]	2 [9]

cyclosporine group [27]. The mean calculated GFR (mL/min per 1.73 m^2) at 12 months was 75.8±20.1 with belatacept-treated patients and 74.4±22.7 in the cyclosporine group. At 60 months, the greatest difference was seen with mean calculated GFR: 77.2±22.7 in the belatacept group and 59.3±15.3 in the cyclosporine group. Three belatacept patients died (two with a function graft, one after graft loss) and two cyclosporine patients died (both with functioning graft). Six cases of biopsy-proven acute rejection were diagnosed in the belatacept group. Two cases were patients on the 4 week dosing schedule and four cases were in the 8 week dosing group. There were no biopsy-proven rejection cases in the cyclosporine group. The most common adverse effects in belatacept patients were nasopharyngitis, urinary tract infection, diarrhea, and upper respiratory infection. There were no new cases of PTLD in this follow-up study. The cardiovascular risk factors favored belatacept over cyclosporine (Table 27.2) [27].

Belatacept is currently undergoing the FDA approval process and the other side effects discussed are from the sister drug abatacept (Orencia®). Gastrointestinal effects, including diverticulitis and

nausea, were reported in 5 % and 10 % of patients. Patients experienced acute infusion-related reactions in roughly 9 % compared with 6 % in placebo, and the reactions included dizziness, hypertension, and headache. Patients reported headache up to 18 % compared with placebo. The product information cites pyelonephritis 0.2–0.5 % and urinary tract infections up to 6 %. Respiratory effects include acute exacerbation of chronic obstructive pulmonary disease 43 %, bronchitis 0.5 %, nasopharyngitis 12 %, pneumonia 0.5 %, respiratory tract infection 37.6 %, and upper respiratory infection 10 % [18].

Drug–drug interactions

Theoretical pharmacokinetic interactions might occur secondary to the immunoglobulin protein; however, it is unlikely to affect small-molecule oxidation or glucuronidation, but might interact with other immunoglobulin clearance. The pharmacodynamic interactions are an increased risk of infections or increased competition of binding sites or targets. The drug interactions discussed below are based on the data from abatacept, as belatacept has not been FDA approved at the time of publication. The combination of TNF antagonists and abatacept (CTLA4-Ig) can have an increased risk of infection if used together and documented to be 43–63% higher than TNF antagonist therapy alone. Controlled clinical trials have demonstrated that the concomitant use of abatacept and TNF antagonists resulted in an increased risk for serious infection and provided no additional benefit. Therefore, concurrent therapy with abatacept and TNF antagonists, such as adalimumab, is not recommended [18].

The administration of live vaccines during or within 3 months following abatacept treatment is not recommended owing to the secondary transmission of infection by the live vaccine. There is a possibility for abatacept to affect host defenses against infections, since the cellular immune response may be altered. It is generally recommended to avoid live vaccines after solid organ transplant, depending on specific transplant centers [18].

Therapeutic drug monitoring

As of the date of this publication, clinical trials have recommended that therapeutic drug monitoring is not necessary owing to the time invariance of belatacept pharmacokinetics, the minimal potential for drug–drug interaction, and the low mean variability in exposure indicating that dose is a good predictor of belatacept [28–31].

Absorption, distribution, metabolism, and excretion

Based on an integrated assessment of the in vitro pharmacokinetics–pharmacodynamics relationship for the inhibition of alloresponse by belatacept and results from an in vivo primate transplant model, target trough concentrations of 20 µg/mL, 5 µg/mL, and 2 µg/mL during month 1, months 2–3, and months 4–6 after transplantation respectively were identified to design the dose regimens in renal

transplantation subjects. Overall, >80% of the renal transplant recipients treated with the recommended dosing regimen (less-intensive (LI) regimen) achieved the intended target trough concentrations in Phase III studies. Data from the Phase III studies also demonstrated that the observed trough concentration of belatacept during months 2–7 was approximately two- to three-fold higher for the more-intensive (MI) regimen than for the LI regimen, consistent with the twofold higher cumulative dose for the MI regimen during months 2–6. Trough concentrations of belatacept were then tapered to similar values during the maintenance phase (beyond month 7), when the dose and frequency of administration were identical for the two regimens [31].

Pharmacogenemoics

Pharmacogenetic strategies can be used as an adjunct to therapeutic drug monitoring in achieving target blood levels of immunosuppressive drugs. There is documented research of CYP 450 3A5 genotype and dosing of immunosuppressive drugs like tacrolimus and UGT1A9 for mycophenophenolate [32]. Pharmacogenemoics might play a role with mutations on B7 or on the binding sites, which at this point in time are not discovered or used in clinical practice. There is research being conducted to understand individual variation in cytokine gene expression and genes encoding surface costimulatory molecules. Hutchings *et al.* are investigating correlations between single nucleotide polymorphisms in genes for IL-6 and IL-10 with cellular expression of B7 costimulatory molecules and associations of race and rejection episodes in kidney transplant recipients [33].

References

1 Durrbach A, Francois H, Jacquet A *et al.* Co-signals in organ transplantation. *Curr Opin Organ Transplant* 2010;15:474–480.

2 Snanoudj R, Frangie C, Deroure B, Francois H, Creput C *et al.* The blockade of T-cell co-stimulation as a

therapeutic stratagem for immunosuppression: focus on belatacept. *Biologics* 2007;1:203–213.

3 Bromley SK, Iaboni A, Davis SJ *et al*. Immunological synapse and CD28–CD80 interactions. *Nat Immunol* 2001;2:1159–1166.

4 Von Kooten C, Banchereau J. Functions of CD40 on B cells, dendritic cells and other cells. *Curr Opin Immunol* 1997;9:330–337.

5 Greenwald RJ, Freeman GJ, Sharpe AH. The B7 family revisited. *Annu Rev Immunol* 2005;23:515–548.

6 Kirk AD, Burkly LC, Batty DS *et al*. Treatment with humanized monoclonal antibody against CD154 prevents acute renal allograft rejection in nonhuman primates. *Nat Med* 1999;5:686–693.

7 Kawai T, Andrews D, Colvin RB *et al*. Thromboembolic complications after treatment with monoclonal antibody against CD40 ligand. *Nat Med* 2000; 6:114.

8 Rangel EB. Belatacept in clinical and experimental transplantation – progress and promise. *Drugs Today* 2010;46:235–242.

9 Larsen CP, Pearson TC, Adams AB *et al*. Rational development of LEA29Y (belatacept), a high affinity variant of CTLA-4-Ig with potent immunosuppressive properties. *Am J Transplant* 2005;5:443–453.

10 Poirier N, Blancho G, Vanhove B. Alternatives to calcinuerin inhibition in renal transplantation: belatacept, the first co-stimulation blocker. *Immunotherapy* 2010;2(5):625–636.

11 Vincenti F, Larsen C, Durrback A *et al*. Costimulation blockade with belatacept in renal transplantation. *N Engl J Med.* 2005;353:770–781.

12 Vincenti F, Charpentier B, Vanrenterghem Y *et al*. A Phase III study of belatacept-based immunosuppression regimens versus cyclosporine in renal transplant recipients (BENEFIT Study). *Am J Transplant* 2010; 10:535–546.

13 Durrbach A, Pestana JM, Pearson T *et al*. A Phase III study of belatacept versus cyclosporine in kidney transplant from the extended criteria donors (BENEFIT-EXT Study). *Am J Transplant* 2010;10:547–557.

14 Larsen CP, Grinyo J, Charpentier B *et al*. Belatacept vs cyclosporine in kidney transplant recipients: two-year outcomes from the BENEFIT study. American Transplant Congress 2010; abstract 142.

15 Durrbach A, Larsen CP, Pestana JM *et al*. Belatacept vs cyclosporine in the ECD kidney transplants: two-year outcomes from the BENEFIT-EXT study. American Transplant Congress 2010; abstract 143.

16 Greene JL, Leytze GM, Emswiler J *et al*. Covaltent dimerization of CD28/CTLA-4 and oligomerization of CD80/CD86 regulate T cell costimulatory interactions. *J Biol Chem* 1996;271:26762–26771.

17 Dumont FJ. Technology evaluation: abatacept, Bristol-Myers Squibb. *Curr Opin Mol Ther* 2004;6:318–330.

18 Orencia® Package Insert. Bristol Myers Squibb, August 2009.

19 Teng GG, Turkiewicz AM, Moreland LW. Abatacept: a costimulatory inhibitor for treatment of rheumatoid arthritis. *Expert Opin Biol Ther* 2005;5(9): 1245–1254.

20 Kremer JM, Westhovens R, Leon M *et al*: Treatment of rheumatoid arthritis by selective inhibition of T-cell activation with fusion protein CTLA4Ig. *N Engl J Med* 2003;349(20):1907–1915.

21 Linsley PS, Greene JL, Brady W *et al*. Human B7-1 (CD80) and By-2(CD86) bind with similar activities but distinct kinetics to CD28 and CTLA-4 receptors. *Immunity* 1994;1:793–801.

22 Snanoudk R, Frangie C, Deroure B *et al*. The blockade of T-cell co-stimulation as a therapeutic stratagem for immunosuppression: focus on belatacept. *Biologics* 2007;1:203–213.

23 Latek R, Fleener C, Lamian V *et al*. Assessment of belatacept-mediated costimulation blockade through evaluation of CD80/86-receptor saturation. *Transplantation* 2009;87:926–933.

24 Zhou Z, Shen J, Kaul S *et al*. Belatacept population pharmacokinetics in renal transplant patients. American Transplant Congress 2010; abstract 1501.

25 Abrams JR, Lebwohl MG, Guzzo CA *et al*: CTLA4IG-mediated blockade of T-cell costimulation in patients with psoriasis. *J Clin Invest* 1999;103(9):1243–1252.

26 Grinyo J, Charpentier B, Pestana JM *et al*. Safety profile of belatacept in kidney transplant recipients from a pooled analysis of Phase II and Phase III studies. American Transplant Congress 2010; abstract 144.

27 Vincenti F, Blancho G, Durrbach A *et al*. Five-year safety and efficacy of belatacept in renal transplantation. *J Am Soc Nephrol* 2010;21:1587–1596.

28 Van Gelder T. Mycophenolate blood level monitoring: recent progress. *Am J Transplant* 2009; 9:1495–1499.

29 Felipe CR, Silva HT, Jr, Machado PGP *et al*. Time-dependent changes in cyclosporine exposure: implications for achieving target concentrations. *Transpl Int* 2003;16:494–503.

30 Kahan BD. Pharmacokinetic considerations in the therapeutic application of cyclosporine in renal transplantation. *Transplant Proc* 1996;28:2143–2146.

31 Bristol-Myers Squibb. Belatacept (BMS-224818), FDA's Cardiovascular and Renal Drugs Advisory Committee Briefing Document for March 2010 Meeting. http://

www.fda.gov/downloads/AdvisoryCommittees/
CommitteesMeetingMaterials/Drugs/Cardiovascular
andRenalDrugsAdvisoryCommittee/UCM201859.pdf.

32 MacPhee IAM. Use of pharmacogenetics to optimize immunosuppressive therapy. *Ther Drug Monit* 2010;32: 261–264.

33 Hutchings A, Guay-Woodfor L, Thomas JM *et al.* Association of cytokine single nucleotide polymorphisms with B7 costimulatory molecules in kidney allograft recipients. *Pediatr Transplant* 2002;6: 69–77.

CHAPTER 28

Combination and Adjuvant Therapies to Facilitate the Efficacy of Costimulatory Blockade

Swetha K. Srinivasan, Helen L. Triemer, and Allan D. Kirk
Emory Transplantation Center, Emory University, Atlanta, GA, USA

Introduction

Organ transplantation has become a widely utilized treatment modality for patients with end-stage organ failure. However, it remains limited by the requirement for continuous immune modification to prevent rejection of the transplanted organs. While great progress has been made in preventing acute T-cell-mediated rejection, no single therapy has been shown to evoke sustained control over alloimmunity. As such, most patients require daily combination therapies of some sort to preserve graft function. These costly drug regimens generally have a narrow therapeutic window such that even strictly adherent patients vacillate between general immune incompetence and alloimmune responsiveness. This results in indolent immune injury to the graft, chronic systemic side effects, or both. Thus, the early benefits of organ transplantation typically give way over a decade to inexorable graft destruction through the effects of recurrent cellular or alloantibody-mediated graft injury, and/or accelerated co-morbid illnesses that are exacerbated by the off-target side effects of the daily drug therapies. Indeed, renal allograft survival has changed only modestly in the last 10 years and remains characterized by steady graft loss and premature death from accelerated cardiovascular, infectious, and malignant disease

[1, 2]. Thus, two primary deficiencies shape modern transplantation: the need for continuous therapy and the relatively nonspecific nature of modern immunosuppressive regimens.

Many signaling pathways have been identified that suppress T cell function and have subsequently been exploited to prevent allograft rejection [3]. However, throughout the development of transplantation, clinicians have recognized that generalized immune suppression is poorly tolerated. This has spurred research into the manner in which T cell responses are initiated and curtailed physiologically in an *antigen-specific* manner, and that research has given rise to a model in which physiologic immune responses are awakened by antigen *stimulation*, but shaped and controlled by accessory *costimulation*. Emanating from the original concepts of Bretscher and Cohn, and subsequent refinements from Lafferty and Cunningham, a "two-signal" model for immune cell activation (an antigen-specific "signal one" and a nonspecific costimulatory "signal two") has now blossomed into a mature understanding of how immune responses augment and contract in response to antigenic stimuli. Indeed, current costimulation biology involves scores of receptor–ligand interactions and numerous interrelated intracellular signaling pathways [4].

Immunotherapy in Transplantation: Principles and Practice, First Edition. Edited by Bruce Kaplan, Gilbert J. Burckart and Fadi G. Lakkis.
© 2012 Blackwell Publishing Ltd. Published 2012 by Blackwell Publishing Ltd.

Although the specifics of costimulatory biology are complex, the fundamental concepts are rather simple. In general, antigen binding through antigen receptors establishes *to what* the immune system will respond, and costimulatory pathway activation determines *how* it will respond, be it augmentation of a protective response, regulation of an inflammatory focus, or contraction after an immune threat is controlled. As such, costimulation pathways are critical in maintaining immune homeostasis and ensuring that responses occur within physiologic boundaries of immune repertoire size, avoiding immune exhaustion or lymphoproliferative disorders. As these pathways have been studied, three points have become clear. First, *costimulatory pathways are critically involved in the initiation of an alloimmune response*. Essentially every costimulatory pathway studied has shown an alloimmune response phenotype. Second, *no single costimulatory pathway completely controls rejection in out-bred adult animals or humans*. There is significant redundancy amongst the pathways involved that has evolved to avoid a single pathogenic mechanism from thwarting protective immunity. Third and importantly, *the influence of costimulation wanes as an immune response matures*. The costimulatory checks and balances required to initiate a new immune response are less relevant once an immune response has been deployed and been proven (through survival) to be beneficial.

As evidence has emerged regarding the relevance of costimulation in alloimmunity, costimulation pathways have increasingly been exploited in preclinical models of transplantation and are now beginning to be targeted in the clinic. In particular, monoclonal antibodies (mAbs) and fusion proteins specific for the extracellular domains of costimulatory receptors and their ligands have emerged as a new class of immunotherapeutic drug. Essentially all costimulation-based therapies have begun their journey to clinical translation in mouse models and subsequently followed a developmental path through preclinical nonhuman primate (NHP) studies to humans. Although human data are emerging, most of the data regarding these agents comes from interpretation of animal studies, and has fostered the realization

that these pathways are important, but not infallible in preventing rejection. Thus, the optimal means of deploying costimulation-based therapies remain to be determined, and the prevailing challenges in drug development relate largely to how best to combine costimulatory agents with other agents. Specifically, efforts are being directed toward the development of combinations that not only provide satisfactory prophylaxis from rejection, but also preserve the antigen-specific potential that has inspired the development of costimulatory blockade (CoB).

At present, two critical costimulatory pathways have been studied in sufficient depth to allow their movement into the clinic: the CD28–CD80/86 pathway and the CD40–CD154 pathway. Additional accessory molecules influencing cell adhesion and facilitating costimulatory interactions have been identified and recognized to have synergistic potential along with these costimulatory pathways; among them are the lymphocyte function associated antigen-1 (LFA-1, CD18/11a), the intracellular adhesion molecule (ICAM, CD54) pathway, and the CD2-leukocyte function antigen (LFA-3, CD58) pathway. Each pathway has a unique temporal, spatial, and functional expression during a T cell response, and an understanding of these nuances appears to be pivotal in developing an optimal antirejection regimen. Similarly, the effects of modifying multiple costimulatory pathways in one patient and the drug–drug interactions between CoB agents and conventional immune therapies such as calcineurin inhibitors (CNIs) are just now unfolding in ways that inform the development of combination therapies. This chapter will provide historical perspective on the bench-to-bedside advancement of CoB, as well as details regarding the structure and mechanism of action of agents that have reached the clinic. It also will discuss potential adjuvant therapies and therapeutic strategies that might bolster the antirejection effect of CoB without eliminating the antigen-specific character of the class. At present, CoB agents have been used in combination with other biologics only in preclinical models. As such, the relevant preclinical NHP trials will be discussed.

History and general pathway biology

The CD28–B7 costimulatory pathway

As early as 1968, the requirement for secondary cell signaling to allow optimal lymphocyte activation was recognized and espoused by Bretscher and Cohn [5]. They described how induction of antibody formation required recognition of two determinants on an antigen and established the associative recognition model, in which a secondary signal was crucial for B cell formation. In 1975, Lafferty and Cunningham extrapolated the two binding site theory to T cells [4]. They speculated that even weak antigen–receptor bonds could lead to strong stimulation through the enhancing effects of a second signal, or T cell costimulation.

Schwartz and colleagues brought about new evidence in support of the two-signal model for T cell activation in 1987 [6]. While studying the details of signal 1, they showed that modified antigen-presenting cells (APCs) that engaged only signal 1 produced inactive T cell clones. In 1989, Janeway showed that costimulation was required for APC activation and that costimulatory molecule upregulation enhanced the process of antigen presentation to T cells [7]. Jenkins and Schwartz later showed that T cell receptor (TCR)–antigen interactions would, in the absence of costimulation, lead to anergy and/or apoptosis, and that this could be prevented if CD28–B7 protein interactions were present [8].

CD28, found on the surface of T cells, was the first costimulation molecule to be identified as pivotal in T cell proliferation and differentiation [9]. CD28 binds the B7 proteins CD80 and CD86, thus increasing interleukin-2 (IL-2) transcription and decreasing the TCR's signaling threshold [10]. In conjunction with TCR stimulation, CD28 ligation dramatically augments cytokine production. In the 1990s, substantial interest was generated in the therapeutic potential in blockade of this pathway with the demonstration by Lenschow et al. that the fusion protein CTLA4-Ig could prevent the rejection of islet xenografts in mice [11]. This was followed by numerous studies in mice and primates demonstrating that organ rejection could be significantly delayed by B7-specific blockade [12].

Paradoxically, the concept of co-*inhibition* was found to involve the same pathway as the original co-*stimulation* molecule with the discovery of CTLA-4 (CD152), a homologue of CD28 [13]. CD152 binds with 10- to 20-fold greater affinity than CD28 to CD80 and CD86. While its expression is absent on resting T cells, it is upregulated on CD28 activated T cells, and dominantly inhibits IL-2 expression, competing with CD28 for B7 molecules and arresting T cells in the G_1 phase of the cell cycle as a means of negative feedback. In what is now recognized as an elegantly efficient means of immune regulation, the process of response initiation is intimately associated with the mechanisms of response termination. Importantly, however, the competitive nature of CD28 and CD152 binding to B7 molecules also means that interference with this pathway has the potential for dose-related immune suppression or immune augmentation depending on the prevailing receptor (CD28 or CD152 respectively) controlling the immune posture at any given time.

The CD40–CD154 costimulatory pathway

An additional major costimulation pathway to be recognized was the CD40–CD154 pathway. Initially described by Paulie et al. and defined by Ledbetter as Bp50 in 1986, CD40 is a member of the TNF receptor superfamily that is constitutively expressed on cells with antigen presentation capabilities such as B cells, macrophages, dendritic cells (DCs), and thymic epithelia [14, 15]. It can be induced on endothelial cells and fibroblasts [16]. It has a significant role in B cell activation and the maturation of DCs, which become 100-fold more potent initiators of T cell responses following CD40-dependent maturation [17, 18]. It is critically involved in the activation of APC-like functions for these cells, and importantly induces B7 molecule expression as well as a number of proimmune cytokines. As such, CD40 ligation facilitates T cell costimulation and in doing so aids in the initiation of T cell responses. CD40 costimulation also provides signals for B cell proliferation, immunoglobulin production and isotype switching, memory B cell development, macrophage effector function, and endothelial cell adhesion molecule upregulation.

CD154 was first defined as the ligand for CD40 by Armitage and coworkers and Noelle *et al.* in 1992 [19–21]. It is expressed as a homotrimeric type II integral membrane protein and a soluble cleaved cytokine. Following signal 1, CD154 expression is enhanced by CD28 signaling [17]. CD154 can be found primarily on activated CD4+ cells, as well as CD8+ cells, B cells, eosinophils, mast cells, basophils, DCs, epithelial cells, fibroblasts, and endothelial cells to a lesser degree [22, 23]. It is produced intracellularly in activated T cells and is rapidly deployed as a homo-trimer to the T cell surface following TCR and CD28 engagement so as to provide positive feedback for local APCs. CD154 is also known to be present in platelets and is released upon platelet degranulation [24]. As such, trauma is intimately related to the delivery of costimulation to the site of injury, and facilitating APC activation in the environment most likely to be proximal to the antigen inciting the tissue injury. The critical and fundamental relationship between trauma, antigen presentation and T and B cell activation mediated through the CD40–CD154 pathway has been made apparent by dramatic effects of organ transplant rejection in rodent and primate models, and the clear influence of platelet-derived CD154 on allograft rejection [23, 25]. This relationship has also made translation of CD154-specific agents for clinical use challenging, in that interference with this pathway has the potential for interference with coagulative homeostasis and thrombosis.

Like the CD28–B7 pathway, enthusiasm for the therapeutic potential of the CD40–CD154 pathway's blockade derived from mouse islet studies, with Parker *et al.* showing that a CD154-specific mAb could prevent islet rejection and when combined with donor-specific transfusion this led to indefinite graft survival with antigen specificity [26]. Larsen and coworkers solidified the synergistic nature of these approaches in mice and Kirk *et al.* translated these findings into a therapeutic approach in primates, with the latter work igniting substantial enthusiasm for the clinical applicability of this approach [27–29].

Adhesion molecule pathways

With time, numerous additional costimulatory pathways have been characterized and most have shown relevance in murine transplant models [30]. As these have yet to present themselves in the clinic, they will not be detailed in this chapter. However, other relevant pathways broadly characterized as adhesion molecule pathways have proven themselves relevant to the discussion of optimal use of costimulatory pathway inhibition. The distinctions between adhesion and costimulatory molecules have become less apparent with time. Both mediate nonantigen-specific interactions that facilitate subsequent T cell activation. In general, costimulatory molecules mediate this through alterations in cell signaling, while adhesion pathways facilitate the geometry of a cell–cell interaction and optimize the TCR–major histocompatibility complex (MHC) immune synapse; however, there are clear examples of cross-over in these mechanisms. Regardless, it has increasingly become apparent that *adhesion and costimulation pathways have synergistic influence on downstream T cell function*. Two pathways are particularly relevant given their therapeutic manipulation in the clinic: the LFA-1 (CD18/11a)–ICAM (CD54) pathway, and the CD2–LFA-3 (CD58) pathway.

First identified by Davignon and Springer, LFA-1 is part of the family of integrin-type adhesion molecules grouped according to their common β-chains (CD18) [31]. LFA-1 has a distinct α-chain (CD11a) and is found on T cells, B cells, macrophages, and neutrophils. It interacts with ICAM and has been shown to play an important role in facilitating APC–T cell adhesion, antibody production, T cell trafficking, and costimulation of T cells [32].

LFA-1 is crucial in promoting the initial interactions between naive T cells and APCs needed for T cell activation and effector maturation. Its adhesive properties are manifested during the initial phases of T cell activation when LFA-1 is localized at the center of the T cell–APC immunological synapse, while the TCR–MHC molecules remain in the periphery [33, 34]. As the synapse matures, the TCRs move to the center of the immunologic synapse, leaving a peripheral ring of LFA-1 that remains for at least 4h surrounding the synapse. This encourages prolonged cell–cell contact, thus promoting optimal T cell activation. Given the profound effect of LFA-1 on determining signal-1 (TCR) strength, its potential to influence the relevance of signal-2 (costimulation) is evident.

LFA-1 is also found on B cells, where it may play a facilitative role in antigen presentation. Normal antibody production requires clustering of B cells, T cells, and DCs. This interaction is inhibited by anti-LFA-1 in culture, suggesting a true role for LFA-1 in this association [35]. In terms of lymphocyte trafficking, LFA-1 has been implicated as vital for lymphocyte transendothelial migration at sites of inflammation. Lymphocyte recruitment at sites of tissue injury appears to be inhibited by anti-LFA-1 therapy, reaffirming its role in destructive immunity [32]. Finally, LFA-1 may transmit costimulatory-like signals. For example, LFA-1–ICAM engagement leads to sustained increases in intracellular calcium, elevated inositol phospholipid hydrolysis and the hyperphosphorylation of the TCR [36]. Whether this constitutes a bona fide costimulatory signal remains controversial. However, absence of the LFA-1–ICAM interaction has been shown to inhibit naive T cell proliferation and cytokine synthesis [37]. It is likely that the LFA-1–ICAM interaction, specifically the β2 subunit of LFA-1, promotes a more vigorous signal 1 by strengthening and lengthening the MHC–TCR interaction and in doing so promotes the effects of other ligand–receptor pairs.

Also of interest with regard to its influence on costimulatory blockade is the CD2–CD58 (LFA-3) pathway. As initially described by Sanchez-Madrid *et al.*, LFA-3 binds to the T cell surface receptor CD2 and promotes intercellular adhesion [38]. The CD2 molecule is a 50 kDa transmembrane glycoprotein expressed on mature T cells, thymocytes, and NK cells that increases adhesion and augments T cell responses between the APC–TCR engagement [39]. The CD2–LFA-3 interaction has been studied with regard to its role in T cell activation, T cell cytokine production, and association with cytotoxicity. Unlike the previously discussed pathways, the relationship between this pathway and its homologue in mice is less direct. In mice, the CD2 ligand is CD48, and downstream effects have a less clear

relationship to the anticipatable effects in humans. Murine studies have demonstrated that the CD2–CD48 interaction is responsible for B-cell-dependent T cell proliferation [40]. In addition, CD2-deficient mice have been shown to be deficient in T cell proliferation and cytokine production [41].

Both the LFA-1 and LFA-3 pathways have been exploited in the clinic to combat psoriasis [42]. Blockade of these pathways has been shown to be effective in controlling refractory T-cell-mediated psoriatic lesions. Interestingly, their clinical efficacy has been associated with their propensity to deplete or modify the function of memory T cells, either removing them from the lesion (anti-LFA-1) or depleting them (CD2-specific therapies) [43]. This latter observation has recently stimulated investigation into its use as a potential adjuvant agent with CoB. Given the reduced influence of CoB as a T cell response matures, agents that target more mature T cell forms present themselves as attractive adjuvant drugs for CoB-based therapeutic regimens.

Molecular structure and specific agents

General structural considerations
In general, all agents that have reached the clinic targeting costimulatory pathways have been either mAbs or fusion proteins. Both of these classes of drug have exceptionally high specificity owing to their specific binding sites derived either from the receptor or ligand itself or an immunoglobulin Fab domain specific for some epitope on the targeted molecule. This means that blockade occurs only in cells expressing the targeted molecule, lessening the potential for off-target side effects. This also eliminates direct drug–drug interactions and facilitates the use of these agents in combination with one another.

Following the landmark work of Köhler and Milstein demonstrating the feasibility of mAb formation, therapeutic mAbs have moved from the products of heterologous hybridoma formation to highly engineered molecules controlled for many important structural features, including binding

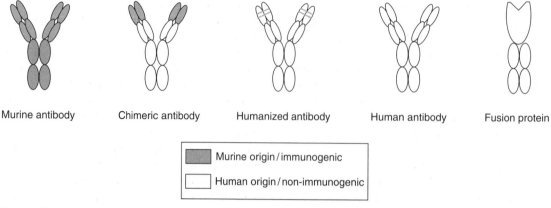

Murine antibody   Chimeric antibody   Humanized antibody   Human antibody   Fusion protein

Murine origin / immunogenic

Human origin / non-immunogenic

Figure 28.1 The general structure of monoclonal antibodies and fusion proteins. Monoclonal antibodies have been engineered to consist of reduced amount of heterologous protein sequence (shown in gray) and as a result have been developed to be less immunogenic when used in humans. Both fully human antibodies and fusion proteins are composed of completely human sequences. This reduces, but does not eliminate, their potential for immunogenicity, since glycosylation can vary from the native conformations of the human molecules (not shown) and novel epitopes can be formed in fusion proteins at the area of fusion between their immunoglobulin domain and their receptor domain.

affinity, isotype, and species of origin [44]. While early mAbs were derived from xenogeneic species (e.g., from mouse cells responding to human proteins) and generated a neutralizing antibody response towards themselves, modern antibodies and fusion proteins including chimeric, humanized, and fully human antibodies have greatly limited these limitations [45]. As such, modern therapeutics all derive from some form of chimeric or protein humanization technology. This ability to evade neutralizing antibodies has been critical in bringing CoB to the clinic, in that it has facilitated the use of CoB agents as maintenance drugs rather than brief induction-phase therapies.

Several forms of engineered molecules are available. Chimeric antibodies are those created by fusing the antigen-binding domain of a heterologous antibody to the human structural regions (e.g., the Fc domain of IgG1) (Figure 28.1). This process reduces the presence of heterologous peptide sequences and affords the opportunity to develop Fc-specific characteristics to a particular antibody (e.g., complement fixation). Humanized antibodies carry this process further by grafting only the complementarity determining region (CDR) of the heterologous antibody to a human antibody

scaffolding. This further reduces the presence of nonhuman peptide sequences, but also risks altering the binding affinity of the parent antibody. This latter drawback has been recently addressed through the development of fully humanized antibodies. These have been developed by engineering mice to express human immunoglobulin gene sequences and thus produce antibodies with a human framework when immunized with human proteins. As this field has advanced, the capacity to create completely engineered human antibodies has emerged, bypassing the need in some cases for an initial immunization altogether. Thus, therapeutic antibodies have progressively become less immunogenic, and been formed with specific effector functions in mind.

An alternative therapeutic strategy to mAbs is displayed with the construction of fusion proteins (Figure 28.1). Like chimeric antibodies, these molecules graft a known protein domain (such as a ligand for an adhesion or costimulation molecule) with the Fc portion of a human immunoglobin (e.g., IgG1). Although artificial, fusion proteins are comprised of human sequences and, as such, retain the function of the target ligand/receptor without

Table 28.1 Monoclonal antibody nomenclature.

Prefix	Target		Source		Suffix
varies	*-vi(r)-*	viral	*-u-*	human	*-mab*
	-ba(c)-	bacterial	*-o-*	mouse	
	-li(m)-	immune	*-a-*	rat	
	-le(s)-	infectious lesions	*-e-*	hamster	
	-ci(r)-	cardiovascular	*-i-*	primate	
	-co(l)-	colonic tumor	*-xi-*	chimeric	
	-me(l)-	melanoma	*-zu-*	humanized	
	-ma(r)-	mammary tumor			
	-go(t)-	testicular tumor			
	-go(v)-	ovarian tumor			
	-pr(o)-	prostate tumor			
	-tu(m)-	miscellaneous tumor			

overt potential for immunogenicity (although immunogenicity can be precipitated by novel domains formed by the protein used or by novel glycosylation patterns inherent in the production cell line). Thus, like humanized antibodies, fusion proteins specifically target ligands of interest with less immunogenicity and more clinically relevant circulating half-lives.

Given the growing number of mAbs and fusion proteins, a specific nomenclature system has been developed. Each therapy is composed of a prefix, several infixes, and a suffix with an intentional etymology (Table 28.1). The suffix -mab is used to designate all medicines that are mAbs, while the suffix -cept signifies a fusion protein. For mAbs, the infix preceding -mab is used to identify the source of the mAb; e.g., either murine (-o), chimeric (-xi), humanized (-zu) or human (-u). Preceding the origin will be an infix indicating the target of this therapy, whether antitumor, antiviral, etc. The prefix is created at the discretion of the inventor. This nomenclature is useful in anticipating the engineering and potential properties of a given agent.

As a result of these engineering methods, numerous drugs have been created with highly specific affinity for their intended receptor and limited immunogenicity. Importantly, while heterologous mAbs were rapidly cleared and thus relegated to brief treatment courses, the reduced immunogenicity of modern agents has permitted their use for indefinite periods of time, opening the

possibility that costimulation pathways could be targeted as a maintenance immunosuppression strategy. Furthermore, the prolonged half-life of these proteins, typically 2–4 weeks, greatly lengthens the dosing interval, potentiating weekly or monthly dosing. This latter point has substantial potential for benefit in terms of medication adherence.

The B7-specific agents

Numerous agents, including antibodies and fusion proteins, have been made available for clinical trials targeting the B7 pathways, and at least one, abatacept, is approved for an immunosuppressive indication. As would be predicted by the relationships between the B7 molecules, CD28 and CD152, agents have been designed with specific intent to suppress immunity (e.g., to combat transplant rejection or autoimmunity) or augment immunity (e.g., for oncologic indications) respectively.

Abatacept is the human form of the fusion protein CTLA4-Ig, and is the most widely used and studied agent for blockade of the CD28–B7 pathway [46]. It consists of an extracellular binding domain of CD152 (CTLA) linked to the modified Fc region of human IgG1. Much like CD152, CTLA4-Ig binds with a higher affinity to CD80/86 on APCs than does CD28, thus serving as a competitive inhibitor of the CD28 pathway [47]. Also, inherent in this approach is the potential to block the negative regulatory influence of CD152, although this presumably would require high local drug concentrations to effectively outcompete native CD152. Abatacept's blockade of both CD80 and CD86 effects have been shown to be superior to mAbs specifically targeting either CD80 or CD86 in NHPs [48].

LEA29Y or belatacept is a variant of CTLA4-Ig with two amino acid substitutions (L104E and A29Y) in the region that binds CD80/86. Belatacept was discovered while screening abatacept variants, and was found to have a fourfold slower off-rate for CD80 and a twofold slower off-rate for CD86 in comparison with abatacept. This enhanced binding has been presumed to be advantageous, making belatacept a preferential agent for B7 blockade. Consistent with this assumption is the finding that belatacept has a 10-fold higher potency at inhibiting T cell proliferation in mixed lymphocyte reaction [49]. Its antirejection effect has been demonstrated in NHP and human transplant models, as discussed below.

MAXY4 is a fusion protein variant of CTLA4-Ig with higher binding specificity to human B7 receptors than abatacept or belatacept. It varies from CTLA4-Ig at the A2408 and A2409 amino acids and is currently being used in preclinical trials to treat autoimmune diseases and transplant rejection. It was created using a proprietary Molecular Breeding™ directed-evolution platform, involving libraries of gene sequences created via DNA shuffling and subsequent scanning for genes of desirable qualities [50, 51]. MAXY4 has been created as a potential next generation of therapeutics with very high binding affinity for CD80/86. It is important to note, however, that, as the affinity of the B7-specific compound increases, its ability to competitively inhibit CD152 binding (in addition to CD28 binding) could lead to a paradoxical immunostimulatory effect. As such, in vivo data and careful attention to the dosing will be required to understand if higher affinity compounds will necessarily produce a better antirejection effect.

Two agents relevant to the CD28–B7 pathway, TGN1412 and Ipilimumab, require mention. Although they have no role in transplantation, they clearly demonstrate the range of biologic effects attributable to manipulation of this pathway.

TGN1412 is a superagonistic anti-human CD28 (IgG4k) mAb that was produced by humanizing a mouse anti-human CD28 IgG1 mAb, 5.11A1 [52]. TGN1412 was shown to bind to CD28 and activate T cells without the need for prior TCR signaling. Moreover, it, and similar CD28 superagonistic mAbs, was shown to preferentially expand immunosuppressive regulatory T cells (Tregs). Unfortunately, when utilized in a Phase I clinical trial done by Parexel International in London, this agent resulted in severe systemic inflammatory responses in all six healthy recipients of the drug, leading to cardiovascular collapse and severe cytokine storm. It was reported that within 16 h of drug administration all recipients became critically ill with pulmonary infiltrates, disseminated intravascular coagulation, and renal failure. It was ultimately concluded that these serious adverse events were caused by biologic effects unforeseen in humans, not predicted by preclinical safety testing [53].

Ipilimumab is a fully humanized IgG1 mAb specific for human CLTA4 (CD152). This antibody has been shown to preferentially bind to human CD152, and thus enhance T cell responses, including tumor-specific T cell responses such as those involved in melanoma immunotherapy [54]. Mostly studied to understand its efficacy in treating melanoma in humans, this agent has also been shown to have effect in treating malignancy after allogeneic bone marrow transplantation.

The CD40–CD154 pathway

Given the critical nature of the CD40–CD154 pathway in transplantation, numerous agents have been developed to inhibit its function. The first of these to reach the clinic was hu5c8, a humanized mAb directed against CD40 ligand or CD154 [28]. It entered trials in idiopathic thrombocytopenic purpura, lupus, and allotransplantation. Although hu5c8 showed remarkable promise in animal models (see below), its appearance in the clinic was too brief to fully define its clinical benefits in these indications. Nevertheless, its use has driven significant advances in the understanding of this pathway. From an efficacy standpoint, promising data emerged in lupus, but the effect in transplantation was disappointing [55]. Although hu5c8 was originally developed to antagonize T-cell-based CD154, it was subsequently shown to influence platelet-derived CD154. This property is a significant part of its antirejection effect [25]. It is perhaps this interaction with platelets that fostered an apparent pro-thrombotic phenotype in patients receiving hu5c8. A 10% incidence of broadly categorized thromboembolic events was noted in early trials with hu5c8 that halted its more extensive evaluation [55]. A second CD154-specific humanized mAb, IDEC-131, was also clearly shown to prevent acute rejection in preclinical models and began Phase I study in lupus in humans. It was pulled from clinical development along with hu5c8 when its parent company merged with that of hu5c8.

In attempts to avoid a potential interaction with platelet-derived CD154 and still inhibit the CD40–CD154 pathway, significant attention has moved toward CD40-specific mAbs. The most advanced of these is 4D11 (ASKP1240), a fully human CD40-specific mAb [56, 57]. This agent is unique, in that it is a fully human antibody derived from mice engineered to express human immunoglobulin gene sequences. This predicts a much improved immunogenicity profile compared with chimeric or humanized constructs. 4D11 blocks the interaction between CD40 and CD154, and preclinical studies (see below) have shown that it significantly delays renal allograft rejection and alloantibody production. Its propensity to deplete CD40-expressing cells appears low. Its relationship to thromboembolism awaits further study. It is presently in Phase I study.

Lucatumumab (HCD122) is a humanized antagonistic anti-CD40 mAb with a dual mechanism of action [58]. CD40 is commonly overexpressed in B cell malignancies and thus presents an attractive target for oncologic therapy. Lucatumumab binds CD40 on tumor cells, thereby inducing apoptosis and preventing proliferation of malignant B cells. It also acts by mediating antibody-dependent cellular toxicity, where an immune effector response kills lucatumumab-bound CD40-expressing malignant cells. This drug is currently being tested in Phase I/II clinical trials for lymphoma and multiple myeloma.

Chi-220 is a chimeric mouse anti-human CD40 mAb that blocks CD154 binding, and has partial agonistic properties [59]. Treatment with Chi-220 has been shown to result in a transient depletion of B cells and activation-induced cell death of CD40-bearing cells. Its partial agonistic effects may prevent the immune augmentation seen with fully agonistic mAbs.

The CD11a–CD54 pathway

Efalizumab is a humanized mAb against the CD11a (LFA-1) molecule, one of the two subunits of the T cell-surface molecule LFA-1 [33]. Binding of efalizumab to its target prevents interaction of LFA-1 and CD52 (ICAM), preventing a critical adhesion event required for lymphocyte diapedesis. As a result, activated T cells are unable to sequester in secondary lymphoid organs or enter inflamed tissues. The result is a therapeutic lymphocytosis, with high lymphocyte counts in sites of antigen presentation and effector function. The actions of efalizumab are reversible and non-T-cell depleting. Until recently, efalizumab was approved for use in psoriasis. However, the appearance of fatal progressing multifocal leukoencephalopathy (PML) in several patients on long-term efalizumab therapy prompted reassessment of its use in this indication and withdrawal from the market. The beneficial effects of efalizumab as an adjuvant agent to B7 blockade (discussed below) have prompted consideration of its short-term use in transplantation, an indication with a broader risk–benefit ratio than psoriasis.

The CD2–CD58 pathway

Alefacept, (also known as ASP0485 or LFA-3-Ig), is a genetically engineered dimeric fusion protein consisting of the CD2 binding portion of LFA-3 and the Fc portion of human IgG1 [60]. CD2 is found on all T cells and increases in density with T cell activation and maturation [61]. As such, it is more highly expressed on those cells actively engaged in an immune response. It inhibits the CD2–LFA-3 interaction, and in doing so it impedes T cell engagement with APCs and endothelium. It also is thought to deplete CD2-expressing cells through complement-mediated lysis. It is currently approved in the USA for treatment of psoriasis, and its efficacy has been linked both clinically in psoriasis and preclinically in transplantation to its predilection for memory effector T cells, those most brightly decorated with CD2 molecules.

General mechanisms of action and transplant-specific biological effects

There are several general mechanisms of action for costimulatory pathway-specific biologics. Indeed, the predominant science behind structural modification defining each agent is driven by a desire to accentuate or suppress a given functional characteristic. The simplest mechanism evoked when conceptualizing the mode of action is steric hindrance. Agents with this property demonstrate competitive inhibition kinetics and their efficacy is driven by the relative affinity compared with the native ligand. Structural modifications can at times generate molecules with an indefinite off-rate, effectively eliminating the potential binding of the native ligand. Given that the mechanism by which the B7 ligands modify an immune response is highly dependent on their abundance and the variable affinity of the CD28 and CD152 receptors, modifications in affinity and avidity have the potential to markedly alter the in vivo effect of a given agent.

Agents possessing Ig Fc domains can evoke methods of action, in addition to competitive steric hindrance, that are reminiscent of antibody binding. MAbs or fusion proteins with mAb Fc tails that can fix complement (e.g., IgG1) have the potential to lyse target-bearing cells and function through a depletional effect. Additional effects can be mediated through receptor cross-linking in the case of divalent proteins, leading to activation or activation-induced apoptosis. Fc tails also facilitate antibody-dependent cellular cytotoxicity (ADCC)-like effects, mobilizing monocytes and other effector cells to the site of drug binding. Cross-linking, or less so mono-valent binding, can also serve as an agonistic ligand and promote target-dependent function. While in vitro studies help define the specific effect of these agents, the true biologic effect requires assessment in vivo, and for human-specific biologics this requires NHP testing or use in humans.

CD28–CD80/86

Blockade of the CD28–B7 protein pathway has been pursued largely to achieve inhibition of the CD28 pathway, but recognizant of the potential to also inhibit CD152 regulation. Although there are

some data suggesting that CD86 may bind preferentially to CD28 whereas CD80 may bind primarily to CTLA4, early experimental experience in NHPs demonstrated that both CD80 and CD86 must be blocked to effectively delay allograft rejection [48]. As such, individual B7-specific mAbs gave way to the clinical development of the fusion protein CTLA4-Ig. Despite exceptional results in mice, use of CTLA4-Ig prolongs the onset of acute rejection in NHPs by only 20–30 days [62,63]. It has not been developed for transplantation, but rather has been registered for the treatment of rheumatoid arthritis, where its efficacy is proven [64].

Given the modest performance in NHPs for transplant, effort was put into development of belatacept for transplantation. As discussed above, belatacept's structural modification gave it a higher affinity for the B7 molecules and a resultant increased potency in inhibiting T cell proliferation and antidonor antibody formation in NHPs [49]. It also achieved prolonged renal allograft survival when used in conjunction with traditional immunosuppressants. The mechanism of action is felt to be steric hindrance, and thus other agents with higher affinity have been explored (see above). However, as the affinity for the B7 ligands increases, the potential for CD152 inhibition grows. Thus, it is unclear whether higher affinity products will be more or less efficacious or safe.

Specific inhibition of CD28 without interfering with CD152 would be a theoretically optimal means of inhibiting an immune response, and could potentially be achieved by developing a CD28-specific mAb. However, divalent mAbs have the potential for cross-linking and signaling, making it possible that CD28-specific mAbs would accelerate immune responsiveness. Such is the case for TGN1412. As described above, TGN1412 was found to have superagonist properties and its use in normal volunteers led to severe cytokine release and shock. Thus, further development in this arena will require agents with single valence or clear antagonistic properties.

Given that rejection occurs in the presence of apparently saturating doses on abatacept or belatacept, significant interest has developed in the mechanisms of costimulation-blockade-resistant rejection (CoBRR). A number of mechanisms have been demonstrated experimentally. It has been shown that CD80/86 double knockout mice are unable to reject cardiac allografts while CD28 knockout mice are able to develop immune responses. This implies that CD28-independent pathways of rejection exist. Kean *et al.* found that NK cells may mediate CoBRR in allogeneic stem cell transplants following non-myeloablative regimens [65]. They described host NK depletion leading to increased donor stem cell survival, increased mixed chimerism, and engraftment of low doses of bone marrow that were otherwise rejected. As the effects of B7 blockade are dependent on the relative concentration of B7, excessive B7 expression, such as that driven by CD40 ligation on APCs, may also promote CoBRR. This has been a theoretical reason to suggest the combination of CD40 blockade with B7 blockade; indeed, this has been successful (discussed below). An additional CoBRR mechanism, specifically to interference with the CD28–B7 pathways, derives from the fact that activated T cells lose CD28 in the terminal stages of effector differentiation [61, 66]. Thus, pre-sensitized individuals with a substantial effector population of CD28-negative cells would be expected to resist the influence of B7 blockade.

The mechanisms by which individuals develop CD28-negative effectors have recently been recognized to extend beyond the realm of prior direct alloantigen exposure. T cells with a memory phenotype develop not only from prior alloantigen exposure, but also through environmental antigen exposure, facilitating the expansion of cells with heterologous cross-reactivity between alloantigens and environmental pathogens. In addition, memory T cells result during homeostatic expansion of T cells after T cell depletion (either physiologic or therapeutic) [67]. Memory cells from any of these sources may lack CD28 or have reduced costimulation requirements, and this has sparked efforts to specifically neutralize memory cells. Strategies in this regard incorporate CNIs and adhesion-specific biologics, as discussed below.

CD40–CD154

As described above, CD154-specific mAbs have been shown to prevent acute rejection in rodent and NHP models. The potential mechanisms at play for this pathway are many, and a dominant pathway

remains undefined. It is likely that the CD40–CD154 pathway is bidirectional. In B cells, the CD40 ligation promotes proliferation and differentiation, while in T cells CD154 cross-linking is known to promote intracellular calcium flux, adhesion molecule expression, and cytokine production, but cannot replace CD28 as a necessary costimulatory ligand [68, 69]. More prominent, however, are the effects of CD40 on APCs, with ligation increasing B7 molecule expression, cytokine production, MHC presentation of antigen, and other TNF receptor-associated factor, and NFκB-related effects. As such, interference with this pathway on either side has the potential to halt T-cell- and B-cell-dependent immunity [17]. All of these effects intuitively could be expected to dampen alloimmunity and the dominant effect of CD40–CD154 pathway interruption remains to be determined. CD154 is also expressed preferentially on activated T cells, and there is evidence suggesting that direct depletion of CD154-expressing cells plays into the effect [17].

While blockade of CD154 with mAbs has been consistently impressive in mice and NHPs, efforts to translate CD154-specific therapies into the clinic have been complicated by unanticipated thrombo-embolic complications. These have been broad in nature, rather than specific or suggestive of a single pro-coagulant mechanism [55]. While they have been presumably due to CD154's expression on thrombin-activated platelets and their role in stabilizing arterial thrombi [70], definitive evidence in this regard remains lacking. Nevertheless, development of CD40–CD154 pathway blockade has gravitated toward CD40-specific mAbs. Murine studies have shown that anti-CD40 mAbs promote graft survival with efficacy similar to anti-CD154, and with comparable synergy to anti-CD154 mAbs in combination with belatacept or CTLA4-Ig.

Subsequently, anti-CD40 agents have been developed for clinical application with promising results. Chi-220, a chimeric anti-human mAb to CD40, has been shown to prolong islet and renal allograft survival in NHPs, as has 3A8 [59]. Potential mechanisms are many and include depletion of peripheral B cells, inhibition of T cell proliferation, steric hindrance of CD154 to CD40, and a partial agonist effect to promote weak signals that increase the cell's susceptibility to anergy.

More recently, 4D11 has shown promise in delaying renal allograft rejection and antibody production in NHPs [56, 57]. In cynomolgus monkeys receiving renal allografts, T-cell-mediated autoimmune responses are suppressed and decreases in peripheral B cell counts are evident. While the drug was well tolerated in general, in a recent report a single animal was found post-mortem to have a cerebral infarct. 4D11 appears to be moving toward clinical trials. Thus, targeting CD40 appears the most likely adjuvant costimulatory strategy to join belatacept in the near term.

CD11a–CD54

The CD11a–CD54 (LFA-1–ICAM) pathway has been studied for the last 20 years; however, interest in targeting this pathway in association with CoB has been recently resurgent. Perhaps the most relevant effect of LFA-1-specific agents is interruption of lymphocyte diapedesis into inflamed tissues. Indeed, treatment with LFA-1-specific antibodies leads to a peripheral lymphocytosis that persists for the duration of treatment. This presumably prevents T cells from infiltrating an allograft, and from gaining access to costimulation-rich APCs in the secondary lymphoid tissue. As such, LFA-1 blockade likely prolongs allograft survival through disruption of T cell adhesive properties and interruption of its lymphocyte trafficking abilities [33]. Further investigation will determine the utility of blockade with this pathway via clinical trials.

Several lines of evidence have developed suggesting a therapeutic role for LFA-1 blockade, particularly when used in combination with other immunosuppressive therapies. Preclinical studies have shown that anti-LFA-1 monotherapy can lead to increased NHP cardiac allograft survival and increased islet cell tolerance in mouse models [71]. Combined with other immunosuppressive agents, anti-LFA-1 has been shown to have an additive potency. Anti-LFA-1 has been shown to inhibit alloantibody and xenoantibody responses, suggesting that LFA-1 blockade may interfere with normal B cell responses [71].

Clinical trials using anti-LFA-1 mAbs began in the 1990s. Early studies using mouse anti-human CD11a antibody showed mixed results in preventing kidney allograft rejection [33]. The most recent therapeutic foray with LFA-1 pathway inhibition has come from the development of efalizumab, a humanized IgG1 LFA-1-specific mAb. This agent has been shown to successfully treat the T-cell-mediated disease psoriasis, and it has been this experience that has encouraged trials in kidney and islet transplantation [72]. A multicenter trial combining efalizumab with cyclosporine, mycophenolate mofetil (MMF), and prednisone showed that low-dose efalizumab suggested a small reduction in acute rejection rates, but a concerning increase in Epstein–Barr virus (EBV)-associated post-transplant lympho-proliferative disorder (PTLD) [72]. These results suggested that efalizumab has potent immunosuppressive properties requiring compensatory reduction in adjuvant therapy. Accordingly, subsequent trials in kidney and islet transplantation were designed with less-intense adjuvant regimens and had promising early results. The development of efalizumab has been significantly delayed of late, as it has been pulled off the market by reports in psoriasis patients treated long term developing the JC-virus-driven PML [33]. Thus, the LFA-1–ICAM pathway has a clear role in immune activation and potential for exploitation in immunosuppressive regimens, but the optimal therapeutic use remains undefined. Nevertheless, these early studies have promoted the further study of LFA-1-based therapies in the transplant arena, and in particular their role in costimulation-based therapies.

CD2–CD58

Blockade of the CD2–CD58 (LFA-3) pathway has been used clinically in treatment of psoriasis. Alefacept, or LFA-3Ig, is thought to eliminate cells with high levels of CD2 expressed on their cell surface and also to antagonize stabilization of the TCR immune synapse [73]. In particular, these effects have been linked to alefacept's ability to mollify the influence of effector memory T cells. By interrupting CD2's interaction with LFA-3, helper T cell adhesion to APCs is disrupted as its subsequent effector T cell engagement with antigen and MHC complex molecules is hindered. Effector T cell elimination also ensues via complement-mediated lysis. Studies in NHPs have shown decreased T cell numbers in treated animals, with a greater reduction in CD8+ cells that was reversed upon withdrawal of LFA-3Ig [61]. Further analysis described this lymphopenia to be the result of substantial effector memory T cell depletion, without alteration in the number of naive T cells. Alefacept's performance in transplant studies has been modest. It has been shown to delay the onset of acute rejection in NHP heart and kidney transplant models by up to 30 days [74, 75].

In considering the transplant-specific effects of all agents, used in isolation, CoB-based agents have been impressive in naive animals with sustained effects that give way to chronic graft loss over time. In sensitized or immunologically mature animals, the effects of CoB have been modest at best. Adhesion-based agents have shown biologic effect, but have not led to graft prolongation that is clinically relevant.

Pharmacodynamic/ pharmacokinetic/therapeutic drug monitoring

Unlike small-molecule inhibitors that have short half-lives, predictable volumes of distribution, and established therapeutic parameters of drug exposure, biologics are difficult to establish a proper metric to associate with efficacy. Their serum concentration provides some evidence of prevalence, but most are presumed to function at the cell surface and in particular in secondary lymphoid organs or sites of inflammation. The receptor occupancy model put forth by Clark *et al.* provides a useful way to conceptualize drug effect [76]. It explains that the activity of a drug at its receptor quantifies the relationship between drug concentration and observed effect [77]. The receptor occupancy theory classically describes the response to ligand A as a function of intrinsic efficacy of the drug to induce a physiologic response, the receptor density, the strength of activation to a tissue response, and an equilibrium constant specific to the drug–receptor complex. With this model, drugs are characterized independent of systemic parameters, and translated to new therapeutic models. It is in this manner that we conceptualize the phamacokinetics and pharmacodynamics of CoB agents. Specifically, consideration must be given not only to the vigor with which an agent binds to its target, but also the dynamics of target expression through the course of an immune response. This is critically important for the agents under consideration in this chapter, as the principal target molecules modulate dramatically as an immune response matures (Figure 28.2).

While CD28 and CD152 molecules play reciprocal roles in the T cell response, the two ligands CD80 and CD86 are also thought to demonstrate distinctive roles in T cell activation. In general,

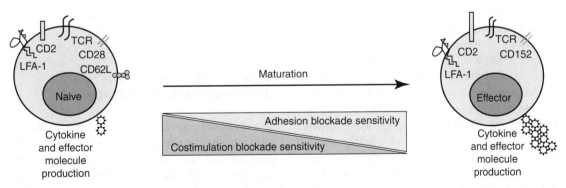

Figure 28.2 Changes in surface molecule expression with T cell maturation. The susceptibility of a T cell to costimulation blockade or adhesion molecule blockade changes during T cell maturation from a naive T cell to an effector T cell due to changes in ligand density and surface molecule expression. In particular, T cell activation leads to loss of CD28, acquisition of CD152, reduced TCR density, and increased density of CD2 and LFA-1.

CD86 is constitutively expressed and rapidly upregulated on APCs, while CD80 is typically expressed after a prolonged stimulation [33]. This may suggest that CD86 is more important in initiating T cell activation and that CD80 may play a more significant role in sustaining the immune response. Recent work also indicates that, at certain times, CD86 may bind preferentially to CD28, whereas CD80 may bind primarily to CTLA4 [78]. All these differences may translate into selective recruitment of CD28 or CD152 at various phases of an alloimmune response. Blockade of the costimulatory signal required to fully activate T cells has been accomplished with the above-mentioned agents, and can be quantified specifically in terms of receptor occupancy. Vincenti and coworkers showed that belatacept saturation of CD80 receptors alone was not sufficient to inhibit in vitro alloresponses [79]. However, higher doses of belatacept that adequately saturated both CD80 and CD86 were able to completely inhibit in vitro alloresponses. This study has come the closest to validating usage of a receptor occupancy assay as a pharmacodynamic marker of belatacept CoB via CD86 saturation. However, there is no clear means of measuring belatacept dosing at present.

Although rigorous receptor occupancy characterization has not been carried out for anti-CD154 and anti-CD40 agents, preliminary data exist to allow us to gauge efficacy and receptor binding affinities. For example, Gilson *et al.* compared the binding affinities of the rat anti-mouse CD40 mAb 7E1G1 and 7E1G2 in vitro with a B cell line M12 [80]. They incubated B cells with increasing concentrations of the 7E1 variants against a known anti-CD40 mouse agonist and later detected bound antibody with fluorescently labeled anti-rat IgG secondary antibody. The results of this study showed similar binding affinity between the variants and the known anti-CD40 agent. This highlights the ambiguity in characterizing efficacy based on receptor occupancy with anti-CD40 and anti-CD154 agents due to the many clonal variants that exist and a lack of data; however, such studies are clearly underway.

A major confounding variable for CD154-based therapies is the massive CD154 reservoir contained within platelets. As platelets degranulate in response to trauma, serum levels of CD154 can increase considerably. As such, the receptor occupancy can be expected to change not only in relation to the drug concentration, but also the physiologic state of the recipient. The relationship between anti-CD154 efficacy and ambient CD154 levels is completely undefined.

Similar fluxes in target concentrations are seen in adhesion-based pathways. Weaver and colleagues measured the effect of cell maturation on CD2 expression and saw a twofold increase in CD2 density on alloresponsive cells as they progressed from naivety to terminal differentiation [61]. Importantly, the highest CD2 density was seen on CD28-negative effector memory cells. Additionally, mixed lymphocyte cultures with CFSE-labeled responder lymphocytes showed an inhibition in proliferation of CD4+ and CD8+ cells with alefacept treatment, in a dose-dependent fashion. This characterization of alefacept's binding affinities is preliminary and is potentially an assay to guide future endeavors using LFA-3 Ig.

LFA-1-specific therapy has been associated with lymphocytosis, a result of the blockade of lymphocyte trafficking to the nodes and peripheral tissues. This lymphocytosis may be a means of assessing drug effect, but will likely be too variable to provide precise dosing guidance. Receptor occupancy may be relevant, although the measurements will be confined to cells in the periphery that presumably will be those mobilized by the drug. The failure to assess nonmobilized cells may overestimate receptor occupancy.

Drug–drug interactions and combination therapy

As discussed above, no single costimulatory pathway has proven completely necessary for allograft rejection, and no CoB agent used alone has been sufficient to continuously prevent rejection in primates. This is not to say that CoB lacks promise as a therapeutic class, but rather that it must be deployed in rational combination with other therapies to be clinically successful. In considering appropriate combination strategies, significant thought should be given to the primary advantage and weakness of CoB: respectively, CoB preserves antigen specificity, but becomes less influential as an immune response matures. Thus, agents paired with CoB should preserve TCR signaling, but are likely to be considered prophylactic as opposed to rescue strategies, and will be less relevant in the situation of prior allosensitization.

CoB with conventional immunosuppression

The pathway to drug registration requires that agents be compared with the existing standard before being introduced to the market. The most direct approach is to use a new agent as a replacement for a known existing agent. Thus, CoB agents largely have been folded into conventional triple immunosuppressive regimens (CNI, MMF, and steroids) as they are prepared for clinical translation, replacing either CNIs or steroids. Prednisone and MMF are two standard maintenance agents that are known to bolster the effect of CNI or sirolimus-based regimens, but they are not sufficient as centerpiece maintenance immunosuppressants. Studies combining CD28–B7 and CD40–CD154 pathway inhibitors with prednisone and or MMF have failed to demonstrate any clear adverse interaction and suggest additive immunosuppressive potency [81, 82]. Knowledge of the pathways targeted by B7-, CD40-, or CD154-specific agents would predict no antagonist relationship between CoB and glucocorticosteroids or purine analogs such as MMF and azathioprine. Accordingly, the Phase II and Phase III studies with belatacept have been in combination with prednisone and MMF using belatacept as a CNI replacement [17, 83].

The relationship between CoB and Tregs, specifically CD4+CD25+ Tregs, remains incompletely defined, as does the influence of CD25-specific mAbs on Treg function. Regardless, many preclinical studies have combined B7-, CD40- or CD154-specific agents with CD25-specific mAbs without apparent adverse effect [84, 85]. NHP studies suggest that the use of CoB with CD25 blockade

(e.g., daclizumab or basiliximab) is at least harmless, but whether CD25-specific mAbs are of benefit has not been rigorously addressed. The clinical trials investigating belatacept have been in combination with basiliximab [83, 86, 87].

The conceptual need to preserve the TCR has complicated the consideration of CoB in combination with CNIs, a class of agent that interrupts TCR signaling. Experimental data suggest that CNIs attenuate the pro-tolerant immunomodulatory effects of CoB and, as such, are best avoided [88]. However, as T cells terminally differentiate and become relatively CoB independent, CNIs appear to be exceptionally good at suppressing their proliferation and function [89]. Thus, CNIs could be expected to reduce both the threat of CoBRR and the potential for antigen-specific immune modulation while inducing the same broad off-target side effects that have inspired CoB in the first place. Most preclinical and all clinical studies investigating CoB-based agents have avoided CNIs; but not unpredictably, this has been associated with an increased acute rejection rate in the CoB arms of these studies [90]. This rate of CoBRR in humans has been higher than that predicted in preclinical work, leading to speculation that adult humans are more prone to CoBRR by virtue of the fact that they are more endowed with heterologously alloreactive, memory-type T cells [67, 91]. Subsequent preclinical work with the CD40-specific mAb 4D11 has used the CNI tacrolimus in the regimen with promising success [56, 57, 92]. Similarly, conversion to CoB-based maintenance following conventional CNI-based immunosuppression has been demonstrated in NHPs [93]. Thus, the immunosuppressive capacity of CoB is likely unaltered by CNIs. However, a means of avoiding CoBRR without the broad systemic effects of CNIs would be desirable, and the ultimate promise of antigen-specific prevention of rejection will likely require CNI avoidance.

The use of the mammalian target of rapamycin (mTOR) inhibitor sirolimus has proven to be an attractive pairing with CoB-based regimens. Conceptually, mTOR inhibition should preserve TCR signaling and promote activation-induced apoptosis in a synergistic manner with CoB. Indeed, murine studies support the use of sirolimus with both CD28–B7 and CD40–CD154 pathway blockade, and specifically demonstrate superiority over CNI pairings [88, 94]. Sirolimus has been used extensively with CD154-specific mAbs with excellent results, including induction of donor-specific tolerance in NHPs treated with sirolimus and IDEC-131 [95]. It has also been combined with CTLA4-Ig with less pronounced synergy [61]. Unfortunately, the use of sirolimus in NHPs has been complicated somewhat by gastrointestinal toxicities and poor oral absorption that have limited their ease of use [96]. Sirolimus has not been paired with CoB in a published clinical work, although trials are ongoing to establish its role in the clinic [97].

Depletional induction agents such as rabbit antithymocyte globulin and alemtuzumab have been considered with CoB-based maintenance therapies. However, murine studies have shown that homeostatic lymphocyte activation induced by profound lymphopenia induces a memory phenotype that is resistant to CoB-based therapies [98]. Indeed, CoB-based regimens that have led to tolerance in an intact mouse have failed in mice recovering from lymphopenia. Depletional induction strategies are difficult to model in NHPs, since human-specific agents work poorly in NHPs and deplete with a different spectrum and dosing range than in humans [99, 100]. There is modest evidence suggesting that depletion can be paired with CoB in NHPs [101, 102]. There are no published clinical studies pairing depletion with CoB, although several studies are being performed [97].

Combined costimulation blockade

Simultaneous inhibition of the CD28–B7 and CD40–CD154 pathways has shown great promise in promoting allograft survival in mice and NHPs [27, 29, 103]. Indeed, combined use of B7-specific agents with either CD40- or CD154-specific agents have proven to be remarkably effective in preventing allograft, and even xenograft, rejection in every model tested to date [59, 80,104–108]. Simultaneous blockade of each pathway has shown significant inhibition of T- and B-cell-dependent immune responses exceeding that achieved with individual pathway blockade.

Many prominent demonstrations of combined B7-specific (abatacept of belatacept) and CD40–CD154-specific therapies have defined the preclinical promise of CoB. Most notably, graft survival in NHPs has extended well beyond the cessation of therapy in most studies, suggesting that pure CoB-based combinations are permissive for physiologic mechanisms that limit autoimmunity and promote self-tolerance. Rejection-free graft survival extending for months to years after the end of therapy has been reported in kidney and islet transplant models using numerous combinations [27, 29, 59, 109].

Unfortunately, no combined CoB approach has been forthcoming in the clinic, and this is likely a function of the logistics of drug development. At present, no company has both CD28–B7 and CD40–CD154 pathway agents available for clinical trials. Furthermore, only one CoB agent, abatacept, has been approved for clinical use and transplantation has not been a targeted area of development for that agent. Thus, the inability to combine multiple investigational agents from multiple companies in a single clinical trial has delayed the obvious combined application of agents targeting these two pathways. This is clearly an area supported by strong preclinical data that will require clinical translation as CoB agents become approved.

Combined costimulation and adhesion blockade

As discussed above, the primary driver of CoBRR is immune memory, specifically cells that through prior antigen exposure of homeostatic expansion have lower costimulation requirements for activation or have lost prominent costimulatory molecules during terminal differentiation. It is in targeting CoBRR that adhesion molecule therapy has emerged as a promising adjuvant agent.

In recent NHP preclinical studies, Weaver et al. showed that alefacept prevents renal allograft rejection when used in concert with the B7-specific agent CTLA4-Ig and specifically related this effect to the depletion of CD28-

negative effector memory T cells [61]. These studies showed that T cells (particularly CD8$^+$ effectors) lose CD28 during terminal effector maturation and could be expected to be resistant to CD28–B7-targeted CoB. Fortunately, CD2 density increases commensurate with the decrease in CD28, making those cells least likely to respond to CD28–B7 blockade as most likely to be eliminated by alefacept (Plate 28.1). This revelation has catalyzed work on the CD2–-LFA-3 costimulatory pathway as a potential target for prevention of acute rejection in kidney transplantation in combination with other CoB-based biologics. Weaver et al.'s usage of alefacept in a regimen with CTLA4-Ig and sirolimus prolonged renal allograft survival in macaques and delayed onset of alloantibody formation [61]. The adjuvant effect of alefacept in B7-targeted CoB may relate to the loss of CD28 on substantial numbers of effector memory T cells. As such, alefacept's pairing with B7-specific agents is mechanistically attractive.

Similar effects have been recently reported using LFA-1 blockade when used in concert with either CD28–B7 or CD40–CD154 inhibition. The potential for synergy between CD40- and LFA-1-based pathways has long been recognized [110]. Blazar et al. showed that the combination of CTLA4-Ig and anti-LFA-1 had increased efficacy in prevention of graft versus host disease in mice after total body irradiation and bone marrow transplantation [111]. Along similar terms, usage of anti-LFA-1 mAb and anti-CD154 mAb showed synergistic suppression of CD4- and CD8-mediated rejection of hepatocytes in mice [112]. Increased survival of skin allografts in mice and prevention of the development of chronic vasculopathy in cardiac allografts in mice has also been shown [113].

These studies have spurred the use of TS-1, an NHP-LFA-1-specific mAb in NHP islet transplantation. In abstracts reported at the 2010 American Transplant Congress, LFA-1-specific treatment has been remarkably effective in preventing CoBRR. Badell et al. have recently reported indefinite islet allograft survival through pairing TS-1 with either belatacept or 3A8 [114]. These data suggest that the relationship between

adhesion blockade and CoB is a synergistic one worthy of translational investigation.

Clinical efficacy/safety

Little can be definitively said about CoB-based regimens with regard to clinical safety and efficacy. The only substantial data in transplantation are from the belatacept Phase II and III studies [83, 90, 115]. A partially blinded, randomized Phase II study was performed to assess the noninferiority of belatacept to CNIs, specifically cyclosporine, in the incidence of acute rejection at 6 months in renal transplant patients. Patients in this study were randomly assigned to groups of high-intensity belatacept, less-intensity belatacept, or cyclosporine in combination with MMF, steroids, and basiliximab. The incidence of acute rejection at 6 months was similar in all three groups. Hypertension, diabetes mellitus, leukopenia, and anemia were found to be higher in the cyclosporine-treated group, whereas hyperlipidemia was found to be higher in the belatacept-treated groups.

As a follow-up, two trials have recently been reported confirming the potential utility of belatacept as a CNI replacement [90, 115]. Both of these pivotal Phase III trials, one in standard-criteria donor kidney recipients and the other in recipients of extended-criteria donor kidneys, have shown that belatacept-treated patients have less hypertension and hyperlipidemia and improved renal function, but, interestingly, a higher incidence of early, reversible, T-cell-mediated rejection. Analysis of these data continues, but the results are consistent with a regimen that (as would be predicted from the preclinical data) mollifies naive T cells but leaves heterologously alloimmune terminal effectors inadequately controlled. These memory-type cells are effective in initiating early rejection, but are too terminally differentiated to sustain a response. Thus, the early clinical experience points to the relationship between memory and CoBRR described above. Also stemming from this experience has been a small number of early cases of EBV-associated lymphoproliferative disorders. While not statistically powered to assess this complication, there is an emerging sense that EBV-specific immunity is hampered by belatacept. Subsequent trials have been designed to avoid EBV naive recipients.

An additional glimpse into the safety of CoB can be derived from the use of abatacept in patients with rheumatoid arthritis (RA). The AIM trial, a Phase III randomized, double-blinded, placebo-controlled trial, showed abatacept to have clinical benefits in RA patients who otherwise had refractory RA [64]. Overall, the efficacy and safety of abatacept in RA is promising, and future studies of its utility in treating patients who have failed rituximab therapy are being conducted, as are trials investigating other rheumatic diseases, such as lupus nephritis and spondyloarthropathies.

Alefacept is now approved as a safe and effective therapy for psoriasis, but its safety in transplantation or in combination with CoB is clinically undefined. The biologic activity, safety, and efficacy of efalizumab (anti-LFA-1) were studied in 38 patients receiving renal transplants in a Phase I–II randomized multicenter trial [82]. This trial added efalizumab to triple immunosuppressive therapy including a CNI, MMF, and steroids. While patients were adequately prophylaxed against rejection, a high incidence of EBV-associated PTLD was seen, indicating that this cocktail was overly immuno-suppressive. There have been no data relating efalizumab to CoB; however, the drug was recently pulled from the psoriasis market in the face of a small number of cases of JC-virus-associated PML. All affected patients had been on prolonged efalizumab therapy, making its relevance to brief treatments in combination with CoB unclear.

In general, CoB is lining up as a therapeutic approach with exceptional mechanistic promise. However, its success as an antirejection therapy will be dependent on its proper use and pairing with other agents. This will undoubtedly be a rich area for translational investigation in the future.

Acknowledgments

ADK is supported by the McKelvey Foundation and the Georgia Research Alliance.

References

1 Meier-Kriesche HU, Schold JD, Srinivas TR, Kaplan B. Lack of improvement in renal allograft survival despite a marked decrease in acute rejection rates over the most recent era. *Am J Transplant* 2004;4(3):378–383.

2 Barocci S, Valente U, Fontana I *et al.* Long-term outcome on kidney retransplantation: a review of 100 cases from a single center. *Transplant Proc* 2009; 41(4):1156–1158.

3 Bach FH, Sachs DH. Current concepts: immunology. Transplantation immunology. *N Engl J Med* 1987;317(8):489–492.

4 Lafferty KJ, Cunningham AJ. A new analysis of allogeneic interactions. *Aust J Exp Biol Med Sci* 1975;53(1):27–42.

5 Bretscher P, Cohn M. A theory of self-nonself discrimination. *Science* 1970;169(950):1042–1049.

6 Jenkins MK, Schwartz RH. Antigen presentation by chemically modified splenocytes induces antigen-specific T cell unresponsiveness in vitro and in vivo. *J Exp Med* 1987;165(2):302–319.

7 Janeway CA, Jr. Approaching the asymptote? Evolution and revolution in immunology. *Cold Spring Harb Symp Quant Biol* 1989;54(Pt 1):1–13.

8 Schwartz RH. A cell culture model for T lymphocyte clonal anergy. *Science* 1990;248(4961):1349–1356.

9 Martin PJ, Ledbetter JA, Morishita Y *et al.* A 44 kilodalton cell surface homodimer regulates interleukin 2 production by activated human T lymphocytes. *J Immunol* 1986;136(9):3282–3287.

10 Hara T, Fu SM, Hansen JA. Human T cell activation. II. A new activation pathway used by a major T cell population via a disulfide-bonded dimer of a 44 kilodalton polypeptide (9.3 antigen). *J Exp Med* 1985; 161(6):1513–1524.

11 Lenschow DJ, Zeng Y, Thistlethwaite JR *et al.* Long-term survival of xenogeneic pancreatic islet grafts induced by CTLA4Ig. *Science* 1992;257(5071):789–792.

12 Harlan DM, Kirk AD. The future of organ and tissue transplantation: can T-cell costimulatory pathway modifiers revolutionize the prevention of graft rejection? *JAMA* 1999;282(11):1076–1082.

13 Brunet JF, Denizot F, Luciani MF *et al.* A new member of the immunoglobulin superfamily – CTLA-4. *Nature* 1987;328(6127):267–270.

14 Paulie S, Ehlin-Henriksson B, Mellstedt H *et al.* A p50 surface antigen restricted to human urinary bladder carcinomas and B lymphocytes. *Cancer Immunol Immunother* 1985;20(1):23–28.

15 Clark EA, Shu G, Ledbetter JA. Role of the Bp35 cell surface polypeptide in human B-cell activation. *Proc Natl Acad Sci U S A* 1985;82(6):1766–1770.

16 Larsen CP, Pearson TC. The CD40 pathway in allograft rejection, acceptance, and tolerance. *Curr Opin Immunol* 1997;9(5):641–647.

17 Larsen CP, Knechtle SJ, Adams A *et al.* A new look at blockade of T-cell costimulation: a therapeutic strategy for long-term maintenance immunosuppression. *Am J Transplant* 2006;6(5 Pt 1):876–883.

18 Van Essen D, Kikutani H, Gray D. CD40 ligand-transduced co-stimulation of T cells in the development of helper function. *Nature* 1995;378(6557):620–623.

19 Armitage RJ, Fanslow WC, Strockbine L *et al.* Molecular and biological characterization of a murine ligand for CD40. *Nature* 1992;357(6373):80–82.

20 Noelle RJ, Roy M, Shepherd DM *et al.* A 39-kDa protein on activated helper T cells binds CD40 and transduces the signal for cognate activation of B cells. *Proc Natl Acad Sci U S A* 1992;89(14):6550–6554.

21 Armitage RJ, Sato TA, Macduff BM *et al.* Identification of a source of biologically active CD40 ligand. *Eur J Immunol* 1992;22(8):2071–2076.

22 Johnson-Leger C, Christenson JR, Holman M, Klaus GG. Evidence for a critical role for IL-2 in CD40-mediated activation of naive B cells by primary CD4 T cells. *J Immunol* 1998;161(9):4618–4626.

23 Kirk AD, Blair PJ, Tadaki DK *et al.* The role of CD154 in organ transplant rejection and acceptance. *Philos Trans R Soc Lond B Biol Sci* 2001;356(1409):691–702.

24 Henn V, Slupsky JR, Grafe M *et al.* CD40 ligand on activated platelets triggers an inflammatory reaction of endothelial cells. *Nature* 1998;391(6667):591–594.

25 Xu H, Zhang X, Mannon RB, Kirk AD. Platelet-derived or soluble CD154 induces vascularized allograft rejection independent of cell-bound CD154. *J Clin Invest* 2006;116(3):769–774.

26 Parker DC, Greiner DL, Phillips NE *et al.* Survival of mouse pancreatic islet allografts in recipients treated with allogeneic small lymphocytes and antibody to CD40 ligand. *Proc Natl Acad Sci U S A* 1995;92(21):9560–9564.

27 Larsen CP, Elwood ET, Alexander DZ *et al.* Long-term acceptance of skin and cardiac allografts after blocking CD40 and CD28 pathways. *Nature* 1996;381(6581):434–438.

28 Kirk AD, Burkly LC, Batty DS *et al.* Treatment with humanized monoclonal antibody against CD154 prevents acute renal allograft rejection in nonhuman primates. *Nat Med* 1999;5(6):686–693.

29 Kirk AD, Harlan DM, Armstrong NN *et al.* CTLA4-Ig and anti-CD40 ligand prevent renal allograft rejection in primates. *Proc Natl Acad Sci U S A* 1997;94(16):8789–8794.

30 Sayegh MH, Turka LA. The role of T-cell costimulatory activation pathways in transplant rejection. *N Engl J Med* 1998;338(25):1813–1821.

31 Davignon D, Martz E, Reynolds T *et al.* Lymphocyte function-associated antigen 1 (LFA-1): a surface antigen distinct from Lyt-2,3 that participates in T lymphocyte-mediated killing. *Proc Natl Acad Sci U S A* 1981;78(7):4535–4539.

32 Van Seventer GA, Shimizu Y, Horgan KJ, Shaw S. The LFA-1 ligand ICAM-1 provides an important costimulatory signal for T cell receptor-mediated activation of resting T cells. *J Immunol* 1990;144(12):4579–4586.

33 Ford ML, Larsen CP. Translating costimulation blockade to the clinic: lessons learned from three pathways. *Immunol Rev* 2009;229(1):294–306.

34 Johnson JG, Jenkins MK. Accessory cell-derived signals required for T cell activation. *Immunol Res* 1993;12(1):48–64.

35 Owens T. A role for adhesion molecules in contact-dependent T help for B cells. *Eur J Immunol* 1991;21(4):979–983.

36 Van Seventer GA, Bonvini E, Yamada H *et al.* Costimulation of T cell receptor/CD3-mediated activation of resting human CD4⁺ T cells by leukocyte function-associated antigen-1 ligand intercellular cell adhesion molecule-1 involves prolonged inositol phospholipid hydrolysis and sustained increase of intracellular Ca^{2+} levels. *J Immunol* 1992;149(12):3872–3880.

37 Zuckerman LA, Pullen L, Miller J. Functional consequences of costimulation by ICAM-1 on IL-2 gene expression and T cell activation. *J Immunol* 1998;160(7):3259–3268.

38 Sanchez-Madrid F, Krensky AM, Ware CF *et al.* Three distinct antigens associated with human T-lymphocyte-mediated cytolysis: LFA-1, LFA-2, and LFA-3. *Proc Natl Acad Sci U S A* 1982;79(23):7489–7493.

39 Wilkins AL, Yang W, Yang JJ. Structural biology of the cell adhesion protein CD2: from molecular recognition to protein folding and design. *Curr Protein Pept Sci* 2003;4(5):367–373.

40 Latchman Y, Reiser H. Enhanced murine CD4⁺ T cell responses induced by the CD2 ligand CD48. *Eur J Immunol* 1998;28(12):4325–4331.

41 Bachmann MF, Barner M, Kopf M. CD2 sets quantitative thresholds in T cell activation. *J Exp Med* 1999;190(10):1383–1392.

42 Aruffo A, Hollenbaugh D. Therapeutic intervention with inhibitors of co-stimulatory pathways in autoimmune disease. *Curr Opin Immunol* 2001;13(6): 683–686.

43 Semnani RT, Nutman TB, Hochman P *et al.* Costimulation by purified intercellular adhesion molecule 1 and lymphocyte function-associated antigen 3 induces distinct proliferation, cytokine and cell surface antigen profiles in human "naive" and "memory" CD4⁺ T cells. *J Exp Med* 1994;180(6):2125–2135.

44 Köhler G, Milstein C. Derivation of specific antibody-producing tissue culture and tumor lines by cell fusion. *Eur J Immunol* 1976;6(7):511–519.

45 Reichert JM, Valge-Archer VE. Development trends for monoclonal antibody cancer therapeutics. *Nat Rev Drug Discov* 2007;6(5):349–356.

46 Bluestone JA, St Clair EW, Turka LA. CTLA4Ig: bridging the basic immunology with clinical application. *Immunity* 2006;24(3):233–238.

47 Weaver TA, Charafeddine AH, Kirk AD. Costimulation blockade: towards clinical application. *Front Biosci* 2008;13:2120–2139.

48 Kirk AD, Tadaki DK, Celniker A *et al.* Induction therapy with monoclonal antibodies specific for CD80 and CD86 delays the onset of acute renal allograft rejection in non-human primates. *Transplantation* 2001;72(3):377–384.

49 Larsen CP, Pearson TC, Adams AB *et al.* Rational development of LEA29Y (belatacept), a high-affinity variant of CTLA4-Ig with potent immunosuppressive properties. *Am J Transplant* 2005;5(3):443–453.

50 Crameri A, Raillard SA, Bermudez E, Stemmer WP. DNA shuffling of a family of genes from diverse species accelerates directed evolution. *Nature* 1998; 391(6664):288–291.

51 Lazetic S, Leong SR, Chang JC *et al.* Chimeric co-stimulatory molecules that selectively act through CD28 or CTLA-4 on human T cells. *J Biol Chem* 2002;277(41):38660–38668.

52 Stebbings R, Poole S, Thorpe R. Safety of biologics, lessons learnt from TGN1412. *Curr Opin Biotechnol* 2009;20(6):673–677.

53 Suntharalingam G, Perry MR, Ward S *et al.* Cytokine storm in a phase 1 trial of the anti-CD28 monoclonal antibody TGN1412. *N Engl J Med* 2006;355(10): 1018–1028.

54 Weber J. Ipilimumab: controversies in its development, utility and autoimmune adverse events. *Cancer Immunol Immunother* 2009; 58:823–830.

55 Boumpas DT, Furie R, Manzi S *et al.* A short course of BG9588 (anti-CD40 ligand antibody) improves serologic activity and decreases hematuria in patients with proliferative lupus glomerulonephritis. *Arthritis Rheum* 2003;48(3):719–727.

56 Imai A, Suzuki T, Sugitani A *et al.* A novel fully human anti-CD40 monoclonal antibody, 4D11, for kidney transplantation in cynomolgus monkeys. *Transplantation* 2007;84(8):1020–1028.

57 Aoyagi T, Yamashita K, Suzuki T *et al.* A human anti-CD40 monoclonal antibody, 4D11, for kidney transplantation in cynomolgus monkeys: induction and maintenance therapy. *Am J Transplant* 2009;9(8): 1732–1741.

58 Robak T. Novel monoclonal antibodies for the treatment of chronic lymphocytic leukemia. *Curr Cancer Drug Targets* 2008;8(2):156–171.

59 Adams AB, Shirasugi N, Jones TR *et al.* Development of a chimeric anti-CD40 monoclonal antibody that synergizes with LEA29Y to prolong islet allograft survival. *J Immunol* 2005;174(1):542–550.

60 Ellis CN, Krueger GG. Treatment of chronic plaque psoriasis by selective targeting of memory effector T lymphocytes. *N Engl J Med* 2001;345(4):248–255.

61 Weaver TA, Charafeddine AH, Agarwal A *et al.* Alefacept promotes co-stimulation blockade based allograft survival in nonhuman primates. *Nat Med* 2009;15(7):746–749.

62 Pearson TC, Alexander DZ, Corbascio M *et al.* Analysis of the B7 costimulatory pathway in allograft rejection. *Transplantation* 1997;63(10):1463–1469.

63 Pearson TC, Alexander DZ, Winn KJ *et al.* Transplantation tolerance induced by CTLA4-Ig. *Transplantation* 1994;57(12):1701–1706.

64 Goeb V, Buch MH, Vital EM, Emery P. Costimulation blockade in rheumatic diseases: where we are? *Curr Opin Rheumatol* 2009;21(3):244–250.

65 Kean LS, Hamby K, Koehn B *et al.* NK cells mediate costimulation blockade-resistant rejection of allogeneic stem cells during nonmyeloablative transplantation. *Am J Transplant* 2006;6(2):292–304.

66 Zhai Y, Meng L, Gao F *et al.* Allograft rejection by primed/memory CD8⁺ T cells is CD154 blockade resistant: therapeutic implications for sensitized transplant recipients. *J Immunol* 2002;169(8):4667–4673.

67 Page AJ, Ford ML, Kirk AD. Memory T-cell-specific therapeutics in organ transplantation. *Curr Opin Organ Transplant* 2009;14(6):643–649.

68 Blair PJ, Riley JL, Harlan DM *et al.* CD40 ligand (CD154) triggers a short-term CD4⁺ T cell activation response that results in secretion of immunomodulatory cytokines and apoptosis. *J Exp Med* 2000;191(4):651–660.

69 Durie FH, Foy TM, Masters SR *et al.* The role of CD40 in the regulation of humoral and cell-mediated immunity. *Immunol Today* 1994;15(9):406–411.

70 Andre P, Prasad KS, Denis CV *et al*. CD40L stabilizes arterial thrombi by a beta3 integrin – dependent mechanism. *Nat Med* 2002;8(3):247–252.

71 Nicolls MR, Gill RG. LFA-1 (CD11a) as a therapeutic target. *Am J Transplant* 2006;6(1):27–36.

72 Vincenti F, Mendez R, Pescovitz M *et al*. A Phase I/II randomized open-label multicenter trial of efalizumab, a humanized anti-CD11a, anti-LFA-1 in renal transplantation. *Am J Transplant* 2007;7(7):1770–1777.

73 Chamian F, Lowes MA, Lin SL *et al*. Alefacept reduces infiltrating T cells, activated dendritic cells, nd inflammatory genes in psoriasis vulgaris. *Proc Natl Acad Sci U S A* 2005;102(6):2075–2080.

74 Dhanireddy KK, Bruno DA, Weaver TA *et al*. Portal venous donor-specific transfusion in conjunction with sirolimus prolongs renal allograft survival in nonhuman primates. *Am J Transplant* 2009;9(1):124–131.

75 Kaplon RJ, Hochman PS, Michler RE *et al*. Short course single agent therapy with an LFA-3-IgG1 fusion protein prolongs primate cardiac allograft survival. *Transplantation* 1996;61(3):356–363.

76 Rang HP. The receptor concept: pharmacology's big idea. *Br J Pharmacol* 2006;147(Suppl 1):S9–S16.

77 Kenakin T. Efficacy in drug receptor theory: outdated concept or under-valued tool? *Trends Pharmacol Sci* 1999;20(10):400–405.

78 Perez N, Karumuthil-Melethil S, Li R *et al*. Preferential costimulation by CD80 results in IL-10-dependent TGF-beta1$^+$-adaptive regulatory T cell generation. *J Immunol* 2008;180(10):6566–6576.

79 Latek R, Fleener C, Lamian V *et al*. Assessment of belatacept-mediated costimulation blockade throu evaluation of CD80/86-receptor saturation. *Transplantation* 2009;87(6):926–933.

80 Gilson CR, Milas Z, Gangappa S *et al*. Anti-CD40 monoclonal antibody synergizes with CTLA4-Ig in promoting long-term graft survival in murine models of transplantation. *J Immunol* 2009;183(3):1625–1635.

81 Larsen CP, Pearson TC, Adams AB *et al*. Rational development of LEA29Y (belatacept), a high-affinity variant of CTLA4-Ig with potent immunosuppressive properties. *Am J Transplant* 2005;5(3):443–453.

82 Vincenti F, Kirk AD. What's next in the pipeline. *Am J Transplant* 2008;8(10):1972–1981.

83 Vincenti F, Larsen C, Durrbach A *et al*. Costimulation blockade with belatacept in renal transplantation. *N Engl J Med* 2005;353(8):770–781.

84 Xu H, Elster EA, Blair PJ *et al*. Effects of combined treatment with CD25- and CD154-specific monoclonal antibodies in non-human primate allotransplantation. *Am J Transplant* 2003;3(11):1350–1354.

85 Jones TR, Ha J, Williams MA *et al*. The role of the IL-2 pathway in costimulation blockade-resistant rejection of allografts. *J Immunol* 2002;168(3):1123–1130.

86 Emamaullee JA, Merani S, Larsen CP, Shapiro AM. Belatacept and basiliximab diminish human anti-porcine xenoreactivity and synergize to inhibit allo-immunity. *Transplantation* 2008;85(1):118–124.

87 Bluestone JA, Liu W, Yabu JM *et al*. The effect of costimulatory and interleukin 2 receptor blockade on regulatory T cells in renal transplantation. *Am J Transplant* 2008;8(10):2086–2096.

88 Li Y, Li XC, Zheng XX *et al*. Blocking both signal 1 and signal 2 of T-cell activation prevents apoptosis of alloreactive T cells and induction of peripheral allograft tolerance. *Nat Med* 1999;5(11):1298–1302.

89 Pearl JP, Parris J, Hale DA *et al*. Immunocompetent T-cells with a memory-like phenotype are the dominant cell type following antibody-mediated T-cell depletion. *Am J Transplant* 2005;5(3):465–474.

90 Vincenti F, Chapentier B, Vanrentherghem Y *et al*. A Phase III study of belatacept-based immunosuppression regimens versus cyclosporine in renal transplant recipients (BENEFIT Study). *Am J Transplant* 2010;10:535–546.

91 Adams AB, Pearson TC, Larsen CP. Heterologous immunity: an overlooked barrier to tolerance. *Immunol Rev* 2003;196:147–160.

92 Kirk AD. 4D11: the second mouse? *Am J Transplant* 2009;9(8):1701–1702.

93 Cho CS, Burkly LC, Fechner JH, Jr, *et al*. Successful conversion from conventional immunosuppression to anti-CD154 monoclonal antibody costimulatory molecule blockade in rhesus renal allograft recipients. *Transplantation* 2001;72(4):587–597.

94 Wells AD, Li XC, Li Y *et al*. Requirement for T-cell apoptosis in the induction of peripheral transplantation tolerance. *Nat Med* 1999;5(11):1303–1307.

95 Preston EH, Xu H, Dhanireddy KK *et al*. IDEC-131 (anti-CD154), sirolimus and donor-specific transfusion facilitate operational tolerance in non-human primates. *Am J Transplant* 2005;5(5):1032–1041.

96 Montgomery SP, Mog SR, Xu H *et al*. Efficacy and toxicity of a protocol using sirolimus, tacrolimus and daclizumab in a nonhuman primate renal allotransplant model. *Am J Transplant* 2002;2(4):381–385.

97 Clinicaltrials.gov [Internet]. Bethesda (MD): National Library of Medicine (US); 2000. Available from: http://clinicaltrials.gov (accessed 2 March 2010).

98 Wu Z, Bensinger SJ, Zhang J *et al*. Homeostatic proliferation is a barrier to transplantation tolerance. *Nat Med* 2004;10(1):87–92.

99 Preville X, Flacher M, LeMauff B *et al.* Mechanisms involved in antithymocyte globulin immunosuppressive activity in a nonhuman primate model. *Transplantation* 2001;71(3):460–468.

100 Kirk AD, Mannon RB, Kleiner DE *et al.* Results from a human renal allograft tolerance trial valuating T-cell depletion with alemtuzumab combined with deoxyspergualin. *Transplantation* 2005;80(8): 1051–1059.

101 Knechtle SJ, Kirk AD, Fechner JH, Jr, *et al.* Inducing unresponsiveness by the use of anti-CD3 immunotoxin, CTLA4-Ig, and anti-CD40 ligand. *Transplant Proc* 1999;31(3B Suppl):27S–28S.

102 Wu G, Pfeiffer S, Schroder C *et al.* Co-stimulation blockade targeting CD154 and CD28/B7 modulates the induced antibody response after a pig-to-baboon cardiac xenograft. *Xenotransplantation* 2005;12(3): 197–208.

103 Montgomery SP, Xu H, Tadaki DK *et al.* Combination induction therapy with monoclonal antibodies specific for CD80, CD86, and CD154 in nonhuman primate renal transplantation. *Transplantation* 2002; 74(10):1365–1369.

104 Li ZL, Tian PX, Xue WJ, Wu J. Co-expression of sCD40LIg and CTLA4Ig mediated by adenovirus prolonged mouse skin allograft survival. *J Zhejiang Univ Sci B* 2006;7(6):436–444.

105 Zhu P, Chen YF, Chen XP *et al.* Mechanisms of survival prolongation of murine cardiac allografts using the treatment of CTLA4-Ig and MR1. *Transplant Proc* 2008;40(5):1618–1624.

106 Rigby MR, Trexler AM, Pearson TC, Larsen CP. CD28/CD154 blockade prevents autoimmune diabetes by inducing nondeletional tolerance after effector t-cell inhibition and regulatory T-cell expansion. *Diabetes* 2008;57(10):2672–2683.

107 Yin D, Ma L, Shen J *et al.* CTLA-41g in combination with anti-CD40L prolongs xenograft survival and inhibits anti-gal ab production in GT-Ko mice. *Am J Transplant* 2002;2(1):41–47.

108 Cardona K, Korbutt GS, Milas Z *et al.* Long-term survival of neonatal porcine islets in nonhuman primates by targeting costimulation pathways. *Nat Med* 2006;12(3):304–306.

109 Pierson RN, 3rd, Crowe JE, Jr, Pfeiffer S *et al.* CD40-ligand in primate cardiac allograft and viral immunity. *Immunol Res* 2001;23(2–3):253–262.

110 Barrett TB, Shu G, Clark EA. CD40 signaling activates CD11a/CD18 (LFA-1)-mediated adhesion in B cells. *J Immunol* 1991;146(6):1722–1729.

111 Blazar BR, Taylor PA, Panoskaltsis-Mortari A *et al.* Coblockade of the LFA1:ICAM and CD28/CTLA4:B7 pathways is a highly effective means of preventing acute lethal graft-versus-host disease induced by fully major histocompatibility complex-disparate donor grafts. *Blood* 1995;85(9):2607–2618.

112 Wang Y, Gao D, Lunsford KE *et al.* Targeting LFA-1 synergizes with CD40/CD40L blockade for suppression of both CD4-dependent and CD8-dependent rejection. *Am J Transplant* 2003;3(10): 1251–1258.

113 Corbascio M, Mahanty H, Osterholm C *et al.* Anti-lymphocyte function-associated antigen-1 monoclonal antibody inhibits CD40 ligand-independent immune responses and prevents chronic vasculopathy in CD40 ligand-deficient mice. *Transplantation* 2002;74(1):35–41.

114 Badell IR, Thompson P, Turner A *et al.* Combination CD28/LFA-1 blockade promotes alloislet survival in nonhuman primates. *Presented at the American Transplant Congress,* San Diego, CA, 30 April–4 May, 2010.

115 Durbach A, Pestana JM, Pearson T *et al.* A phase III study of belatacept versus cyclosporine in kidney transplants from extended criteria donors (BENEFIT-EXT Study). *Am J Transplant* 2010;10:547–557.

CHAPTER 29

Intravenous Immunoglobulin (IVIG) a Modulator of Immunity and Inflammation with Applications in Solid Organ Transplantation

Stanley C. Jordan[1], Mieko Toyoda[2], Joseph Kahwaji[1], Alice Peng[1], and Ashley A. Vo[1]

[1] Comprehensive Transplant Center, Cedars-Sinai Medical Center, Los Angeles, CA, USA
[2] Transplant Immunology Laboratory, Cedars-Sinai Medical Center, Los Angeles, CA, USA

Introduction

Immunoglobulin molecules, B cells and T cells are the primary effectors of the adaptive immune system [1]. Hypogammaglobulinemia can occur as a result of congenital or acquired conditions. However, the clinical features usually consist of an increased tendency for upper respiratory infections and increased susceptibility to autoimmune diseases [1, 2]. This counterintuitive relationship between immune deficiency and increased risk for autoimmune and inflammatory disorders suggest that IgG molecules may serve a dual role: first as mediators of sterilizing immunity and second as natural regulators of immunity and inflammation.

The use of passive antibody therapy to treat human diseases began more than a century ago with the use of horse anti-diphtheria toxin to treat severe cases of diphtheria [3, 4]. The remarkable story of intravenous immune globulin (IVIG) therapy began in 1980 with the introduction of the first products suitable for intravenous administration aimed at patients with primary and secondary immune deficiencies [1–4]. However, the anti-inflammatory and immune modulatory actions of IVIG were rapidly recognized with resultant broader applications to autoimmunity and systemic inflammatory conditions.

Although licensed for immunoglobulin replacement therapy, IVIG has also achieved broad utility in a number of other conditions, including Guillain–Barré syndrome, Kawasaki disease, and chronic inflammatory demyelinating polyneuropathy. Licensed indications account for less than 50 % of the current worldwide usage. IVIG use in desensitization protocols and for treatment of antibody-mediated rejection (AMR) has emerged as a new area of use. The question of dosing for effect is often posed. For example, IVIG is used at doses of ~500 mg/kg monthly for hypogammaglobulinemia. However, the required dose for anti-inflammatory effects, especially treatment of AMR, is 1–2 g/kg [1, 5–9]. It is easy to explain the beneficial effects of IVIG when used for IgG replacement. Here, one is relying on the presence of natural antibodies that can recognize foreign antigens as well as antibodies in high titer directed against common bacterial, viral, and fungal pathogens the donors have been vaccinated against or exposed to and developed sterilizing immunity. This is felt to be the "strength in numbers" advantage of the IVIG production process, which relies on extraction of IgG from the

Immunotherapy in Transplantation: Principles and Practice, First Edition. Edited by Bruce Kaplan, Gilbert J. Burckart and Fadi G. Lakkis.
© 2012 Blackwell Publishing Ltd. Published 2012 by Blackwell Publishing Ltd.

plasma of thousands of donors [1]. The difficulty arises in explaining how the pooled IgG product administered in the higher doses is capable of modulating immunity and inflammation and downregulating production of deleterious auto- and allo-antibodies of the same molecular class (IgG) [1, 3, 4, 9, 10].

Despite its success in treatment of a variety of autoimmune, hematologic, and now transplant-related conditions, the mechanisms responsible remain incompletely understood. Although there are many excellent reviews [1, 3, 4, 9, 10] of the mechanisms of action of high-dose IVIG and their applicability to the treatment of autoimmune diseases, this review will focus on the mechanisms of action relevant to immune modulation in solid organ transplantation and developing a rational therapeutic strategy for use in desensitization and treatment of AMR. In addition, we will discuss issues pertinent to safety and costs of IVIG use in transplant patients.

Complement activation and immune injury to allografts

Complement activation is now recognized as an important factor responsible for allograft dysfunction and loss during AMR. This is evidenced by the presence of C4d in allografts undergoing AMR [11]. Complement activation occurs by any one of four pathways: The classic pathway by antibody and immune complexes, the alternative pathway, the mannose-binding lectin/mannose-binding lectin-associated serine protease (MBL/MASP) pathway, and, importantly, the recently discovered extrinsic protease pathway [12–17] that results in complement activation after ischemia/reperfusion (I/R) injury independent of antibody/immune complex activation.

The natural functions of the complement system include cell lysis of invading foreign organisms by polymerization of C5b-9 and disruption of the integrity of the phospholipid bilayer, opsonization by C3b, as well as activation of the inflammation cascade in response to the generation of anaphylatoxins (C3a, C5a) [12]. The complement system plays a significant role in promoting antibody-mediated immune responses by aiding in antigen presentation to lymphocytes [18, 19]. C3a, C4a, and C5a are termed anaphylatoxins (inflammatory peptides promoting anaphylaxis) and induce the release of inflammatory mediators from mast cells and phagocytes, which tend to enhance inflammatory responses. Complement factor 5 (C5) is cleaved by C5 convertase (C3b) to produce C5a and complement factor 5b (C5b). C5a is considered the most potent inflammatory peptide of the complement system. It binds to the C5a receptor (C5aR) and promotes the secretion of proinflammatory cytokines from neutrophils, monocytes, and macrophages [12, 19].

C5b sequentially binds to complement factors 6–8 to form C5b–C8, which catalyzes the polymerization of C9 to form the membrane attack complex (MAC) [12, 19]. The MAC inserts itself into foreign bacteria or target tissues such as endothelial cells of mismatched donor organs and causes lysis of target cells. It appears that the major inflammatory effects of C5a and C5b–C9 MAC are largely responsible for the inflammation and tissue damage associated with complement activation (Plate 29.1).

The expression of complement proteins was, until recently, thought to be restricted largely to cells of the immune system. However, in recent years, studies have demonstrated widespread localization of these complement proteins and complement receptors throughout tissues and cell types outside the immune system, including the kidney [20]. The importance of these findings and identification of complement activation pathways induced by I/R injury suggest that complement activation by nonimmune mechanisms may be an important mediator of I/R injury in allografts, as has been recently demonstrated for experimental models of ischemic brain injury [12, 21, 22].

IVIG inhibits complement activation and complement-mediated inflammation

Immunoglobulin molecules are known for their ability to activate complement as part of the body's defense mechanism against invading pathogens [1–4]. However, the concept that immunoglobulin molecules can also inhibit complement activation and "scavenge" anaphylatoxins and active complement components has only recently been recognized [12, 19–22]. Recent data show that pre-incubation of C3a/C5a with F(ab)$'_2$ fragments of IgG results in binding and inhibition of inflammatory activity [19]. The Fc fragment of IgG molecules also shows significant ability to bind to C3b and C4b. Data from an experimental model of stroke injury shows that animals pretreated with IVIG or treated within 1–2h post I/R injury showed significant reductions in infarct size compared with control animals. These investigators showed that the major mediator of I/R injury in the brain was complement and that IVIG was a powerful scavenger of C3b produced in the ischemic brain [19–23]. IVIG treatment has also shown efficacy in limiting antibody-mediated complement activation in several other experimental models [19–23]. These observations have clear implications for the prevention and treatment of AMR. Plate 29.1 shows the complement activation cascade and points where IVIG and other complement modifers are known to interact to inhibit complement activation or scavenge activated complement components. These agents are likely to play an important role in the prevention and management of AMR and possibly I/R injury.

Modification of cell-mediated immunity by IVIG

The noted beneficial effects of IVIG in autoimmune diseases and transplantation have long been attributed to the neutralizing effects on circulating auto- and allo-antibodies [1–4]. However, the beneficial effects of this "neutralization" are noted to extend well beyond the half-life of the administered IVIG. This phenomenon was observed by our group in highly human leukocyte antigen (HLA)-sensitized transplant patients who underwent desensitization with IVIG alone as part of a multicenter, placebo-controlled trial [9]. In a retrospective analysis of anti-HLA class I and class II antibodies from patients who received transplants versus those who did not, those who responded well to the IVIG and received transplants had prolonged suppression of anti-HLA antibody levels for up to 24 months post-treatment. This observation and others [1–5] suggest that IVIG has the ability to regulate long-term auto- and allo-immune responses through interactions with immune cells in the treated patients. For many years, these "interactions" with immune cells were poorly understood, but recent data [1, 3–5] have more clearly defined IVIG's ability to regulate inflammation and deleterious immunity at the cellular level.

IVIG is now recognized to have the ability to interact with multiple cell types that constitute the adaptive and innate immune system. When considered together, these findings represent a major advancement in explaining the beneficial effects of IVIG in disorders caused by intense cellular immune activation, which is particularly relevant to solid organ transplantation [1, 3, 4].

IVIG interaction with Fc receptors: a new paradigm for regulation of cell-mediated immunity

Although numerous mechanism of action of IVIG have been attributed to the F(ab)$'_2$ (antigen-binding) fragments of IgG [1, 3, 5, 19, 23], more recent data strongly suggest a more critical role for the Fc fragments [24–29]. Among the recently identified pathways, the interaction of IVIG with the FcRn or neonatal Fc receptor expressed on endothelium is of interest. The FcRn is an HLA class-I-like molecule with a β2 microglobulin subunit. This receptor is important for recycling IgG molecules in the plasma, thus increasing the half-life of circulating IgG. The interaction of IgG molecules given at high doses is thought to saturate the FcRn and inhibit the binding of native IgG, thus decreasing half-life and increasing degradation of pathogenic antibody. This is especially important if there are high titers of deleterious auto- or allo-antibodies [1, 3, 30, 31].

Fc receptors exist on many immune cells and can exert either activating or suppressive functions. A summary of the activating and suppressive

Table 29.1 Human Fc receptor patterns of expression and function.

Fc receptor type	Cellular expression	Function	Effect of IVIG
FcRn	Expressed on endosomal compartment of intestinal epithelium, vascular endothelium and macrophages	Regulates serum IgG levels by binding pinocytosed IgG in endosomes and recycling to surface	Saturates FcRn increasing degradation of pathogenic auto-allo-antibodies
FcγRI (CD64)	Macrophages, monocytes, neutrophils, eosinophils and DC	Activating FcR	Saturates FcγRI and blocks cellular activation by inflammatory antibodies/immune complexes
FcγRIIa (CD32)	Macrophages, monocytes, neutrophils, eosinophils and DCs	Activating FcR contains activating ITAM motif in cytoplasmic domain	Saturates FcγRIIa and blocks cellular activation by inflammatory antibodies/immune complexes
FcγRIIb (CD32) Isoform of FcγRIIa	Macrophages, monocytes, neutrophils, eosinophils, DCs and B cells	Inhibits immune activation induced by activating FcR. Has inhibitory ITIM motif in cytoplasmic domain	IVIG induces inhibitory FcγRIIb in human and animal models of inflammation. Thought to be primary immune regulatory pathway
FcγRIII (CD16) Two isoforms: FcγRIIIa/b	Macrophages, monocytes, DC and NK cells (FcγRIIIa) Neutrophils (FcγRIIIb)	Activating Fc receptors	Inhibition of FcγRIIIa/b expression by IVIG-induced FcγRIIb Inhibition of ADCC in NK cells by high-dose IVIG binding to CD16

Fc receptors is shown in Table 29.1. A comprehensive analysis of FcR function and animal models of regulation by IVIG is beyond the scope of this review, but the reader is referred to several excellent reviews of this topic [1, 32, 33]. Briefly, after the inhibitory effect of IVIG on FcRn endocytosis of pathogenic auto-/allo-antibodies, two major hypotheses have emerged that might help explain the beneficial effects of IVIG on regulating cellular immunity. First, high-dose IVIG can bind to activating FcγRs and prevent binding of auto-/allo-antibody immune complexes, thus preventing immune activation at multiple levels (see Table 29.1). Second, and probably more important, is the recent evidence that IVIG actually induces the critical inhibitory receptor FcγRIIb on immune cells [1, 3, 31, 32]. Ravetch and coworkers [25–29] have shown that the beneficial effects of IVIG can actually be recapitulated by recombinant IgG Fc fragments. These investigators feel the anti-inflammatory activity of IVIG results from a minor population of the pooled IgG molecules that contains terminal α2,6-sialic acid linkages on their

Fc-linked glycans. They have also shown that the anti-inflammatory properties can be recapitulated with a fully recombinant preparation of appropriately sialylated IgG Fc fragments. More importantly, the authors have recently demonstrated that these sialylated Fcs require binding to a specific C-type lectin, SIGN-R1 (specific ICAM-3 grabbing non-integrin-related1), expressed on macrophages in the splenic marginal zone. In their experiments, splenectomy, loss of SIGN-R1+ cells in the splenic marginal zone, blockade of the carbohydrate recognition domain (CRD) of SIGN-R1, or genetic deletion of SIGN-R1 abrogated the anti-inflammatory activity of IVIG or sialylated Fc fragments. They also found that a human orthologue of SIGN-R1, DC-SIGN, displays a similar binding specificity to SIGN-R1 but differs in its cellular distribution, potentially accounting for some of the species differences observed in IVIG efficacy. These studies are important since they are the first to identify a receptor for sialylated Fcs. These researchers have also made a very important case for the efficacy of recombinant sialylated Fcs as potential therapeutic agents that could eventually replace IVIG, as their experiments show that enhancement of the sialylated Fc population shows equal efficacy to IVIG in significantly reduced dose levels [27–29]. To date, these experiments have only been conducted in mice and their application to human disease is still questionable [10]. In fact, recent data by Baray and coworkers [34, 35] suggest that the regulatory effects of IVIG directed at human dendritic cells (DCs) are independent of interactions with DC-SIGN and do not require sialylation of Fc fragments since F(ab)′$_2$ fragments convey inhibition as well. Similar data have also been reported by Aubin *et al.* [36]. Despite these concerns, this body of work represents a major advancement in our understanding of how IVIG works to regulate cellular effectors of inflammation and may point the way for development of more focused immunotherapeutic agents in the future [37].

Regulation of innate immune responses by IVIG

IVIG regulation of DC activation and function

DC activation is critical to a number of inflammatory disorders and allograft rejection. Several investigators [34–39] have shown that IVIG inhibits DC maturation by inhibition of CD80/86 expression and down regulation of HLA class I/II expression. Recent data also suggests that IVIG inhibits DC activation through inhibition of CD40 expression [35]. In addition, data by Aubin *et al.* [36] have shown in vivo and in vitro models that IVIG inhibits primary immune responses to T-cell-dependent antigens. This was associated with a reduction in antigen-specific T cells and antibody levels 28 days after immunization. These investigators also found that IVIG inhibition of T cell activation and antibody production were mediated by a direct interference of IVIG with DC activation [36]. This consequently inhibits the ability of DCs to activate T cells. IVIG also abrogates the ability of mature DCs to secrete IL-12 and increases the secretion of the regulatory cytokine IL-10. Others have also shown that IVIG suppresses

DC-mediated activation and proliferation of auto-/allo-reactive T cells [38, 39]. It also appears that IVIG can induce DCs to express regulatory activity in adoptive transfer models of autoimmunity [3]. Since the expression of HLA class I/II and CD80/86 are critical for antigen presentation to T cells, inhibition of DC activation by high-dose IVIG could provide an explanation for the powerful immune regulatory actions of IVIG. It is also of interest that IVIG administered at a lower dose (150 mg/kg) exerts a stimulatory effect on DCs in patients with common variable immunodeficiency syndrome (CVID), upregulating CD1a, CD80/86, and CD40 [40]. Activation of immune responses by DCs and the subsequent effects of IVIG are shown in Plate 29.2a and b.

IVIG regulation of monocyte and macrophage function

IVIG has demonstrable effects on monocytes and macrophages. These include the inhibition of pro-inflammatory cytokines and adhesion molecules and induction of cytokine inhibitors (IL-1 receptor antagonist) [41]. Recently, Abe *et al.* [41] examined gene expression in patients with Kawasaki disease (KD) before and after high-dose IVIG infusion. Here, the immunomodulatory effects of IVIG were likely mediated by suppression of an array of immune activation genes in monocytes and macrophages. Gill *et al.* [42] showed that IVIG has direct inhibitory effects on leukocyte recruitment in vitro and in vivo through inhibition of selectin and integrin functions. Others have also demonstrated a potent effect of IVIG on suppression of vaso-occlusion by inhibition of leukocyte adhesion in a mouse model of sickle cell disease [43].

IVIG regulation of adaptive immune responses

Effect on B cells and T cells

Using the mixed lymphocyte culture system, we have shown that IVIG can significantly inhibit T cell activation and reduce the expression of CD40, CD19, ICAM-1, CD86, and MHC-class II on APCs in the mixed lymphocyte reaction [44]. The primary effect is on B cells, and we have demonstrated that IVIG induces significant B cell apoptosis in vitro through Fc receptor-dependent mechanisms. Our group has also shown that IVIG inhibits IgG production in vitro and inhibits γ-IFN and IL-6 gene expression in activated human peripheral blood cells [45]. In addition, Park-Min *et al.* [24] showed that IVIG interacts with FcγRIII on immune cells to downregulate γIFN receptors thus preventing γIFN signaling. A recent paper by Kessel *et al.* [46] showed that IVIG markedly enhances the differentiation, expansion, and effector functions of CD25+/CD4+/Fox-P3+ regulatory T cells. This exciting data suggest a novel mode of action of IVIG that could be used to activate and expand T regulatory cell populations for suppression of inflammation in human transplantation. De Groot *et al.* also recently presented data that may further clarify the immunomodulatory actions of IVIG [47]. These investigators showed that IgG Fc-derived peptides were potent stimulators of natural T regulatory cell development ("Tregitopes"). These peptides have significant homology with HLA class II molecules, suggesting that Fcs have the ability to interact with CD4+ T cells and regulate their function. In vitro and in vivo experiments showed that the Fc-derived Tregitopes reduced inflammatory cytokine production and effector functions of antigen-activated human peripheral blood mononuclear cells while inducting a significant T-reg profile. Mouse models of inflammation were also significantly modified. The authors suggest that this may be a critical pathway for the immunomodulatory and anti-inflammatory actions of IVIG. A summary of the important regulatory effects of IVIG on cellular immunity are shown in Plate 29.2a and b and Plate 29.3.

Experience with IVIG in kidney transplantation

Renal transplantation has long been recognized as the treatment of choice for end-stage renal disease (ESRD), as it offers improved quality of life and survival [48–50]. As a result, the demand for donor kidneys continues to outpace the supply and the ongoing organ shortage crisis persists. Currently, there are more than 82,000 ESRD patients on the deceased donor (DD) waiting list, and almost 30,000 new patients register annually, yet fewer than 16,680 kidney transplants were performed in 2009 (based on OPTN data as of 5 November 2009) [51]. As the demand for organs continues to exceed the supply, the number of days spent waiting for a kidney transplant increases exponentially, particularly for patients that are difficult to match secondary to having broadly reactive HLA-specific alloantibodies or difficult to match blood types.

The disparity in waiting time experienced by these patients is a by-product of an organ allocation policy adopted in the context of an ongoing organ shortage crisis, which dictates that DD kidneys are allocated to blood-type-compatible recipients who have a negative complement-dependent cytotoxic cross-match with their donor. A positive cross-match (+CMX) indicates the presence of donor-specific alloantibodies (DSAs) in the serum of a potential recipient, and is associated with a rate of graft loss that exceeds 80 % [52–54]. Alloantibodies develop following exposure to foreign HLA molecules, usually through pregnancy, transfusion, and/or transplantation. Similarly, anti-ABO blood group antibodies or isoagglutinins develop in response to exposure to foreign blood groups, resulting in immediate graft loss [55]. Given the distribution of blood types in the USA, any potential donor–recipient pair has a 35 % probability of being blood type incompatible.

While local and national efforts to increase organ donation have had some success, the increase is unlikely to provide a large enough donor pool capable of supplying an ABO compatible and a perfectly matched donor for every potential recipient. The scarcity of donor organs has contributed to the disenfranchisement of this group of highly sensitized ESRD patients. Thus, in an effort to optimize organ availability and offer the benefit of renal transplantation to these patients, several transplant centers have developed protocols to overcome sensitization and blood group incompatibilities.

As a result of these efforts, it is now possible to perform successful renal transplantation in the presence of blood group incompatibilities and +CMX. Two main desensitization regimens are currently utilized: low-dose IVIG with plasmapheresis (PP) and high-dose IVIG. Low-dose IVIG/PP has been used successfully in live-donor renal ABO-incompatible (ABOi) and +CMX transplantation [55–60], while high-dose IVIG has been used to desensitize both living-donor +CMX and highly HLA-sensitized (HS) DD recipients from the waitlist [10, 61–65]. In the following sections, each desensitization protocol will be discussed in the context of its clinical relevance and efficacy with regard to controlling the alloimmune response. In addition to the standard desensitization protocols, several treatment adjuncts exist and their merits will be discussed.

Desensitization for ABOi transplantation

Initial outcomes following ABOi transplantation were poor. It was not until the mid 1980s, when Alexandre *et al.* published their series of 20 successful ABOi renal transplants, that the procedure was thought feasible [66]. Their success was attributed to the addition of splenectomy to their desensitization protocol, which included PP, azathioprine, antilymphocyte globulin, and steroids [67]. The need for splenectomy as part of a successful protocol for ABOi renal transplantation was further supported by the work of Tanabe *et al.* [68].

Subsequently, with the recognition of qualitative and quantitative differences in antigen expression between A1 and A2 individuals – specifically, the more favorable A2 phenotype is characterized by a lower density of antigen expression and fewer available epitopes for antibody binding [69–72] – the need for splenectomy as part of a successful desensitization protocol was questioned. Early reports indicated that successful engraftment across a blood group barrier was possible without splenectomy. However, the grafts suffered from unacceptably high rates of AMR [56]. It was not until the development of an anti-CD20 monoclonal antibody that splenectomy-free protocols were developed [73, 74]. Sonnenday *et al.* demonstrated the ability of anti-CD20 to provide adequate transient protection during engraftment, thus

coining the phrase "medical splenectomy." The six patients reported in the series were treated with the Johns Hopkins standard PP/IVIG desensitization protocol; in addition, each patient received a single dose of anti-CD20 monoclonal antibody on the final pre-transplant day of PP/IVIG [73].

As a result of new and more powerful maintenance immunosuppression therapies with B cell anti-proliferative properties including mycophenolate mofetil, the recognition that accommodation occurs after ABOi transplantation [75], and the ability of post-transplant PP to reduce the risk of rejection by controlling anti-agglutinin titers, excellent results after ABOi renal transplantation are possible. In a single series of 60 ABOi transplants performed at Johns Hopkins, Montgomery *et al.* [76] recently reported excellent 1, 3, and 5 year graft survival rates that compared favorably with the outcomes reported by the US Organ Procurement Transplantation Network (UNOS). Only 15% of patients experienced rejection episodes and the graft function was excellent at 5 years of follow-up. These investigators felt that protocols using PP and low-dose IVIG should allow the wide implementation of ABOi transplantation, a therapy that would greatly increase the number of kidney transplants performed in the USA.

At Cedars-Sinai Medical Center, we have adopted a protocol for ABOi transplants that employs administration of rituximab 1 g 2 weeks prior to initiation of PP, PP every other day × 5 followed by high-dose IVIG (2 g/kg × 1). Our aim is to reduce anti-A/B titers to <1:8 prior to transplantation. This protocol also yields excellent results in 22 patients treated [77]. Thus, the use of PP + IVIG in high dose or low dose has made ABOi transplantation possible, something that was thought to be a distant goal only a few years ago.

Immunomodulation with IVIG: desensitization of highly HS patients

Data from our group and others suggest that IVIG therapy given to highly sensitized patients results in reduced allosensitization, reduced I/R injuries, fewer acute rejection episodes, and higher successful long-term allograft outcomes for cardiac and renal allograft recipients [7, 10, 61–65, 78]. We and others have confirmed that pretreatment with IVIG results in reductions of anti-HLA antibodies and is effective in treatment of allograft rejection episodes [7, 10, 63]. We have also shown that IVIG is effective in reducing anti-HLA antibody levels and significantly improving transplant rates in highly HS patients in a controlled clinical trial [10].

The high-dose IVIG protocol developed at Cedars-Sinai evolved from our experience in treating a highly sensitized child in 1991 [79]. This experience eventually led to the development of a controlled clinical trial of IVIG in highly sensitized patients awaiting transplantation.

The NIH-IG02 study was a multicenter, controlled clinical, double-blinded trial of IVIG versus placebo in highly sensitized patients awaiting kidney transplantation. The study was designed to determine whether IVIG could reduce panel-reactive antibody (PRA) levels and improve rates of transplantation without concomitantly increasing the risk of graft loss in this difficult-to-transplant group. This study represents the only controlled clinical trial of a desensitization therapy.

Data from this trial was published [10]. Briefly, IVIG was superior to placebo in reducing anti-HLA IgG levels ($p = 0.007$, IVIG versus placebo) and improving rates of transplantation. The 3 year follow up shows the predicted mean time to transplantation was 4.8 years in the IVIG group versus 10.3 years in the placebo group ($p = 0.05$). With a median follow-up of 3 years post-transplant, the viable transplants functioned normally with a mean (±SE) serum creatinine of 1.68 ± 0.28 (IVIG) versus 1.28 ± 0.13 mg/dL for placebo ($p = 0.29$). Allograft survival was also superior in the IVIG group at 3 years. Based on data generated from the NIH-IG02 trial, we developed the following approach to desensitization at our center. For IVIG alone, we usually give four doses of IVIG monthly (2 g/kg, maximum dose 140 g) until a negative or acceptable (<225 channel shifts by flow cytometry CMX (FCMX)) is obtained. We have also adapted this to use for highly sensitized DD transplant candidates who have been on the UNOS waitlist for >5 years, have a PRA of >30%, and who receive frequent offers for kidneys from donors with whom they have a +CMX. Outcomes for patients transplanted after desensitization with high-dose IVIG at our institution are outlined below.

Between January 1994 and May 2008, 169 HS patients underwent desensitization and transplantation using high-dose IVIG±rituximab, and/or PP and were available for evaluation. Our early experience (1994–2005) was with IVIG 2 g/kg monthly×4 alone. CMXs were often positive at the time of transplant (FCMX+). The average PRA was 52%; 39% were retransplants; 42% were DD and 58% were living donor. We examined the 1-, 3-, and 5-year graft patient survival rates, mean serum creatinine values of those with functioning grafts, and causes of graft loss. Of the 169 HS patients, 150 patients (91.5% death-censored graft survival) had functioning grafts at 1 year; 14 grafts had failed, 2 were lost to follow-up, and 3 had death with functioning grafts. Of 84 patients with 3 years of follow-up, there were 64 functioning grafts (83.1%). At 5 years, 76.7% had functioning grafts, 10 had failed (four lost to rejection, one lost to thrombosis, four lost to noncompliance and poor follow-up, one loss attributed to chronic nephropathy). The average serum creatinine concentrations of the functioning grafts at 1 year, 3 years, and 5 years were 1.36 ± 0.51 mg/dL, 1.43 ± 0.52 mg/dL, and 1.60 ± 0.78 mg/dL respectively. Patient survivals were 97.6%, 96.4% and 89.6% at 1 year, 3 years, and 5 years respectively. The 1-, 3-, and 5-year outcomes for patients undergoing desensitization with high-dose IVIG compares with the reported UNOS graft survivals for patients with PRAs of 0–9% and 10–79% versus the poorer outcomes for patients with PRAs of >80% [80]. Late failures were due to noncompliance or death with functioning graft. Overall, we conclude, desensitization therapy with high-dose IVIG offers HS patients an opportunity for successful long-term graft survival. However, it is important to realize that the advent of newer, more sensitive assays for detection of anti-HLA antibodies may make it more difficult to demonstrate a beneficial reduction in anti-HLA antibody that is permissive for transplantation after desensitization.

Low-dose IVIG and PP

An alternative to high-dose IVIG is a combination therapy with low-dose IVIG (100 mg/kg) and PP. PP/IVIG is limited, however, to live donor kidney transplantation, as DSAs will rebound within days of discontinuing therapy, which poses a problem when the timing of the transplant is not determined, as is the case with DD transplantation. The components of the therapy are thought to act in concert such that PP removes circulating DSAs while IVIG inhibits the function of residual DSAs and limits the production of endogenous alloantibody.

Montgomery *et al.* first demonstrated the utility of PP/IVIG as preemptive therapy to remove DSAs in sensitized patients prior to renal transplantation [59]. In the initial series, four patients (three with flow +CMX; one with cytotoxic +CMX) were successfully desensitized prior to receiving a kidney from their live donor. Each patient was started on immunosuppression consisting of tacrolimus and mycophenolate mofetil on the first day of PP, and received PP with replacement of 1–1.5 plasma volumes using either 5% albumin or fresh frozen plasma. Immediately following each PP procedure, patients received 100 mg/kg IVIG. Induction therapy on the day of transplant included humanized monoclonal anti-IL-2 receptor antibody (daclizumab, Roche Pharmaceuticals, Nutley, NJ) and a steroid bolus with rapid post-operative taper. Since that report, 138 +CMX patients have been successfully desensitized and transplanted with a 10-year death-censored graft survival of 89% (R. Montgomery, 2009, unpublished data). Further, Montgomery and Zachary have demonstrated that the kinetics of antibody removal is consistent and that the number of treatments necessary to reduce DSAs to a level that is safe for transplantation can be estimated from the starting titer [81].

IVIG + rituximab for desensitization

For patients who do not respond to IVIG alone or who have high-titer anti-HLA antibodies, our group (Cedars-Sinai Medical Center) developed a new protocol. The protocol involves the use of IVIG (2 g/kg) followed by two weekly doses of rituximab (anti-CD20, anti-B cell) chimeric monoclonal antibody (1 g). Another 2 g/kg dose of IVIG is given 1 week after the final dose of rituximab. This protocol reduces the time of desensitization using the high-dose IVIG protocol from 16 weeks to 4–5 weeks. In a Phase I/II trial of this protocol we were able to transplant 80% of highly HS patients studied (16/20). Rejection episodes occurred in 50%, while patient and graft survival at 1 year were 100% and 94% respectively. Patients who received DD transplants waited 144±89 months (range: 60–324 months) on the transplant waitlist before receiving desensitization with IVIG and rituximab, but waited only 4.9±5.9 months (range: 1.5–18 months) after treatment for a transplant [82]. Our subsequent experience using IVIG + single-dose rituximab in 76 highly HS patients confirms our previous observations. The AMR rate was 25% with patient and graft survival of 98% and 89% for both living donor/DD recipients at 24 months post-transplant [83].

IVIG for treatment of AMR

Our group was the first to report on the use of IVIG for treatment of AMR in kidney and heart allograft recipients with AMR [7]. Although this experience in now more than a decade old, it was useful in showing that AMR episodes could respond to IVIG and pulse methylprednisolone, although the mechanisms of action were not appreciated at that time. The first patient treated with high-dose IVIG for resistant rejection (1994) had failed OKT3 therapy and two courses of pulse methyl-prednisolone. The features of AMR were not appreciated at that time, but the patient was noted to develop a positive post-transplant complement-dependent cytotoxicity (CDC) cross-match with donor cells that showed in vitro inhibition with IVIG. The decision to treat with high-dose IVIG was based on this observation and the patient's unresponsiveness to other treatments. The patient had a dramatic response to the IVIG treatment with serum creatinine decreasing from 3.0 mg/dL to 1.0 mg/dL over 3–4 days. The patient had no further AMR episodes and has a serum creatinine of 1.7 mg/dL 15 years post-transplant. At that time, we felt this represented a new approach to cross-match positive rejection episodes and other patients were treated with high-dose IVIG for severe rejection episodes associated with cross-match positivity as described [7, 84]. Other groups have also described the benefits of high-dose IVIG in treating resistant AMR episodes [8, 9, 85]. IVIG + pulse methyl-prednisolone with/without plasma exchange was used as our primary treatment for AMR until 2004 [84]. Lefaucheur *et al.* [86] recently reported on a retrospective comparison of high-dose IVIG alone (12 patients) versus IVIG + rituximab + plasma exchange (12 patients) for treatment of AMR. The IVIG-alone group was treated between January 2000 and December 2003, while the patients receiving combined therapy were treated from January 2004 to December 2005. The investigators found that the combined therapy was superior to IVIG alone in providing improved graft survival at 36 months (91.7% combined versus 50% IVIG alone, *p* = 0.02) and providing long-term sup-pression of DSA levels. Although, this is not a randomized study and the number of patients is small, these findings would support our own observations that led us to change our approach to treatment of AMR in 2004. What these obser-vations suggest is that combination therapies (IVIG + rituximab) appear to offer superior outcomes in terms of modification of DSA levels and improving long-term allograft survival.

Optimal treatment of AMR probably requires a combination of rituximab with PP and low-dose IVIG or with high-dose IVIG (1–2 g/kg) owing to the inability of rituximab to deplete CD20-negative plasma cells that continue to produce DSAs and mediate graft injury.

Our center has extensive experience with HS patients who received kidney transplants after desensitization with IVIG and rituximab [82, 87]. Recently, we evaluated 123 HS patients transplanted after desensitization (7/06–2/09). Twenty-two patients developed AMR post-transplant, usually within the first month. All were treated with a combination of steroids (10 mg/kg daily × 3), IVIG 2 g/kg (maximum dose 140 g × 1), and rituximab (375 mg/m^2 × 1). Some patients also received PP and two underwent splenectomy. Six of twenty-two patients, 27%, lost their allograft to severe AMR, usually within 1 month. Thus, a 73%

survival rate for severe AMR was seen in this high-risk group [88].

Kaposztas *et al.* reported 2-year outcomes in their recent retrospective study looking at 54 patients treated for AMR [89]. Group A had 26 patients that underwent treatment with PP and rituximab and Group B had 28 patients who received PP without rituximab. Patients that had low serum IgG levels also received IVIG. The 2-year graft survival was significantly better in the group that received rituximab (90% versus 60%), with the difference attributed to rituximab. A trend toward improved graft survival was also seen in those that received IVIG (*p* = 0.050). This retrospective study has one of the largest cohorts reported to date and supports the use of rituximab for the treatment of AMR with good short-term allograft survival; however, many patient variables were not consistent between the groups. Mulley *et al.* [90] recently reported a case series of seven patients with refractory AMR that responded to treatment with a single low-dose of rituximab (500 mg). All patients had recovery of renal function with patient and graft survivals at a mean 21 months follow-up of 100%. Three patients had significant viral infections, but all recovered. Recent data from experimental primate islet transplants show that the addition of B cell depletion to standard immunosuppression results in significant prolongation of islet allograft survival with inhibition of alloantibody responses [91]. In addition, Kessler *et al.* [92] recently reported the complete reversal of an AMR episode of an islet transplant using the combination of IVIG + rituximab. Complete ablation of DSAs was also noted in association with allograft recovery.

Complications and cost of IVIG therapy

Unlike the use of IVIG in immunodeficiency, patients who are highly HLA sensitized require higher doses (1–2 g/kg per dose) to achieve a beneficial outcome. The use of higher doses and concentrations of IVIG products results in higher rates of infusion-related complications that were,

Table 29.2 IVIG-related adverse event (AE) and significant adverse event (SAE).

	Carimune (n=98)	Gamimune-N (n=76)	Polygam (n=105)
% AE or SAE	n=8 (SAE)	N/A	n=5 (SAE)
Gender	3 male/5 female	N/A	2 male/3 female
Age range (years)	39–79	15–75	34–77
Type of AE/SAE			
thrombotic	0	0	5 (4.7%); P<0.01
ARF[a]	8 (8.2%); P<0.001	0	0
other (headache)	49 (50%)	39 (52%)	52 (50%)
Doses	2 g/kg=7 patients	2 g/kg	2 g/kg=4 patients
	1 g/kg=1 patient		1 g/kg=1 patient

[a]ARF: acute renal failure.

at first, not anticipated and were poorly understood. We have recently reviewed the complications associated with IVIG infusions in patients with normal renal function and those on dialysis [10, 93, 94]. Briefly, the safety of IVIG infusion (2 g/kg) doses given over a 4 h hemodialysis session, monthly × 4 versus placebo (0.1% albumin) in equivalent doses was studied in the IG02 trial [33]. There were more than 300 infusions in each arm of the study using Gamimune N 10% versus placebo. Adverse events were similar in both arms of the study (24 IVIG versus 23 placebo). The most common adverse event in the IVIG arm was headache (52% versus 24%, p=0.056). This usually abated with reduction in infusion rate and acetaminophen. Thus, we concluded from this double-blind placebo-controlled trial that high-dose IVIG infusions during hemodialysis are safe.

A retrospective analysis of infusion-related adverse events associated with various IVIG products, including Polygam®, Carimune®, Gamunex®, and Gammagard® Liquid, found that adverse events could be related to differences in excipient content and osmolality [93]. These are reviewed below. Table 29.2 shows the incidence of IVIG-related side effects experienced at our center with various products. The commonest side effects encountered included acute renal failure with sucrose-containing products, thrombotic episodes with hyperosmotic products containing saline as an excipient, and hemolysis with isosmolar liquid products [93, 94].

IVIG and acute myocardial infarction (AMI)

Five cases of AMI (p<0.01) were seen in patients who received Polygam 10%. All five patients had risk factors for cardiac disease. Each patient developed symptoms during or shortly (3–5 h) after IVIG infusion, which included shortness of breath and chest pain. The diagnosis of AMI was confirmed by electrocardiogram and/or troponin elevations. Polygam's excipient is a sodium chloride solution with an approximate osmolality of 1250 mOsm/L at 10%. The salt-based high-viscosity vehicle of this product was likely responsible for initiation of the thrombotic event seen (AMI). Other patients were noted to develop thrombosis of dialysis fistulas. This product is no longer used at most centers in the USA.

IVIG and acute renal failure (ARF)

Eight cases of ARF (p<0.001) were seen in patients who received Carimune®, a sucrose-containing IVIG. All eight patients had identifiable risk factors for ARF. Renal biopsy done in one patient was notable for acute tubular necrosis and marked vacuolization of proximal tubular cells that were attributed to IVIG/sucrose. Shortly after the infusion, the patient's serum creatinine rose to 7.4 mg/dL and dialysis was required. The use of high-dose IVIG products that contain sucrose should be avoided in post-transplant patients or those with other risk factors that might predispose to acute renal failure. Most sucrose-containing IVIG products have now been replaced by newer isosmolar IVIGs.

IVIG and hemolytic anemia

Acute hemolyis following IVIG administration was very rare until the development of more refined IVIG products produced by chromatography techniques. These products contain higher titers of pathogen-specific antibodies than lyophilized products where protein degradation likely occurs. These chromatographically derived IVIG products contain anti-blood group antibodies (i.e., anti-A/B) since they are derived from the plasma of thousands of donors in higher titers than seen with previous products. Administration of these products has been associated with episodes of clinically relevant hemolysis [94, 95]. We have shown that titers of anti-A vary from different IVIG products, with the liquid, isosmolar products having the highest titers and most common association with clinical hemolysis episodes (Figure 29.1).

We recently reported a series of 18 cases of IVIG-induced hemolytic anemia in our highly HLA sensitized ESRD patients following IVIG infusions on dialysis. All patients had a positive direct antiglobulin test. Average pre- and post-IVIG hemoglobin values were 11.6 g/dL and 7.8 g/dL respectively. Blood transfusions were required by

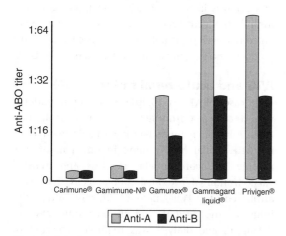

Figure 29.1 The anti-A and anti-B blood group antibody titers in various IVIG products. Note the higher titers are found in the newer isosmolar liquid products (Gamunex®, Gammagard Liquid®, and Privigen®). (Titers performed by the Cedars-Sinai Medical Center Blood Bank.)

83% of patients. All cases of hemolysis were observed in patients that received liquid preparations of IVIG (Gamunex 10%, Gammagard® Liquid 10%, and Privigen® 10%). Liquid IVIG preparations have higher anti-A/B titers than lyophilized preparations do. Since most IVIG manufacturers are now switching to liquid IVIG products with concentrations of 10%, we feel that more episodes of acute hemolysis are likely, and this should be a consideration in patients receiving IVIG in high doses who are A, B, or AB blood group positive.

Cost of IVIG therapy in transplant patients

IVIG is an expensive therapy that raises questions from insurers and hospitals regarding the justification of costs for this and other drugs used for desensitization. The ultimate question relates to the cost effectiveness of IVIG for desensitization. Currently, a four-dose course of IVIG for a 70 kg person at 2 g/kg would cost ~ US$55 000. However, one must compare this with the cost of maintaining patients on chronic hemodialysis. According to USRDS 2008 data, the cost of hemodialysis per patient was $71 889 per year in 2006. This compared with $53 327 per year for peritoneal dialysis and $24 951 per year for a transplant recipient. These are estimates for Medicare and may not include hospitalization cost or outpatient surgery cost (i.e., fistulae surgeries) for these patient groups [96, 97].

In the IG02 study [10], the calculated cost saving was ~ US$300 000/patient transplanted versus those who remained on dialysis for the 5 years of the study. Data from USRDS (2003) also confirm that a considerable cost saving to Medicare is seen in highly sensitized patients transplanted versus those who remain on dialysis [78].

A recent meta-analysis compiled by the Canadian Blood Services concluded that sensitized patients receiving IVIG to decrease donor-specific sensitization prior to kidney transplantation have a better survival and decreased mortality than dialysis patients, and that desensitization from all studies examined is considered cost effective [97].

IVIG's relevance to clinical transplantation

Experience with high-dose IVIG and PP/low-dose IVIG desensitization protocols among highly sensitized and ABOi patients has established these strategies as safe and viable alternatives to prolonged periods of dialysis while waiting for a compatible DD organ. It is clear that ABO incompatibility and positive donor-specific cross-matches should no longer be considered contraindications to renal transplantation [10, 81–87]. It is clear that IVIG remains critical to all of the above protocols and has made an important contribution to improving the opportunities for and success of organ transplants for highly sensitized patients. Advances in the clinical management of highly HS patients preceded the advancements in our understanding of the mechanism of action of IVIG. In the past 2 years, there have been important and significant advances in this understanding and how this could lead to a better application of IVIG in our transplant patient population.

One important area is in the treatment of AMR. Here, the anti-inflammatory and immunomodulatory actions of IVIG appear to have a clear benefit in the management of this severe complication of transplantation. However, we know that other agents are often necessary. These would include PP and possibly B cell depletion with rituximab [84, 86].

Summary

With functions as diverse as providing sterilizing immunity from infections, inhibiting and scavenging activated complement fragments, modifying cell-mediated immune responses, and blocking antibody-mediated injury to allografts, IVIG will probably have an important role in clinical transplantation for many years to come.

Acknowledgments

The Rebecca Sakai Memorial Fund and the Joyce Jillson Fund for Transplant Research. We also want to express our gratitude to the entire staff of the Transplant Immunotherapy Program at Cedars-Sinai Medical Center for their hard work and dedication.

References

1 Nimmerjahn F, Ravetch J. Anti-inflammatory actions of intravenous immunoglobulin. *Annu Rev Immunol* 2008;26:513–533.

2 Brandt D, Gershwin ME. Common variable immune deficiency and autoimmunity. *Autoimmun Rev* 2006;5:465–470.

3 Tha-In T, Bayry J, Metsellar H *et al.* Modulation of the cellular immune system by intravenous immunoglobulin. *Trends Immunol* 2008;29:608–615.

4 Hartnug H-P. Advances in the understanding of the mechanisms of action of IVIg. *J Neurol* 2008;255:3–6.

5 Clynes R. Protective mechanisms of IVIG. *Curr Opin Immunol* 2007;19:646–651.

6 Jordan SC, Toyoda M, Vo A. Intravenous immunoglobulin a natural regulator of immunity and inflammation. *Transplantation* 2009;88:1–6.

7 Jordan SC, Quartel AW, Czer LS *et al.* Posttransplant therapy using high-dose human immunoglobulin (intravenous gammaglobulin) to control acute humoral rejection in renal and cardiac allograft recipients and potential mechanism of action. *Transplantation* 1998;66(6):800–805.

8 Casadei DH, del C Rial M, Opelz G *et al.* A randomized and prospective study comparing treatment with high-dose intravenous immunoglobulin with monoclonal antibodies for rescue of kidney grafts with steroid-resistant rejection. *Transplantation* 2001;71: 53–58.

9 Luke PP, Scantlebury VP, Jordan ML *et al.* Reversal of steroid and anti-lymphocyte antibody-resistant rejection using intravenous immunoglobulin (IVIG) in renal transplant recipients. *Transplantation* 2001; 72:419–422.

10 Jordan SC, Tyan D, Stablein D *et al.* Evaluation of intravenous immunoglobulin as an agent to lower allosensitization and improve transplantation in highly-HLA sensitized adult patients with end stage renal disease: report of the NIH IG02 trial. *J Am Soc Nephrol* 2004;15:3256–3262.

11 Colvin RB. Antibody-mediated renal allograft rejection: diagnosis and pathogenesis. *J Am Soc Nephrol* 2007;18(4):1046–1056.

12 Arumugam TV, Woodruff TM, Lathia JD *et al*. Neuroprotection in stroke by complement inhibition and immunoglobulin therapy. *Neuroscience* 2009; 158(3):1074–1089.

13 Thurman JM. Holers VM. The central role of the alternative complement pathway in human disease. *J Immunol* 2006;176:1305–1310.

14 Arumugam TV, Shiels IA, Woodruff TM *et al*. The role of the complement system in ischemia–reperfusion injury. *Shock* 2004;21:401–409.

15 Degan SE, Thiel S, Jensenius JC. New prespectives on mannan-binding lectin-mediated complement activation. *Immunobiology* 2007;212:301–311.

16 Wills-Karp M. Complement activation pathways: a bridge between innate and adaptive immune responses in asthma. *Proc Am Thorac Soc* 2007;4:247–251.

17 Huber-Lang M, Sarma JV, Zetoune FS *et al*. Generation of C5a in the absence of C3: a new complement activation pathway. *Nat Med* 2006;12:682–687.

18 Kemper C, Atkinson JP. T-cell regulation: With complements from innate immunity. *Nat Rev Immunol* 2007;7:9–18.

19 Basta M. Ambivalent effect of immunoglobulin on the complement system: activation versus inhibition. *Mol Immunol* 2008;45:4073–4079.

20 Thurman J. Triggers of inflammation after renal ischemia/reperfusion injury. *Clin Immunol* 2007;123:7–13.

21 Arumugam TV, Tang SC, Lathia JD *et al*. Intravenous immunoglobulin (IVIG) protects the brain against experimental stroke by preventing complement-mediated neuronal cell death. *Proc Natl Acad Sci U S A* 2007;104:14104–14109.

22 Arumugam TV, Selvaraj PK, Woodruff TM, Mattson MP. Targeting ischemic brain injury with intravenous immunoglobulin. *Expert Opin Ther Targets* 2008;12: 19–29.

23 Basta M, Van Goor F, Luccioli S *et al*. F(ab)′$_2$-mediated neutralization of C3a and C5a anaphylatoxins: a novel effector function of immunoglobulins. *Nat. Med* 2003;9:431–438.

24 Park-Min KH, Serbina NV, Yang W *et al*. Fc gamma RIII-dependent inhibition of interferon-gamma responses mediates suppressive effects of intravenous immune globulin. *Immunity* 2007;26(1):67–78.

25 Sameulsson A, Towers TL, Ravetch JV. Anti-inflamatory activity of IVIG mediated through the inhibitory Fc receptor. *Science* 2001;29:484–486.

26 Kaneko Y, Nimmerjahn F, Madaio M, Ravetch J. Pathology and protection in nephrotoxic nephritis is determined by selective engagement of specific Fc receptors. *J Exper Med* 2006;203:789–797.

27 Anthony RM, Nimmerjahn F, Ashline DJ *et al*. Recapitulation of IVIG anti-inflammatory activity with a recombinant IgG Fc. *Science* 2008;320(5874):373–376.

28 Kaneko Y, Nimmerjahn F, Ravetch J. Anti-inflammatory activity of immunoglobulin G resulting from Fc sialylation. *Science* 2006;313:670–673.

29 Anthony RM, Wermeling F, Karlsson MC, Ravetch JV. Identification of a receptor required for the anti-inflammatory activity of IVIG. *Proc Natl Acad Sci U S A* 2008;105(50):19571–19578.

30 Ghetie V, Ward ES. Multiple roles for the major histocompatibility complex class I-related receptor FcRn. *Annu Rev Immunol* 2000;18:739–766.

31 Roopenian DC, Akilesh S. FcRn: the neonatal Fc receptor comes of age. *Nat Rev Immunol* 2007;7: 715–725.

32 Nimmerjahn F, Ravetch JV. Fcγ receptors: old friends and new family members. *Immunity* 24:19–28.

33 Ravetch JV, Clynes RA. 1998. Divergent roles for Fc receptors and complement in vivo. *Annu Rev Immunol* 2006;16:421–432.

34 Bayry J, Lacroix-Desmazes S, Carbonneil C *et al*. Inhibition of maturation and function of dendritic cells by intravenous immunoglobulin. *Blood* 2003; 101:758–765.

35 Bayry J, Bansal K, Kazatchkine MD, Kaveri SV. DC-SIGN and alpha 2,6-sialylated IgG Fc interaction is dispensable for the anti-inflammatory activity of IVIg on human dendritic cells. *Proc Natl Acad Sci U S A* 2009; 106(9):E24.

36 Aubin E, Lemieux R, Bazian R. Indirect inhibition of in vivo and in vitro T-cell response by IVIG due to impaired antigen presentation. *Blood* 2010;115(9): 1727–1734.

37 Kaveri S, Lacroix-Desmazes S, Bayry J. The antinflammatory IgG. *N Engl J Med* 2008;359:307–309.

38 Tha-In T, Metselaar HJ, Tilanus HW *et al*. Superior immunomodulatory effects of intravenous immuno-globulins on human T-cells and dendritic cells: comparison to calcineurin inhibitors. *Transplantation* 2006;81: 1725–1734.

39 Smed-Sörensen A, Moll M, Cheng TY *et al*. IgG regulates the CD1 expression profile and lipid antigen presenting function in human dendritic cells via FcγRIIa. *Blood* 2008;111:5037–5046.

40 Durandy A, Kaveri S, Kuiipers T *et al*. Intravenous immunoglobulin – understanding properties and mechanisms. *Clin Exp Immunol* 2009;158:2–13.

41 Abe J, Jibiki T, Noma S *et al*. Gene expression profiling of the effect of high-dose intravenous Ig in patients with Kawasaki disease. *J Immunol* 2005;174(9):5837–5845.

42 Gill V, Doig C, Knight D *et al.* Targeting adhesion molecules as a potential mechanism of action for intravenous immunoglobulin. *Circulation* 2005;112: 2031–2039.

43 Turhan A, Jenab P, Bruhns P *et al.* Intravenous gammaglobulin prevents venular vaso-occlusion in sickle cell mice by inhibiting leukocyte adhesion and the interactions between sickle erythrocytes and adherent leukocytes. *Blood* 2004;103:2397–2400.

44 Toyoda M, Pao A, Petrosian A, Jordan SC. Pooled human gammaglobulin modulates surface molecule expression and induces apoptosis in human B cells. *Am J Transplant* 2003;3:156–166.

45 Toyoda M, Zhang XM, Petrosian A *et al.* Inhibition of allospecific responses in the mixed lymphocyte reaction by pooled human gammaglobulin. *Transplant Immunol.* 1994;2(4):337–341.

46 Kessel A, Ammuri H, Peri R *et al.* Intravenous immunoglobulin therapy affects T-regulatory cells by increasing their suppressive function. *J Immunol* 2007;179:5571–5575.

47 De Groot AS, Moise L, McMurry JA *et al.* Activation of natural regulatory T cells by IgG Fc-derived peptide "Tregitopes". *Blood* 2008;112(8):3303–3311.

48 Evans RW, Manninen DL, Garrison LPJ *et al.* The quality of life of patients with end-stage renal disease. *N Engl J Med* 1985;312:553–559.

49 Port FK, Wolfe RA, Mauger EA *et al.* Comparison of survival probabilities for dialysis patients vs cadaveric renal transplant recipients. *JAMA* 1993;270: 1339–1343.

50 Russell JD, Beecroft ML, Ludwin D, Churchill DN. The quality of life in renal transplantation – a prospective study. *Transplantation* 1992;54:656–660.

51 Organ Procurement and Transplantation Network. Scientific registry of transplant recipients. http://www. optn.org/data/ (accessed 18 June 2008).

52 Kissmeyer-Nielsen F, Olsen S, Petersen VP, Fjeldborg O. Hyperacute rejection of kidney allografts, associated with pre-existing humoral antibodies against donor cells. *Lancet* 1966;2:662–665.

53 Patel R, Terasaki PI. Significance of the positive cross-match test in kidney transplantation. *N Engl J Med* 1969;280:735–739.

54 Williams GM, Hume DM, Hudson RPJ *et al.* "Hyperacute" renal-homograft rejection in man. *N Engl J Med* 1968;279:611–618.

55 Starzl TE, Marchioro TL, Holmes JH *et al.* Renal homografts in patients with major donor-recipient blood group incompatibilities. *Surgery* 1964;55: 195–200.

56 Gloor JM, DeGoey SR, Pineda AA *et al.* Overcoming a positive crossmatch in living-donor kidney transplantation. *Am J Transplant* 2003;3:1017–1023.

57 Gloor JM, Lager DJ, Moore SB *et al.* ABO-incompatible kidney transplantation using both A2 and non-A2 living donors. *Transplantation* 2003;75:971–977.

58 Montgomery RA, Cooper M, Kraus E *et al.* Renal transplantation at the Johns Hopkins Comprehensive Transplant Center. *Clin Transpl* 2003:199–213.

59 Montgomery RA, Zachary AA, Racusen LC *et al.* Plasmapheresis and intravenous immune globulin provides effective rescue therapy for refractory humoral rejection and allows kidneys to be successfully transplanted into cross-match-positive recipients. *Transplantation* 2000;70:887–895.

60 Schweitzer EJ, Wilson JS, Fernandez-Vina M *et al.* A high panel-reactive antibody rescue protocol for cross-match-positive live donor kidney transplants. *Transplantation* 2000;70:1531–1536.

61 Glotz D, Antoine C, Julia P *et al.* Intravenous immunoglobulins and transplantation for patients with anti-HLA antibodies. *Transpl Int* 2004;17:1–8.

62 Glotz D, Antoine C, Julia P *et al.* Desensitization and subsequent kidney transplantation of patients using intravenous immunoglobulins (IVIG). *Am J Transplant* 2002;2:758–760.

63 Jordan SC, Pescovits M. Presensitization: the problem and its management. *Clin J Am Soc Nephrol* 2006;1: 421–432.

64 Jordan SC, Vo A, Bunnapradist S *et al.* Intravenous immune globulin treatment inhibits crossmatch positivity and allows for successful transplantation of incompatible organs in living-donor and cadaver recipients. *Transplantation* 2003;76:631–636.

65 Tyan DB, Li VA, Czer L *et al.* Intravenous immunoglobulin suppression of HLA alloantibody in highly sensitized transplant candidates and transplantation with a histoincompatible organ. *Transplantation* 1994;57:553–562.

66 Alexandre GP, Squifflet JP, De Bruyere M *et al.* Present experiences in a series of 26 ABO-incompatible living donor renal allografts. *Transplant Proc* 1987;19: 4538–4542.

67 Alexandre GP, Squifflet JP, De Bruyere M *et al.* Splenectomy as a prerequisite for successful human ABO-incompatible renal transplantation. *Transplant Proc* 1985;17:138–143.

68 Tanabe K, Takahashi K, Sonda K *et al.* Long-term results of ABO-incompatible living kidney transplantation: a single-center experience. *Transplantation* 1998;65: 224–228.

69 Breimer ME, Samuelsson BE. The specific distribution of glycolipid-based blood group A antigens in human kidney related to A1/A2, Lewis, and secretor status of single individuals. A possible molecular explanation for the successful transplantation of A2 kidneys into O recipients. *Transplantation* 1986;42:88–91.

70 Clausen H, Levery SB, Nudelman E *et al.* Repetitive A epitope (type 3 chain A) defined by blood group A1-specific monoclonal antibody TH-1: chemical basis of qualitative A1 and A2 distinction. *Proc Natl Acad Sci U S A* 1985;82:1199–1203.

71 Economidou J, Hughes-Jones NC, Gardner B. Quantitative measurements concerning A and B antigen sites. *Vox Sang* 1967;12:321–328.

72 Nelson PW, Helling TS, Pierce GE *et al.* Successful transplantation of blood group A2 kidneys into non-A recipients. *Transplantation* 1988;45:316–319.

73 Sonnenday CJ, Warren DS, Cooper M *et al.* Plasmapheresis, CMV hyperimmune globulin, and anti-CD20 allow ABO-incompatible renal transplantation without splenectomy. *Am J Transplant* 2004; 4:1315–1322.

74 Tyden G, Kumlien G, Fehrman I. Successful ABO-incompatible kidney transplantations without splenectomy using antigen-specific immunoadsorption and rituximab. *Transplantation* 2003;76:730–731.

75 Warren DS, Zachary AA, Sonnenday CJ *et al.* Successful renal transplantation across simultaneous ABO incompatible and positive crossmatch barriers. *Am J Transplant* 2004;4:561–568.

76 Montgomery RA, Locke JE, King KE *et al.* ABO incompatible renal transplantation: a paradigm ready for broad implementation. *Transplantation* 2009; 87(8):1246–1255.

77 Sivakumaran P, Vo AA, Villicana R *et al.* Therapeutic plasma exchange for desensitization prior to transplantation in ABO-incompatible renal allografts. *J Clin Apher* 2009;24(4):155–160.

78 Jordan SC, Vo A, Peng A *et al.* Intravenous gammaglobulin (IVIG): a novel approach to improve transplant rates and outcomes in highly HLA-sensitized patients. *Am J Transplant* 2006;6(3): 459–466.

79 Jordan SC, Tyan DB. Intravenous gamma globulin (IVIG) inhibits lymphocytotoxic antibody in vitro. *J Am Soc Nephrol* 1991;2:803.

80 Peng A, Vo A, Villicana R *et al.* Long term graft and patient outcomes in highly-HLA sensitized (HS) deceased donor (DD) kidney transplant (KT) recipients desensitized with high dose (HD) IVIG. *Am J Transplant* 2008;8(Suppl s2):303.

81 Montgomery RA, Zachary AA. Transplantation patients with a postitive donor-specific crossmatch: a single center's perspective. *Pediatr Transplant* 2004;8:535–542.

82 Vo A, Lukovsky M, Toyoda M *et al.* Rituximab and intravenous immune globulin for desensitization during renal transplantation. *N Engl J Med* 2008;359:242–251.

83 Vo AA, Toyoda M, Kahwaji J *et al.* Use of intravenous immune globulin and rituximab for desensitization of highly-HLA sensitized patients awaiting kidney transplantation. *Transplantation* 2010;89(9):1095–1102.

84 Jordan SC, Vo A, Tyan D *et al.* Current approaches to treatment of antibody-mediated rejection. *Pediatr Transplant* 2005;9:408–415.

85 Lefaucheur C, Suberbielle-Boissel C, Hill GS *et al.* Clinical relevance of preformed HLA donor-specific antibodies in kidney transplantation. *Am J Transplant* 2008;8:324–331.

86 Lefaucheur C, Nochy D, Andrade J *et al.* Comparison of combination plasmapheresis/IVIG/anti-CD20 versus high dose IVIG in the treatment of antibody-mediated rejection. *Am J Transplant* 2009;9:1099–1107.

87 Jordan SC, Reinsmoen R, Peng A. Advances in diagnosing and managing antibody mediated rejection. *Pediatr Nephrol* 2010;25(10):2035–2045.

88 Vo A, Cao K, Lai C-H *et al.* Characteristics of patients who develop antibody-mediated rejection (AMR) post-transplant after desensitization with IVIG + rituximab: analysis of risk factors and outcomes. *Am J Tranplant* 2009;9:334 (abstract #494).

89 Kaposztas Z, Podder H, Mauiyyedi S *et al.* Impact of rituximab therapy for treatment of acute humoral rejection. *Clin Transplant* 2009;23:63–73.

90 Mulley WR, Hudson FJ, Tait BD *et al.* A single low-fixed dose of rituximab to salvage renal transplants from refractory antibody-mediated rejection. *Transplantation* 2009;87:286–289.

91 Lui C, Noorchashm H, Sutter JA *et al.* B lymphocyte-directed immunotherapy promotes long-term islet allograft survival in nonhuman primates. *Nat Med* 2007;13:1295–1298.

92 Kessler L, Parissiadis A, Bayle F *et al.* Evidence for humoral rejection of a pancreatic islet graft and rescue with rituximab and IV immunoglobulin therapy. *Am J Transplant* 2009;9:1961–1966.

93 Vo A, Lukovsky M, Toyoda M *et al.* Safety and adverse event profiles of intravenous gammaglobulin products used for immunomodulation: a single center experience. *Clin J Am Soc Nephrol* 2006;1(4): 844–852.

94 Kahwaji J, Barker E, Pepkowitz S *et al.* Acute hemolysis after high-dose intravenous immunoglobulin therapy in highly-HLA sensitized patients. *Clin J Am Soc Nephrol* 2009;4:1993–1997.

95 Coghill J, Comeau T, Shea T *et al.* Acute hemolysis in a patient with cytomegalovirus pneumonitis treated with intravenous immunoglobulin (IVIG). *Biol Blood Marrow Transplant* 2006;12(7);786–788.

96 US Renal Data System, USRDS 2008 Annual Data Report: Atlas of Chronic Kidney Disease and End-Stage Renal Disease in the United States. Bethesda, MD: National Institutes of Health, National Institute of Diabetes and Digestive and Kidney Diseases; 2008, pp. 223–238.

97 Shehata, N, Palda AV, Meyer R *et al.* The use of immunoglobulin therapy for patients undergoing solid organ transplantation: an evidence-based practice guideline. *Transfus Med Rev* 24(1 Suppl 1):S7–S27.

Index

Immunotherapy in Transplantation: Principles and Practice, First Edition. Edited by Bruce Kaplan, Gilbert J. Burckart and Fadi G. Lakkis.
© 2012 Blackwell Publishing Ltd. Published 2012 by Blackwell Publishing Ltd.